EMERGENCY MEDICINE SECRETS

EMERGENCY MEDICINE SECRETS

Vincent J. Markovchick, M.D., FACEP

Director, Emergency Medical Services
Denver General Hospital
Associate Professor of Surgery
Division of Emergency Medicine, Department of Surgery
University of Colorado Health Sciences Center
Denver, Colorado

Peter T. Pons, M.D., FACEP

Associate Director, Emergency Medical Services
Denver General Hospital
Assistant Professor of Surgery
Division of Emergency Medicine, Department of Surgery
University of Colorado Health Sciences Center
Denver, Colorado

Richard E. Wolfe, M.D., FACEP

Staff, Emergency Medical Services
Denver General Hospital
Assistant Professor of Surgery
Division of Emergency Medicine, Department of Surgery
University of Colorado Health Sciences Center
Denver, Colorado

HANLEY & BELFUS, INC./Philadelphia
MOSBY/St. Louis • Baltimore • Boston • Chicago • London
  Philadelphia • Sydney •Toronto

Publisher: HANLEY & BELFUS, INC.
                210 S. 13th Street
                Philadelphia, PA 19107
                (215) 546-7293
                FAX (215) 790-9330

North American and worldwide sales and distribution:

                MOSBY
                11830 Westline Industrial Drive
                St. Louis, MO 63146

In Canada: Times Mirror Professional Publishing, Ltd.
                130 Flaska Drive
                Markham, Ontario L6G 1B8
                Canada

EMERGENCY MEDICINE SECRETS   ISBN 1-56053-051-0

Library of Congress catalog card number   92-71699

Last digit is the print number: 9 8 7 6 5 4 3 2

DEDICATION

The three editors dedicate this book to Peter Rosen, M.D. As our mentor and role model, he has inspired us to strive toward excellence in medicine and education.

> To my parents, Anna and Nicholas, for their lifelong love and encouragement
>
> VJM

> To my wife, Kathy, whose love, support, and patience make everything worthwhile
>
> PTP

> To Alice, whose untiring support is the foundation on which I pursue my academic aspirations
>
> REW

Special acknowledgment to Phyllis Parrington for her exceptional organizational and secretarial skills and her ability to maintain a sense of humor throughout this endeavor.

CONTENTS

XVII. BEHAVIORAL EMERGENCIES

XVIII. COST CONTAINMENT AND RISK MANAGEMENT

XIX. MEDICAL CONTROL AND DISASTER MANAGEMENT

CONTRIBUTORS

Charles M. Abernathy, M.D.
Professor of Surgery, University of Colorado School of Medicine, Denver, Colorado

Jean T. Abbott, M.D., FACEP
Assistant Professor, Division of Emergency Medicine, University of Colorado School of Medicine, Denver, Colorado

Olivia Vynn Adair, M.D.
Assistant Professor, Department of Cardiology, University of Colorado School of Medicine, Denver, Colorado

Stephen L. Adams, M.D.
Associate Chief, Division of Emergency Medicine, Northwestern University Medical School, Chicago, Illinois

Roger M. Barkin, M.D., M.P.H.
Chairman, Department of Pediatrics, Rose Medical Center; Professor, Department of Surgery, Division of Emergency Medicine, University of Colorado School of Medicine, Denver, Colorado

F. Keith Battan, M.D.
Assistant Professor of Pediatrics, University of Colorado School of Medicine, Denver, Colorado

Marc J. Bayer, M.D.
Department of Emergency Medicine, UCSF School of Medicine, San Francisco, California

James E. Bodenhamer, M.D.
Staff Emergency Physician, Department of Emergency Medicine, St. Anthony Hospital, Denver, Colorado

Joan Bothner, M.D.
Assistant Professor of Pediatrics, University of Colorado School of Medicine, Denver, Colorado

Andrea M. Brault, M.D.
Resident, Department of Emergency Medicine, University of California at Irvine, Orange, California

Russell U. Braun, M.D.
Assistant Clinical Professor of Medicine, UCSF School of Medicine, San Francisco, California

Jeffrey Brent, M.D., Ph.D.
Assistant Professor, Division of Emergency Medicine, University of Colorado School of Medicine, Denver, Colorado

Elizabeth Brew, M.D.
Department of Surgery, University of Colorado School of Medicine, Denver, Colorado

Michael W. Brunko, M.D., FACEP
Assistant Clinical Professor of Surgery, University of Colorado School of Medicine,
Denver Coloardo

Richard W. Brunton, D.D.S.
Chief Resident, Dentistry and Oral-Maxillofacial Surgery, Denver General Hospital,
Denver, Colorado

James H. Bryan, M.D., Ph.D.
Department of Emergency Medicine, University of California at Irvine, Orange,
California

Charles B. Cairns, M.D.
Assistant Professor, Division of Emergency Medicine, University of Colorado School of
Medicine, Denver, Colorado

Stephen V. Cantrill, M.D.
Associate Director, Emergency Medical Services, Denver General Hospital, Denver,
Colorado

Michael A. Casillas, D.D.S
Resident, Dentistry and Oral-Maxillofacial Surgery, Denver General Hospital, Denver,
Colorado

Steven M. Chernow, M.D.
Division of Emergency Medicine, University of Colorado School of Medicine, Denver,
Colorado

Mark E. Copeland, M.D.
Senior Resident, Denver Affiliated Residency in Emergency Medicine, Denver, Colorado

Daniel F. Danzl, M.D., FACEP
Professor and Chair, Department of Emergency Medicine, University of Louisville School
of Medicine, Louisville, Kentucky

Marc A. Davis, M.D.
Emergency Medical Services, Denver General Hospital, Denver, Colorado

Robert J. Doherty, M.D.
Instructor, Division of Emergency Medicine, University of Maryland School of Medicine,
Baltimore, Maryland

Steven Dominguez, M.D.
Division of Emergency Medicine, UCLA School of Medicine, Los Angeles, California

Pamela M. Downey, M.D., FRCP
Residency Program Director, Emergency Medicine, University of Calgary Faculty of
Medicine, Calgary, Alberta, Canada

Thomas R. Drake, M.D.
Clinical Instructor in Emergency Medicine, Denver General Hospital, Denver, Colorado

Ellen M. Dugan, M.D.
Assistant Professor, Department of Emergency Medicine, Georgetown University School
of Medicine, Washington, D.C.

Michael P. Earnest, M.D.
Professor of Neurology and Preventive Medicine, University of Colorado School of Medicine, Denver, Colorado

Joanne Edney, M.D.
Attending Physician, Denver General Hospital, Denver, and Longmont United Hospital, Longmont, Colorado; Medical Director, Mountainview Fire Protection District

Lisa S. Emmans, M.D.
Resident, Denver Affiliated Residency in Emergency Medicine, Denver, Colorado

Kim Marie Feldhaus, M.D.
Emergency Medical Services, Denver General Hospital, Denver, Colorado

Bernard J. Feldman, M.D.
Chairman, Department of Emergency Medicine, Christ Hospital and Medical Center, Oak Lawn, Illinois; Head, Section of Emergency Medicine, and Associate Professor, Department of Family Medicine, Rush Medical College, Chicago, Illinois

Carl M. Ferraro, M.D., FACEP
Assistant Professor of Clinical Emergency Medicine, University of Illinois College of Medicine, Chicago, Illinois

Marsha Ford, M.D., FACEP
Director, Toxicology Division, Carolinas Medical Center, Charlotte, North Carolina

Peter O. Fried, M.D.
Program Director, Department of Emergency Medicine, Christ Hospital and Medical Center, Oak Lawn, Illinois; Assistant Professor, Rush Medical College, Chicago, Illinois

Stanley J. Galle, Jr., M.D., FACEP
Medical Director, Emergency Department, Saint Joseph Hospital, Denver, Colorado

Benjamin A. Gitterman, M.D.
Associate Professor of Pediatrics and Preventive Medicine, University of Colordo School of Medicine; Director, Ambulatory Pediatric Services, Denver Health and Hospitals, Denver, Colorado

Loi E. Graham, M.D.
Department of Emergency Medicine, Vancouver General Hospital, Vancouver, British Columbia, Canada

Wayne F. Guerra, M.D.
Chief Resident, Emergency Medicine, Denver General Hospital, Denver, Colorado

Kent N. Hall, M.D.
Assistant Professor, Department of Emergency Medicine, Medical College of Wisconsin, Milwaukee, Wisconsin

Glenn C. Hamilton, M.D.
Professor and Chair, Department of Emergency Medicine, Wright State University School of Medicine, Dayton, Ohio

Linda L. Hanson, M.D.
Attending Physician, Department of Emergency Medicine, St. Joseph's Hospital, Denver, Colorado

Eugene Hardin, M.D., FACEP
Associate Professor of Emergency Medicine, Charles R. Drew University of Medicine,
Los Angeles, California

Alden H. Harken, M.D.
Professor and Chairman, Department of Surgery, University of Colorado School of
Medicine, Denver, Colorado

Ann Harwood-Nuss, M.D., FACEP
Professor, Division of Emergency Medicine, University of Florida Health Science Center,
Jacksonville, Florida

Edward P. Havranek, M.D.
Assistant Professor of Medicine, University of Colorado School of Medicine, Denver,
Colorado

Philip L. Henneman, M.D., FACEP
Associate Professor of Medicine, UCLA School of Medicine, Los Angeles, California

Jeffrey S. Hill, M.D.
Chief Resident, Emergency Medicine, Denver General Hospital, Denver, Colorado

Robert S. Hockbeger, M.D.
Associate Clinical Professor of Medicine, UCLA School of Medicine, Los Angeles; Chair,
Department of Emergency Medicine, Harbor–UCLA Medical Center, Torrance,
California

Benjamin Honigman, M.D.
Associate Professor of Surgery, Division of Emergency Medicine, University of Colorado
School of Medicine, Denver, Colorado

John M. Howell, M.D., FACEP
Associate Professor of Emergency Medicine, Georgetown University School of Medicine,
Washington, D.C.

David S. Howes, M.D., FACEP
Assistant Professor of Medicine, University of Chicago Pritzker School of Medicine,
Chicago, Illinois

Richard L. Hughes, M.D.
Assistant Professor of Neurology, and Director, University of Colorado Affiliated
Hospitals Stroke Project, Denver, Colorado

D. Michael Hunt, M.D., FACEP
Assistant Professor of Emergency Medicine, George Washington University School of
Medicine, Washington, D.C.

Grant D. Innes, M.D., FRCP(C)
Clinical Research Coordinator, Department of Emergency Medicine, Royal Columbian
Hospital, Vancouver, British Columbia, Canada

Eric Isaacs, M.D.
Department of Emergency Medical Services, UCSF School of Medicine, San Francisco,
California

R. Scott Israel, M.D.
Department of Emergency Medicine, University of Oregon Health Sciences University School of Medicine, Portland, Oregon

Kenneth C. Jackimczyk, M.D.
Residency Director, Department of Emergency Medicine, Maricopa Medical Center, Phoenix, Arizona

Andrew M. Johanos, M.D.
Chief Resident, Emergency Medicine, Denver General Hospital, Denver, Colorado

Robert C. Jorden, M.D., FACEP
Clinical Professor of Emergency Medicine, University of Arizona College of Medicine, Tucson, Arizona

Lisa Josephson, M.D.
Clinical Instructor in Emergency Medicine, University of California at Irvine, Orange, California

Nicholas J. Jouriles, M.D.
Assistant Director, Emergency Medicine Residency, Metro Health Medical Center; Assistant Professor, Case Western Reserve University School of Medicine, Cleveland, Ohio

Juliana Karp, M.D.
Chief Resident, Emergency Medicine, Denver General Hospital, Denver, Colorado

Eugene E. Kercher, M.D., FACEP
Assistant Clinical Professor, Department of Medicine, UCLA School of Medicine, Los Angeles, California

Richard Kingsland, M.D.
Department of Emergency Medicine, University of California, San Diego, School of Medicine, San Diego, California

Kristi L. Koenig, M.D.
Assistant Professor of Medicine, UCSF School of Medicine, San Francisco, California

Michael A. Kohn, M.D.
Chief Resident, Denver Affiliated Residency in Emergency Medicine, Denver, Colorado

Mickey Kolodny, M.D., FACEP
Clinical Instructor, Emergency Department, Charles R. Drew University of Medicine, Los Angeles, California

Ken Kulig, M.D., FACEP
Associate Clinical Professor, Division of Emergency Medicine, University of Colorado School of Medicine, Denver, Colorado

Mark I. Langdorf, M.D., MHPE, FACEP
Associate Clinical Professor and Residency Director, Department of Emergency Medicine, University of California at Irvine, Orange, California

Louis J. Ling, M.D.
Associate Medical Director, Academic Affairs, Hennepin County Medical Center, Minneapolis, Minnesota

John Longano, M.D.
Division of Emergency Medicine, Northwestern University Medical School, Chicago, Illinois

Atkinson W. Longmire, M.D., FACEP
Fellow in Emergency Medicine, Vanderbilt University School of Medicine, Nashville, Tennessee

Steven R. Lowenstein, M.D., M.P.H.
Associate Professor of Medicine, Surgery, and Preventative Medicine and Biometrics; Associate Director, Division of Emergency Medicine, University of Colorado School of Medicine, Denver, Colorado

David J. Magid, M.D.
Resident, Denver Affiliated Residency in Emergency Medicine, Denver, Colorado

A. Roy Magnusson, M.D., FACEP
Director, Emergency Medicine Residency, and Assistant Professor of Emergency Medicine, Department of Emergency Medicine, Oregon Health Sciences University School of Medicine, Portland, Oregon

Catherine A. Marco, M.D.
Assistant Professor of Emergency Medicine, Johns Hopkins University School of Medicine, Baltimore, MD

Vince Markovchick, M.D.
Director, Emergency Medical Services, Denver General Hospital, Associate Professor of Surgery, Division of Emergency Medicine, University of Colorado School of Medicine, Denver, Colorado

John A. Marx, M.D., FACEP
Chair, Department of Emergency Medicine, Carolinas Medical Center, Charlotte; Clinical Professor, Department of Emergency Medicine, University of North Carolina at Chapel Hill School of Medicine, Chapel Hill, North Carolina

Alex M. Maslanka, M.D.
Emergency Medical Services, Denver General Hospital, Denver, Colorado

James Mathews, M.D.
Chief, Division of Emergency Medicine, and Associate Professor of Medicine, Northwestern University Medical School, Chicago, Illinois

John McGoldrick, M.D.
Attending Emergency Physician, Denver General Hospital, Denver, Colorado

Thomas McLaughlin, D.O.
Director, Emergency Services, U.S. Air Force Academy Hospital, Colorado Springs, Colorado

Robert McNamara, M.D., FACEP
Associate Professor and Residency Program Director, Department of Emergency Medicine, Medical College of Pennsylvania, Philadelphia, Pennsylvania

Harvey W. Meislin, M.D., FACEP
Professor and Chief, Section of Emergency Medicine, and Director, Emergency Services, University Medical Center, University of Arizona School of Medicine, Tucson, Arizona

Cheryl Melick-Casanova, M.D.
Attending Physician, Department of Emergency Medicine, Swedish Medical Center, Englewood, Colorado

Merle Miller, M.D.
Emergency Medical Services, Denver General Hospital, Denver, Colorado

Elizabeth L. Mitchell, M.D.
Assistant Professor, Division of Emergency Medicine, University of Colorado School of Medicine, Denver, Colorado

James C. Mitchiner, M.D.
Program Director, Emergency Medicine Residency Program, St. Joseph Mercy Hospital; Clinical Instructor, Department of Surgery, University of Michigan Medical School, Ann Arbor, Michigan

Ernest E. Moore, M.D.
Chief of Surgery, Denver General Hospital; Professor and Vice-Chairman of Surgery, University of Colorado School of Medicine, Denver, Colorado

Gregory P. Moore, M.D., FACEP
Associate Residency Director, Methodist Hospital, Indianapolis, Indiana

Peter Moyer, M.D., FACEP
Associate Professor, Boston University School of Medicine; Director, Emergency Department, Boston City Hospital, Boston, Massachusetts

Michael F. Murphy, M.D., FRCPC
Assistant Professor, Department of Anesthesia, Dalhousie University Faculty of Medicine, Halifax, Nova Scotia, Canada

Edward Newton, M.D., FACEP
Assistant Professor and Residency Director, Department of Emergency Medicine, Los Angeles County and USC Medical Center, Los Angeles, California

Denise Norton, M.D.
Resident in Surgery, University of Colorado School of Medicine, Denver, Colorado

Gary J. Ordog, M.D., FACEP
Associate Professor of Emergency Medicine, UCLA School of Medicine and Charles R. Drew University of Medicine, Los Angeles, California

Polly E. Parsons, M.D.
Associate Professor of Medicine, University of Colorado School of Medicine, Denver, Colorado

Peter T. Pons, M.D., FACEP
Associate Director, Emergency Medical Services, Denver General Hospital; Assistant Professor of Surgery, Division of Emergency Medicine, University of Colorado School of Medicine, Denver, Colorado

Thomas B. Purcell, M.D.
Adjunct Assistant Professor of Medicine, UCLA School of Medicine, Los Angeles, California

Roy Purssell, M.D.
Clinical Associate Professor, Division of Emergency Medicine, University of British Columbia Faculty of Medicine, Vancouver General Hospital, Vancouver, British Columbia, Canada

Mark A. Radlauer, M.D.
Emergency Medical Services, Denver General Hospital, Denver, Colorado

Stacie L. Ranniger, M.D.
Assistant Professor of Surgery, University of Colorado School of Medicine, Denver, Colorado

Robert A. Read, M.D.
Assistant Professor of Surgery, University of Colorado School of Medicine, Denver, Colorado

Jedd Roe, M.D.
Attending Faculty, Emergency Medical Services, Denver General Hospital; Associate Director, Paramedic Division, Denver Department of Health and Hospitals, Denver, Colorado

Peter Rosen, M.D.
Director of Education, Department of Emergency Medicine; Director, Emergency Medicine Residency Program; Adjunct Professor of Medicine and Surgery; Assistant Director, Department of Emergency Medicine, University of California, San Diego, School of Medicine, La Jolla, California

Douglas A. Rund, M.D., FACEP
Professor and Chairman, Department of Emergency Medicine, Ohio State University College of Medicine, Columbus, Ohio

Ricciardettu P. Scalzi, M.D.
Attending Physician, Emergency Department, Scottsdale Memorial Hospital, Scottsdale, Arizona

Jeffrey J. Schaider, M.D.
Associate Residency Director, Department of Emergency Medicine, Cook County Hospital; Assistant Professor of Clinical Emergency Medicine, University of Illinois College of Medicine, Chicago, Illinois

Robert D. Schmidt, M.D.
Assistant Director, Emergency Medical Services, St. Anthony Hospital, Denver, Colorado

Robert E. Schneider, M.D., FACEP, FACS
Residency Director, Emergency Medicine, Carolinas Medical Center, Charlotte, North Carolina

Elaine Norman Scholes, M.D.
Associate Professor of Pediatrics, University of Colorado School of Medicine, Denver, Colorado

Sarah K. Scott, M.D.
Lutheran Hospital, Wheatridge, Colorado

Donna Seger, M.D., FACEP, ABMT
Assistant Professor of Emergency Medicine and Medicine, Vanderbilt University School
of Medicine, Nashville, Tennessee

Lee W. Shockley, M.D., FACEP
Assistant Professor, Department of Surgery, University of Colorado School of Medicine,
Denver, Colorado

Barry Simon, M.D.
Assistant Clinical Professor of Medicine, UCSF School of Medicine, San Francisco,
California

Corey M. Slovis, M.D., FACP, FACEP
Professor and Chairman, Department of Emergency Medicine, Vanderbilt University
School of Medicine, Nashville, Tennessee

Rodney W. Smith, M.D., FACEP
Clinical Assistant Professor of Emergency Medicine, Indiana University School of
Medicine, Indianapolis, Indiana

Daniel W. Spaite, M.D., FACEP
Associate Professor of Emergency Medicine, Arizona Emergency Medicine Research
Center, University of Arizona College of Medicine, Tucson, Arizona

Phyllis H. Stenklyft, M.D.
Assistant Professor of Surgery and Pediatrics, Division of Emergency Medicine,
University of Florida Health Science Center, Jacksonville, Florida

Ernest Stremski, M.D.
Assistant Professor, Department of Pediatrics, Division of Emergency Medicine/
Toxicology, Medical College of Wisconsin, Milwaukee, Wisconsin

Harold Thomas, Jr., M.D.
Assistant Professor of Emergency Medicine, Bowman-Gray School of Medicine, Winston-
Salem, North Carolina

Alexander T. Trott, M.D.
Professor of Emergency Medicine, University of Cincinnati College of Medicine,
Cincinnati, Ohio

Daryl M. Turner, M.D.
Senior Emergency Medicine Resident, Division of Emergency Medicine, University of
Florida Health Science Center, Jacksonville, Florida

Robert S. Van Hare, M.D.
Staff Physician, Emergency Department, Overlake Hospital Medical Center, Bellevue,
Washington

Laurie Vande Krol, M.D.
Instructor, Division of Emergency Medicine, University of Colorado School of Medicine,
Denver, Colorado

W. Peter Vellman, M.D.
Director, Emergency Medical Services, St. Anthony Hospital, Denver, Colorado

David J. Vukich, M.D., FACEP
Associate Professor and Chief, Division of Emergency Medicine, University of Florida
Health Center, Jacksonville, Florida

Jonathan Wasserberger, M.D., FACEP
Associate Professor of Emergency Medicine, UCLA School of Medicine and Charles R.
Drew University of Medicine, Los Angeles, California

Diana R. Williams, M.D.
Assistant Clinical Professor of Emergency Medicine, University of Illinois College of
Medicine, Chicago, Illinois

Richard E. Wolfe, M.D.
Staff, Emergency Medicine Services, Denver General Hospital; Assistant Professor,
Division of Emergency Medicine, University of Colorado School of Medicine, Denver,
Colorado

Allan B. Wolfson, M.D., FACEP, FACP
Associate Professor of Medicine, Division of Emergency Medicine, University of
Pittsburgh School of Medicine, Pittsburgh, Pennsylvania

William F. Young, Jr., M.D., FACEP
Assistant Chief, Emergency Medicine, Valley Medical Center, Fresno; Assistant Clinical
Professor, Department of Medicine, UCSF School of Medicine, San Francisco,
California

Richard D. Zallen, D.D.S., M.D.
Director of Dentistry and Oral Maxillofacial Surgery, Denver General Hospital;
Professor of Dentistry, Division of Oral Maxillofacial Surgery, University of Colorado
School of Dentistry, Denver, Colorado

Andrew B. Ziller, M.D.
Staff Physician, Emergency Department, Rose Medical Center, Denver, Colorado

PREFACE

Emergency medicine, the newest medical specialty, has only just begun to acquire its own body of literature. It encompasses the breadth of all other specialties but has distinct aspects of its own, such as prehospital care. In order to complement the achievements of the pioneering educators and clinicians of our field, Emergency Medicine joins the ranks of the more established specialties in The Secrets Series®. The art of emergency medicine is the ability to evaluate, diagnose, and treat—often with minimal data and time. Knowing the questions and answers that routinely confront the physician on the front line of medicine is the first step in surviving in the chaotic atmosphere of the emergency department. The use of the Socratic method is well recognized by most bedside teachers as a way to actively involve the student in the learning process. Through the questions and answers contained here, we have attempted to emphasize the information needed for the decisive and safe practice of emergency medicine. We hope that this book will stimulate the student to seek further knowledge from the comprehensive textbooks and the scientific literature of our field.

Vincent J. Markovchick, M.D., FACEP
Peter T. Pons, M.D., FACEP
Richard E. Wolfe, M.D., FACEP

I. Decision Making in Emergency Medicine

1. DECISION MAKING IN EMERGENCY MEDICINE

Vince Markovchick, M.D., FACEP

1. Is there anything unique about emergency medicine?
Although there is significant crossover between emergency medicine and all other clinical specialties, emergency medicine has unique aspects, such as the approach to patient care and the decision-making process.

2. Describe the conventional method of evaluating a patient.
A comprehensive history, physical examination, "routine" laboratory diagnostic studies, special diagnostic procedures, and the formulation of a problem-oriented medical record and rational course of therapy constitute the "ideal" approach to patient care because it is so comprehensive.

3. Why is the conventional methodology not ideal in the setting of an emergency department (ED)?
Even though in retrospect only 10–20% of patients presenting to an ED truly have emergent problems, it must be presumed that every patient who comes to an ED has an emergent condition. Therefore, the first and most important question that must be answered is, *What is the life threat?* The conventional approach does not ensure an expeditious answer to this question. Time constraints also impede the use of conventional methodology in the ED.

4. How do I identify the life-threatened patient?
Three components are necessary to quickly identify the life-threatened patient:
1. A chief complaint
2. A complete and accurate set of vital signs in the field and in the ED
3. An opportunity to visualize, auscultate, and touch the patient

5. What is so important about the chief complaint?
The chief complaint, which sometimes cannot be obtained directly from the patient but must be obtained from family members, observers, emergency medical technicians (EMTs), or others at the scene, will immediately help categorize the general type of problem (e.g., cardiac, traumatic, respiratory, etc.).

6. Why are vital signs important?
Vital signs are the most reliable, objective data that are immediately available to ED personnel. Vital signs and the chief complaint, when used as triage tools, will identify the vast majority of life-threatened patients. It is essential that one be totally familiar with normal vital signs for all age groups.

7. What are the determinants of (normal) vital signs?

Age, underlying physical condition, medical problems (e.g., hypertension), and current medications (e.g., beta blockers) are important considerations in determining normal vital signs for a given patient. For example, a well-conditioned, young athlete who has just sustained major trauma and arrives with a resting, supine pulse of 80 must be presumed to have significant blood loss because his normal pulse is probably in the 40–50 range.

8. Why do I need to compare field vital signs with ED vital signs?

Most prehospital care systems with a level of care beyond basic transport also provide therapy to patients. Because this therapy usually makes positive changes in the patient's condition, the patient may look deceptively well upon arrival in the ED. For example, a 20-year-old female with acute onset of left lower quadrant abdominal pain, who is found to be cool, clammy, and diaphoretic, with a pulse of 116 and a blood pressure of 78 palpable, and who receives 1500 cc of IV fluid en route to the ED, may arrive with normal vital signs and no skin changes. If one does not read and pay attention to the EMT's description of the patient and the initial vital signs, the presumption may be made that this is a stable patient.

9. When are "normal" vital signs abnormal?

This is where the chief complaint comes in. For example, a 20-year-old male who states he has asthma and has been wheezing for hours arrives in the ED with a respiratory rate of 14. An asthmatic who is dyspneic and wheezing should have a respiratory rate of at least 20–30/min. Thus a "normal" respiratory rate of 14 in this setting indicates the patient is fatiguing and is in respiratory failure. This is a classic example of when "normal" is extremely abnormal.

10. Why do I need to visualize, auscultate, and touch the patient?

In many instances, these measures help to identify the life threat (e.g., is it the upper airway, lower airway, or circulation?). Touching the skin is important in order to determine whether shock is associated with vasoconstriction (hypovolemic or cardiogenic) or with vasodilatation (septic, neurogenic, or anaphylactic). Auscultation will identify life threats associated with the lower airway (e.g., bronchoconstriction, tension pneumothorax).

11. Once I have identified the life threat, what do I do?

Do not go on. Stop immediately and intervene to reverse the life threat. For example, if the initial encounter with the patient identifies upper airway obstruction, take whatever measures are necessary to alleviate upper airway obstruction such as suctioning, positioning, or intubating the patient. If the problem is hemorrhage, volume restoration and hemorrhage control (when possible) are indicated.

12. Okay, I've identified and stabilized or ruled out an immediate life threat in the patient. What else is unique about the approach?

The differential diagnosis formulated in the ED must begin with the most serious condition possible to explain the patient's presentation and work down from there. An example is a 60-year-old male who presents with nausea, vomiting, and epigastric pain. Instead of assuming the condition is caused by a gastrointestinal disorder, one must consider that the presentation could represent an acute myocardial infarction (MI) and take the appropriate steps to stabilize (i.e., start an IV and place the patient on O_2 and a cardiac monitor) the patient and rule out an MI (an adequate history, physical exam, and EKG).

13. Why does formulating a differential diagnosis sometimes lead to problems?

The natural tendency in formulating a differential diagnosis is to think of the most common or statistically most probable condition to explain the patient's initial presentation to the

ED. If one does this, one will be right most of the time but may overlook the most serious, albeit usually most uncommon, problem. Therefore, the practice of emergency medicine involves some degree of healthy paranoia in that one must consider the most serious condition possible, and, through a logical process of elimination, rule it out and thereby arrive at the correct and generally more common diagnosis.

14. Is a diagnosis always possible or necessary with information I can obtain in the ED?
Of course not. Sometimes it takes days, weeks, or months for the final diagnosis to be made. It is unreasonable to expect that every patient evaluated in the ED should or must have a diagnosis made in the ED. If you have an obsessive-compulsive personality with a need to be absolutely certain before you can act to stabilize or treat a patient, then the ED is an unhealthy work environment for you.

15. Suppose I can't make the diagnosis. What do I do?
If is advisable to be intellectually honest and admit to the patient and write in the medical record the inability to make a diagnosis. As stated earlier, it is the role of the ED physician to rule out serious or life-threatening causes of a patient's presentation and not to arrive at the definitive diagnosis. For example, a patient who presents with acute abdominal pain, who has had an appropriate history, physical exam, and diagnostic studies performed, and who in your best judgment does not have a life-threatening or acute surgical problem, should be so informed. The discharge diagnosis would be abdominal pain of unknown etiology. This avoids the trap so often encountered of labeling the patient with a benign diagnosis such as gastroenteritis that is often not supported by the medical record. More importantly, it avoids giving the patient the impression that there is a totally benign process occurring and will help to avoid the medical (and legal) problem of the patient presenting 3 days later with a ruptured appendix (see ch. 113, p. 431).

16. What is the most important question to ask a patient who presents with a chronic, recurrent condition?
What's different now? This question should be asked of all patients who have a chronic condition that brings them to an ED. The classic example is migraine headache. The patient with a chronic, recurrent migraine headache who is not asked this question may, on this presentation, have had an acute subarachnoid bleed. Such a patient may not volunteer that this headache is different from the pattern of chronic migraines unless asked.

17. How do I decide if the patient needs hospitalization?
Obviously the medical condition is the first factor to consider. The question that must be answered is, "Is there a medical need that can be fulfilled only by hospitalization?" For example, does the patient need oxygen therapy or cardiac monitoring? Another factor to weigh in the decision regarding hospitalization is whether the patient can be safely observed in the outpatient setting. For example, a patient who has sustained head trauma and needs to follow head trauma precautions at home, and who is either homeless or lives alone, cannot be safely discharged. Unfortunately, ability to pay is also sometimes inappropriately used in ED disposition decisions.

18. If the patient does not need admission, how do I arrange a satisfactory disposition?
Every patient seen in the ED must be referred to a physician or back to the ED for follow-up care. Failure to do so constitutes patient abandonment. Appropriate and specific follow-up instructions should be given to all patients.

19. What do you mean by specific follow-up instructions?
All follow-up instructions must include specific mention of the most serious potential complication of the patient's condition. For example, a patient who is being discharged

home with the diagnosis of a probable herniated L4, 5 intervertebral disc should always be instructed to return immediately if any bowel or bladder dysfunction develops. This takes into account the most serious complication of a herniated lumbar disc, which is a central mid-line herniation with bowel or bladder dysfunction, and constitutes an acute neurosurgical emergency.

20. What about the chart?
The chart must reflect the answers to the preceding questions in this chapter. It need not list the entire differential diagnosis but one should be able to ascertain from reading the chart that the more serious diagnoses were indeed considered. It also must contain appropriate follow-up instructions.

2. MANAGEMENT OF CARDIAC ARREST AND RESUSCITATION

Charles B. Cairns, M.D., and Steven R. Lowenstein, M.D., M.P.H.

1. What are the ABCs of resuscitation?
Airway, breathing, and circulation.

2. How should cardiopulmonary resuscitation (CPR) be performed?
The ABCs should guide and steady the resuscitation of all critically ill patients, including all cardiac arrest victims.
   1. Activate the emergency medical services (EMS) if out of hospital or the cardiac arrest response in hospital.
   2. Open the airway by performing a head tilt/chin lift or a head tilt/jaw thrust maneuver. These maneuvers cause anterior displacement of the mandible and lift the tongue and epiglottis away from the glottic opening. Tidal volumes are adequate with either maneuver. To improve airway patency, suction the mouth and oropharynx and insert an oropharyngeal or nasopharyngeal airway.
   3. Assist breathing by performing mouth-to-mouth, mouth-to-mask, or bag-valve-mask breathing. The recommended technique will depend on the clinical setting, the equipment available, and the rescuer's skill and training. Although these techniques can sustain ventilation and oxygenation indefinitely in ideal situations (for example, in the OR), in the emergency setting they are suboptimal. Air leaks at the face mask result in inadequate lung ventilation. Furthermore, insufflation of the stomach, followed by emesis and aspiration, is an ever-present threat. To reduce these risks, deliver slow, even breaths, pausing for full deflation between breaths, and avoid excessive peak inspiratory pressures. Use the Sellick maneuver (continuous application of digital pressure to the cricoid cartilage) in order to compress the esophagus and reduce the risk of vomiting and aspiration.
   4. After opening the airway and initiating rescue breathing, check for spontaneous circulation by palpating for a carotid or femoral pulse. If the patient is pulseless, begin chest compressions. Compress the chest smoothly and forcefully 80 to 100 times per minute. If there are two rescuers, interpose one artificial breath after every five chest compressions. If only one rescuer is available, the recommended sequence is 15 compressions, followed by 2 breaths.

3. What are the exceptions to the rule of the ABCs?

1. **Monitored cardiac arrest.** When a patient in a monitored setting experiences sudden ventricular tachycardia or ventricular fibrillation, the first priority is immediate electrical defibrillation.

2. **Traumatic arrest.** In traumatic cardiac arrest, closed-chest CPR is usually ineffective. In trauma, the etiology of the arrest may be a tension pneumothorax, cardiac tamponade, or exsanguinating hemorrhage from the thorax or abdomen. An immediate thoracotomy, not CPR, is indicated. In addition, in the setting of significant craniofacial trauma or forceful deceleration, a fracture or dislocation of the cervical spine may be present. Where an injury to the neck is suspected, a jaw thrust (and never a head tilt) should be used to open the airway.

4. What is the mechanism of blood flow during CPR?

Two basic models explain the mechanism of blood flow during CPR. In the **cardiac pump model** the heart is squeezed between the sternum and spine. Chest compression results in systole, and the atrioventricular valves close normally, assuring unidirectional, antegrade flow. During the relaxation phase (diastole), intracardiac pressures fall, the valves open, and blood is drawn into the heart from the lungs and vena cavae.

In the **thoracic pump model** the heart is considered a passive conduit. Chest compression results in uniformly increased pressures throughout the heart and thorax. Forward blood flow is achieved selectively in the arterial system, because the stiff-walled arteries resist collapse and because retrograde flow is prevented in the great veins by one-way valves. Aspects of both models have been substantiated in animal models, and both pumps probably contribute to blood flow during CPR.

5. Is blood flow to the brain and heart adequate during CPR?

In both models blood flow to the brain is a function of the aortic-to-jugular venous pressure difference during systole (the compression phase of CPR). The cerebral flow measured experimentally is approximately 30% of normal. Blood flow to the heart occurs during the relaxation phase of CPR and is a function of the aortic-to-right atrial pressure difference in diastole. Unfortunately, net myocardial flow via the coronary arteries is essentially nil during closed-chest CPR, and even retrograde coronary artery flow has been demonstrated.

6. What is the role of pharmacologic therapy during CPR?

The immediate goal of pharmacologic therapy is to improve myocardial blood flow, the key physiologic parameter conducive to the return of spontaneous circulation. Alpha-adrenergic agonists, such as epinephrine, augment the aortic to right atrial diastolic gradient by increasing arterial vascular tone. Although pure alpha-adrenergic agents, such as methoxamine and norepinephrine, also increase arterial pressure and myocardial blood flow, none has been shown to be superior to epinephrine.

7. What are the most common causes of cardiopulmonary arrest?

Most cardiopulmonary arrests in both prehospital and hospital settings are caused by ventricular fibrillation (VF), which usually occurs in patients with ischemic heart disease. Yet, drug toxicity, electrolyte disturbances (hyperkalemia), and prolonged hypoxemia are also important inciting factors.

A significant proportion (30–50%) of cardiac arrests are brady-asystolic at the onset. Common causes of this rhythm are hypoxia or acidemia. Another important cause of brady-asystole is heightened vagal tone, which may be precipitated by drugs, anesthetic agents, inferoposterior myocardial infarction (Bezold-Jarisch reflex) or invasive procedures.

Electromechanical dissociation (EMD) is the third common arrest rhythm. The most common etiology of EMD is prolonged arrest itself; typically, after 8 minutes or more of VF, electrical defibrillation is futile and induces a slow, wide-complex EMD, which is usually irreversible and known as pulseless idioventricular rhythm. EMD may also present as an inciting, rather than a terminal, rhythm. Examples are tension pneumothorax, cardiac tamponade, exsanguination, anaphylaxis or pulmonary embolus (discussed below).

8. Briefly list the reversible causes and immediate treatment of cardiopulmonary arrest.
  1. **Hyperkalemia.** Treatment induces calcium chloride, sodium bicarbonate, and an insulin-glucose infusion.
  2. **Anaphylaxis.** Rapid tracheal intubation and administration of crystalloid and epinephrine are the cornerstones of resuscitation.
  3. **Cardiac tamponade.** A pericardiocentesis or subxyphoid pericardiorraphy are life-saving.
  4. **Tension pneumothorax.** Immediate decompression is mandatory.
  5. **Hypovolemia.** Treatment includes immediate IV administration of crystalloid solutions. In traumatic arrest, blood products (whole blood or packed cells) should be given concomitantly with crystalloid.
  6. **Torsade de pointes.** Treatment includes cardioversion, followed by magnesium, isoproterenol, and rapid ventricular pacing.
  7. **Toxic cardiopulmonary arrests.** Carbon monoxide poisoning occurs after prolonged exposure to smoke or inhalation of the exhaust from incomplete combustion. High flow and hyperbaric oxygen, along with management of acidosis, are the cornerstones of treatment. Cyanide poisoning occurs surprisingly often, especially during fires involving other synthetic materials. The antidote is intravenous sodium nitrite and sodium thiosulfate. Tricyclic antidepressant drugs act as type IA antiarrhythmic agents and cause cardiac conduction slowing, ventricular arrhythmias, hypotension, and seizures. Vigorous alkalinization and seizure control are required.
  8. **Primary asphyxia.** In addition to anaphylaxis, obstructive asphyxia may occur after foreign body aspiration, inflammatory conditions of the hypopharynx (epiglottitis or retropharyngeal abscess), or cervicofacial trauma. The latter results in edema or hematoma formation, subcutaneous emphysema, or laryngeal or tracheal disruption. Treatment includes establishment of a patent airway, endotracheal intubation (orally or by cricothyrotomy), and assisted ventilation with 100% oxygen.

9. How should ventricular fibrillation be treated?
The essential ingredient is speed; the prognosis dims with every minute of delay. An initial defibrillation dose of 200 joules is recommended to minimize myocardial damage and to prevent the development of post-countershock pulseless bradyarrhythmias. Recent studies of animals suggest that in prolonged cardiac arrest, augmentation of myocardial blood flow with epinephrine prior to countershock may improve defibrillation success.

10. What about persistent ventricular fibrillation?
  1. Perform endotracheal intubation and assure adequate ventilation.
  2. Administer magnesium sulfate (2–5 mg IV), which may be an effective antifibrillatory agent.
  3. Administer epinephrine (dosage is controversial, see question #16) to augment aortic diastolic blood pressure and improve myocardial perfusion.
  4. Administer lidocaine (1 mg/kg) or procainamide (20–30 mg/min up to maximum of 17 mg/kg). Bretylium tosylate (5–10 mg/kg) is an alternative antidysrhythmic agent. However, neither lidocaine nor any other drug has proved efficacious in improving defibrillation success rates or in restoring a perfusing rhythm in patients in ventricular fibrillation.

11. Is pulseless idioventricular rhythm treatable?
Delayed electrical countershock frequently results in asystole or a pulseless idioventricular rhythm (PIVR), which most often is untreatable and results in death. In animal experiments,

high-dose epinephrine (0.1–0.2 mg/kg) has helped to restore cardiac contractility and pacemaker activity and may improve the outcome in post-countershock brady-asystole. In the prehospital setting, PIVR may be a transient rhythm following defibrillation. A recent review of such cases revealed a hosptial discharge rate of 8%.

12. How should asystole be treated?

Asystole should be treated according to a three-step approach.

    1. Confirm the absence of cardiac activity (a flat-line EKG may be recorded because of technical mistakes). Verify the absence of pulses at the carotid or femoral artery. Check for loose or disconnected battery cables and monitor leads. Finally, rotate the monitoring leads 90° and increase the amplitude to detect occult, fine, ventricular fibrillation.

    2. Atropine should be administered to counter hypervagotonia, which may accompany inferoposterior myocardial infarction, acidosis, drug administration, or hypoxia.

    3. Administer epinephrine.

    4. Consider aminophylline, 250 mg, for refractory asystole.

13. Is electrical defibrillation or pacemaker therapy used for asystole?

Electrical defibrillation should be reserved for cases in which differentiation between asystole and fine ventricular fibrillation is difficult; in these ambiguous situations, defibrillation should be employed after administration of epinephrine. Pacemaker therapy is often attempted for asystole but is seldom effective in restoring a pulsatile rhythm.

14. What are the appropriate routes of drug administration?

Intravenous administration is the preferred route of drug therapy during cardiopulmonary arrest. If a central venous catheter is in place, then the most distal port should be used. Otherwise, use of a peripheral vein catheter will result in a slightly delayed onset of action, although the peak drug effect is similar to that for the central route. Intracardiac administration should be reserved for cases of open cardiac massage. A number of drugs (epinephrine, atropine, lidocaine) are absorbed systemically after endotracheal administration, yet the effectiveness of this route during CPR is suspect. Pulmonary blood flow, and hence systemic absorption, is minimal during CPR. Recent studies in animals suggest that comparable hemodynamic responses occur only with endotracheal doses of epinephrine 10 times that of the intravenous doses. Virtually every drug used for resuscitation can be administered in conventional doses via the intraosseous route. This method is useful in pediatric patients, when an intravenous line cannot be established rapidly.

15. When may prehospital resuscitation efforts be terminated?

According to the most recent advanced cardiac life support (ACLS) guidelines, prehospital resuscitation can be discontinued by EMS authorities when the patient is nonresuscitable after an adequate trial of ACLS, including:

    1. Successful endotracheal intubation.

    2. Intravenous access has been achieved and rhythm-appropriate medications and countershocks have been administered.

    3. Persistent asystole or agonal electrocardiographic patterns are present.

    4. No reversible causes are identified.

    5. A valid no-CPR order is presented to the rescuers.

CONTROVERSIES

16. What is the appropriate dose of epinephrine?

For: The conventional dose of epinephrine (0.5–1.0 mg IV every 5 minutes) was derived empirically from animal studies and then applied arbitrarily to humans. No dose-response studies were performed. Indeed, the "standard" 1-mg dose of epinephrine actually reduces myocardial blood flow in experimental studies and has never been proved to be efficacious in human cardiac arrest. A number of recent animal experiments and human trials indicate that "high-dose" epinephrine (0.1–0.2 mg/kg) results in higher rates of return of spontaneous circulation, compared to standard doses. These preliminary and limited clinical trials have not demonstrated any evidence of detrimental side effects.

Against: Although recent human trials may have demonstrated a higher rate of return of spontaneous circulation with "high-dose" epinephrine, no trial has demonstrated improved neurologic recovery. Until a well-designed study is performed, current therapy should remain standard. This is especially true because the result of high-dose treatment may be an increased number of neurologically impaired survivors.

17. Is sodium bicarbonate indicated in the routine management of cardiopulmonary arrest?

For: When cardiopulmonary arrest occurs, acidemia follows. Even if CPR is performed "correctly," tissue perfusion is suboptimal and metabolic acidosis occurs. In addition, and more importantly, alveolar hypoventilation (respiratory acidosis) occurs. Buffering is necessary to counter the pernicious effects of acidemia. A severe fall in pH interferes with the vascular and myocardial responses to adrenergic drugs and endogenous catecholamines and reduces cardiac chronotropy and inotropy. In addition, acidosis leads to ventricular irritability and a lower threshold for ventricular fibrillation. Finally, below a pH of 7.2, myocardial contractile function may decline, resulting in refractory EMD.

While the primary treatment of the acidemia of cardiac arrest is adequate ventilation, metabolic acidosis often progresses inexorably. Sodium bicarbonate is the only buffer commonly available, and its use has traditionally been recommended when the pH falls to a life-threatening range, usually below 7.2. Sodium bicarbonate may be particularly useful in attenuating post-resuscitation myocardial dysfunction.

Against: The primary treatment of the acidemia of cardiac arrest is adequate ventilation, which in clinical and animal studies correlates with survival. In addition, the metabolic acidosis is usually unimportant in the first 15 to 18 minutes of resuscitation. If ventilation is maintained, the arterial pH usually remains above 7.2; moderate acidosis in this range does not interfere with defibrillation, shifts the oxyhemoglobin dissociation curve to the right, may actually augment cardiac contractility, and protects against, rather than precipitates, EMD.

Sodium bicarbonate is a poor buffering agent for cardiac resuscitation. Sodium bicarbonate causes volume overload, hyperosmolarity, hypernatremia, and hyperkalemia, even when used as recommended. Iatrogenic alkalosis may cause arrhythmias, cerebral vasoconstriction, lactic acid production, and a left shift of the oxygen hemoglobin saturation curve, further limiting tissue oxygen delivery. Most important, the bicarbonate ion, after combining with hydrogen ion, generates new carbon dioxide. Biologic membranes are highly permeable to carbon dioxide (but are much more slowly permeable to sodium bicarbonate). Therefore, administration of sodium bicarbonate causes a paradoxical intracellular acidosis. Recent studies indicate that intramyocardial hypercarbia causes a profound decline in cardiac contractile function and will lead to failure of resuscitation. Myocardial PCO_2 in human resuscitation may reach levels in excess of 250 mmHg, further highlighting the risks of administering carbon dioxide–generating agents such as sodium bicarbonate. Within the myocardial cell, hypercapnia impairs contractility and results in refractory EMD.

18. So, do I administer bicarbonate or not?

Sodium bicarbonate is not recommended because no buffer therapy is needed in the first 15 minutes of arrest (so long as adequate lung ventilation is maintained), and because the optimal acid-base status for resuscitation has not been established. Only restoration of the spontaneous circulation—not a buffering agent—can reverse the development of intramyocardial hypercarbia.

19. Is there a role for routine administration of calcium during CPR?
For: Adequate levels of ionized calcium are necessary for effective cardiovascular function. In the setting of ionized hypocalcemia, administration of calcium chloride improves cardiovascular hemodynamics. Recent human and animal trials have confirmed that ionized calcium levels fall precipitously during prolonged (>7.5 minutes) cardiac arrest. The only prospective, double-blinded study of calcium administration in cardiac arrest suggested that "high-dose" calcium ($CaCl_2$ 500–1000 mg IV) may facilitate restoration of circulatory function, especially when the QRS complex is wide.
Against: Calcium overload is thought to play an important role in ischemia and reperfusion cell injury, and increases in intracellular calcium are associated with cell death. There is no evidence that calcium administration increases neurologic recovery or hospital discharge rates.

20. When is administration of calcium indicated?
Current ACLS guidelines suggest that calcium should be administered only to patients with hyperkalemia, calcium antagonist overdose, or hypocalcemia.

BIBLIOGRAPHY

1. American Heart Association: Guidelines for cardiopulmonary resuscitation (CPR) and emergency cardiac care (ECC). JAMA 268:2172, 1992.
2. Brown CG, Martin DR, Pepe PE, et al: A comparison of standard-dose and high-dose epinephrine in cardiac arrest outside the hospital. N Engl J Med 327:15, 1992.
3. Cairns CB, Niemann JT, Pelikan PCD, Shama J: Ionized hypocalcemia during prolonged cardiac arrest and closed-chest CPR in a canine model. Ann Emerg Med 20:1178, 1991.
4. Callaham ML: High-dose epinephrine therapy and other advances in treating cardiac arrest. West J Med 152:697, 1990.
5. Eisenberg MS, Bergnen L, Haustrom A: Epidemiology of cardiac arrest and resuscitation in a suburban community. JACEP 8:2, 1979.
6. Hoffman JR, Stevenson CW: Postdefibrillation idioventricular rhythm   a salvageable condition. West J Med 146:188, 1987.
7. Niemann JT, Cairns CB, Shama J, et al: Treatment of prolonged ventricular fibrillation: Immediate countershock versus high-dose epinephrine and CPR prior to countershock. Circulation 95:281, 1992.
8. Paradis NA, Martin GB, Rosenberg J, et al: The effect of standard and high-dose epinephrine on coronary perfusion pressure during prolonged cardiopulmonary resuscitation. JAMA 265:1139, 1991.
9. Urban P, Scheidegger D, Buchmann B, Barth D: Cardiac arrest and blood ionized calcium levels. Ann Intern Med 109:110, 1988.
10. Viskin S, Belhassen B, Roth A, et al: Aminophylline for bradyasystolic cardiac arrest refractory to atropine and epinephrine. Ann Intern Med 118:279, 1993.

3. AIRWAY MANAGEMENT

Barry Simon, M.D.

1. Do I really need to know about airway management?
In clinical medicine, expeditious airway management saves lives.

2. How is the adequacy of ventilation assessed?
First, look at the patient. Cyanosis suggests profound hypoxia. Diaphoresis and somnolence indicate hypercapnia and respiratory acidosis. Measure the respiratory rate and assess the

tidal volume by placing your hand over the endotracheal tube or the patient's mouth. If you're still concerned, use a pulse oximeter. Mild to moderate hypoxia can be monitored with pulse oximetry, which measures arterial oxygen saturation. If there is question of inadequate ventilation, an arterial blood gas or measurement of end-tidal CO_2 should be considered.

3. Why do patients need their airway managed?
Airway management is indicated for many reasons. **Assisted ventilation** can help to decrease intracranial pressure or correct hypercarbia and acidosis. **Oxygenation** may also be needed in patients with severe lung disease or injury who are unable to maintain an acceptable PaO_2. **Overcoming or preventing airway obstruction** is imperative in patients with neck trauma, epiglottitis, or smoke inhalation. **Prevention of aspiration** in patients with altered mentation is best accomplished with endotracheal intubation. **Administration of intratracheal drugs** through the endotracheal tube is indicated in a resuscitation until an intravenous line can be established.

4. What is the most common cause of airway obstruction?
The tongue obstructs the airway far more commonly than do foreign bodies or edema. With decreasing level of consciousness, the supporting muscles in the floor of the mouth lose tone and the tongue falls posteriorly, obstructing the oropharynx. The fastest, least invasive treatment modality is the head tilt/chin lift maneuver. A nasopharyngeal or oral airway should be inserted in a patient with ongoing upper airway obstruction unrelieved by repositioning the patient.

5. What is an EOA?
The esophageal obturator airway, or EOA, is a 34-cm-long plastic tube with a mask at the proximal end and a balloon at the distal end. This device is placed blindly in the esophagus and the balloon is inflated to prevent air from entering the stomach and vomitus from entering the airway.

6. What are the indications for the EOA?
The EOA is acceptable only in a prehospital setting when assisted ventilation is needed and the providers are not trained or authorized to perform endotracheal intubation.

7. Is the EOA safe?
Not really. The greatest danger is the risk of inadvertent intubation of the trachea. A more common complication is aspiration because the EOA does not protect the trachea from secretions, bleeding, and emesis. Esophageal rupture has been reported in patients who have attempted to vomit with an EOA in place.

8. What are the relative contraindications to blind nasotracheal intubation (BNTI)?
Apnea is the most important contraindication, as the chance of esophageal intubation is unacceptably high. Because epistaxis complicates BNTI in one-third of cases, the procedure is contraindicated in patients with coagulopathies. Other routes of intubation are advisable in patients with maxillary facial or severe nasal fractures, as a false passage, severe epistaxis, or rarely cranial placement may occur. Hematomas, epiglottitis, and infections of the upper neck are relative contraindications because of the risk of sudden airway obstruction or laryngospasm.

9. Name some complications of BNTI.
Hypoxia may occur during the intubation process. Besides epistaxis and esophageal intubation, there are acute complications such as avulsion of the turbinates, avulsion of the vocal cords, and pharyngeal perforations with retropharyngeal dissection. Significant elevation in

intracranial pressure with coughing may precipitate uncal herniation in head-injured patients. Sinusitis may occur several days later from obstruction of the paranasal ostia.

10. What is rapid-sequence intubation?

Rapid-sequence intubation is a method of safely paralyzing and intubating a patient with a full stomach. Because all emergency patients are at high risk for aspiration, the airway must be secured as quickly as possible. Paralysis with succinylcholine dramatically facilitates visualization and tube placement, and reduces complications that occur with attempts to intubate an awake, struggling patient.

11. Don't you need to be an anesthesiologist to perform rapid-sequence intubation?

No. The basics can be remembered as the 5 Ps: preparation, preoxygenation, priming, pressure, and paralysis. **Prepare** by having all the necessary drugs and tools available. This includes checking the balloon, suction, and light on the laryngoscope. **Preoxygenate** in order to avoid bagging the patient while the airway is unprotected. **Prime** with induction drugs and other agents that might be needed to lower intracranial pressure. Apply **pressure** (Sellick's maneuver) after loss of consciousness to prevent regurgitation and aspiration. **Paralyze** with succinylcholine and intubate.

Rapid-sequence Intubation

1. Preoxygenate with 100% oxygen (no positive-pressure)
2. Prepare equipment (suction, ETT, bag, mask, laryngoscope, etc.)
3. Pretreat with a defasciculating dose (.01 mg/kg) of vecuronium or pancuronium
4. Prime with thiopental, 3–4 mg/kg rapid IVP
5. Apply Sellick maneuver (cricoid pressure) as consciousness is lost
6. Follow thiopental immediately with 1–2 mg/kg of succinylcholine to paralyze
7. Intubate the trachea and verify position
8. Release cricoid pressure

Alternative

Rapid-sequence Intubation

1. Preoxygenate with 100% oxygen (no positive-pressure ventilation)
2. Prepare equipment (suction, ETT, bag, mask, laryngoscope, etc.)
3. Prime with thiopental, 3–4 mg/kg rapid IVP
4. Paralyze with vecuronium, 2.5 mg/kg IVP
5. Apply Sellick maneuver (cricoid pressure) as consciousness is lost
6. Intubate the trachea and verify position
7. Release cricoid pressure

12. How do I "preoxygenate" a patient prior to intubation?

Bag-valve-mask ventilation is the only option in the apneic patient, even though this will increase the risk of aspiration by raising gastric pressure. If a patient is making effective respiratory efforts, then he or she should receive passive oxygenation via a nonrebreather mask on 100% oxygen.

13. What is Sellick's maneuver?

Sellick described a method of applying pressure over the cricoid cartilage to help prevent aspiration. Pressure should be equivalent to the amount of force it takes to cause discomfort when pressing over the bridge of one's nose. Pressure is applied after loss of consciousness and is maintained until the endotracheal tube balloon is inflated and tube placement is confirmed.

14. How do I remember the size of the endotracheal tube for children?
The easiest way is to carry a card in your wallet. However, the following formula works for ages 2 to 20:

$$\text{Tube size} = \frac{(\text{age in years} + 16)}{4}$$

Infants under 2 years can usually accept a tube about the size of their small finger.

15. Why is succinylcholine the most common paralyzing agent in rapid-sequence induction?
No other neuromuscular blocking agent has as rapid an onset of action (45–60 seconds) or as brief a duration of activity (4–7 minutes). This provides added safety, with the return of spontaneous respiration within 7 minutes.

16. What are the theoretical risks of succinylcholine?
Despite its significant benefits, it has many undesirable characteristics, some of which may be dangerous. It increases intragastric, intraocular, and intracranial pressure. Life-threatening hyperkalemia may occur in patients with neuromuscular disease, or 3 to 4 days after major burns and trauma. Severe muscle contractions cause delayed pain and at times rhabdomyolysis. Rarely, it can precipitate malignant hyperthermia.

17. Are there any alternative paralytics?
Vecuronium has been suggested as an alternative to succinylcholine. It has few complications and when used in large doses has an onset of action nearly as fast as succinylcholine. Its duration of action is greater than 45 minutes when used in rapid-sequence doses. Pancuronium is an alternative but is a poor choice for rapid-sequence induction because of its slow onset of action. Newer nondepolarizing drugs with properties similar to succinyl-choline should be available in the near future.

18. Are there any contraindications to rapid-sequence induction?
Yes. Paralyze a patient only when you are sure you can intubate. A difficult airway with anatomic distortion (e.g., patients with penetrating neck trauma or epiglottitis) is a relative contraindication. Rapid-sequence intubation should also be avoided in patients who cannot be preoxygenated (e.g., those with severe COPD or asthma).

19. How do I manage patients who have contraindications to rapid-sequence induction?
Nasotracheal intubation is a good alternative in patients with pulmonary disease. If unsuccessful, or if there is a contraindication, oral awake intubation with an induction agent such as ketamine will allow the patient to maintain both a certain degree of ventilation and airway protection during the procedure. Ketamine should not be used in head-injured patients, as it dramatically increases intracranial pressure.

20. What alternatives are left if these standard techniques fail?
   1. **Cricothyrotomy,** a surgical airway through the cricothyroid membrane, can be performed rapidly, although it is often complicated by hemorrhage and is contraindicated in children under the age of 8.
   2. **Tracheostomy** is more time consuming but is the surgical airway of choice in children and tracheal injury.
   3. **Fiberoptic intubation** allows visualization of the cords and trachea but is technically difficult and time consuming.

4. In **tactile intubation,** the practitioner uses the index and middle fingers to palpate the epiglottis and guide the tube through the cords. The patient needs to be comatose or heavily sedated, and the success rate is lower than with rapid sequence intubation.

5. **Retrograde intubation** involves placing a wire through cricoid membrane and securing it through the mouth. The wire is then used as a guide to pass the endotracheal tube.

6. **Percutaneous transtracheal ventilation** involves inserting a catheter into the trachea and ventilating the patient with high-pressure oxygen. These two last techniques are rarely used and require prior training or special equipment.

21. Once the patient is intubated, how do I determine if the endotracheal tube is correctly placed?
The single best method of confirming placement is to actually see the tube pass through the cords. Monitoring of oxygen saturation and the use of capnography or colorimetric end-tidal CO_2 devices are useful adjuncts. Other findings are helpful but are **not** definitive: the tube fogs and clears with ventilation; breath sounds are heard in both axillas but not over the stomach; chest expansion is noted and symmetric.

22. Doesn't the chest radiograph confirm placement in the trachea?
No. Although the chest radiograph is helpful in ruling out bronchial intubation, the tube can easily be placed in the esophagus and appear to be in the trachea just proximal to the carina.

4. SHOCK

Robert D. Schmidt, M.D.

1. Define shock.
Shock is a clinical syndrome defined by an inadequate blood flow and transport of oxygen to organs and tissues. It also has been defined as a reduction of blood flow by diminished cardiac output or maldistributed output such that potential irreversible tissue damage occurs.

2. What needs to be done immediately in a patient in clinical shock?
The ABCs (airway, breathing, circulation) and a set of vital signs should be included in the primary survey of all seriously ill or injured patients. Patients should be given supplemental oxygen, have large-bore intravenous access, and have cardiac monitoring. In trauma patients, any obvious external hemorrhage should be controlled.

3. Name the three pathophysiologic classifications of shock and give examples of each class.
Blood flow is determined by three entities: blood volume, vascular capacitance and resistance, and pump function. Thus there are three pathophysiologic classifications of shock: hypovolemic, vasogenic, and cardiogenic. Examples of causes of hypovolemic shock are gastrointestinal bleeds, ruptured aortic aneurysm, and severe diabetic ketoacidosis. Examples of vasogenic include septic shock, anaphylactic shock, neurogenic shock, and shock from pharmacologic causes. Cardiogenic shock includes acute myocardial infarction with shock, cardiomyopathies, valvular abnormalities (especially severe aortic stenosis and regurgitation), arrhythmias, and pulmonary embolism. Pulmonary embolism can be included as a separate classification—obstructive—but presents similarly to cardiogenic causes.

4. Clinically how do you determine a patient's class of shock?

In addition to history, one of the most helpful bedside tests is feeling the skin of the extremities. Warm skin with shock is helpful in distinguishing vasogenic causes. If the skin is cool, then cardiogenic or hypovolemic shock is most likely.

5. What are the body's compensatory responses to volume loss?

The loss of blood volume causes a decrease in cardiac output. A reflex tachycardia occurs in order to maintain an adequate blood pressure. This decreased cardiac output also causes a release of epinephrine and norepinephrine, mediated by baroreceptors, by a reflex known as the sympathoadrenal reaction. These catecholamines increase cardiac output through improved contractility, elevated pulse rate, and increased venous tone. They elevate blood pressure through arteriole constriction by increased systemic vascular resistance. The arterioles with the greatest amount of receptors and the greatest sensitivity to catechols are in the skin, muscles, kidney, and gastrointestinal tract. This causes shunting of blood to the heart and brain, which have a low concentration of these receptors. The increase in arteriolar tone in the periphery decreases capillary hydrostatic pressure, causing a net movement of fluid into the vascular space. Decreased renal blood flow reduces urinary output and fluid loss.

6. How sensitive are supine vital signs in determining volume loss?

Not very sensitive. The body can compensate for up to 15% intravascular volume loss before developing tachycardia. It may take 30% volume loss to have a significant loss in blood pressure.

7. Are orthostatic vital signs a sensitive indicator of hypovolemia? What determines a positive orthostatic test?

To know what is considered abnormal you must first know what is normal. Studies of orthostatic changes in healthy "euvolemic" people have shown an average increase in pulse from 12.6 to 17.9 with a large standard deviation. Therefore, an increase of 20 bpm in pulse as a determinant of hypovolemia is nonspecific because many normal individuals are in this category. Using an increase of 30 bpm as a specific indicator for hypovolemia, orthostatics are not sensitive until there has been a 20% intravascular volume loss. Blood pressure changes are not helpful because they may be drastic even in healthy people. The development of symptoms (e.g., dizziness) upon standing does not occur in healthy individuals and is considered abnormal.

8. What is normal central venous pressure (CVP)?

Normal CVP is 5–12 cm H_2O.

9. What are the four determinants of CVP?

Intravascular volume, intrathoracic pressure, right ventricular function, and venous tone all affect CVP. To reduce variability caused by intrathoracic pressure, CVP should be measured at end expiration.

10. Define sepsis.

It is the condition associated with the presence of pathogenic microorganisms or their toxins in the blood. Shock from sepsis occurs from gram-negative bacteria in the greatest majority of cases but also occurs from gram-positive bacteria, viruses, protozoa, and fungi.

11. Who is at risk for sepsis?

Patients at the extremes of age, burn victims, patients who have undergone recent abdominal and genitourinary procedures, diabetics, cancer patients, and patients pharmacologically immunosuppressed from chemotherapeutics and steroids.

12. What are the causes of shock from sepsis?

Endotoxin is a strong antigenic stimulus that causes the release of vasoactive substances such as histamine, prostaglandins, and bradykinin, resulting in peripheral venous and arteriolar dilatation. Histamine and bradykinin also increase endothelial permeability, causing intravascular volume loss of fluid in the periphery.

13. What are the classic changes in systemic vascular resistance (SVR) and cardiac output in septic shock?

In classic "warm" septic shock, the SVR is much reduced and cardiac output is increased. The increase in cardiac output is a compensatory mechanism by the body in response to the loss in vascular resistance. It is not completely compensatory because of a myocardial depressant factor released in sepsis.

14. How can septic shock appear like cardiogenic shock?

In hypodynamic or "cold" septic shock, seen more frequently in the elderly, there are two causes for reduced cardiac output. First, the myocardial depressant factor decreases the cardiac index. Second, in progressive sepsis, there are increases in pulmonary capillary resistance. These factors cause a significant decrease in cardiac output and appear like right-sided congestive heart failure. Cold septic shock is associated with a high mortality.

15. What are the primary goals in the treatment of septic shock in the emergency department (ED)?

The goals of treatment are to maximize tissue oxygenation, improve hemodynamic dysfunction, correct underlying metabolic abnormalities, and treat the infection.

16. What specific treatments are important in septic shock?

Supplemental oxygen should be given to any septic patient. All patients in septic shock will have intravascular volume loss and require aggressive volume resuscitation. If blood pressure and tissue perfusion, measured by mental status and urine output, do not improve with volume, dopamine is an excellent initial pressor agent in septic shock. Severe acidosis may restrict the effectiveness of dopamine, and norepinephrine (Levophed) may be a better choice. Septic shock is an indication for starting antibiotics in the ED. Antibiotic choice should depend on the suspected source of the infection. Regardless of source, gram-negative coverage is essential with an aminoglycoside or a third-generation cephalosporin.

17. What is the utility of the Killip classification?

The Killip classification is based on clinical criteria that correlate the degree of pump dysfunction with acute mortality in a patient with myocardial infarction. Class I has no evidence of left ventricular failure and has a 5% mortality. Class II has bibasilar rales, an S3 gallop, and a 15–20% mortality. Class III patients have pulmonary edema and a 40% mortality. Class IV patients are in cardiogenic shock defined by: (1) systolic blood pressure less than 90 mmHg, (2) peripheral vasoconstriction, (3) oliguria, and (4) pulmonary vascular congestion. They have a mortality of 80%. It has been reported that necrosis of 35–70% of the left ventricle is indicative of patients dying with cardiogenic shock.

18. How do I approach the patient with a myocardial infarction and cardiogenic shock?

With all forms of shock, supplemental oxygen should be delivered. Arrhythmias must be treated. If there is no pulmonary edema, volume can be given in aliquots of 200–300 cc boluses, particularly if there is EKG evidence of right ventricular (RV) infarction. Dopamine and dobutamine are the pressors of choice for improvement of hemodynamics. Dobutamine is likely to be a better choice, except in RV infarct. This is particularly true if there is evidence of pulmonary edema, since dobutamine reduces left ventricular end-diastolic pressure (LVEDP), whereas dopamine increases LVEDP. Thrombolytic agents have been shown to improve survival in relationship to the amount of tissue in jeopardy; thus the early administration of these agents must be considered.

19. How does pulmonary embolism (PE) cause shock?

Massive PE causes shock on the basis of reduced cross-sectional area of the pulmonary outflow tract. This occurs at a reduction of 50% or more of the cross-sectional area in normal individuals. With this large acute reduction in area, the pulmonary artery systolic pressure maximum of 40 mmHg is reached, blood flow is then reduced, and shock ensues.

20. What is the treatment of shock secondary to a massive PE?

Massive PE should be treated similarly to cardiogenic shock from myocardial infarction with oxygen (intubation if necessary), volume, and pressors. Thrombolytics have not been studied well enough in massive PE to show improved survival. However, their use has been demonstrated to improve hemodynamics with reduced tricuspid regurgitation, reduced RV dilatation, and improved cardiac output in patients with massive PE.

21. How do I approach the patient with hemorrhagic shock?

Be on a hunt for the source of blood loss. A chest radiograph is key in looking for widened mediastinum, pneumothorax, and hemothorax. A pelvic radiograph to search for fractures is important because pelvic fractures can cause rapidly progressive shock and death from hemorrhage. Peritoneal lavage and CT scan are sensitive procedures for intraperitoneal hemorrhage, but in shock from trauma a peritoneal lavage is the procedure of choice because it can be performed in minutes. Obtaining a baseline hematocrit and sending a sample to the blood bank for cross-matching are critical initial lab tests.

22. What is the approach to fluid and blood resuscitation in hemorrhagic shock?

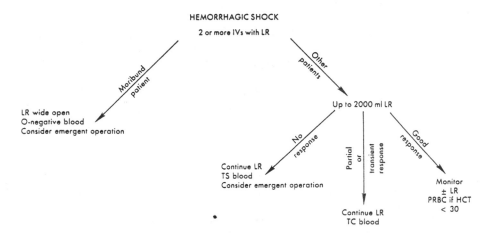

Fluid resuscitation of hemorrhagic shock. LR, lactated Ringer's solution; TS, type specific; TC, typed and crossmatched blood; PRBC, packed red blood cells; HCT, hematocrit. (From Mannix FL: Hemorrhagic shock. In Rosen P, et al (eds): Emergency Medicine: Concepts and Clinical Practice, 2nd ed. St. Louis, Mosby–Year Book, Inc., 1988, p 179.

23. What is neurogenic shock? How do I initially treat it?

With acute spinal cord injuries, sympathetic tone is lost in regions distal to the lesion, causing arteriolar and venous dilatation. In addition, bradycardia may be seen with cervical lesions, resulting from reduced sympathetic stimulation to the sinus node. Any degree of hypovolemia from other injuries can cause extremely low blood pressures. Neurogenic shock should be managed with volume (up to a liter of crystalloid in the face of no blood loss), atropine if bradycardia is present, and an alpha agonist (dopamine or ephedrine) for refractory hypotension.

24. Name four causes of traumatic cardiogenic shock.
Pericardial tamponade, myocardial contusion, tension pneumothorax, and air gas embolism from bronchial tears.

25. When should pericardial tamponade be suspected?
Acute pericardial tamponade occurs in about 2% of penetrating chest trauma and is more common with stab wounds than gunshot wounds. Tamponade is rare after blunt trauma. Beck's classic triad of distended neck veins, decreased arterial pressure, and muffled heart sounds occurs only in about a third of patients. A high CVP in the face of tachycardia and hypotension in penetrating trauma is reliable for tamponade. Examination and chest radiograph will exclude tension pneumothorax.

CONTROVERSIES

26. Is rapid crystalloid administration helpful or harmful in treating hemorrhagic shock?
For: Aggressive crystalloid infusion clearly improves circulatory hemodynamics (blood pressure, pulse, and urine output), thus preventing irreversible shock and allowing time to get the patient to definitive care.
Against: Rapid crystalloid infusion decreases the blood's oxygen-carrying capacity and may increase via hemodilution the rate of hemorrhage in a patient with an ongoing source for hemorrhage. Therefore, aggressive volume resuscitation should not be commenced until definitive resuscitative measures, i.e., administration of red blood cells and immediate control of the hemorrhage, have been carried out.

27. Does hypertonic saline resuscitation have any place in shock resuscitation?
Hypertonic saline (3%–7.5% sodium chloride), alone or with the additives dextran and mannitol, restores extracellular volume faster than isotonic saline. Hypertonic saline has also been shown to have beneficial hemodynamic effects because of a positive inotropic effect. A recent multicenter study comparing outcomes of patients with post-traumatic hypotension, treated with small volumes of either hypertonic or isotonic saline in the field, demonstrated no statistical difference in overall survival between the two groups.

BIBLIOGRAPHY

1. Bresler MJ: Future role of thrombolytic therapy in emergency medicine. Ann Emerg Med 18:1331, 1989.
2. Chatterjee K: Myocardial infarction shock. Crit Care Clin 1:3:563, 1985.
3. Dhainaut JF, et al: Right ventricular dysfunction in patients with septic shock. Intens Care Med 14:488, 1988.
4. Donahue AM: Central venous pressure measurement. In Roberts JR, Hedges JR (eds): Clinical Procedures in Emergency Medicine. Philadelphia, W.B. Saunders, 1991, pp 332–338.
5. Luce JM: Pathogenesis and management of septic shock. Chest 91:883, 1987.
6. Mannix FL: Hemorrhagic shock. In Rosen P, et al (eds): Emergency Medicine: Concepts and Clinical Practice, 2nd ed. St. Louis, Mosby–Year Book, Inc., 1988, p 179.
7. Mattox KL, et al: Prehospital hypertonic saline-dextran infusion for post-traumatic hypotension: The USA multicenter trial. Ann Surg 213:482, 1991.
8. Schmidt RD, Wolfe R: Shock. In Rosen P, et al (eds): Emergency Medicine: Concepts and Clinical Practice, 3nd ed. St. Louis, Mosby–Year Book, Inc., 1992, pp 163–172.
9. Shamji FM, Todd TRJ: Hypovolemic shock. Crit Care Clin 1:3:609, 1985.
10. Wilson RF: The pathophysiology of shock. Intens Care Med 6:89, 1980.

II. Primary Complaints

5. ALTERED MENTAL STATUS AND COMA

Kenneth Jackimczyk, M.D.

1. What is coma? What terms should be used to describe altered sensorium?

Coma is a depressed mental state in which verbal and physical stimuli cannot elicit useful responses. Other terms such as lethargic, stuporous, or obtunded mean different things to different observers and should be avoided. You may be "alert but confused" as you read this chapter. It is best to describe the mental functions the patient can perform, e.g., the patient is oriented to person, place and time, knows the president, and can count backwards from twenty.

2. What causes coma?

Mental alertness is maintained by the cerebral hemispheres in conjunction with the reticular activating system (RAS). Coma can be produced by diffuse disease of both cerebral hemispheres (usually a metabolic problem), disease in the brain stem that damages the RAS, or a structural CNS lesion that causes pressure on the RAS.

3. How can I remember the causes of coma and altered mental status?

When you are faced with a patient who is acutely ill, sometimes your own brain doesn't function very well. At those times, it is helpful to use a mnemonic. Henry has devised a good one for coma: TIPS–Vowels, that is TIPS–AEIOU.

TIPS
T	Trauma, temperature
I	Infection (CNS and systemic)
P	Psychiatric
S	Space-occupying lesions, stroke, subarachnoid hemorrhage, shock

VOWELS
A	Alcohol and other drugs
E	Endocrine, exocrine, electrolytes
I	Insulin (diabetes)
O	Oxygen (lack of), opiates
U	Uremia

4. What important historical facts should be obtained from the patient with altered mental status or coma?

This seems like a stupid question, because the patient with altered consciousness cannot give you a reliable history and the comatose patient cannot give any history at all! You should question prehospital personnel carefully and attempt to contact the patient's friends or family. Ask about the onset of symptoms (acute or gradual), recent neurologic symptoms (headache, seizure, or focal neurologic abnormalities), drug or alcohol abuse, recent trauma, prior psychiatric problems, and past medical history (neurologic disorders, diabetes, renal failure, or cardiac disease). If you're having trouble getting historical information, search the patient's belongings for pill bottles, check the patient's wallet for telephone numbers or names of friends, and review previous medical records.

5. How can I perform a brief, directed physical examination on the patient with altered consciousness?

The goal of the physical examination is to differentiate structural focal CNS problems from diffuse metabolic processes. Pay special attention to vital signs, general appearance, mental status, eye findings, and the motor exam. Vital signs and eye findings are so important they are discussed elsewhere in this chapter.

The general appearance should be noted prior to examining the patient. Are there signs of trauma? Is there symmetry of spontaneous movements?

Mental status should be quickly assessed. Ask four sets of progressively more difficult questions: (1) orientation to person, place, and time; (2) name the president; (3) count backwards from twenty (if done correctly ask for serial 3's or 7's); and (4) recent recall of three unrelated objects.

Motor examination is performed to determine the symmetry of motor tone or strength and response of deep tendon reflexes.

6. What is the Glascow coma scale?

The Glascow coma scale is a simple reproducible scoring system used in trauma patients to define the level of coma. It is useful for standardizing assessments among multiple observers, and for monitoring changes in the degree of coma. The score is determined by eliciting the best response obtained from the patient in three categories: eye opening, verbal response, and motor response. It is not sensitive enough to detect subtle alterations of consciousness in the noncomatose patient. It is also somewhat disconcerting to have a point system where inanimate objects get a score of three points.

Glascow Coma Scale

OBSERVATION		POINTS
Eye Opening	Spontaneous	4
	To verbal command	3
	To pain	2
	No response	1
Best Verbal Response	Oriented/converses	5
	Confused conversation	4
	Inappropriate words	3
	Incomprehensible sounds	2
	No response	1
Best Motor Response	Obeys	6
	Localizes pain	5
	Flexion withdrawal	4
	Decorticate posture	3
	Decerebrate posture	2
	No response	1
Total Points		3–15

7. How important is measuring the temperature of the comatose patient?

Vital signs often provide clues to the etiology of coma. A core temperature must be obtained. An elevated temperature should lead you to investigate the possibility of meningitis, sepsis, heat stroke, or hyperthyroidism. Hypothermia can be due to environmental exposure, hypoglycemia, or rarely addisonian crisis. Do not assume that an abnormal temperature is the result of a neurogenic cause until you eliminate other causes.

8. What about the other vital signs? What is their significance?
I wouldn't pose two questions discussing the vital signs if they weren't important. Check the cardiac monitor. Bradycardia or dysrhythmias can alter cerebral perfusion and cause altered sensorium. Carefully count respirations. Tachypnea may indicate the presence of hypoxemia or a metabolic acidosis, and diminished respiratory efforts may require assisted ventilation. Do not assume that hypotension has a CNS cause. Look for hypovolemia or sepsis as an etiology for hypotension, but remember that adults (in contrast to infants) cannot become hypovolemic from intracranial bleeding alone. Hypertension may be a result of increased intracranial pressure, but uncontrolled hypertension may also cause encephalopathy and coma.

9. What is Cushing's reflex?
Cushing's reflex is an alteration of vital signs—increased blood pressure and decreased pulse—secondary to increased intracranial pressure.

10. What is decorticate and decerebrate posturing?
Posturing may be seen with noxious stimulation in the comatose patient with severe brain injury. Decorticate posturing refers to hyperextension of the legs with flexion of the arms and elbows. Decorticate posturing results from damage to the descending motor pathways above the central midbrain. Decerebrate posturing is a more grave sign and refers to hyperextension of both the upper and lower extremities. Decerebrate posturing reflects damage to the midbrain and upper pons. If you have trouble remembering which position is which, think of the upper extremities in flexion with the hands over the heart ("cor") in de-"cor"-ticate posturing.

11. What information can be obtained from the eye examination of the comatose patient?
The eyes should be examined for **position**, **reactivity**, and **reflexes**.

When the eyelids are opened, note the **position** of the eyes. If the eyes flutter upward, exposing only the sclera, suspect psychogenic coma. If the eyes exhibit bilateral roving movements that cross the midline, you know that the brainstem is intact.

Pupil **reactivity** is the single best test to differentiate metabolic coma from coma caused by a structural lesion, because it is relatively resistant to metabolic insult and is usually preserved in a metabolic coma. Pupil reactivity may be subtle, necessitating use of a bright light in a dark room.

Testing of the eye **reflexes** is the single best method for determining the status of the brainstem. Two methods can be used: (1) oculocephalic (doll's eyes) or (2) oculovestibular (cold calorics). Oculocephalic testing requires rapid twisting of the neck, which is a "bad idea" in the unconscious patient because occult cervical trauma may be present. Oculovestibular testing is easy to perform and can be done without manipulating the neck. The ear canal is irrigated with 50 cc of ice water. A normal awake patient has two competing eye movements: rapid nystagmus away from the irrigated ear and slow tonic deviation toward the cold stimulus. Remember the mnemonic COWS, Cold Opposite Warm Same, which refers to the direction of the fast component.

← **Rapid Nystagmus**

Cold water irrigation

Slow tonic deviation →

A patient with psychogenic coma will have normal reflexes and exhibit rapid nystagmus. The comatose patient with an intact brainstem will lack the nystagmus phase and the eyes will slowly deviate toward the irrigated ear. If the eyes do anything else, grab Plum and Posner to figure out where the lesion is located, but it is not a good sign.

Plum F, Posner JB: The Diagnosis of Stupor and Coma, 3rd ed. Philadelphia, F.A. Davis Co., 1982.

12. I want to impress the attendings. Do you have any tips on physical examination that will let me assume my rightful position as star student?

- If a confused patient is suspected of being postictal, look in the mouth. A tongue laceration supports the diagnosis of a seizure.
- Put on gloves and inspect the scalp. Occult trauma is often overlooked and you may find a laceration or dried blood. An old scar on the scalp may tip you off to a post-traumatic seizure disorder.
- Do not be fooled by a "positive blink test" in a patient with suspected psychogenic coma. When you rapidly flick your hand at a comatose patient who has open eyes, air movement may stimulate a corneal reflex in a patient who is truly comatose.
- Do not be misled by the odor of alcohol. Alcohol has almost no detectable odor, which is why closet alcoholics drink vodka at work. Other spirited liquors such as brandy have a strong odor. The comatose executive who "smells drunk" may actually have had a sudden subarachnoid hemorrhage and spilled brandy on his shirt.

13. Which x-rays should be obtained in the comatose patient?

A cervical spine series must be obtained in any comatose patient with suspected trauma, since physical examination is unreliable. A chest radiograph may be helpful if hypoxemia or pulmonary infection is suspected. Skull series have been supplanted by CT scan and are rarely indicated.

14. Which laboratory tests should be obtained in the patient with a significantly altered level of consciousness?

Obtain a rapid blood glucose (Dextrostix) and correct hypoglycemia if it is found. If alcohol intoxication is suspected, determine the alcohol level with either a Breathalyzer or serum blood alcohol. If hypoglycemia or alcohol intoxication are not found to be the cause of the patient's confusion, further tests are warranted. A complete blood count, electrolytes, BUN, glucose, and arterial blood gases are obtained. Toxicologic screens may be done in the patient with a suspected ingestion, but remember that they are expensive and do not routinely detect every possible ingested substance. Liver function tests, ammonia level, calcium level, and thyroid function studies may be helpful in selected patients.

15. When should I do a CT scan?

Although CT scans have revolutionized the practice of neurology, they are not indicated in every comatose patient. A good history and physical examination combined with a few simple laboratory tests will be adequate in most cases seen in the emergency department, because drug abuse and alcohol abuse are common. If, however, a structural lesion is suspected, then a CT scan should be ordered immediately. If a patient with a suspected metabolic coma begins to worsen, or does not improve after a period of observation, a CT scan should be obtained at that time.

16. When should a lumbar puncture (LP) be performed?

The indications and timing of LP depend on two questions: (1) Is CNS infection suspected? (2) Is there a suspicion of a structural lesion causing increased intracranial pressure?

If meningitis is suspected and there is no indication of increased intracranial pressure, LP should be performed immediately. In the patient with acute trauma or evidence of increased intracranial pressure, CT scan is the diagnostic study of choice and LP is contra-indicated. Patients with a history consistent with a focal CNS infection should have an immediate CT; if it is negative, an LP should be done. If CT cannot be rapidly obtained in such a patient, antibiotic therapy should be instituted. Patients suspected of having a sub-arachnoid hemorrhage (SAH) should have a CT scan, but if it is negative an LP should be done to look for RBCs or xanthochromia, since CT is not 100% sensitive in diagnosing SAH.

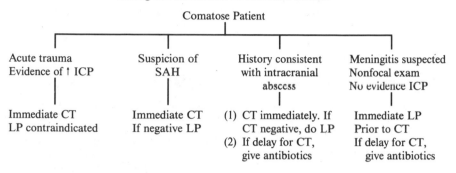

Timing and Indications for Lumbar Puncture

Comatose Patient

Acute trauma Evidence of ↑ ICP	Suspicion of SAH	History consistent with intracranial abscess	Meningitis suspected Nonfocal exam No evidence ICP
Immediate CT LP contraindicated	Immediate CT If negative LP	(1) CT immediately. If CT negative, do LP (2) If delay for CT, give antibiotics	Immediate LP Prior to CT If delay for CT, give antibiotics

17. How are the arterial blood gases (ABGs) used in the comatose patient?
ABGs should be obtained in all comatose patients. They may provide a clue to the etiology of coma, since hypoxemia and derangements of acid-base balance can alter mental status. ABGs are also useful in monitoring the treatment of intracranial pressure in intubated patients. Hyperventilation to a CO_2 of 25–28 causes cerebral vasoconstriction and dimin-ishes intracranial pressure.

18. Okay. I have made the diagnosis of coma. How do I treat it?
Emergency medicine requires simultaneous assessment and treatment. A brilliant diagnosis is useless in a dead patient. Start with the ABCs: airway, breathing, circulation and C spine. Intubate patients with apnea or labored respirations, patients who are likely to aspirate or who need gastric lavage, and any patient who is thought to have increased intracranial pressure. Maintain cervical spine precautions until the possibility of trauma has been excluded. Hypotension should be corrected so that cerebral perfusion pressure can be maintained.

Once the ABCs have been addressed, check a Dextrostix; if the glucose is low, treat hypoglycemia with D50W. It is better to do a fingerstick glucose rather than to give glucose empirically. Next give 100 mg of thiamine and 2 mg of naloxone intravenously. Flumazenil, a benzodiazepine antagonist, can be given as a diagnostic test if a benzodiazepine overdose is suspected, but is to be avoided in any patient with a seizure disorder or cyclic antidepressant ingestion. In suspected drug overdose, gastric lavage is performed. Activated charcoal, 50–100 gm, should be instilled after lavage.

The patient with increased intracranial pressure should be intubated and hyperventilated. Mannitol, 1–2 gm/kg IV, is given.

19. I think my patient is faking it. How can I tell if this is psychogenic coma?
First of all, be grateful. A patient in psychogenic coma is better than one who is angry and combative. Approach the patient incorrectly and you can awaken your patient to a hostile alert state.

Perform a careful neurologic examination. Open the eyelids. If the eyes deviate upward and only the sclera show (Bell's phenomenon), you should suspect psychogenic coma. When the eyelids are opened in a patient with true coma, the lids will close slowly and incompletely.

It is difficult to fake this movement. Lift the arm and drop it toward the face; if the face is avoided, this is most likely psychogenic coma. Next talk to the patient in a calm, caring tone. Often reassurance will awaken the patient. If this does not work, you may want to check some simple lab tests, including a Dextrostix. If the patient remains comatose, irritating but nonpainful stimuli such as tickling the feet with a cotton swab may elicit a response. Remember that this is not a test of wills between you and the patient. Repeated painful stimulation will get the patient angry and ruin attempts at therapeutic intervention, and there is no indication for such maneuvers.

If all else fails, perform cold caloric testing. The presence of nystagmus confirms the diagnosis of psychogenic coma. What do you do then? It's time to pick up a copy of *Psychiatry Secrets*.

BIBLIOGRAPHY

1. Henry GL: Coma and altered states of consciousness. In Tintinalli JE, et al (eds): Emergency Medicine: A Comprehensive Study Guide, 3rd ed. New York, McGraw-Hill, 1992, pp 150–158.
2. Henry GL, Little N: Neurologic Emergencies. New York, McGraw-Hill, 1985.
3. Huff JS: Coma. In Rosen P, et al (eds): Emergency Medicine: Concepts and Clinical Practice, 2nd ed. St. Louis, C.V. Mosby Co., 1988, pp 249–269.
4. Jorden RC: Initial evaluation of the patient with altered mental status. Top Emerg Med 13:1–9, 1991.
5. Plum F, Posner JB: The Diagnosis of Stupor and Coma, 3rd ed. Philadelphia, F.A. Davis, 1982.
6. Ropper AH: Coma in the Emergency Room. In Earnest M (ed): Neurologic Emergencies. New York, Churchill Livingstone, 1983, pp 79–102.

6. FEVER

James H. Bryan, M.D., Ph.D., and Kristi L. Koenig, M.D.

> Humanity has but three great enemies: fever, famine, and war; of these, by far the greatest, by far the most terrible, is fever.
>
> Sir William Osler

1. Is it important to read this chapter?
Yes, but of course every author says that. Fever accounts for 6% of all adult and 20% of all pediatric visits to the emergency department (ED). In addition, failure to properly diagnose and treat fever results in a substantial number of malpractice suits.

2. What is fever?
A true fever is caused by elevation of the hypothalamic set point. This causes the body to attempt to generate heat (e.g., by shivering) in order to elevate the body's core temperature. In other forms of elevated temperature (e.g., burns, heat stroke or exhaustion, malignant hyperthermia), the body attempts to cool itself to maintain a normal temperature.

3. Is a fever good for anything, or is my body just trying to make me miserable?
This is a matter of debate. Most investigators believe that fever is beneficial in fighting disease. Induction of high fever has been used in experimental cancer treatments. Higher temperatures increase the activity of neutrophils and lymphocytes and decrease the levels of serum iron, a substrate that many bacteria need to reproduce. While the only proven benefit

of fever has been in inhibiting neurosyphilis and disseminated gonorrhea, it appears that fever also inhibits coxsackieviruses and polioviruses. Other studies, however, indicate that fever may actually be detrimental in patients with tetanus, streptococci, or pneumococci. In addition, endotoxin reportedly has increased activity at higher temperatures.

4. What temperature constitutes a fever?
This varies with age. Most pediatricians consider 38°C (100.4°F) rectally to constitute a fever in children. In adults, a temperature of 38.3°C (100.9°F) is considered a fever.

5. Does it matter which method I use to take a temperature?
Yes. There are large variations between the methods used, especially in children. Rectal temperatures are considered to be the most accurate representation of core temperatures. Both oral and tympanic temperatures tend to be, on the average, 0.7°C less than rectal temperatures. In addition, oral temperatures can vary as much as 1.6°C, depending on the location of the probe in the mouth and respiratory rate. Axillary temperatures are approximately 0.7°C below oral temperatures, are notoriously inaccurate, and miss many significant fevers.

6. What about subjective fevers? Can parents accurately judge whether their child has a fever without using a thermometer?
Not really. Parents who say their child is febrile are correct only about 50% of the time. You might as well flip a coin.

7. Does a higher temperature indicate a more serious illness?
Not necessarily. While children with bacteremia are more likely to have hyperpyrexia, many less serious diseases such as viral illnesses are also associated with high fevers. In addition, many elderly patients are unable to mount a fever in response to serious infections. However, studies have shown that 90% of febrile patients over age 60 require hospitalization.

8. Is it true that fevers caused by viruses respond better to acetaminophen than fevers caused by serious bacterial infections?
No. There is no clinically significant difference in response to acetaminophen between viral and bacterial illnesses.

9. If my patient is febrile, should I always attempt to lower the temperature?
This is controversial. As noted above, fever may actually be beneficial in fighting some infections. In addition, aggressive cooling measures such as sponge baths and cooling blankets may actually increase, rather than decrease, a patient's discomfort. Antipyretics may also mask a fever and delay the diagnosis of recurrent or new bacterial infections. However, most physicians consider using antipyretics in patients who are uncomfortable because of fever. You should strongly consider using antipyretics in pregnant women, children at risk for febrile seizures, and patients with preexisting cardiac compromise who would not tolerate the increased metabolic demands of a fever.

10. I slept through a lot of my lectures. Are there causes of fever other than infection?
Yes. While infections are definitely the most common causes of fever, there are numerous other endogenous and exogenous etiologies. Neoplastic diseases (e.g., leukemia, lymphoma, solid tumors) and collagen vascular diseases (e.g., giant cell arteritis, polyarteritis nodosa, systemic lupus erythematosus, rheumatoid arthritis) are the second and third most common causes of fever, respectively. Other causes include central nervous system lesions (e.g., stroke, intracranial bleed, trauma), factitious fever (often in health care professionals), drugs, and environmental heat exposure.

11. Which drugs can cause fevers?

While any drug is capable of producing a "drug fever," the most common are listed in the table below. Of these, penicillin and penicillin analogues are the most frequent causative agents. The fever usually begins 7–10 days after initiation of drug therapy. There is an associated rash or eosinophilia in about 20% of cases. In addition to "drug fevers," cocaine, amphetamines, and tricyclic antidepressants may produce fevers acutely. "Drug fever" should always be a diagnosis of exclusion.

Drugs Commonly Associated with "Drug Fevers"

Antibiotics	Anticonvulsants	NSAIDs
INH	Carbamazepine	Ibuprofen
Nitrofurantoin	Phenytoin	Salicylates
Penicillins/cephalosporins	Cardiac drugs	Others
Rifampin	Hydralazine	Barbiturates
Sulfonamides	Methyldopa	Cimetidine
Anticancer drugs	Nifedipine	Iodides
Bleomycin	Phenytoin	
Streptozocin	Procainamide	
	Quinidine	

12. What is the difference between an FUO and a UFO?

FUO stands for fever of unknown or undetermined origin, whereas a UFO is an unidentified flying object. Although you might see a patient with a prior diagnosis of FUO in your ED, you probably will not see a UFO. An FUO is defined as a fever greater than 38.3°C (100.9°F) documented on several occasions during a period greater than 3 weeks with an uncertain diagnosis after 1 week of evaluation in the hospital. Thus, if this is the patient's initial evaluation for fever, even if you cannot identify a source, the ED diagnosis would *not* be FUO. The most common causes of FUO are occult infection and malignancy, each accounting for approximately 30% of cases.

13. How do I evaluate a patient with a fever?

A thorough history and physical examination (H&P) are the most important aspects of the evaluation. Associated symptoms (e.g., cough, shortness of breath, pain, dysuria), duration of fever, ill contacts, history or risk of immunocompromise (e.g., AIDS, diabetes, alcohol or drug abuse), travel, and current medications are all important in determining both the etiology and seriousness of a fever. Although the physical examination may locate the source of the fever, the most important aspect of the examination is the general appearance of the patient. Specifically, does the patient look "toxic" or "well"? The exam may also reveal mental status changes or rashes that might be indicative of more serious systemic diseases. In addition, do not forget to look closely at the vital signs.

14. What about the vital signs? Doesn't everyone with a fever have an increased pulse and respiratory rate?

Patients with fever usually have increased pulse and respirations, but it is important to look at the magnitude of the increase. The pulse should increase about 10 bpm for each 0.6°C (1°F) increase in temperature. Classically, a "pulse-temperature dissociation" occurs in certain diseases such as typhoid, malaria, legionnaire's disease, and mycoplasma. This means that the patient will present with fever and a relative bradycardia (i.e., there is less than a 10 bpm increase in pulse per 0.6°C increase in temperature). In early septic shock, tachycardia inappropriate for the degree of fever is often seen. Hyperventilation out of proportion to fever is characteristic of pneumonia and gram-negative bacteremia.

15. What about laboratory tests? Which tests should I order?
The H&P should direct you to the appropriate tests. If the H&P are inconclusive, consider ordering some simple screening tests. A minimum workup should include a complete blood count (CBC) with differential, a urinalysis, an erythrocyte sedimentation rate (ESR), and a chest x-ray. Clinical judgment will determine other specific diagnostic studies such as lumbar puncture, fluid aspiration, IVP, CT scans, etc.

16. How valuable is the white blood cell (WBC) count?
While the absolute WBC count or band count is neither sensitive nor specific, some sources state that a normal WBC count and differential have a high negative predictive value (i.e., normal values imply that serious disease does not exist). Elderly patients, however, may present with serious infections in the face of a normal WBC and differential. Low WBC counts are indicative of immunocompromise, viral illnesses, or septicemia. The neutrophil morphology is of greater importance than the CBC. Toxic granulations, Döhle bodies, and/or cytoplasmic vacuolization are indicative of more serious bacterial infections.

17. What about the ESR?
While an increase in ESR (>30) is very sensitive, it is not specific. Therefore, it may imply that an infection exists, but will not help to determine the source.

18. How do I approach the child under 2 years of age with a fever?
See chapter 66, p. 247.

BIBLIOGRAPHY

1. Alpert G, Hibbert E, Fleisher GR: Case-control study of hyperpyrexia in children. Pediatr Infect Dis J 9:161, 1990.
2. Baker MD, Fosarelli PD, Carpenter RO: Childhood fever: Correlation of diagnosis with temperature response to acetaminophen. Pediatrics 80:315, 1987.
3. Banco L, Veltri D: Ability of mothers to subjectively assess the presence of fever in their children. Am J Dis Child 138:976, 1984.
4. Baraff LJ: Management of the febrile child: A survey of pediatric and emergency medicine residency directors. Pediatr Infect Dis J 10:795, 1991.
5. Brusch JL, Weinstein L: Fever of unknown origin. Med Clin North Am 72:1247, 1988.
6. Harwood-Nuss A, Linden CH, Luten RC, et al (eds): The Clinical Practice of Emergency Medicine. Philadelphia, J.B. Lippincott, 1991.
7. Muma BK, Treloar DJ, Wurmlinger K, et al: Comparison of rectal, axillary, and tympanic membrane temperatures in infants and young children. Ann Emerg Med 20:41, 1991.
8. Sinkinson CA, Brusch JL, Fitzgerald FT: How to evaluate patients having fever without localizing signs or symptoms. Emerg Med Reports 10:177, 1989.
9. Styrt B, Sugarman B: Antipyresis and fever. Arch Intern Med 150:1589, 1990.

7. CHEST PAIN

Thomas McLaughlin, D.O., and Glenn C. Hamilton, M.D.

1. Why is the etiology of chest pain often difficult to determine in the emergency department (ED)?
1. Various disease processes in a variety of organs may result in chest pain.
2. The severity of the pain is often unrelated to its life-threatening potential.

3. The location of the pain perceived by the patient frequently does not correspond with its source.

4. Physical findings, laboratory assays, and radiologic studies are often unavailable or nondiagnostic in the ED.

5. More than one disease process may be present.

2. Is the location of the pain diagnostic of its etiology?
No. Somatic fibers from the dermis are numerous and enter the spinal cord at a single level, resulting in sharp, localized pain. Visceral afferent fibers from internal organs of the thorax and upper abdomen are less numerous. They enter the spinal cord at multiple levels from T1–T6, resulting in a pain that is dull, aching and poorly localized. Connections between the visceral and somatic fibers may result in the visceral pain being perceived as originating from somatic locations such as the shoulder or arm.

3. Identify six life-threatening causes of acute chest pain that must be considered first when evaluating a patient in the ED.
Myocardial infarction, unstable angina, aortic dissection, pulmonary embolism, pneumothorax, and esophageal rupture.

4. Name some other conditions that may present as chest pain.
Stable angina, valvular heart disease, pericarditis, pneumonia, pleurisy, reflux esophagitis, esophageal spasm, thoracic outlet syndrome, musculoskeletal pain, peptic ulcer disease, cholecystitis, pancreatitis, herpes zoster, anxiety, hyperventilation.

5. What is the safest initial approach to patients presenting with chest pain?
With few exceptions, all patients with acute chest pain should be approached with the assumption of a life-threatening etiology. Therefore prior to any diagnostic studies, supplemental oxygen, intravenous access, and cardiac monitoring should be initiated.

6. How do I begin to assess the patient with chest pain?
An accurate history is the most important component of the evaluation. Factors to be considered include the onset, quality, location, pattern of radiation, and duration of the pain as well as associated symptoms. Precipitating factors such as exertion, movement, or inspiration, as well as relieving factors such as rest, nitroglycerin, antacids, or body position, may also provide clues to the origin of the pain.

Classic Patterns of Chest Pain

ETIOLOGY	QUALITY	LOCATION	RADIATION	DURATION	ASSOC. SYMPTOMS	ONSET
Myocardial infarction	visceral	retrosternal	neck, jaw, shoulder, arm	>15 min	nasea vomiting diaphoresis dyspnea	variable
Angina	visceral	retrosternal	neck, jaw, shoulder, arm	5–15 min	nausea diaphoresis dyspnea	gradual
Aortic dissection	severe	retrosternal	interscapular tearing	constant	nausea dyspnea diaphoresis	sudden
Pulmonary embolism	pleuritic	lateral	—	constant	dyspnea apprehension	sudden

Table continued on next page.

Classic Patterns of Chest Pain (Continued)

ETIOLOGY	QUALITY	LOCATION	RADIATION	DURATION	ASSOC. SYMPTOMS	ONSET
Pneumothorax	pleuritic	lateral	neck, back	constant	dyspnea	sudden
Pericarditis	sharp stabbing	retrosternal	back, neck, shoulder, arm	constant	dyspnea dysphagia	variable
Esophageal rupture	boring	retrosternal epigastric	post thorax	constant	diaphoresis dyspnea (late)	sudden
Esophagitis	aching boring	retrosternal	interscapular jaws, neck, shoulder	min-hours	dysphagia	variable
Esophageal spasm	visceral	retrosternal	interscapular	min-hours	dysphagia	variable
Musculo-skeletal	sharp aching superficial	localized	—	variable	dyspnea	variable

7. What are the major risk factors associated with ischemic heart disease?
Age greater than 40, male sex, family history, cigarette smoking, hypertension, hypercholesterolemia, and diabetes mellitus.

8. Is radiating pain significant?
Radiation of chest pain is suggestive but not diagnostic of cardiac ischemia. Visceral pain, including aortic, esophageal, gastric, and pulmonary processes, may also present with radiation of pain to the neck, shoulder, or arm. Chest pain that radiates to the arm and neck does increase the likelihood of acute myocardial infarction, however. In one study of patients admitted with chest pain and subsequently diagnosed with myocardial infarction, 71% had pain radiating to the arms and/or neck. Similar radiation of pain occurred in only 39% of those admitted with chest pain who did not have myocardial infarction.

9. How does the patient's appearance correlate with the origin of chest pain?
Catastrophic illnesses often result in anxiety, diaphoresis, and an ill appearance. Splinting may be due to pulmonary embolism, pleurisy, pneumothorax, or musculoskeletal chest pain. Levine's sign, which consists of a patient placing a clenched fist over the sternum to describe the pain, is frequently associated with ischemic heart disease. Kussmaul's sign is a paradoxical filling of the neck veins during inspiration and suggests a right ventricular infarction, massive pulmonary embolism, or pericarditis.

10. How are vital signs helpful?
Assessment of the vital signs may provide valuable information. A blood pressure difference between the upper extremities of greater than 20 mmHg or a loss or reduction of lower extremity pulses is indicative of a dissecting aortic aneurysm. Tachypnea may be due to the hypoxia of pulmonary embolism or pneumonia or secondary to pain. An elevated temperature usually indicates an inflammatory or infectious process such as pericarditis or pneumonia.

11. What physical examination findings may help differentiate among the causes of acute chest pain?
Isolated physical findings are rarely diagnostic of the origin of chest pain, but when used in context with the history, they may be extremely valuable. Palpation may reveal localized tenderness and reproduce musculoskeletal pain, but 5–10% of patients with chest pain

partially or fully reproduced by palpation have ischemic heart disease. Cardiac auscultation may reveal a new murmur of aortic insufficiency suggestive of aortic dissection or a new murmur of mitral regurgitation secondary to papillary muscle dysfunction from an inferior wall myocardial infarction. A pericardial friction rub is suggestive of pericarditis. Mediastinal air from esophageal rupture results in a crunching sound called Hammon's sign. Decreased breath sounds or hyperresonance may indicate a pneumothorax.

12. How is the EKG helpful in ischemic heart disease?

An EKG provides documentation of cardiac ischemia or infarction when positive. It may be normal initially in 20% of patients in the ED who are later diagnosed as having an acute myocardial infarction. An EKG is also necessary to fulfill the criterion for the administration of thrombolytic agents: ST segment elevation of greater than or equal to 1 mm in two continuous leads. Questions have been raised about emergency physician's accuracy in identifying ST-T changes in the EKG. Comparison with old EKGs may reveal subtle but significant changes.

13. What chest x-ray abnormalities occur in diseases causing chest pain?

Chest x-rays of patients presenting with chest pain are frequently normal but may be diagnostic, as in a pneumothorax. Aortic dissection may show a widened mediastinum and/or a 4–5-mm separation between the calcified intima and lateral edge of the aortic knob. Pulmonary embolism may show an elevated hemidiaphragm or a wedge-shaped pulmonary infiltrate. Esophageal rupture frequently presents with mediastinal air and pleural effusion.

14. Are cardiac enzymes useful in the evaluation of chest pain in the ED?

Cardiac enzyme determination is usually not helpful in the ED setting for two reasons. (1) Creatine kinase elevations do not occur until 4–6 hours following the onset of an acute infarction. Lactic dehydrogenase (LDH) and serum glutamate oxaloacetate transaminase (SGOT) elevations occur even later. (2) Even in a patient with protracted chest pain, the actual infarction may have occurred just prior to evaluation. Isoenzyme determinations, although having a specificity of 98%, have traditionally showed similar limitations, resulting in a sensitivity of only 35%. Recently developed rapid and more sensitive CK-MB assays may allow for serial CK-MB determinations in the ED. Elevation of CK-MB levels between samples 2–4 hours apart may help to identify patients with acute myocardial infarction, particularly in the elderly population. Studies are currently ongoing.

15. Are other clinical laboratory studies useful in the evaluation of acute chest pain?

With the exception of ABGs in the workup of pulmonary embolus, routine laboratory studies have little or no use in the evaluation of chest pain.

16. Are there any bedside tests that may help to identify the origin of acute chest pain?

Several bedside tests may be helpful but are rarely diagnostic in themselves. Relief with nitroglycerin occurs in both angina and esophageal spasm, whereas acute myocardial infarction and unstable angina may remain unrelieved. Antacids or a "GI cocktail" consisting of viscous lidocaine and an antacid will frequently resolve esophageal pain but will also relieve pain in 10% of patients with angina. Pain from pericarditis is frequently worse in the supine position and relieved when leaning forward. Pain from esophageal disease is worsened with changes in position such as leaning forward or lying down. Musculoskeletal pain is also worsened with movement.

17. What additional radiologic diagnostic studies may be useful?

A dissecting aortic aneurysm may be diagnosed by a thoracic arteriogram, a rapid-sequence CT scan, or a transesophageal echocardiogram. A suspected pulmonary embolism may be confirmed by a ventilation-perfusion scan or pulmonary angiography. Esophageal rupture may be diagnosed by an esophagogram with a water-soluble contrast material.

18. Approximately 3% of patients with symptoms of chest pain due to acute myocardial infarction are discharged to home. What factors have been associated with failure to make the diagnosis?

1. Younger age group of patients
2. Failure to obtain an accurate history
3. Incorrect interpretation of the EKG
4. Failure to recognize atypical presentations
5. Hesitance to admit patients with vague symptoms
6. Reliance on laboratory assays, i.e., cardiac enzymes
7. Insufficient experience or training

BIBLIOGRAPHY

1. Aghababian RV, Umali CB: Chest pain. In Rosen P, et al (eds): Diagnostic Radiology in Emergency Medicine. St. Louis, Mosby–Year Book, 1992.
2. American College of Emergency Physicians: Clinical Policy for Management of Adult Patients Presenting with Chief Complaint of Chest Pain, with No History of Trauma. Dallas, 1990.
3. Callahan ML (ed): Current Practice of Emergency Medicine, 2nd ed. Philadelphia, B.C. Decker, 1991.
4. Gibler WB, Teichman S, Christensen R, Lewis LM: Early detection of acute myocardial infarction using serial CK-MB sampling in the ED: Results of the CK-MB Project Pilot Trial (abstract). Ann Emerg Med 20:953, 1991.
5. Hamilton GC, Sanders AB, Strange GR, Trott AT (eds): Emergency Medicine: An Approach to Clinical Problem Solving. Philadelphia, W.B. Saunders, 1991.
6. Hindes R, Kowey PR: Emergency department evaluation of the patient with chest pain. Curr Top Emerg Med 1:1, 1985.
7. Jayes RL, Larsen GG, Beshansky JR, et al: Physician electrocardiogram reading in the emergency department: Accuracy and effect on triage decisions. Findings from a multicenter study. J Gen Intern Med 7:387–392, 1992.
8. McCarthy BD, Wong JB, Selker HP: Detecting acute cardiac ischemia in the emergency department. J Gen Intern Med 5:365–373, 1990.
9. Nowakowski JF: Use of cardiac enzymes in the evaluation of acute chest pain. Ann Emerg Med 15:354–360, 1986.
10. Roberts R, Henderson RD, Wigle ED: Esophageal disease as a cause of severe retrosternal chest pain. Chest 67:523–526, 1975.

8. ABDOMINAL PAIN

Thomas Purcell, M.D.

1. What is the difference between visceral and somatic pain? How is this of practical importance?

Evolving patterns of pain frequently reveal the source and give an idea of the extent to which the process has advanced. Early, the patient may describe a deep-seated, dull pain (visceral pain) emanating from inflammation or stretching of the smooth muscle of hollow viscera or the capsule of solid organs. This pain is poorly localized but generally falls somewhere along the midline of the abdomen. Later, as inflammation progresses to the parietal peritoneum, the pain becomes better localized, lateralized over the involved organ, and sharper in intensity (somatic or parietal pain). A clear understanding of the process enables the clinician to more precisely identify both cause and rate of progression of pathology.

2. What is the difference between localized and generalized peritonitis?
As the peritoneum adjacent to a diseased organ becomes inflamed, palpation or any abdominal movement causes stretching of the sensitized peritoneum and, consequently, pain localized at that site (localized peritonitis). If irritating material (pus, blood, gastric contents) spills into the peritoneal cavity, the entire peritoneal surface may become sensitive to stretch or motion, and any movement or palpation may provoke pain at any or all points within the abdominal cavity (generalized peritonitis).

3. Which tests for peritoneal irritation are best?
Rebound tenderness is the traditional physical finding for peritonitis. However, in a patient with likely generalized peritonitis (obvious distress, an excruciating pain every time the ambulance hits a bump), the standard tests for rebound tenderness are unnecessarily harsh. Asking the patient to cough will generally supply adequate peritoneal motion to give a positive test. On the other hand, when in every respect the exam is normal, one highly sensitive test for peritoneal irritation is the heel-drop jarring (Markle) test. The patient is asked to stand, rise up on tiptoe with knees straight, and then forcibly drop down on both heels with an audible thump. Among patients with appendicitis, this test was found to be 74% sensitive, compared with 64% for the standard rebound test.

4. Why is it important to establish the temporal relationship of pain to vomiting?
Generally, pain preceding vomiting is suggestive of a surgical process, whereas vomiting before onset of pain is more typical of a nonsurgical condition. Epigastric pain that is relieved by vomiting suggests intragastric pathology or gastric outlet obstruction.

5. What is the relationship of peritoneal inflammation to loss of appetite?
Anorexia and nausea and vomiting are directly proportional to the severity and extent of peritoneal irritation. The presence of appetite does not rule out a surgically significant inflammatory process such as appendicitis. For example, a retrocecal appendicitis with limited peritoneal irritation may be associated with minimal gastrointestinal upset.

6. What are the pitfalls in evaluating elderly patients with acute abdominal pain?
Advanced age may blunt the manifestations of acute abdominal disease. Pain may be less severe, fever is often less pronounced, and signs of peritoneal inflammation such as muscular guarding and rebound tenderness may be diminished or even absent. Elevation of white blood cell (WBC) count is less sensitive in the elderly: in patients older than 65 requiring immediate surgery, 39% have a WBC count over 10,000 compared with 71% of patients younger than 65. Nevertheless, the overall incidence of surgical pathology among patients over 65 years old admitted for abdominal pain is high, from 33% to 39%, compared to 16% among patients under 65. Elderly patients often do not exhibit the same degree of abnormality in vital signs or physical findings as do those in younger age groups.

7. What other factors should be sought in the history that may significantly alter the presentation of patients with abdominal pain?
Symptoms and physical findings in patients with schizophrenia and diabetes may be significantly muted. In addition, the use of narcotics, steroids, or antibiotics may substantially alter signs as well as laboratory results.

8. What is the significance of obstipation?
Frequently the patient will give a history of constipation; even more characteristic, however, is obstipation—the inability to pass either stool or flatus. Inability to pass flatus for more than 8 hours despite a perceived need is highly suggestive of obstruction.

9. What vital sign is most closely associated with the degree of peritonitis?
Tachycardia is universal with advancing peritonitis. The initial pulse has less importance than serial observations do. An unexplained rise in pulse may be an early clue that early surgical exploration is indicated.

10. Does the duration of abdominal pain help in categorizing etiology?
In general, severe abdominal pain that persists for 6 hours or more is likely to be caused by surgically correctable problems. Similarly, patients with pain of less than 48 hours' duration have a significantly higher incidence of surgical disease than do those with pain of longer duration.

11. What are the most commonly missed surgical causes of abdominal pain?
An analysis of 100 consecutive cases of abdominal pain revealed that among patients wrongfully discharged from the emergency department (ED), the two most commonly missed diagnoses were appendicitis and acute intestinal obstruction.

12. Is there a place for narcotic analgesics in the management of acute abdominal pain of uncertain etiology?
For fear of masking vital symptoms or physical findings, conventional surgical wisdom proscribes the use of narcotic analgesics until a firm diagnosis is established. In recent years, however, some authors have suggested that pain medication may be administered to selected patients with stable vital signs because the analgesic effect may be readily reversed at any time following the administration of naloxone. Further, although inconclusive, there are data to suggest that evaluation of acute abdominal disease may be even facilitated once severe pain has been relieved and the patient can cooperate more fully. Prior to administration of narcotic analgesics, surgical consultation should be obtained and all appropriate consent forms for anticipated treatment completed. Patients who have received narcotics for pain control should be discouraged from leaving the ED against medical advice.

13. Which are the most useful preliminary lab tests to order?
A complete blood count with differential WBC count is generally recommended along with urinalysis. The initial hematocrit helps to define antecedent anemia, and serial measurements may reveal ongoing hemorrhage. An elevated WBC count suggests significant pathology but is nonspecific. Elevated urinary specific gravity reflects dehydration, and an increased urinary bilirubin in the absence of urobilinogen points toward total obstruction of the common bile duct. Pyuria, hematuria, and positive dipstick for glucose and ketones may reveal nonsurgical causes for abdominal pain.

Amylase, considered a key test by some, may be added but is nonspecific. In addition to indicating pancreatitis, amylase may be elevated with biliary obstruction, cholecystitis, posterior perforation of a peptic ulcer, bowel obstruction or inflammation, and salpingitis. Any female with childbearing capability should receive a pregnancy test. Serum electrolytes, glucose, blood urea nitrogen, and creatinine are indicated if there is clinical hypovolemia due to copious vomiting or diarrhea, tense abdominal distention, or delay of several days after onset of symptoms, and especially if the patient is likely to require emergency general anesthesia. An EKG should be obtained if the patient is older than 40.

14. Are x-rays always indicated?
No. Plain films of the abdomen have the highest yield when used in the evaluation of patients with suspected bowel obstruction, intussusception or ileus, free air, intra-abdominal mass, renal calculi, gallbladder disease, aortic aneurysm, past history of abdominal surgery or tumor, or severe or generalized abdominal pain and tenderness.

Conversely, among patients with uncomplicated peptic ulcer disease or massive hematemesis, pain present for more than 1 week, strangulated abdominal wall hernias, or other obvious clinical indications for laparotomy, plain films probably add little.

15. Which plain films are most useful?
Traditional teaching holds that plain abdominal films should include a supine view plus either an upright view, a left lateral decubitus view (if unable to stand), or all three. The supine view of the abdomen is the most informative and worthwhile abdominal film. The upright film is superior for visualizing (a) air-fluid levels associated with ileus and obstruction and (b) biliary air. If the patient is unable to stand, the left lateral decubitus (left side down) view may be substituted when looking for either obstruction or free air.

The erect chest x-ray is most sensitive for detection of free intraperitoneal air and may also demonstrate basal pneumonia, ruptured esophagus, elevated hemidiaphragm, air-fluid levels associated with subdiaphragmatic or hepatic abscess, pleural effusion, and pneumothorax. Ironically, in the evaluation of patients with abdominal pain, the upright chest film, taken alone, has been shown to be more useful than films of the abdomen itself.

16. Are air-fluid levels within the intestine always abnormal?
It is commonly taught that air-fluid levels (AFL) when seen on an upright abdominal film are "pathognomonic" for small bowel obstruction. However, a study of 300 normal patients showed that the average number of AFLs was 3–5, with some films demonstrating as many as 20. Although typically less than 2.5 cm in length, some ranged up to 10 cm. Significantly, most of the AFLs were found in the large bowel; only 14 of 300 normal patients studied demonstrated AFLs in the small bowel. The authors suggested that before AFLs are used as the sole criterion for the diagnosis of paralytic ileus or mechanical obstruction, one should see more than two AFLs within the dilated loops of the small bowel.

Gammill SL, Nice CM: Air fluid levels: Their occurrence in normal patients and their role in the analysis of ileus. Surgery 71:771–780, 1972.

17. A 7-year-old child presents with acute abdominal pain with a history of several similar bouts over the past 5 months. Physical examination is unremarkable. What is the most likely etiology?
In children over the age of 5, abdominal pain that is intermittent and of over 3 months' duration is on a functional basis in over 95% of cases, especially in the absence of such objective findings as fever, delayed growth patterns, anemia, gastrointestinal bleeding, or lateralizing pain and tenderness.

18. A patient with severe abdominal pain is found to be in diabetic ketoacidosis (DKA). How does the emergency physician decide whether the abdominal pain is a manifestation of the DKA or whether a surgical condition has precipitated DKA?
Patients with established DKA often present to the ED with severe abdominal pain. Physical examination reveals a dehydrated, hyperpneic patient with generalized abdominal tenderness and guarding, which may progress to boardlike rigidity. Bowel sounds usually are reduced or absent, and rebound tenderness may be noted. Although the precise mechanism of abdominal pain and ileus in patients with DKA is not well understood, hypovolemia, hypotension, and a total body potassium deficit probably contribute. An acute surgical lesion may initiate DKA; nevertheless, most patients have no such pathology. Symptoms characteristically resolve as medical treatment restores the patient to biochemical homeostasis. In any event, treatment of the DKA must precede any surgical intervention due to the extremely high intraoperative mortality among patients not so stabilized.

BIBLIOGRAPHY

1. Brewer RJ, Golden GT, Hitch DC, et al: Abdominal pain: An analysis of 1,000 consecutive cases in a university hospital emergency room. Am J Surg 131:219–223, 1976.
2. Buchman TG, Zuidema GD: Reasons for delay of the diagnosis of acute appendicitis. Surg Gynecol Obstet 158:260–266, 1984.
3. Farrell MK: Abdominal pain. Pediatrics 74(Suppl):955–957, 1984.
4. Greene CS: Indications for plain abdominal radiography in the emergency department. Ann Emerg Med 15:257–260, 1986.
5. Markle GB: Heel-drop jarring test for appendicitis (letter). Arch Surg 120:243, 1985.
6. Podgorny G: Abdominal pain and analgesia. Ann Emerg Med 10:10, 1981.
7. Schwartz SI: Manifestations of gastrointestinal disease. In Schwartz SI (ed): Principles of Surgery, 5th ed. New York, 1989.
8. Silen W: Cope's Early Diagnosis of the Acute Abdomen, 17th ed. New York, Oxford University Press, 1987.
9. Zoltie N, Cust MP: Analgesia in the acute abdomen. Ann R Coll Surg Engl 68:209–210, 1986.

9. NAUSEA AND VOMITING

Juliana Karp, M.D.

1. Vomiting! Do I really need to read this chapter when there are so many more interesting chapters in this book?

Yes! One of the most common and harmful mistakes made in the emergency department (ED) is assuming that nausea and vomiting is due to gastroenteritis without thinking of and ruling out more serious causes. Besides, vomiting is one of the most common presenting complaints in the ED.

2. What causes vomiting?

The act of vomiting is a highly complex act involving a vomiting center in the medulla. This center may be excited in three ways.

1. Via vagal and sympathetic afferents from the peritoneum, gastrointestinal (GI), biliary, and genitourinary tracts, pelvic organs, heart, pharynx, head, and vestibular apparatus
2. By impulses coming from sites higher in the central nervous system
3. Via the chemoreceptor trigger zone located in the floor of the fourth ventricle

3. Can vomiting itself lead to potential complications?

Absolutely, some of which are life threatening: severe dehydration, metabolic alkalosis, severe electrolyte depletion (particularly sodium, potassium, and chloride ions), esophageal or gastric bleeding, and esophageal perforation or tear (Mallory-Weiss tear).

4. Name the common GI disorders that cause vomiting.

Gastroenteritis, gastric outlet obstruction, gastric retention, alcoholic gastritis, pancreatitis, hepatitis, small bowel obstruction, appendicitis, and cholecystitis.

5. What are common causes of vomiting other than GI disorders?

Infections (pneumonia, meningitis, sepsis), metabolic disturbances (diabetic ketoacidosis, uremia), toxicologic (digoxin, theophylline, aspirin, iron), neurologic (hydrocephalus, cerebral edema), renal calculi, ovarian or testicular torsion, pregnancy, ruptured ectopic pregnancy, labyrinthitis, and never forget myocardial ischemia!

6. Can the character of the vomit help you to make a diagnosis?

Sometimes, especially with GI disorders. In acute gastritis, vomit is usually stomach contents mixed with a little bile. In biliary or ureteral colic, the vomit is usually bilious. In sympathetic shock (acute torsion of abdominal or pelvic organ), it is common for the patient to retch frequently but vomit very little. In intestinal obstruction, the character of vomit varies—first gastric contents, then bilious material, with progression to brown feculent material that is pathognomonic of small bowel obstruction. Vomiting of blood is a whole different story. See chapter 32, p. 119.

7. What else do I need to ask the patient?

1. **Associated signs and symptoms** such as pain, fever, jaundice, bowel habits. Think of hepatitis or biliary obstruction with jaundice. Always remember that gastroenteritis is uncommon without diarrhea.

2. **Relationship of vomiting to meals.** Vomiting that occurs soon after a meal is common with gastric outlet obstruction from peptic ulcer disease. Vomiting after a fatty meal is common with cholecystitis. Vomiting of food eaten more than 6 hours earlier is seen with gastric retention.

3. **Do not always focus on the GI system.** Ask about medications and possible drug use, headache and other neurologic symptoms, and last menstrual period. Inquire about cardiac risk factors, especially in older patients.

8. What do I look for on the physical exam?

Physical exam is helpful but can be unreliable. Look for signs of dehydration. Check for bowel sounds, which are increased in gastroenteritis and absent with obstruction or serious abdominal infections. Abdominal tenderness may or may not be present in a variety of disorders, but a rigid abdomen points to peritonitis, a surgical emergency. Women of childbearing age with vomiting and abdominal or pelvic pain require a pelvic examination. Always remember the neurologic exam.

9. Are laboratory tests indicated?

This question must be answered on an individual basis. In general, order tests based on physical exam findings. However, diabetics and elderly patients can "hide" serious infections and metabolic disturbances. Be careful with these patients.

10. When should I order an x-ray?

Again, this must be judged on an individual basis. Abdominal radiography is usually nonspecific but may show free air with perforation of an abdominal viscus or dilated bowel with obstruction. A chest film can be useful in cases of protracted vomiting to rule out aspiration or pneumomediastinum. Remember that lobar pneumonia with diaphragmatic irritation may cause vomiting with abdominal pain and few respiratory symptoms.

11. How should I treat the vomiting patient?

1. First, always remember to protect the airway. Patients with altered mental status should be placed on their side to prevent aspiration.

2. Intravenous fluids are usually indicated for rehydration; normal saline or lactated Ringer's solution is preferred.

3. Nasogastric suction can be both therapeutic and diagnostic and is always indicated when there is a suspicion of a GI bleed.

4. Medications to relieve nausea and vomiting must be used judiciously, especially in patients with altered mental status, hypotension, or uncertain diagnosis.

5. Figure out why the patient is vomiting!

12. What medications should I use?

Antiemetic Medications

GENERIC NAME	TRADE NAME	INDICATION	DOSE
Meclizine	Antivert	Vertigo and motion sickness	25 mg PO qid
Diphenhydramine HCl	Benadryl	Motion sickness	25–50 mg PO or IV qid
Prochlorperazine	Compazine	Nausea, vomiting, anxiety	10 mg PO, IM, or IV qid 25 mg PR bid
Phosphorated carbohydrate	Emetrol	Nausea and vomiting	1–2 tbs PO q 15 min (not to exceed 5 doses)
Promethazine HCl	Phenergan	Nausea, vomiting, motion sickness, anxiety	12.5–50 mg PO or IV qid
Metoclopramide HCl	Reglan	Nausea, vomiting, gastro-esophageal reflux, gastroparesis	5–10 mg PO or IV dosage varies
Chlorpromazine	Thorazine	Nausea, vomiting, anxiety	10–25 mg PO qid 25 mg IM qid 100 mg PR qid
Trimethobenzamide HCl	Tigan	Nausea and vomiting	250 mg PO tid or qid 200 mg PR tid or qid 200 mg IM tid or qid
Scopolamine	Transderm Scop	Nausea, vomiting, motion sickness	1 patch q 3 days
Hydroxyzine pamoate	Vistaril	Nausea, vomiting, anxiety	25–100 mg PO or IM tid-qid
Ondansetron HCl	Zofran	Nausea and vomiting with chemotherapy	Dosage varies

BIBLIOGRAPHY

1. Fuchs S, Jaffe D: Vomiting. Pediatric Emerg Care 6:162–170, 1990.
2. Harwood-Nuss A, et al (eds): The Clinical Practice of Emergency Medicine. Philadelphia, J.B. Lippincott, 1991.
3. Rosen P, et al (eds): Emergency Medicine: Concepts and Clinical Practice, 3rd ed. St. Louis, Mosby–Year Book, 1992.
4. Silen W (ed): Cope's Early Diagnosis of the Acute Abdomen. New York, Oxford University Press, 1987.

10. HEADACHE

Laurie Vande Krol, M.D.

1. How common are headaches? How often do people go to see a doctor for one?

Seventy percent of the U.S. population report having had a headache and 5% have seen a doctor for one. Greater than 1% of all office and emergency department (ED) visits are for headaches.

2. When someone has a headache, what exactly is it that hurts?

The brain cannot feel pain, nor can the pia or arachnoid mater, the skull, or the choroid plexus. Many structures in the head can feel pain, however. These include the scalp skin and vessels, scalp muscles, parts of the dura mater, dural arteries, intracerebral arteries, cranial nerves V, VI, and VII, and the cervical nerves. Irritation of any of these may result in pain, i.e., a headache.

3. What true emergencies may present as a headache?

There are four categories: infectious, traction, extracranial, and inflammatory disorders. Infections include meningitis, sinusitis, mastoiditis, dental infections, and intracranial abscesses. Displacement or traction of pain-sensitive structures of the brain may result from tumors, pseudotumor cerebri, or intracranial bleeds (epidural, subdural, subarachnoid, and intraparenchymal). Extracranial causes of pain include cranial neuralgias, glaucoma, optic neuritis, temporomandibular joint syndrome, and cervical spine disorders. Inflammatory causes include temporal arteritis and other vasculitides such as polyarteritis nodosa. Untreated, any of these disorders may result in serious sequelae.

4. What are the most common causes of headache for which patients seek treatment?

Fortunately, none of the most serious of causes is very common. Muscle contraction (tension) and vascular (migraine) headaches have a much higher incidence. Although painful, these disorders do not have life-threatening sequelae.

5. Are there clinical clues to distinguish tension and migraine headaches from those caused by more ominous conditions?

Yes. Tension and migraine headaches tend to be recurrent and similar from one episode to the next. A headache that is described as a "first" or "worst" headache, or even just different from prior headaches, requires close evaluation. A sudden, severe onset, commonly described as "the worst headache I have ever had," is classic for a subarachnoid hemorrhage. Likewise, the dull, boring headache that is unremitting over days to weeks and awakens one from sleep causes concern for an intracranial mass lesion or depression. Although focal neurologic signs are often present before the onset of a classic migraine, those that are atypical for the patient warrant concern. Finally, associated fever requires evaluation for infection, tumor, or drug use.

6. How do you evaluate the patient complaining of headache?

As with all stable patients, start with the history. Time of onset, age of patient, location in the head, nature, severity, associated symptoms, and exacerbating and relieving factors are important. Investigate a relationship to occupational or family stress. Past medical history, including recent health and prior headache history, may be useful. Ask which prescription or nonprescription medications have recently been started, changed, or stopped. Inquire about familial illnesses, especially a family history of migraines. Discuss sleep habits, vegetative symptoms of depression, smoking, and use of cocaine or other drugs.

7. Does the physical examination add any information?

Absolutely. The history should give you a good idea of what the problem is. The physical findings can support or refute your hypothesis. Vital signs are important. A fever may reflect infection. Hypertension may cause headache. Abnormal pulse or respirations may be due to infection or toxins. However, all vital signs may be altered in the face of severe pain. On the head examination, palpate temporal arteries, sinuses, temporomandibular joints, and the scalp for tenderness. Check the neck for nuchal rigidity. A thorough neurologic examination is vitally important. This includes evaluation of the mental status, cranial nerves, fundi, peripheral motor reflexes, sensation, deep tendon reflexes, and cerebellar function.

8. What diagnostic tests are necessary?

Computed tomography (CT) or magnetic resonance imaging (MRI) will show most mass lesions and intracranial hemorrhages. However, meningitis and 5–15% of subarachnoid bleeds will be missed. Thus if the imaging study is normal, it is necessary to perform a lumbar puncture to rule out these two entities.

9. What if the cerebrospinal fluid comes back looking bloody?

You can tell a traumatic tap from a subarachnoid bleed by comparing the red blood cell counts in different tubes. With a traumatic tap, the blood should clear over time, and thus an early tube would have more cells than a later one. The presence of xanthochromia, heme pigment tinting of the fluid, occurs after blood has been in contact with the cerebrospinal fluid for hours to days, and thus would indicate an intracranial bleed.

10. What are migraine headaches?

Although the public may refer to any severe headache as a migraine, a migraine is a specific type of headache. True migraines are familial, affecting women twice as often as men. The first headache usually occurs in the second or third decade. These headaches are typically described as unilateral, severe, and throbbing, and are commonly associated with photophobia and nausea. However, early and late in the course the headache may be non-throbbing. Variations on all of the symptoms occur, but each patient tends to experience a similar constellation of symptoms in each headache.

11. Distinguish between classic and common migraines.

Migraines are described as consisting of two phases: a prodrome and a headache. The prodrome occurs in approximately 35% of migraine sufferers. It most commonly consists of visual symptoms such as scotomata, zigzag lines, or flashing lights. Other symptoms include paresthesias, visual and auditory hallucinations, and focal neurologic symptoms. When these occur, the headache is described as a classic migraine. When none occurs, the headache is called a common migraine.

12. What causes a migraine?

Some stress or stimulus activates the overlapping immune, complement, and coagulation systems. This first causes vasospasm of the vascular system at the base of the brain, resulting in local anoxia and acidosis. This produces the migraine prodrome. In response to local metabolic demands, the parenchymal and cranial arteries dilate, promoting release of vasoactive substances that produce edema, a lowered pain threshold, and a pounding headache.

13. Can migraine headaches be prevented?

To some degree, the motivated patient can prevent headaches. Patients need regular sleep and low stress levels at work and home. They should avoid foods that contain tyramine or other vasoactive substances such as cheese, chocolate, monosodium glutamate, alcohol, and fermented foods.

14. How do you treat a migraine headache?

There are multiple different medications and regimens to treat migraines (see table below). This should alert you that no single one is completely effective. Classically, an ED patient with a migraine was given a shot of narcotics and antiemetics and sent home to sleep. Most migraines are aborted with deep sleep. However, concerns of complications of narcotic use, including incomplete efficacy, respiratory depression, and narcotic abuse, make this mode of treatment unsatisfactory. More recently, antiemetics with or without corticosteroids or vasoconstricting ergot derivatives have been shown to have a good success rate. Recent research has also revived interest in serotonin agonists for migraine relief.

Emergency Department Pharmacotherapy of Migraine Headaches

MEDICATION	DOSE*
Antihistamines	
Dimenhydrinate (Dramamine)	25 mg IV
Ergot alkaloids	
Ergotamine tartrate	0.25–0.5 mg SQ or IM
Dihydroergotamine (DHE)	1 mg IV
Narcotics	
Butorphanol (Stadol)	2 mg IV
Meperidine (Demerol)	25 mg IV
	50–100 mg IM
Nonsteroidal anti-inflammatory agents	
Ketorolac	30–60 mg IM
Phenothiazines	
Chlorpromazine (Thorazine)	25 mg IV
Prochlorperazine (Compazine)	10 mg IV
Promethazine HCl (Thorazine)	25–50 mg IM or IV
Steroids	
Dexamethasone (Decadron)	4–10 mg IV
	16 mg IM
Serotonin agonists	
Sumatriptan	6–8 mg SQ
Other	
Metoclopramide (Reglan)	10 mg IV
Hydroxyzine HCl (Vistaril)	25–50 mg IM

*Assumes average size adult patient

15. How are cluster headaches different from migraines? How are they treated?

These are nonfamilial headaches affecting men predominantly. Excruciating unilateral pain lasting 30–90 minutes occurs multiple times a day for weeks, followed by a pain-free interval during which time no headache can be elicited. During the attacks, autonomic signs of rhinorrhea and lacrimation frequently occur on the same side of the face. Attacks may be induced by smoking or alcohol. In the ED, oxygen will relieve 90% of cluster headaches within 15 minutes. Other treatments include corticosteroids, calcium channel blockers, lithium, and methysergide.

16. How are muscle contraction (tension) headaches different from migraines?

A tension headache is a steady, nonthrobbing ache or tightness, whereas a migraine tends to be a unilateral throbbing. The tension headache may be bitemporal, occipital, or a "band" around the head. Pressure on the scalp increases painful sensations. However, there is a great deal of symptom overlap in atypical presentations of both types of headaches. Often, a clinical distinction is not possible.

17. How does one treat tension headaches?

Once other causes of headache have been investigated, treatment starts with reassurance and education. Because these headaches are usually chronic, treatment should be with nonaddictive analgesics. Biofeedback and acupuncture may be beneficial. All patients with this diagnosis should be screened for mood disorders, as depression is a common cause of tension headaches.

18. Which toxin may bring in entire families complaining of headache?

Improperly vented exhaust from stoves, furnaces, and automobiles may cause exposure to carbon monoxide. This colorless, odorless gas binds hemoglobin in preference to oxygen.

Family members complain of recurring headache, dizziness, and nausea that are worst upon awakening in the morning and improve after leaving the home. The treatment is high-flow oxygen for mild cases and hyperbaric oxygen for severe cases. Investigation of the source must not be overlooked.

19. Why is temporal arteritis an important diagnosis to consider?
This inflammatory disorder may involve not only the temporal artery but many others, including the ophthalmic artery. If not treated early, blindness may occur. This disorder should be suspected in older patients complaining of a temporal throbbing or burning. They may also report pain with chewing. The temporal region is usually tender to palpation and the erythrocyte sedimentation rate (ESR) is markedly elevated. The definitive diagnosis is made by biopsy of the artery. However, treatment with prednisone should not be delayed until the biopsy is done.

20. What is a "sentinel bleed"?
An intracranial aneurysm may leak a small amount of blood into the subarachnoid space, causing a moderate to severe headache. If this warning headache is ignored, the aneurysm may rupture and cause devastating neurologic damage or death. In the evaluation of a headache, the lumbar puncture will detect even a small amount of blood in the subarachnoid space. Expedient surgery may prevent a catastrophic intracranial hemorrhage.

BIBLIOGRAPHY

1. Bell R, Montoya D, Snualb A, Lee MA: A comparative trial of three agents in the treatment of acute migraine headache. Ann Emerg Med 19:1079–1082, 1990.
2. Edmeads J: Emergency management of headache. Headache 28:675–679, 1988.
3. Diamond S, Dalessio DJ: The Practicing Physician's Approach to Headache, 3rd ed. Baltimore, Williams and Wilkins, 1982.
4. Freitag FG, Diamond M: Emergency treatment of headache. Med Clin North Am 75:749–761, 1991.
5. Jones J, Sklar D, Dougherty J, White W: Randomized double-blind trial of intravenous prochlorperazine for the treatment of acute headache. JAMA 261:1174–1176, 1989.
6. Kerner KF: Management of headache in the emergency department. Top Emerg Med 4:19–34, 1982.
7. Klapper JA, Stanton JS: The emergency treatment of acute migraine headache: A comparison of intravenous dihydroergotamine, dexamethasone, and placebo. Cephalalgia 11(Suppl 11):159–160, 1991.
8. Moskowitz MA: Basic mechanisms in vascular headache. Neurol Clin 8:801–815, 1990.
9. Pradalier A, Clapin A, Dry J: Treatment review: Non-steroidal anti-inflammatory drugs in the treatment and long term prevention of migraine attacks. Headache 28:550–557, 1988.
10. Silberstein SD, Silberstein MM: New concepts in the pathogenesis of migraine headache. Pain Management 3:297–302, 1990.

11. SYNCOPE

William F. Young Jr., M.D., FACEP

1. What is syncope?
Syncope is a sudden temporary loss of consciousness with the inability to maintain postural tone. Because it is a symptom, not a disease, there are a wide variety of causes, both benign and life threatening. Although many authorities and clinical research studies differentiate syncope from coma, head trauma, shock, and seizures, these entities initially may present much the way syncope does.

2. Is syncope a commonly seen problem in emergency medicine?

Syncope accounts for about 3% of emergency room visits and 1–6% of general hospital admissions. The evaluation of syncope is costly, averaging about $2500 per inpatient admission according to a 1982 study.

3. There seem to be a lot of entities that can lead to loss of consciousness. Can you narrow them down?

The causes of syncope can be divided into three broad categories: central nervous system (CNS) dysfunction (HEAD), cardiac pumping dysfunction (HEART), and loss of vascular tone or volume (VESSLS).

Causes of Syncope

H	Hypoxia, hypoglycemia		
E	Epilepsy		
A	Anxiety	V	Vasovagal
D	Dysfunction of brain stem	E	Ectopic pregnancy (hypovolemia)
		S	Situational
H	Heart attack	S	carotid Sinus sensitivity
E	Embolism of pulmonary artery	L	Low systemic vascular resistance
A	Aortic obstruction	S	Subclavian steal
R	Rhythm disturbance		
T	Tachycardia (ventricular)		

The CNS dysfunctions are usually due to loss of vital nutrients such as oxygen or glucose but can also be caused by ischemia and seizure. The cardiac dysfunctions consist of either obstructions, such as pulmonary embolism and aortic stenosis, or dysrhythmias. Ventricular tachycardia constitutes about half of the cardiac causes of syncope, with sick sinus syndrome, bradycardia, and conduction blocks accounting for most of the remaining cardiac causes. The vascular causes include loss of systemic vascular resistance or circulating volume, including vasovagal syncope: the common faint. Cough, defecation, and micturition syncope represent the situational causes, although these may be caused by dysrhythmias.

4. What determines blood pressure?

Blood pressure = systemic vascular resistance × heart rate × stroke volume, where stroke volume is the difference between ventricular filling (volume status) and emptying (contractility). A decrease in any of the components not compensated by the others will cause hypotension and may cause syncope.

5. Do strokes present as syncope?

Vertebrobasilar insufficiency may present as syncope with signs of brain stem dysfunction such as ataxia, diplopia, or vertigo. Strokes due to carotid artery disease rarely cause true syncope, because there is no rapid return to normal consciousness, and focal neurologic deficits occur.

6. What are the odds of determining the cause of a patient's syncopal episode?

In up to 50% of patients, no cause is found despite extensive and expensive workups.

7. What are the priorities in evaluating a patient with syncope?

Fortunately, the vast majority of patients with syncope rapidly return to a normal mental status and have stable vital signs. However, the priorities are as follows: (1) Obtain vital signs and evaluate and treat for immediate life threats (the infamous ABCs). (2) Oxygen, intravenous access, and cardiac and blood pressure monitoring should be started on patients who have abnormal vital signs, persistent altered level of consciousness, chest pain, dyspnea, abdominal pain, or significant history of cardiac disease. (3) Assess for any trauma secondary to fall. Elderly patients are more likely to suffer head trauma secondary to syncope, which initially may represent a greater life threat than the cause of the syncope.

8. Now that immediate life threats have been ruled out, what is next?
Perform a detailed history and directed physical exam, followed by risk assignment. Then selectively obtain specific tests and determine whether hospital admission is indicated.

9. Which components of the history are important?
The single most important historical clue is the patient's recollection of events just prior to the syncope. Abrupt, sudden loss of consciousness without warning is a strong indicator of a cardiac cause, especially a rhythm disturbance. Similarly, syncope associated with effort is associated with cardiac obstructive causes or dysrhythmias. Patients who have vasovagal syncope often have premonitory symptoms of dizziness, yawning, nausea, and diaphoresis, and the event occurs during a period of some psychosocial stress. However, one should ask for clues to hypovolemia, such as thirst, postural dizziness, decreased oral intake, melena, or unusually heavy menstrual bleeding. Syncope after micturition, cough, head turning, defecation, swallowing, or meals suggests situational syncope. Previous episodes of syncope, upper-extremity exertion (e.g., subclavian steal syndrome), and presence of cardiac risk factors should be determined. Some medications can cause syncope, so list all of the patient's medications.

10. How do you know it wasn't a seizure?
A witness is invaluable, but sometimes not available. Recovery from syncope is usually rapid, whereas a victim of a seizure awakens slowly with prolonged confusion. Both may have trauma. Victims of dysrhythmias and vasovagal faints often exhibit myoclonic jerks that many bystanders interpret as a seizure, so ask for specifics. Sometimes, you just have to make your best guess or simultaneously evaluate for both seizure and syncope.

11. What is a "directed physical"?
You are unlikely to detect an important physical finding unless you look for it. Be a detective. In a patient with syncope, carefully examine for "head, heart, and vess'ls" causes, with the patient's history as a guide. For example, assume the patient with abrupt-effort syncope has aortic stenosis or hypertrophic cardiomyopathy, and **look for** the narrow pulse pressure, systolic murmur, or change in murmur with Valsalva. Examine the head carefully for trauma, bruits, and focal neurologic signs. Check blood pressure in both arms, looking for subclavian steal. Orthostatic vital signs are critical, and if positive, a search for occult blood loss or autonomic insufficiency is necessary. A complete neurologic exam is imperative.

12. How are orthostatic vital signs measured and evaluated?
All patients with syncope who have stable vital signs should have orthostatic vital signs. First, the blood pressure and pulse are taken in the supine position. Then the patient is asked to stand for 1 minute. Extreme dizziness, syncope, or a rise in pulse of 30 bpm is sensitive for a 1,000-cc volume loss. (Find the source.) A systolic blood pressure drop of over 30 mm Hg with or without a pulse increase is evidence of orthostatic hypotension, which may represent autonomic insufficiency or volume loss. Be aware that 25% of normal, healthy patients older than 65 years have a drop in systolic blood pressure of 20 mm Hg or more on standing. In addition, the test is not sensitive for volume losses of less than 1,000 cc.

13. Are tests needed to assist in diagnosis?
In the vast majority of cases, no. The history is the critical component, and historical clues can aid in directing the exam and determining a cause. In one study, a detailed history and

physical were sufficient to make the diagnosis in 55% of patients who had syncope that could be categorized. The addition of a specific confirmatory test (such as cardiac echo) based on the history and physical added 8%. The only other consistently useful tests were an electrocardiogram (EKG), adding 12%, and Holter monitor, adding 21%. Computed tomography (CT), electroencephalography (EEG), and radionuclide brain scanning have extremely poor yield without a focal abnormality on neurologic exam.

14. What about laboratory testing?
Fingerstick glucose testing is easy and cheap and may detect hypoglycemia. Electrolytes are rarely helpful, although a low serum bicarbonate may indicate a major motor seizure. Complete blood counts are frequently performed but are usually not helpful in eliciting a diagnosis.

15. Who needs an EKG?
An abnormal EKG is found in 50% of victims of syncope but is diagnostic in only 12%. Nevertheless, unless an obvious cause is found during the history taking and the physical, an EKG should be obtained, because it is not invasive and, if diagnostic, may preclude more expensive or invasive testing. Check the paramedics' run sheet: dysrhythmia was discovered there 20% of the time in one study. An EKG should be considered in any patient who has a sudden (no warning) episode of syncope or who has syncope while in the sitting or recumbent position.

16. What should you look for on the EKG?
Check for the presence of ischemia, infarction, dysrhythmias, preexcitation, long Q-T intervals, and conduction abnormalities. Left ventricular hypertrophy may be a clue to aortic stenosis, hypertension, or cardiomyopathy.

17. What is the role of ambulatory cardiac monitoring?
If the history suggests a cardiac etiology, ambulatory monitoring is indicated—it leads to finding the cause of syncope in 21% of cases. In high-risk patients, such monitoring should be done in the hospital. Unfortunately, there is no consensus concerning the significance of the majority of dysrhythmias found on monitoring, and the cost-effectiveness of this modality needs to be further examined.

18. What factors help in assigning the patient to a high- or low-risk group?
Those who have significant cardiac risk factors, exertional syncope, age >70, recurrent syncope, aortic outflow obstruction, or a history suggestive of cardiac dysrhythmia are at greatest risk. Patients with a cardiac cause of syncope have a 5-year mortality rate of 50% and have often died suddenly. Patients under the age of 30 or who have a history of vasovagal syncope have very low risk.

19. Shouldn't all patients with syncope be admitted to make sure that something doesn't "turn up" during admission?
This would become prohibitively expensive. Patients for whom there is a high index of suspicion for a cardiac cause should be strongly considered for admission and expeditious workup. However, in low-risk patients, admission and comprehensive evaluation are unwarranted. Most causes of syncope are either evident on initial evaluation or are elusive, even with extensive testing with electrophysiologic studies, EEG, CT, and other modalities.

20. Who is the best candidate for electrophysiologic studies?
A patient with structural heart disease with recurrent unexplained syncope is the best candidate for such study because the diagnostic yield is reasonable, and treatment of the discovered abnormalities is often successful.

BIBLIOGRAPHY

1. Day SC, Cook EF, Funkenstein H, et al: Evaluation and outcome of emergency room patients with transient loss of consciousness. Am J Med 73:15, 1982.
2. Eagle KA, Black HR, Cook EF, et al: Evaluation of prognostic classifications for patients with syncope. Am J Med 79:455, 1985.
3. Kapoor WN: Evaluation and outcome of patients with syncope. Medicine 69:160, 1990.
4. Kapoor WN, Karpf M, Maher Y, et al: Syncope of unknown origin: The need for a more cost-effective approach to its diagnostic evaluation. JAMA 247:2687, 1982.
5. Kapoor WN, Karpf M, Wieand S, et al: A prospective evaluation and follow-up of patients with syncope. N Engl J Med 309:197, 1983.
6. Kapoor W, Snustad D, Peterson J, et al: Syncope in the elderly. Am J Med 80:419, 1986.
7. Knopp R, Claypool R, Leonardi D: Use of the tilt test in measuring acute blood loss. Ann Emerg Med 9:29, 1980.
8. Lipsitz LA: Syncope in the elderly. Ann Intern Med 99:92, 1983.
9. Martin GJ, Adams SL, Martin HG, et al: Prospective evaluation of syncope. Ann Emerg Med 13:499, 1984.
10. Manolis AS, Linzer M, Salem D, et al: Syncope: Current diagnostic evaluation and management. Ann Intern Med 112:850, 1990.
11. Schaal SF, Boudoulas H, Nelson SD, Lewis RP: Syncope. Curr Probl Cardiol 17:207–264, 1992.

12. VERTIGO AND DIZZINESS

James E. Bodenhamer, M.D.

1. What is WADAO?

A common and usually confusing syndrome that strikes a sense of uneasiness in most clinical practitioners, WADAO is an acronym for weak and dizzy all over.

2. How is vertigo different from dizziness?

Vertigo is the illusion or hallucination of motion when there is none. Patients may describe their vertiginous symptoms as spinning, rotating, whirling, rocking, or tilting. Dizziness is an imprecise term used to describe various peculiar symptoms such as faintness, giddiness, light-headedness, or unsteadiness.

3. Which three systems regulate equilibrium and spatial orientation?

1. The **visual system** (eyes and eye muscles),
2. The **proprioceptive system** (posterior columns, tendons, joints, and muscles), and
3. The **statokinetic system** (ear, labyrinth, eighth cranial nerve, brain stem, cerebellum, and cerebral cortex).

Disturbance in any of these can result in dizziness; however, abnormalities in the statokinetic system alone can cause vertigo.

4. How do I approach the work-up of a patient with dizziness?

First, you need to rule out syncope or vertigo. One study found that 43% of patients complaining of dizziness had a peripheral vestibular disorder (vertigo) and 21% had cardiovascular etiologies such as dysrhythmias or hypovolemia. Although the differential diagnosis of dizziness is extensive, a careful history and physical examination will often make the diagnosis.

Differential Diagnosis of Dizziness

Visual disturbances	Other
Glaucoma	Hyperventilation
Refraction problems	Anemia
Ocular muscle abnormalities	Hypoxia
Proprioceptive dysfunction	Medication-related
Pellagra	Post-traumatic
Chronic alcoholism	Psychogenic
Pernicious anemia	Endocrinologic
Tabes dorsalis	

5. What pertinent physical findings should I look for?

A general physical exam should include particular attention to the pulse, blood pressure, and cardiovascular system, with note of any arrhythmias. The presence of bruits suggests atherosclerotic disease and should be sought in patients suspected of having vertebrobasilar insufficiency. Orthostatic vital signs are essential. A rectal examination should be performed to rule out occult gastrointestinal hemorrhage. Examination of external auditory canals, tympanic membrane, and hearing is mandatory. A complete neurologic examination is warranted, with special attention to cranial nerves and cerebellar function. Every patient with vertigo should be tested for positional nystagmus. This is usually performed by having the patient change from a sitting to supine position while quickly turning the paient's head to one side. This maneuver should be repeated turning the head to the other side. Attention should be paid to the presence and direction of nystagmus, the latency of response, and any associated symptoms (e.g., reproduction of vertigo, nausea, vomiting).

6. What is the importance of nystagmus in the vertiginous patient?

If a patient's symptoms are due to an organic vestibular dysfunction, then every episode of vertigo should be accompanied by nystagmus. If a patient complains of vertigo but has no nystagmus, then a psychogenic origin is likely.

7. How does nystagmus help differentiate peripheral vertigo from central vertigo?

Vertiginous patients with peripheral disease will typically have horizontal or horizonto-rotary nystagmus. The nystagmus will be unidirectional and observed in both eyes. It will be most pronounced at the onset and gradually subside over several hours to several days. Additionally, visual fixation will suppress the nystagmus; thus the nystagmus will be more pronounced with the eyes closed (visible or palpated through the closed lid). The most common cause of peripheral vertigo is benign paroxysmal positional vertigo. When afflicted patients are tested for positional nystagmus, they demonstrate latent (1 to 2 seconds) horizonto-rotary nystagmus toward the inferior ear that is associated with severe, short-lived, fatigable vertigo, as well as nausea and vomiting.

Central nystagmus, seen in patients with central vertigo, may be in any direction and may involve only one eye. Vertical and unilateral nystagmus typically represents brainstem disease. Central nystagmus may be continuous and is not visually suppressed. Central lesions may occasionally cause positional nystagmus; however, the nystagmus may last as long as the new position is maintained, and these patients rarely complain of vertigo while nystagmus is present.

8. Other than nystagmus, are there ways to differentiate peripheral vertigo from central vertigo?

Vertigo due to peripheral etiologies generally has an acute, sudden, often violent onset and is frequently associated with nausea and vomiting, hearing abnormalities, and diaphoresis.

Central vertigo classically has an insidious onset with rather mild vertiginous symptoms. Neurologic abnormalities may be found on exam.

9. What are common causes of peripheral vertigo?
Obstruction of the external auditory canal, acute or chronic otitis media, Menière's disease, benign paroxysmal positional vertigo, acute labyrinthitis, and vestibular neuronitis.

10. What is Menière's disease?
Menière's disease is associated with a triad of symptoms: vertigo, tinnitus, and deafness. It usually occurs between the ages of 30 and 60 years. Etiology is unclear, but some believe it is due to extravasation of endolymph into the perilymphatic space. Symptoms last 1–2 hours and are often recurrent.

11. How do I diagnose benign positional vertigo (BPV)?
BPV is more common in the elderly, occurs only with change in position, and lasts only 1–2 minutes. Patients who continually change positions may report that their symptoms last longer. Symptoms are reproducible by testing for positional nystagmus (see question #5). Typically BPV is a self-limited disease, lasting weeks to months, but may be recurrent.

12. What is an acoustic neuroma?
Acoustic neuroma is a tumor that begins from sheath cells typically of the vestibular portion of the eighth cranial nerve in the internal auditory canal. Most patients with acoustic neuroma give a vague, undramatic history of unsteadiness associated with hearing loss or tinnitus. As the neoplasm enlarges, cranial nerve or cerebellar dysfunction may be present. CT imaging can be helpful, but even moderate-sized tumors may be missed on routine scanning.

13. What are the common causes of central vertigo?
Posterior fossa tumors, vascular insufficiency of the vertebrobasilar system, temporal lobe epilepsy, basilar artery migraine, multiple sclerosis, and closed head injuries (inner ear or central vestibular nuclei trauma).

14. Are laboratory tests useful in a vertiginous patient?
In general, they are not. However, if a patient has a history of diabetes or an age greater than 45 years, blood glucose and EKG should be checked. Other tests include a serum pregnancy test in a young dizzy female and a hematocrit in any patient with a history worrisome for anemia. CT and MRI should be considered in patients in whom a central disease is suspected.

15. What is the symptomatic treatment of vertigo?
Treatment should be directed at the underlying cause. Symptomatic therapy for vertigo should include antiemetics, sedatives, and/or vestibular suppressants such as benzodiazepines, antihistamines, and drugs with anticholinergic properties. Droperidol (2.5–5 mg) is a potent neuroleptic, antiemetic, and sedative with vestibular suppressant effects; therefore, it is ideal therapy for acute vertigo. Intravenous diazepam in 2–10-mg doses is also effective for an acute attack. A number of regimens have been used for outpatient treatment: transdermal scopolamine; meclizine hydrochloride (Antivert), 25 mg every 8 hours; promethazine hydrochloride (Phenergan), 25 mg every 6 hours; and diphenhydramine hydrochloride (Benadryl), 25–50 mg every 6 to 8 hours. Patients suspected of having peripheral vertigo should be referred to an otolaryngologist, and those suspected of having central vertigo require follow-up with a neurologist or neurosurgeon.

BIBLIOGRAPHY

1. Baldwin RL: Droperidol in the treatment of vertigo. South Med J 76:1271–1272, 1983.
2. Busis SN: Diagnostic evaluation of the patient presenting with vertigo. Otolaryngol Clin North Am 6:3–23, 1973.
3. Frederic MW: Central vertigo. Otolaryngol Clin North Am 6:267–285, 1973.
4. Herr RD, Zun L, Mathews JJ: A direct approach to the dizzy patient. Ann Emerg Med 18:664–672, 1989.
5. Mohr DN: The syndrome of paroxysmal positional vertigo: A review. West J Med 145:645–650, 1986.
6. Nolte J (ed): The Human Brain: An Introduction to Its Functional Anatomy. St. Louis, CV Mosby, 1981, pp 144–163.
7. Schultz KE: Vertigo and syncope. In Rosen P, et al (eds): Emergency Medicine: Concepts and Clinical Practice, 2nd ed. St. Louis, Mosby–Year Book, 1988, pp 1773–1802.
8. Shiffman F, Dancer J, Rothballer AB, et al: The diagnosis and evaluation of acoustic neuromas. Otolaryngol Clin North Am 6:189–228, 1973.
9. Slater R: Vertigo: How serious are recurrent and single attacks? Postgrad Med 84:58–67, 1988.
10. Toglia JU: Diagnosis and treatment of vertigo and dizziness. Med Times 109:29–32, 1981.

13. SEIZURES

Kent N. Hall, M.D.

1. What is a seizure? What is its significance?

Seizures are the result of excessive or chaotic discharge from cerebral neurons. Although most clinicians call the resulting effect (jerking movements, staring, etc.) a "seizure," the seizure is the neuronal activity itself. The observable manifestation is called "seizure activity."

The importance of seizures is obvious. Something is interfering with the normal functioning of a group of neurons. The hyperactivity of the neurons causes a buildup of metabolic by-products, resulting in a harmful effect on the neurons. Neurons are dependent on aerobic metabolism. When the need for oxygen (cell metabolism) outstrips the availability of oxygen ("oxygen debt"), the neuron is injured. If this situation is prolonged, cell death results.

2. How do I recognize a seizure?

This is not as obvious as it may seem. Seizures can manifest themselves in a variety of ways, depending on the size and location of the area of the brain involved. A list of types of seizures by manifestation is given in the table below. Generally seizures fall into three categories: focal, generalized, and focal with secondary generalization. A focal seizure is confined to a particular area of the brain and thus affects only a given area of the body. A generalized seizure manifests itself by seizure activity that involves the entire body. A focal seizure with secondary generalization initially involves a part of the brain, but spreads to encompass the entire brain. The initial manifestation is isolated to a particular body area, but spreads to encompass the entire body. A high index of suspicion is necessary to recognize the more "atypical" seizure activity for what it truly is. When a seizure has occurred but has stopped prior to your seeing the patient, you should look for secondary signs of seizures, which include incontinence of urine or feces and biting of the tongue or buccal mucosa.

Classification of Seizures

TYPE	MANIFESTATION
Generalized	
Tonic clonic (grand mal)	Loss of consciousness followed immediately by tonic contraction of muscles, then clonic contraction of muscles (jerking) that may last for several minutes. A period of disorientation (postictal period) occurs after the tonic-clonic activity.
Absence (petit mal)	Sudden loss of awareness with cessation of activity or body position control. The period usually lasts for seconds to minutes and is followed by a relatively short postictal phase.
Atonic (drop attacks)	Complete loss of postural control with falling to the ground, sometimes causing injury. Usually occurs in children.
Partial of Focal	
Simple partial	Multiple patterns are possible depending on the area of the brain affected. If the motor cortex is involved, the patient will have contraction of the corresponding body area. If nonmotor areas of the brain are involved, the sensation may include paresthesias, hallucinations, déjà vu, etc.
Complex partial	Usually there is loss of ongoing motor activity with minor motor activity, such as lip smacking, walking aimlessly, etc.
Partial with Secondary Generalization	Initial manifestations are the same as partial. However, there is progression of the activity to involve the entire body, with loss of postural control and possibly tonic-clonic muscle activity.

3. What is the initial approach to a patient who is having a seizure?

Start with the ABCs (airway, breathing, circulation). In other words, address the vital signs—*all* the vital signs. Your first attention should be toward the patient's airway. Multiple techniques are available for opening or obtaining an airway. These have been addressed in other chapters of this book. Supplemental oxygen should be administered because of the increased oxygen demand caused by the excessive muscle action. Evaluation of the cardiovascular status with determination of blood pressure and capillary refill and subsequent correction with fluids (normal saline or lactated Ringer's) addresses "C." Attention to the temperature and prompt response to an abnormality is also important.

4. How do I stop the seizures?

If a seizure lasts longer than 5 minutes, immediate intervention is indicated. In traditional medicine the usual sequence is diagnosis, then treatment. Often in emergency medicine, it is necessary to diagnose and treat simultaneously. This is one of those times. Do not wait until after taking a history, doing a complete physical examination, and ordering ancillary tests before addressing the seizure activity. **Seizures damage the brain; the longer they are allowed to continue, the more damage occurs.**

Benzodiazepines are the drugs of choice for treating prolonged seizures (status epilepticus). Diazepam was traditionally the preferred drug. The dosage is 5–10 mg IV push repeated until a total of 20 mg is given or the seizure stops. It has been supplanted more recently by lorazepam. The dosage of this agent is 2–4 mg IV push up to a total of 10–15 mg. The preference of lorazepam over diazepam is because of its longer antiepileptic action (45–60 min vs. 15–30 min) and longer half-life (6–8 hr vs. 3–4 hr). If multiple doses of a benzodiazepine do not stop the seizure, or if benzodiazepines are contraindicated in the patient, a loading dose of a primary anticonvulsant (see below) should be administered.

5. Once the seizure has stopped, how do I keep it from recurring?

This question brings us to another class of drugs, the anticonvulsants. The drugs most often used to stop seizures or keep seizures from recurring, along with their doses and routes of administration, are listed below. Anticonvulsants not only keep seizures from recurring in the emergency department (ED), but also are used to stop seizures that are resistant to the benzodiazepines.

Anticonvulsants

NAME	DOSE	ROUTE OF ADMINISTRATION
Phenytoin	15–18 mg/kg	IV

Should not be given faster than 50 mg/min; patient should be on a cardiac monitor; stop infusion if toxicity noted (prolongation of QRS >50% of baseline, hypotension).

Phenobarbital	Up to 10 mg/kg	IV

Should not be given faster than 60 mg/min; dose can be repeated once at 30 minutes if no effect; maximum total dose is 600 mg acutely; beware of respiratory depression, especially if the patient has received diazepam.

Paraldehyde	12 ml of 10% solution	Orally by NG
	4–8 ml of 10% solution	Retention enema

Severe metabolic acidosis can occur; hypotension with right heart failure is reported.

6. Name the causes of seizures.

The more common causes by age of patient are listed below. Immediately reversible causes that physicians should be especially vigilant for and that rapidly respond to treatment include hypoglycemia and hypoxia (secondary to narcotic overdose). Therefore, an initial Dextrostix and empirical administration of naloxone is indicated. Note the similarity of causes of seizures in the very young and very old.

Causes of Seizures

Infant
> Birth trauma (hypoxia, intracranial trauma), infection (brain abscess, meningitis), electrolyte abnormalities (hyponatremia, hypocalcemia, hypomagnesemia), congenital malformations (intracerebral cysts, hydrocephalus), and genetic disorders (inborn errors of metabolism, pyridoxine deficiency)

Child
> Febrile seizure, idiopathic seizure, trauma, infection (meningitis)

Adolescent
> Trauma, idiopathic, drug or alcohol related (acute intoxication or withdrawal), arteriovenous malformation

Young Adult
> Trauma, alcohol related (acute intoxication or withdrawal), brain tumor

Older Adult
> Brain tumor, stroke, intracerebral hemorrhage, alcoholism, metabolic derangements (hyponatremia, hypernatremia, hypocalcemia, hypoglycemia, uremia, hepatic failure)

7. Is the history really important?

The history is vitally important! Use the mnemonic COLD to be sure you have covered the aspects of the seizure activity itself:

C   Character (what type of seizure activity was there)
O   Onset (when did it start, what was the patient doing)
L   Location (where did the activity start)
D   Duration (how long did it last)

Other important points include the patient's past medical history (especially previous seizure history), current medications, and history of recent or remote trauma.

8. Besides the neurologic examination, what other parts of the physical are important and why?

A complete head-to-toe examination is important. The examination is often normal, but on occasion may give clues to an underlying problem. Specifically, examination of the skin might reveal lesions consistent with meningococcemia or other infectious problems. Examination of the head is important to look for trauma. If nuchal rigidity is found, meningitis or subarachnoid hemorrhage should be suspected. A heart murmur, especially if records indicate none was heard before, might indicate subacute bacterial endocarditis with resultant embolization as the cause of the seizure.

The neurologic examination is very important. Focal neurologic findings, such as focal paresis after the seizure (Todd's paralysis), are virtually pathognomonic of a focal cerebral lesion (tumor, abscess, cerebral contusion) as the cause of the seizure. Evaluation of the cranial nerves and the eye grounds can indicate increased intracranial pressure.

9. How do I complete the work-up of the patient with a history of seizures?

After history and physical examination come ancillary tests. Seizure patients often undergo multiple ancillary tests, few of which result in a change in treatment or disposition. Studies have shown that the single most important laboratory test to perform is an anticonvulsant level, usually the one the patient is *supposed* to be taking. If the level is subtherapeutic, then the patient should be given a loading dose of this medication to achieve a therapeutic level.

10. What if the patient has never had a seizure before?

If this is a new-onset seizure, the use of ancillary tests becomes more important. However, the yield is still quite low. A screen for metabolic derangements (sodium, calcium, glucose, magnesium) is important. In the ED, a CT scan of the head (without contrast) to look for intracranial bleeding or other immediately life-threatening problems is warranted. Toxicologic screens should be obtained if clinically indicated.

11. What is the appropriate disposition of a patient with a recurrence of seizures?

If there are no abnormal findings on history or physical examination, the patient can be discharged with follow-up by the primary care physician or neurologist. If the anticonvulsant level is normal or the history suggests a change in seizure activity (increased frequency, different type), the patient should be evaluated as a new seizure patient. This may include admission if follow-up is not assured or if findings during the work-up indicate the need for hospitalization.

12. Does the fact that the patient has a first-time seizure make a difference in management and/or disposition?

Almost all patients with new-onset seizures should be treated with anticonvulsants in the ED. Exceptions include children with febrile seizures and patients with alcohol- or cocaine-related seizures. In any event, discussion of the case with a neurologist is warranted prior to the patient leaving the ED.

The disposition of the patient with a first-time seizure and a negative work-up in the ED is controversial. The conservative approach is to admit all such patients for inpatient evaluation. However, recently there has been a movement toward discharge to home when good follow-up care is available. If contact has been made with the patient's primary physician or neurologist, and close follow-up can be arranged, the patient may be discharged to home. In going over the discharge instructions, the physician should emphasize to the patient not to drive, use any machinery, or be around high places (construction, open areas, etc.). Further, the patient should be started on an anticonvulsant as described above.

13. Are afebrile children with seizures different from adults with seizures?

Children are different in two very important ways. First, the causes of seizures are different. Infants rarely have seizures without an underlying problem, either structural or metabolic. Primary epilepsy initially manifests in the 2–18 year age range. A full work-up must always be performed, especially in the patient with a first seizure.

Second, the anticonvulsant of choice for neonates is phenobarbital at a dose of 10–15 mg/kg IV slow push. The benzodiazepines are second-line agents in this age group. Obviously, before the phenobarbital is going to work, any underlying metabolic derangement must be appropriately addressed.

14. What is a febrile seizure? How is it different from other seizures of childhood?

Febrile seizures are associated with a rapid increase in temperature and usually occur in children between the ages of 6 months and 2 years. A simple febrile seizure is defined as that occurring in a patient in the appropriate age range, lasting less than 5 minutes, without focal findings and with a complete return to baseline mental status within 15 minutes. In fact, if the seizure does not meet these diagnostic criteria, an intracranial process (tumor, infection) must be ruled out.

15. What is the appropriate disposition and follow-up?

In a simple febrile seizure, the patient can be discharged after an adequate evaluation. No anticonvulsants need to be prescribed. However, the underlying problem causing the fever should be addressed, and appropriate follow-up with the primary care physician should be arranged. If the patient has a complex febrile seizure (focal seizure activity, duration greater than 15 minutes, or age outside the above age range, but the seizure is associated with a fever), then close follow-up by a pediatric neurologist should be considered. The decision to admit this patient can be made in consultation with the pediatrician or neurologist, but is not mandatory in all cases.

16. What is a pseudoseizure? How is it diagnosed?

Pseudoseizures are seizure-like activity with no underlying abnormal electrical activity in the brain. They are difficult to diagnose in the ED. Maneuvers that have been shown to work *in some cases* include suggesting to the patient that the seizure will stop soon or attempting to distract the patient with loud noises or bright lights during the "seizure" activity. The diagnosis can be made electrically if the patient is hooked up to an EEG machine (not customary in the ED). During the pseudoseizure, no abnormal electrical activity will be seen. Similarly, measurement of serum prolactin 20 minutes after the "seizure" will help to differentiate a true seizure from a pseudoseizure. In true seizures, the prolactin level is elevated at least two times, whereas in pseudoseizures the prolactin remains in the normal range. Obviously, neither of these methods is available in the ED. Because pseudoseizures often occur in patients with underlying "true" seizure disorders, the diagnosis is rarely made in the ED.

17. What is the significance of the anion gap in the diagnosis of grand mal seizure?

An increased transient (less than 1 hour duration) anion gap is good indirect evidence that a grand mal seizure has occurred. This is determined by blood samples drawn as close to the time of seizure as possible. Thus field blood samples are ideal for this study.

18. Are lumbar punctures and head CT scans indicated in the work-up of febrile seizures?
Lumbar punctures should be performed in any patient with clinical signs of meningitis and should be strongly considered in all patients under 12–18 months of age. CT scans are rarely helpful and are seldom useful, but should be obtained if there is any question or antecedent trauma, focal neurologic findings, or focal seizures.

BIBLIOGRAPHY

1. Barsan B, et al: Emergency Drug Therapy. Philadelphia, W.B. Saunders, 1991.
2. Gabor AJ: Lorazepam versus phenobarbital: Candidates for drug of choice for treatment of status epilepticus. J Epilepsy 3:3, 1990.
3. Mitchell WG, et al: Lorazepam is the treatment of choice for status epilepticus. J Epilepsy 3:7, 1990.
4. Pritchard PB: The effect of seizures on hormones. Epilepsia 32(Suppl 6):S46, 1991.
5. Rosen P, et al (eds): Emergency Medicine: Concepts and Clinical Practice, 3rd ed. St. Louis, Mosby–Year Book, 1992.
6. Tintinalli JE, et al (eds): Emergency Medicine: A Comprehensive Study Guide, 3rd ed. New York, McGraw-Hill, 1992.
7. Treiman DM: The role of benzodiazepines in the management of status epilepticus. Neurology 40(Suppl 2):32, 1990.
8. Turnbull TL, et al: Utility of laboratory studies in the emergency department patient with new-onset seizure. Ann Emerg Med 19:373, 1990.
9. Wilson JD, et al: Harrison's Principles of Internal Medicine. New York, McGraw-Hill, 1991.

14. ANAPHYLAXIS

Vince Markovchick, M.D.

1. What is anaphylaxis?
Anaphylaxis is a systemic immediate hypersensitivity reaction of multiple organ systems to an antigen-induced IgE-mediated immunologic mediator release in previously sensitized individuals.

2. What are the most common causes?
Ingestion, inhalation or parenteral injection of antigens that sensitize predisposed individuals. Common antigens include drugs (e.g., penicillin), foods (shellfish, nuts, egg whites), insect stings (hymenoptera) and bites (snakes), diagnostic agents (ionic contrast media), and physical and environmental agents (exercise and cold).

3. What are the most common "target" organs?
The most common organ systems involved are the skin (urticaria, angioedema), mucous membranes (edema), upper respiratory tract (edema and hypersecretions), lower respiratory tract (bronchoconstriction), and cardiovascular system (vasodilatation).

4. What are the most common signs and symptoms?
The clinical presentation ranges from mild to life threatening. Mild manifestations that occur in most people include urticaria and angioedema. Life-threatening manifestations involve the respiratory or cardiovascular systems. Respiratory signs and symptoms include acute upper airway obstruction presenting with stridor or lower airway manifestations of

bronchospasm with diffuse wheezing. Cardiovascular collapse presents in the form of syncope, hypotension, tachycardia, and arrhythmias.

5. What is the role of diagnostic studies?
There is no role for diagnostic studies in anaphylaxis because diagnosis and treatment are based solely on clinical signs and symptoms. There is a role for skin testing either prior to administration of an antigen or in follow-up referral to determine exact allergens involved.

6. What is the differential diagnosis?
Anaphylaxis may be confused with septic and cardiogenic shock, asthma, croup and epiglottitis, vasovagal syncope, and myocardial or any acute cardiovascular or respiratory collapse of unclear etiology.

7. What is the most common form of anaphylaxis? How is it treated?
Urticaria, either simple or confluent, is the most benign and, fortunately, the most common clinical manifestation. This is thought to be due to a capillary leak mediated by histamine release. It may be treated by the administration of antihistamines (PO, IM or IV) or epinephrine (subcutaneous).

8. What is the initial treatment for life-threatening forms of anaphylaxis?
1. Upper airway obstruction with stridor and edema should be treated with high-flow nebulized oxygen, racemic epinephrine, and IV epinephrine. If airway obstruction is severe or increases, endotracheal intubation or cricothyrotomy should be performed.

2. Acute bronchospasm should be treated with epinephrine. Mild to moderate wheezing in patients with a normal blood pressure may be treated with .01 mg/kg of 1:1000 epinephrine administered subcutaneously or IM. If the patient is in severe respiratory distress or has a "quiet" chest, IV epinephrine should be administered via a drip infusion: 1 mg epinephrine in 250 cc D5W at an initial rate of 1 μg/min.

3. Cardiovascular collapse presenting with hypotension should be treated with a constant infusion of epinephrine, titrating the rate to attain a systolic BP of 100 mm Hg or mean arterial pressure of 80 mm Hg.

4. For patients in full cardiac arrest, administer 0.1–0.2 mg/kg of 1:10,000 epinephrine slow IV push or via endotracheal tube. In addition, immediate endotracheal intubation or cricothyrotomy should be performed.

9. What are the adjuncts to initial epinephrine and airway management?
If intubation is unsuccessful and cricothyrotomy is contraindicated, percutaneous trans-tracheal jet ventilation via needle cricothyrotomy should be considered, especially in small children. Intravenous diphenhydramine (2 mg/kg) should be administered to all patients. Simultaneous administration of H2 blocker such as cimetidine, 300 mg IV, may be helpful. Aerosolized bronchodilators such as metaproterenol are useful if bronchospasm is present. Corticosteroids are usually given but do not have an immediate positive effect. For refractory hypotension, pressors such as norepinephrine or dopamine may be administered. Glucagon, 1 mg IV q 5 min, may be helpful in "epinephrine-resistant" patients who are on long-term beta-adrenergic blocking agents such as propranolol.

10. What are the complications of bolus IV epinephrine administration?
When epinephrine 1:10,000 is administered via IV push in patients who have an obtainable blood pressure or pulse, there is significant potential for overtreatment and the potentiation of hypertension, tachycardia, chest pain, and ventricular arrhythmias. Extreme care must be exercised in elderly patients and in those with underlying coronary artery disease. It is

much safer to administer IV epinephrine by a controlled titratable drip infusion with continuous monitoring of cardiac rhythm and blood pressure.

11. Is there a role for prophylactic treatment in anaphylaxis? How is this performed?

When the potential benefits of treatment or diagnosis outweigh the risks (e.g., administration of antivenom for life- or limb-threatening snake bites), informed consent should be obtained if the patient is competent. Pretreatment with IV Benadryl and corticosteroids should be carried out. An IV epinephrine infusion should be prepared. The patient should be in an ICU setting with continuous monitoring of blood pressure, cardiac rhythm, and oxygen saturation. Full intubation and cricothyrotomy equipment should be at the bedside. Administration of the antigen (e.g., rattlesnake antivenom) should be started very slowly with a physician at the bedside who is capable of immediately administering IV epinephrine and managing the airway. Nonionic contrast medium for diagnostic imaging studies should be administered to patients with a history of anaphylaxis to ionic contrast material.

12. What about steroids?

Because corticosteroids have an onset of action of approximately 4–6 hours after administration, they have limited or no benefit in the initial acute treatment of anaphylaxis. However, the administration of hydrocortisone (250–1,000 mg IV) or methylprednisolone (125–250 mg IV), followed by a tapering dose over 7–10 days, is an acceptable regimen following the resolution of the initial anaphylactic episode.

13. What is the disposition of a patient who initially responds to aggressive treatment?

Even though the majority of patients will respond positively to early, aggressive treatment and may even become asymptomatic, all patients with true anaphylactic reactions should be admitted to either an ED observation unit or the hospital for short-term observation. Patients who continue to have life-threatening symptoms (e.g., bronchospasm, hypotension, or upper airway obstruction) should be admitted to an ICU.

14. What is the prehospital treatment of anaphylaxis?

Patients who are known to be at high risk (e.g., previous anaphylactic reaction to hymenoptera) should be prescribed and educated in the self-administration of epinephrine at the first sign of anaphylactic symptoms. In addition, self-administration of oral diphenhydramine is indicated for the treatment of mild reactions such as urticaria or concomitant with the administration of epinephrine.

BIBLIOGRAPHY

1. Jacobs RL, et al: Potentiated anaphylaxis in patients with drug-induced beta-adrenergic blockage. J Allergy Clin Immunol 68:125, 1981.
2. Lee ML: Glucagon in anaphylaxis (letter). J Allergy Clin Immunol 69:331, 1981.
3. Lindzon RD, Silvers WS: Anaphylaxis. In Rosen P (ed): Emergency Medicine: Concepts and Clinical Practice, 3rd ed. St. Louis, C.V. Mosby, 1992, pp 1042–1065.
4. Lucke WC: Anaphylaxis. Emergindex, Vol. 67, Denver, Micromedex Inc., 1991.
5. Lucke WC, Thomas H: Anaphylaxis: Pathophysiology, clinical presentations and treatment. J Emerg Med 1:83–95, 1983.
6. Phanuphak P, Schocket A, Kohler PF: Treatment of chronic idiopathic urticaria with combined H_1 and H_2 blockers. Clin Allergy 8:429, 1978.
7. Roberts JR, Greenberg MI: Endotracheal epinephrine in cardiorespiratory collapse. JACEP 8:515–519, 1979.
8. Silverman JH, Van Hook C, Haponik EF: Hemodynamic changes in human anaphylaxis. Am J Med 77:341–344, 1984.
9. Weiszer I: Allergic emergencies. In Patterson R (ed): Allergic Diseases: Diagnosis and Management. Philadelphia, J.B. Lippincott, 1980, pp 374–394.

15. LOW BACK PAIN

Robert S. Hockberger, M.D., FACEP

1. Can I skip this chapter?

Not if you anticipate a career that involves caring for adults. Low back pain (LBP) is the fourth most common adult ambulatory complaint in the United States following the common cold, minor trauma, and headache. Four out of five people over 25 years of age will have at least one incapacitating episode of LBP during their life. LBP is the number one cause of restricted activity in patients under 45 years and ranks number three (after heart disease and arthritis) in patients over 45 years. The cost of diagnosis, treatment, disability, lost productivity, and litigation due to LBP exceeds $20 billion yearly, making it the third most expensive medical disorder in the United States following heart disease and cancer.

2. What are the causes of LBP?

Most cases of LBP are musculoskeletal, involving principally an injury or strain of the ligaments/muscles of the lower back and lumbar disc disease. However, certain nonmusculoskeletal diseases present with the complaint of LBP, including renal disease, pancreatic disease, perforated peptic ulcer, retrocecal appendicitis, and ruptured abdominal aortic aneurysm. In addition, malignancies and infections involving the spinal column usually present with LBP.

3. When should I suspect malignancy as a cause of LBP? How should it be evaluated?

Patients under 50 years of age develop primary tumors of the spine (usually benign), and patients over 50 years of age who develop malignancies (particularly thyroid, breast, lung, kidney, and prostate cancer) frequently develop metastases to the spinal column. Patients at risk include those with known malignancy or signs and symptoms suggestive of malignancy and patients who have had LBP for over 1 month, particularly when treatment with nonsteroidal anti-inflammatory medications (NSAIDs) has proved ineffective. Evaluation of such patients should include lumbosacral spine x-rays and an erythrocyte sedimentation rate (ESR). If either test is abnormal, a bone scan should be obtained and the patient referred for further evaluation.

4. When should a spinal column infection be suspected? How should it be evaluated?

Patients at greatest risk for vertebral body or disc space infections include children, immunosuppressed patients (particularly diabetics), intravenous drug abusers, and patients who have recently undergone back surgery. They usually present with LBP associated with fever and localized vertebral bony tenderness. However, fever is absent in up to one-third of cases. Lumbosacral spine x-rays are often normal (particularly if pain has been present for less than several weeks), but the ESR is usually elevated. Abnormal x-rays or an elevated ESR should result in hospitalization for a bone scan and definitive care.

5. What does it mean when a patient with LBP also has leg pain?

Patients with LBP may have pain that is *referred* down a leg as the result of inflammation of the sciatic nerve or that *radiates* down a leg as the result of nerve root impingement (usually from a herniated lumbar disc or narrowing of a vertebral foramina from spinal stenosis). Referred pain is usually dull and poorly localized, does not radiate distal to the knee, and is not associated with a positive straight-leg raising (SLR) test or neurologic impairment of the lower extremities. Alternatively, nerve root impingement results in sharp, well-localized radicular pain that frequently (but not always) radiates distal to the knee, is invariably associated with a positive SLR test, and may be associated with neurologic impairment.

56

6. How should the SLR test be performed? What does it mean?

With the patient lying supine on the examining table, the physician should slowly raise the patient's involved leg off the bed (flexing the leg at the hip while keeping the knee straightened) until the patient complains of discomfort. Most healthy adults will not complain of discomfort or will have only mild discomfort from the stretching of the hamstring muscles after the leg is elevated over 60 degrees. Some patients with low back strain complain of discomfort at the site of injury during the SLR test, but radicular symptoms will not occur. A *positive SLR test* occurs when leg elevation results in pain that radiates down the involved leg and infers nerve root impingement from a herniated lumbar disc or lateral spinal stenosis. A *positive crossed-SLR test* occurs when elevation of the uninvolved leg causes pain to radiate down the involved leg. When such pain is present, it is a very sensitive and specific sign for disc herniation.

7. How extensive must the patient's history and physical examination be?

Include in the history the patient's age (infections and malignancies are more common in the very young and very old), known medical problems, and previous episodes of LBP; the nature of the injury; the duration of symptoms and response to treatment (if any); the presence or absence of radicular symptoms; and any history of bowel or bladder dysfunction (evidence of impingement on the cauda equina). Physical examination should determine the degree of patient distress and limitation of spinal movement, the presence of "trigger points" of maximal tenderness, evidence of paravertebral muscle spasm, and results of neurologic exam of the lower extremities (motor, sensory, and reflex evaluation).

8. Whom should I irradiate?

For some reason, everyone (patients *and* doctors) loves x-rays. Unfortunately, they are expensive (we spend approximately $1 billion per year on lumbosacral spine films in the U.S.), result in gonadal radiation, and are rarely of help in directing initial diagnosis and treatment. Lumbosacral spine films should be obtained in patients with acute LBP who are suspected of having a spinal column malignancy or infection, in patients who have experienced significant trauma or who are in marked physical distress, and in patients who exhibit a neurologic deficit. Otherwise, x-rays should be reserved for patients who fail to improve with initial management.

9. Who should receive a CT scan or MRI evaluation?

CT and MRI should be used acutely to evaluate patients with suspected disc herniation who present with lower extremity motor paralysis or bowel/bladder dysfunction (evidence of massive central disc herniation). Such patients should be hospitalized because they frequently require urgent neurosurgical intervention. CT or MRI should also be used to evaluate patients with *any* evidence of neurologic impairment that can possibly be due to nerve impingement from a spinal epidural metastasis or an epidural abscess. The former requires high-dose radiation therapy, the latter usually surgical drainage in addition to intravenous antibiotics.

10. Who should be hospitalized for treatment?

With the exception of previously discussed patients who require emergency CT or MRI, there are no "standard" indications for hospitalization. Hospitalize patients with suspected disc herniation who are in significant physical distress and/or exhibit evidence of motor impairment of the lower extremities, because their failure to respond to aggressive conservative management may necessitate surgical intervention.

11. How should patients be treated in the emergency department (ED)?

Quickly. There is no need to await definitive diagnosis prior to providing pain relief. Patients who have trigger points frequently benefit from local injection with a steriod–local anesthetic combination. Other patients should be given oral or parenteral NSAIDs, and a cold pack applied locally to injured muscles and ligaments. Occasionally, parenteral narcotics are necessary to provide adequate analgesia.

12. What is the best initial outpatient treatment for LBP?

Most patients profit from bed rest (except for bathroom privileges) for 2–3 days in order to rest injured muscles and ligaments. The period can extend to 7–10 days for those with suspected disc herniation. A firm mattress is best.

Cryotherapy (cold application) should be administered four or five times a day. Instruct patients to use crushed ice placed in a self-sealed plastic bag and wrapped in a towel, maintaining the cold application for at least 30 minutes.

Most patients benefit from oral NSAIDs, but some require opioids to produce adequate analgesia during the first few days. Sedatives and muscle relaxants probably do little to actually "relax" injured muscles, but because of their sedating effects, they are helpful in improving patient compliance with instructions for bed rest.

13. What are appropriate aftercare instructions?

All patients with suspected disc disease and those with low back strain who do not improve within 1 week should be seen by a physician for follow-up evaluation. All patients should be instructed to return immediately if they develop any bowel or bladder dysfunction or if they have increasing progressive weakness or radicular pain.

14. What happens to patients with LBP once they leave the ED?

The prognosis for patients having a first episode of LBP (once you have considered and eliminated the possibility of underlying disease) is quite good; 70% are better by one week, 80% by two weeks, and 90% by one month. This is probably why most studies comparing medical management, chiropractic manipulation, and other treatment modalities rarely find significant differences in outcome, because almost everyone gets better no matter what you do. Those who do not improve with conservative management may have underlying disease (inflammatory disorders, malignancy, infections, or disc disease) that was not apparent at the time of initial evaluation or, alternatively, may suffer from nonmedical conditions such as psychiatric disorders, drug dependence, or job dissatisfaction.

BIBLIOGRAPHY

1. Blackburn WD, Alarcon GS, Ball GV: Evaluation of patients with back pain of suspected inflammatory nature. Am J Med 85:766, 1988.
2. Butt WP: Radiology for back pain. Clin Radiol 40:6, 1989.
3. Byrne TN: Spinal cord compression from epidural metastases. N Engl J Med 327:614, 1992.
4. Deyo RA, Bigos SJ, Maravilla KR: Diagnostic imaging procedures for the lumbar spine. Ann Intern Med 111:865, 1989.
5. Deyo RA: Cancer as a cause of back pain: Frequency, presentation and diagnostic strategies. J Gen Intern Med 3:230, 1988.
6. Deyo RA: Conservative therapy for low back pain: Distinguishing useful from useless therapy. JAMA 250:1057, 1983.
7. Deyo RA: How many days of rest for acute low back pain? A randomized clinical trial. Am J Med 85:766, 1988.
8. Deyo RA: Patient satisfaction with medical care for acute low back pain. Spine 11:28, 1986.
9. Deyo RA, Rainville J, Kent DL: What can the history and physical examination tell us about low back pain? JAMA 268:760, 1992.
10. Frymoyer JW: Back pain and sciatica. N Engl J Med 318:291, 1990.
11. Hockberger RS: Acute low back pain. In Callahan ML (ed): Decision Making in Emergency Medicine. Philadelphia, B.C. Decker, 1990, p 292.
12. King PA: Evaluating the child with back pain. Pediatr Clin North Am 33:1489, 1986.
13. Shiqing X: Significance of the straight-leg raising test in the diagnosis and clinical evaluation of lower lumbar intervertebral disc protrusion. J Bone Joint Surg 69A:517, 1987.
14. Singer J: Predicting outcome in acute low back pain. Can Fam Phys 33:655, 1987.
15. Swezey RL, Crittenden JO, Swezey AM: Outpatient treatment of lumbar disc sciatica. West J Med 145:43, 1986.

III. Nontraumatic Illness

16. NONTRAUMATIC OCULAR EMERGENCIES

Ricciardetto P. Scalzi, M.D., and Gregory P. Moore, M.D., FACEP

1. What do I need to know to prescribe ophthalmologic drugs properly?
These medications come in ointment and liquid form. Ointment has a longer duration of action because it does not dissipate through the tear duct. Therefore, it only needs to be applied every 4–6 hours, making its use more convenient in pediatric patients. A disadvantage in adults is decreased vision due to the solid substance moving around on the cornea. Eye drops are absorbed more rapidly and act for shorter periods of time; thus they must be administered every 2–4 hours but cause no visual problems. They are difficult to insert into the eye in noncompliant children.

Ophthalmologic drugs have all the side effects of their oral counterparts and care should be taken when dispensing them. Great care should be taken when prescribing beta-blocker drops to asthmatics, vasoconstrictors to those with cardiac disease, and anticholinergics to those with contraindications.

2. Ophthalmologic drug pearls:
1. Never give a patient a topical anesthetic at discharge. The lack of sensation predisposes patients to self-injury (it doesn't hurt when they rub it), and these medications retard epithelial healing.

2. Never use atropine eye drops. They cause dilatation of the pupil and loss of accommodation for up to 2–3 weeks.

3. Never use steroids in the eye without ophthalmologic consultation. The result can be disastrous if the current problem is due to herpes simplex.

4. Sulfacetamide stings, decreasing patient compliance.

5. Neomycin should be avoided, as it causes a hypersensitivity reaction in 5–15% of cases.

6. Having patients close their eyes tightly or squeeze the bridge of their nose after installing drops increases the local concentration of medication by blocking drainage through the tear duct.

7. The lowest concentration of antibiotics generally are the most effective (e.g., sulfa 10% concentration is better than 30%).

3. Tell me all I need to know about conjunctivitis.
1. Bacterial causes are pneumococcus, *H. influenzae*, and staphylococcus. Treat accordingly.

2. If associated with preauricular node, think adenovirus.

3. Viral conjunctivitis is usually bilateral with watery discharge. Bacterial conjunctivitis is usually purulent and unilateral. There is so much overlap, however, that all bets are off. Probably should treat all with 5–7 days of antibiotics.

4. In neonate, suspect gonococcal etiology.

5. In either a neonate or adult with venereal disease, suspect chlamydia.

6. If there are giant papilla under upper lid, suspect allergy to soft contact lenses.

7. With itching, tearing, and possibly chemosis (conjunctival edema), suspect allergy and treat with topical decongestant.

4. What is endophthalmitis?

Endophthalmitis is infection within the orbit itself. It is usually seen as a collection of pus in the anterior chamber (hypopyon) that resembles a dependent meniscus similar to the blood collection in a hyphema. Antecedent causes include conjunctivitis with organisms capable of penetrating the cornea (e.g., gonococcus), corneal ulcers and penetrating trauma from any cause. Aggressive treatment should be initiated immediately with ophthalmologic consultation and includes intravenous and/or subconjunctival antibiotics and tetanus prophylaxis, and may include anterior chamber paracentesis and/or operative debridement.

5. What is the difference between periorbital and orbital cellulitis?

Periorbital (or preseptal) cellulitis is soft tissue infection of anterior eye structures usually localized to the eyelids and conjunctivae. Orbital cellulitis represents a deeper and more serious infection (behind the septum) that involves posterior eye structures and may form an abscess. Both tend to be unilateral and may be preceded by trauma as well as upper respiratory, sinus, or dental infections. Orbital cellulitis is most often due to direct spread from ethmoid sinusitis, whereas periorbital cellulitis is usually due to hematogenous spread of bacteria.

6. What is the difference clinically between periorbital and orbital cellulitis?

The two may be difficult to distinguish clinically, especially in children. Periorbital cellulitis tends to cause local eyelid symptoms, occasionally ocular discharge, and may be associated with fever or leukocytosis. Visual acuity and pupillary reflexes are normal.

Orbital cellulitis may present with all of the above plus proptosis, fever, and pain with extraocular movements. The latter is possibly the most consistent finding. Decreased visual acuity, loss of sensation in V1 and V2 (CNV), and increased intraocular pressure are more uncommon findings.

Treatment should include antibiotics (usually IV) that cover staphylococcal, streptococcal and Hemophilus organisms. In unclear cases, CT scan of the orbits may provide the definitive differentiation.

7. How are papillitis and papilledema different?

Although clinically these two processes appear very similar, **papillitis** (specifically optic neuritis) is focal demyelination of the optic nerve resulting in a hyperemic nerve head developing over hours to days. The average age of onset is 31. An association with multiple sclerosis has been made in 35% of cases. **Papilledema** is swelling of the optic disc due to increased intracranial pressure. It is usually bilateral but may be asymmetric and may be due to brain abscess or tumor, intracranial bleeding, meningitis/encephalitis, hydrocephalus, severe hypertension, or pseudotumor cerebri.

Papillitis vs. Papilledema

	PAPILLITIS	PAPILLEDEMA
Pupil reactivity	Slow	Normal
Visual acuity	Decreased	Normal
Pain	Present	Absent
Usual localization	Unilateral	Bilateral
Fundus	——— Blurred disc margins ———	

8. Describe the differences in presentation and treatment of central retinal artery and central retinal vein occlusion.

Occlusion of the retinal artery or its branches results in a dilated nonreactive pupil on the affected side and a milky to pale retina with a "cherry red spot" at the macula (macular blood supply is from the choroid layer of the orbit). The funduscopic exam of a central retinal vein occlusion is described as a "blood-splashed fundus" because of the multiple hemorrhages present. Both occur in the atherosclerotic middle-aged or elderly hypertensive population and present as sudden painless loss of vision. Efforts to decrease intraocular pressure (see question #10), rebreathing CO_2, and globe massage may be useful acutely for arterial occlusions, but prognosis for both entities remains poor.

9. How is iritis differentiated from acute angle closure glaucoma in a patient with red eye?

Iritis vs. Glaucoma

	IRITIS	GLAUCOMA
Symptoms	Pain, headache, and photophobia	May also have abdominal pain, nausea and vomiting
Pupil	Small, concentrated redness around pupil (ciliary flush)	Dilated, unresponsive
Anterior chamber	Cell and flare on slit-lamp (like snow falling)	Hazy, corneal edema (steamy)
Etiology	Often unknown: usually trauma, inflammatory bowel, connective tissue disease	Blockage of aqueous outflow by iris that is dilated by entering dark room or by anticholinergic drugs
Diagnosis	Indicative slit-lamp findings	Elevated intraocular pressure (usually over 50)

10. How are they treated?

Iritis is treated with pain medication, a cycloplegic to dilate the iris and prevent adhesions between the iris and the lens (posterior synechiae), and topical steroids (only after consulting an ophthalmologist!).

Acute glaucoma is treated with emergent consultation, intravenous mannitol or glycerol to decrease intraocular pressure by osmotic diuresis, topical pilocarpine or timolol to decrease pupil size, and acetazolamide IV to decrease aqueous production.

11. And if I don't have a slit lamp to evaluate red eye?

Topical application of anesthetic drops should decrease or eradicate pain due to abrasion or conjunctivitis (not so with iritis or glaucoma). Shining a light into the normal eye should make the opposite eye hurt if the patient has iritis (due to consensual movement of the inflamed affected contralateral iris). This test may be more sensitive than the slit-lamp exam.

12. Name four toxins that can cause painless loss of vision.

Methanol, quinine, ergot preparations, and salicylates.

13. List the causes of a unilateral dilated pupil (anisocoria).

Normal finding (20% of population)
Antecedent cause (e.g., surgery, trauma, etc.)
Traumatic mydriasis or miosis
Unilateral use of topical drugs
Horner's syndrome
Intracranial third nerve palsy
 (brainstem herniation)
Nebulized anticholinergics

14. What do I do if someone presents with their eyelids stuck together from super glue?

Mineral oil is nontoxic to the eye and will often dissolve the glue. Acetone may also be used but is very irritating when it gets into the eye. If neither is successful, the patient should apply mineral oil frequently to the lid margin and consult an ophthalmologist. The lids may take several days to separate.

BIBLIOGRAPHY

1. Au YK: Pain elicited by consensual pupillary reflex: A diagnostic test for acute iritis. Lancet 2(8258):1254, 1981.
2. Clark RB: Common ophthalmologic problems. In Rosen P, et al (eds): Emergency Medicine: Concepts and Clinical Practice, 2nd ed. St. Louis, Mosby–Year Book, 1988.
3. Hulbert MFG: Efficacy of eyepad in corneal healing after corneal foreign body removal. Lancet 337(8742):643, 1991.
4. Leitman MN: Manual for Eye Examination and Diagnosis. Oradell, NJ, Medical Economics Company, 1988.
5. Mathews J, Zun ED: Ophthalmologic emergencies and ocular trauma. Emerg Clin North Am vol. 6, no. 1, Feb. 1988.
6. Ostler HB: Risk of tetanus from corneal injuries. JAMA 260:553, 1988.
7. Sclera DP: Topical anesthesia of the eye as a diagnostic test. Ann Emerg Med 18:1209, 1989.
8. Shingleton BJ: A clearer look at ocular emergency. Emerg Med May 15, 1989.

17. NONTRAUMATIC ENT EMERGENCIES

D. Michael Hunt, M.D.

EPISTAXIS

1. What are the most common causes of nosebleeds?

Nosebleeds can appear spontaneously, usually in association with dry nasal mucosa (from a deviated septum or rhinitis sicca) or infection. Minor local trauma from nose picking or direct blows to the nose are also frequent causes. Less commonly detected sources include foreign bodies, tumors, coagulopathies, exposure to anticoagulant drugs such as aspirin or Coumadin or to toxic or caustic materials (including chronic cocaine exposure), and even endocrine disorders such as endometriosis.

2. Doesn't hypertension cause epistaxis?

Not as an acute event. The hypertensive patient who presents with a nosebleed typically has hypertension as a chronic condition and has developed atherosclerosis, which makes the blood vessels relatively fragile and more likely to be disrupted when exposed to any of the above conditions.

3. Does bleeding originate from any one particular source?

A majority of nosebleeds, approximately 90%, originate from the anterior portion of the nose, a rich vascular network on the anterior portion of the septum known as Kiesselbach's plexus, or Little's area. The blood supply for most of this region is derived from the external carotid system. From a practical standpoint, a nosebleed with a source that can be directly visualized is considered "anterior." Posterior bleeds arise from either the external or internal carotid artery branches and tend to be more difficult to control. The hemorrhage tends to be more severe and is seen more frequently in the elderly. Atraumatic bleeding almost always comes from an isolated, unilateral source, and when it appears from both nares, it is due to blood passing behind the nasal septum.

4. What are the key historical questions to ask the patient?

Is there a prior history of nosebleeds? How about a past medical history of hypertension, excessive alcohol use, bleeding disorders, or other underlying conditions? Was any trauma (even nose picking) involved? On which side did the bleeding start? Any recent sinus infections or surgeries? How about Coumadin or aspirin use? Questions about steps taken by the patient to stop the bleeding or the amount of blood lost are inconsequential. Would the patient be in your emergency department if home treatment was successful? Patient estimates of blood loss are often exaggerated. If excessive hemorrhage is not reflected in the vital signs, it will be apparent during the physical examination.

5. Is there one key point to the successful management of nosebleeds?

There are two key considerations. The first issue to address is that of preparation. Because epistaxis rarely presents as a life-threatening condition that demands rapid institution of the ABCs of resuscitation, there is almost always time to assemble the necessary equipment and supplies for treatment (see below). While obtaining the history, have the patient pinch the nose firmly or place a nasal clamp on the patient with firm pressure on the septum. The patient and the examiner should both be gowned. Additionally, the examiner should wear disposable gloves, mask, and eye protection. The second key point is to identify the source of the hemorrhage. Once that is accomplished, the battle is half won.

Supplies for Examination and Treatment of Nosebleeds

EXAMINATION	STABILIZATION	TREATMENT
Protective garb	Bayonet forceps	Silver nitrate cautery sticks
Head lamp or mirror	Cotton pledgets	Electrocautery (if available)
Nasal speculum	4% Topical lidocaine	Gelfoam (or similar material)
Cotton swabs	1% Injectable lidocaine	½″ Petroleum-impregnated gauze
Fraser tip suction	with epinephrine	Antibiotic ointment
Emesis basin	4% Topical cocaine	Foley catheter or commercial balloon
4×4 Gauze	Topical vasoconstrictor	Rolled 4×4 gauze with silk suture

6. How do I treat it?

As mentioned, identify the source. Using the nasal speculum, suction and water moistened cotton swabs; remove the existing clots until the bleeding site is seen. Insert a medicated pledget with topical cocaine or xylocaine with epinephrine for 5 to 10 minutes to allow vasoconstriction and anesthesia to occur. Remove the pledget and begin with simple methods. If the source is in Kiesselbach's plexus and is less than 1 cm², use silver nitrate or electrocautery with additional submucosal anesthetic infiltration. Alternatively, a small piece of Gelfoam, Avitene, or similar substance may be moistened with a vasoconstrictor and applied to the bleeding site. If these methods are unsuccessful, it is time for an anterior nasal pack. Stair-step application of ½″ antibiotic-coated petroleum gauze in an anterior-posterior direction should be performed with nasal speculum and bayonet forceps until the nasal cavity is filled from the floor, superiorly. Sponge-like Merocel packs that are coated with antibiotic ointment and reconstituted with saline after insertion are easy to apply and are frequently effective. If inspection of the posterior pharynx demonstrates no continued bleeding after the vasoconstriction wears off (about 30 minutes), the patient may be discharged.

7. What are the important discharge instructions?
The pack should be removed in 24–48 hours. If the pack stays in place longer than that time, systemic antibiotics (penicillin) should be initiated to prevent sinusitis. The patient should avoid activities or ingestions that may transiently increase blood pressure (sneezing, bending over, caffeine, etc.). If recurrences fail to respond to direct pressure at home for 10 minutes, the patient should seek medical attention. Bleeding from desiccated nasal mucosa can be prevented by regular applications of petroleum or antibiotic ointment and use of room humidifiers.

8. How do I diagnose posterior epistaxis?
If a properly placed anterior pack fails, then the patient has a posterior bleed, and more aggressive treatment is required. Posterior packs are accomplished with rolled 4×4-inch gauze, a Foley catheter, or Nasostat or other commercially available balloon product. A unilateral anterior pack is still required in conjunction with a posterior pack.

9. Do I send a patient home with a posterior pack?
No. All patients who require a posterior pack or who otherwise have persistent bleeding must be admitted to the hospital.

10. Didn't you forget to mention laboratory studies?
No. It's just that most patients don't need them. The exceptions are patients on Coumadin or with suspected coagulopathies, and those who are hemodynamically unstable or require admission.

FOREIGN BODIES

11. How should a foreign body be removed from the ear?
First, identify it. Often, patients present only with a sensation of fullness, pain, discharge, or altered hearing. Middle ear symptoms may predominate if the tympanic membrane is ruptured. "Spontaneous" foreign bodies in adults are almost always insects. Foreign bodies introduced by the adult patient are usually cotton, but in children might be anything that could conceivably fit in the external auditory canal (EAC).

12. Now will you tell me how to remove it?
A number of instruments can assist in extraction:

Foreign body (alligator forceps)	Fraser tip suction	Ear curette
Right-angle probe	Irrigation syringe	Water-Pik
Tissue forceps	Adson forceps	Skin hook
Cyanoacrylate glue	Fogarty biliary catheter	Day hook

If a live insect is in the EAC, it should first be killed by instilling 2% lidocaine (which is quicker and less messy than mineral oil) before intact or segmental removal. If the tympanic membrane is intact and space exists between the EAC and the object, a stream of liquid can be directed behind the foreign body to force it out. A mixture of water and isopropyl alcohol as an irrigation solution tends to cause less swelling of organic matter and evaporates quicker. Direct instrument manipulation or suction will remove most other objects. Occasionally, cyanoacrylate glue on the end of a suture or a small balloon-tipped catheter will do the trick.

13. Is there any special consideration to be given to ear foreign bodies?
The skin of the EAC is exquisitely sensitive to touch. Use topical anesthesia and be gentle. For children, sedation may be required.

14. What about patient disposition?

Uncomplicated removal requires no follow-up. Minor EAC abrasions heal quickly. Any associated infection should be treated. If the tympanic membrane is ruptured or the patient has additional complaints, an otolaryngologist should be consulted. Difficult extractions, including those related to lack of patient cooperation, require specialist involvement as well.

15. Are nasal foreign bodies any different from those in the ear?

Yes. Because almost all objects are placed there by the patient, the foreign body is usually inanimate and the patient is usually a child. Also, because the nasal cavity is larger than the EAC, a wider variety of objects may be encountered and the presentation is typically painless.

16. How do these patients present?

Unless the patient or a witness reports the insertion of a foreign body, the chief complaint is that of unilateral, malodorous nasal discharge. The discharge may be thin and mucoid, serosanguinous, or, most often, purulent.

17. Is there any special trick to removing foreign bodies from the nose?

Prepare a 50/50 mixture of a topical vasoconstrictor and 4% topical lidocaine and spray it into the involved nostril with an atomizer or spray bottle. This will anesthetize the sensitive nasal mucosa and reduce congestion to facilitate removal. Once this is done, a simple measure such as occluding the unaffected nostril and having the patient blow forcefully can expel the object.

18. And if this doesn't work?

The general measures listed for foreign body removal from the ear can be applied in this situation. Because the nasal opening and cavity are larger, a greater number and larger instruments, such as a Kelly clamp, bayonet forceps, or Foley catheter can be used, but instrument manipulation remains the mainstay for foreign body removal.

19. Is any additional treatment necessary after removal?

Because nasal foreign bodies are so frequently seen in conjunction wiith sinusitis and otitis media, the presence of such infections should be documented and treated with appropriate antibiotics and decongestants.

20. "I think I've got something stuck in my throat." How is the patient with this complaint managed?

The fact that the patient can talk is a good sign. Airway foreign body or compromise must be addressed and ruled out. The patient should be asked about the nature of the foreign body, the duration of the sensation, the ability to swallow liquids or solids, and the perceived location of the object. Patient estimates of location are surprisingly accurate.

21. How should I organize my search for the object?

Direct visualization can identify sharp objects such as fish bones that may become impaled in the posterior pharynx or the base of the tongue. Indirect or fiberoptic laryngoscopy, in conjunction with local anesthesia, can pinpoint objects stuck in the vallecula, epiglottis, or pyriform sinus.

22. If the physical exam does not reveal the foreign body, what should be done next?

Soft tissue density lateral radiographs of the neck and/or chest x-ray studies should be obtained. Both large and sharp, angulated objects tend to lodge in the esophagus. The next step involves the use of a water-soluble radiographic contrast material with a water-soluble agent such as Gastrografin if esophageal perforation is a possibility. Barium should be avoided initially because it may interfere with subsequent endoscopy. Esophagoscopy should be considered in patients with persistent symptoms or when the diagnosis is in doubt.

23. What is the management?
Objects that can be visualized directly can be removed with bayonet forceps or a Kelly clamp. Smooth objects in the esophagus can be removed by placing the patient in extreme Trendelenburg position, passing a Foley catheter beyond the object, expanding the balloon, and withdrawing the catheter. Intravenous glucagon (0.5–2.0 mg) may relax the lower esophageal sphincter, allowing a distal obstruction to pass. Calcium channel blockers and sublingual nitroglycerin have also been advocated for their ability to produce similar results. Papain-containing agents should not be used. Sharp objects should be removed endoscopically. Repeat esophagography should be performed when the removal involves sharp or impaled objects, prolonged or aggressive manipulation or if perforation is a consideration.

24. Any parting words on the subject?
Well, there's good news and bad news. Some 80–90% of foreign bodies will pass through the GI tract without significant problems. The bad news is that the remainder will require surgical removal. These latter objects tend to be sharp or long (>6.5 cm) and are among the 1% that cause perforation. A special case should be made for disk or button batteries. As most are prone to leakage, every effort should be made to remove them if localized to the esophagus. Otherwise, the location in the GI system should be followed until elimination is confirmed.

SINUSITIS

25. What is sinusitis? What are the common causes?
Sinusitis is an inflammation of the paranasal sinuses, including the maxillary, ethmoid, frontal, and sphenoid sinuses. It is the consequence of ostia occlusion, most commonly due to local mucosal swelling from a viral upper respiratory infection. Allergies, trauma, or mechanical obstruction from tumors, foreign bodies, or abnormal anatomy may also cause the occlusion that leads to bacterial overgrowth and excess mucus production. When symptoms last less than 3 weeks, the process is characterized as acute.

26. How do I make the diagnosis?
Patients often have headache, fever, facial tenderness and pain, nasal congestion or purulent discharge, maxillary dental pain, anosmia, and halitosis. Patients may also relate a history of nocturnal coughing, post-nasal drip, and sore throat. Depending on the location of the infection, pain may intensify with bending forward or lying supine. The physical examination is often unrewarding but one should attempt to elicit pain with palpation and percussion over the affected region. Anterior rhinoscopy with a head lamp and nasal speculum reveals the presence of pus, foreign bodies, masses, or anatomic abnormalities. Decreased transillumination of the maxillary and frontal sinuses with a strong point light source may indicate the need for further diagnostic studies.

27. Which other diagnostic studies should I pursue?
Plain sinus radiographs, especially good Waters, Caldwell, and lateral views, can demonstrate air-fluid interfaces or chronic mucosal thickening. A CT scan is superior in defining disease but, in the acute setting, is appropriately reserved for when orbital or intracranial involvement or other complications are suspected. Ultrasonography has low sensitivity and specificity but can be used if radiation exposure is contraindicated. Nasal endoscopy is an excellent modality for identifying disease but is employed only by an otolaryngologist and rarely on an emergent basis.

28. How is sinusitis treated?

There are two therapeutic goals: to open the ostia to facilitate drainage and to eliminate the infection. The former is accomplished with a variety of topical and/or systemic decongestants. The use of vasoconstrictor sprays such as phenylephrine hydrochloride (Neo-Synephrine) or oxymetazoline HCl (Afrin) can provide immediate relief but should be used no longer than 3–4 days because of the propensity for rebound edema. Oral agents such as phenylpropanolamine or pseudoephedrine allow for more prolonged treatment and affect deeper tissues not penetrated by the topical sprays. Antihistamines are reserved for patients with specific allergic indications. The appropriate initial antibiotic is either ampicillin (500 mg every 6 hours) or amoxicillin (500 mg every 8 hours) for 10–14 days. Patients with penicillin allergies should be started on erythromycin, trimethoprim-sulfamethoxazole, or cephalexin. Failure to improve within 7 days should prompt a change in antibiotic therapy.

29. Which patients need referral and admission?

If there is no improvement after two complete courses of antibiotics, the patient should be referred to an otolaryngologist. Complications arising during the course of therapy can be classified as local, orbital, and intracranial. Patients with sinusitis who demonstrate evidence of orbital or CNS involvement should be treated as medical emergencies. Locally, mucoceles and osteomyelitis can develop. Extension of any infection into the surrounding tissues must be halted immediately. Orbital complications are the most frequent, especially in children, and run the gamut from cellulitis to abscess formation. Cavernous sinus thrombosis, resulting from the direct spread of infection through valveless veins, is imminently life-threatening. It is heralded by a toxic appearance, high fever, third and sixth nerve palsies, retinal engorgement, and bilateral chemosis and proptosis. Other intracranial complications demanding aggressive intensive therapy include meningitis, subdural empyema and brain abscesses.

BIBLIOGRAPHY

1. Druce HM: Diagnosis of sinusitis in adults: History, physical examination, nasal cytology, echo, and rhinoscope. J Allergy Clin Immunol 90(Part 2):436–441, 1992.
2. Fritz S, Kelen GD, Silvertson KT: Foreign bodies of the external auditory canal. Emerg Med Clin North Am 5:183–192, 1987.
3. Jones NS, Lannigan FJ, Salama NY: Foreign bodies in the throat: A prospective study of 388 cases. J Laryng Otolaryngol 105:104–108, 1991.
4. Josephson GD, Godley FA, Stierna P: Practical management of epistaxis. Med Clin North Am 75:1311–1320, 1991.
5. Padgham N: Epistaxis: Anatomical and clinical correlates. J Laryng Otolaryngol 104:308–311, 1990.
6. Parretta LJ, Denslow BL, Brown CG: Emergency evaluation and management of epistaxis. Emerg Med Clin North Am 5:265–277, 1987.
7. Pons PT: Foreign bodies. In Rosen P, et al (eds): Emergency Medicine: Concepts and Clinical Practice, 3rd ed. St. Louis, Mosby-Year Book, 1992.
8. Stafford CT: The clinician's view of sinusitis. Otolaryngol Head Neck Surg 103(Part 2):870–875, 1990.
9. Stair TO: Otolaryngologic disorders. In Rosen P, et al (eds): Emergency Medicine: Concepts and Clinical Practice, 3rd ed. St. Louis, Mosby-Year Book, 1992.
10. Taylor RB: Esophageal foreign bodies. Emerg Med Clin North Am 5:301–311, 1987.
11. Wagenmann M, Naclerio RM: Complications of sinusitis. J Allergy Clin Immunol 90(Part 2):552–554, 1992.
12. Werman HA: Removal of foreign bodies of the nose. Emerg Med Clin North Am 5:253–263, 1987.

18. DENTAL AND ORAL SURGICAL EMERGENCIES

Richard D. Zallen, D.D.S., M.D., Richard W. Brunton, D.D.S., and Michael A. Casillas, D.D.S.

1. How are teeth numbered?

In the adult, teeth are numbered from the upper right side, with the third molar being designated as tooth number 1, the upper right second molar is number 2, the upper right first molar is number 3, the next two bicuspids are numbers 4 and 5, the upper right canine is number 6, the upper right lateral incisor is number 7, the upper right central incisor is number 8, the upper left central incisor is number 9, and the rest of the upper left side is completed, with the upper left third molar being number 16. From here, you drop down to the lower left third molar, which is number 17, and continue on to the third molar on the right side, which is number 32.

Upper Right	Upper Left
1, 2, 3, 4, 5, 6, 7, 8,	9,10,11,12,13,14,15,16
Lower Right	Lower Left
32,31,30,29,28,27,26,25,	24,23,22,21,20,19,18,17

In the younger person with deciduous teeth (baby teeth), the upper right second molar is A, the first molar is B, the cuspid is C, the lateral incisor is D, the central incisor is E, the upper left central incisor is F, and the rest of the upper left side is completed, with the upper second molar being J. From here, drop down to the lower left second molar, which is K, and continue on to the second molar on the right side, which is T.

Upper Right	Upper Left
A, B, C, D, E,	F, G, H, I, J
Lower Right	Lower Left
T, S, R, Q, P,	O, N, M, L, K

Children between the ages of 6 and 13 are in a mixed dentition stage with some adult and some deciduous teeth. Their teeth are numbered and lettered as the above two diagrams illustrate.

2. What are the types of tooth fractures? Is treatment required?

The two basic types of tooth fracture are those of the crown or the root. Fractures of the crown that affect only the enamel generally require no emergent treatment. Fractures that include the dentin and/or the pulp should be treated by placement of CaOH paste over the fracture. Root fractures require stabilization to adjacent teeth with dental resin, ligature wire, or Erich arch bars.

3. How should an avulsed tooth be transported?

The best transport medium is the patient's own saliva. The patient should transport the tooth in the mouth if possible. Alternative transport media include milk, saliva, saline, or a wet handkerchief. The tooth should be handled as little as possible and only by the crown.

4. When should an avulsed tooth be reimplanted?

The best time for reimplantation is within 2 hours. Primary teeth should not be reimplanted. Patients with advanced periodontal disease, gross caries, or poor oral hygiene are poor candidates for reimplantation.

5. Should antibiotics be prescribed for an alveolar housing fracture or a reimplanted tooth?
Yes. A 5-day course of penicillin is recommended. In allergic patients, erythromycin is the drug of choice.

6. What are the concerns with electrical burns to the mouth?
Electrical burns are deceptive. The ultimate extent of tissue damage is greater than is present on initial exam, and the full extent of the injury may not be appreciated for 4–7 days. Wound contracture may produce microstomia. Close observation is warranted because of the possibility of delayed arterial hemorrhage.

7. How should a tongue laceration with profuse bleeding be treated?
Initially, packing with gauze and applying pressure should allow visualization of the source of bleeding. Injection of a local anesthetic with 1:100,000 epinephrine will aid with vasoconstriction. Clamping, ligating and/or using electrocautery will help to control the larger bleeders. If minor bleeding persists, the laceration should be closed in a layered fashion utilizing resorbable sutures for deep approximation and silk for surface approximation.

8. How should a through-and-through lip laceration be closed?
Initial debridement of the wound may require surgical and saline peroxide debridement. Mucosal preparation with pHisoHex is recommended. The mucosa is then sutured with resorbable suture. Reprepping from the outside is recommended. A layered closure is then done, using resorbable sutures for deep tissue approximation and nylon for skin. Prophylactic antibiotic coverage with penicillin for 5 days is recommended.

9. How should human or animal bites of the mouth be treated?
Human bites are best managed with copious irrigation, surgical debridement, and prophylactic antibiotics. Penicillin is the drug of choice. Wounds should be closed primarily if possible, although delayed primary closure is a viable option in some cases. Animal bites are handled much in the same way. Antibiotics are recommended and may vary depending on species. Patients bitten by animals with suspected rabies must be treated aggressively, including irrigation with quaternary ammonia compounds with 70% alcohol, rabies post-exposure prophylaxis, and tetanus prophylaxis.

10. When should antibiotics be used in management of dental infections?
An acute dentoalveolar abscess usually requires antibiotic therapy, with penicillin being the drug of choice. Adjunctive therapy should include endodontic treatment or extraction of the offending tooth and incision and drainage. The patient should be followed closely, usually within 24 hours.

11. What are some nondental etiologies of orofacial pain?
Pain can originate from the temporomandibular joint, muscles of mastication, salivary glands, nose and paranasal sinuses, blood vessels (arteritis), nerves, and oral ulcers.

12. When should a patient with a dental abscess be admitted to the hospital?
Criteria for admission should be based on history and physical findings: size and location of the swelling, rapidity of onset, dysphagia, dyspnea, fever, malaise, trismus, and age, state of hydration, laboratory evaluation, and immune status of the patient.

13. What are the risks of regional dental anesthesia?
Toxicity, allergy, syncope, muscle trismus, needle tract infection, intraarterial or intravenous injection, hematomas, and transient Bell's palsy from accidental injection into the area of the parotid gland. Broken needles rarely occur.

14. What is ANUG? How is it treated?

Acute necrotizing ulcerative gingivitis is an acute infection of the gingiva. ANUG typically presents with blunted interdental papilla, which represents areas of necrosis, gingival bleeding, pain, fetid oris, gingival swelling, and lymphadenopathy. ANUG responds well to local debridement and irrigation. Antibiotics should be used only in refractory cases, and penicillin is the drug of choice.

15. Why is a lateral pharyngeal abscess of great concern?

A lateral pharyngeal abscess occurs between the pharyngeal mucosa and the superior constrictor muscle. Presenting symptoms usually include dysphagia, pain, trismus, and fever. Medial bulging of the lateral pharyngeal wall frequently occurs, causing displacement of the uvula to the opposite side. This infection is potentially life threatening because of airway obstruction, and requires urgent incision and drainage.

16. What is Ludwig's angina?

It is an infection of the submandibular, sublingual, and submental spaces bilaterally. A dental etiology is present in 90% of the cases. Treatment consists of maintaining the airway, removal of the cause, incision and drainage, IV antibiotics (high-dose penicillin is the drug of choice), and hydration.

17. How are aphthous ulcers and herpetic lesions differentiated in the oral cavity?

Recurrent aphthous ulcers, also known as "canker sores," occur as a single circular ulcer and usually are less than 1 cm in diameter. The lesion has a central yellow area surrounded by a prominent band of erythema. Herpetic lesions usually present as clusters of small vesicles that eventually coalesce. Recurrent aphthous ulcers may occur anywhere in the oral cavity except the lips, hard palate, and attached gingiva. Recurrent herpes, on the other hand, occurs exclusively in these areas. Both types of lesion can be quite painful.

18. How are oral cavity ulcers treated?

Recurrent aphthous ulcers are symptomatically treated with therapy that ranges from topical corticosteroids, to antibiotics, to anesthetic mouth rinses. A Kaopectate, Benadryl, and Xylocaine suspension has been shown to provide relief in cases of multiple recurrent aphthous ulcers. The treatment of herpes simplex virus is aimed at palliation of pain. Topical acyclovir, when used during the prodromal stage, has been shown to decrease size and time to resolution of the lesions.

19. How is post-extraction hemorrhage evaluated and treated?

The patient's past medical history and current medications should be thoroughly reviewed. Evaluation must include good lighting and suction to evaluate the alveolus for a bleeding source. Application of a gauze dressing over the extraction site will stop most bleeding episodes. Other available agents are absorbable gelatin sponges, Surgicel, bone wax, and topical thrombin. A carefully placed suture often helps to stop the bleeding. Refractory bleeding should be further evaluated with appropriate laboratory studies.

20. What is the classification of mandibular fractures?

The best clinical classification is by anatomic region: symphysis (midline and parasymphyseal), body, angle, ascending ramus, condyle, and alveolar housing. Another classification describes the specific type of fracture: simple, compound, comminuted, multiple, greenstick, or pathologic.

21. How do you radiologically examine a patient for a mandibular fracture?

The x-rays of choice are: panographic, Townes, posteroanterior, lateral oblique right and left, dental periapical, CT scan (rarely), and temporomandibular (rarely).

22. How do you clinically examine a patient for a mandibular fracture?

The main diagnostic criteria are a history of trauma, abnormal mandibular movements elicited by bimanual palpation, step deformities or changes in the occlusion, and soft tissue trauma, including laceration, hematoma, and loose teeth.

23. What is a lasso ligature?

A lasso ligature is used when a mandibular fracture is located between two teeth. It is a 24-, 25-, or 26-gauge wire that is placed around one or two teeth adjacent to the fracture. The wire is tightened so as to bring the fracture into closer alignment. This helps to relieve pain, stop bleeding, and prevent the continued flow of saliva into the fracture site.

24. When are antibiotics indicated for a mandibular fracture?

Antibiotics are indicated in all mandibular fractures except subcondylar fractures that are not compounded into the external auditory canal. Penicillin is the drug of choice.

25. What is a mandibular contrecoup fracture?

It is a fracture away from the site of trauma. A classic example is trauma to the parasymphysis area with unilateral or bilateral subcondylar fracture.

26. What are the immediate clinical problems associated with a fractured mandible?

The immediate problems are airway compromise, bleeding, pain, fracture displacement, displaced or aspirated teeth, lacerations, trimus, and subcutaneous emphysema.

27. What is a dry socket? How is it treated?

A dry socket is a painful post-extraction tooth socket usually in the mandibular third molars but may also affect other sockets. It starts 2–3 days following the extraction and may last for several days (5–10). It is treated by irrigating any debris out of the socket and placing a sedative dressing in the socket.

BIBLIOGRAPHY

1. Alling C, Osbon D (eds): Maxillofacial Trauma. Philadelphia, Lea & Febiger, 1988.
2. Flynn T: Odontogenic infections. Oral Maxillofacial Surg Clin North Am 3:311, 1991.
3. Fonseca R, Walker R (eds): Oral and Maxillofacial Trauma. Philadelphia, W.B. Saunders, 1991.
4. Josell S, Abrams R: Managing common dental problems and emergencies. Pediatr Clin North Am 38:1325, 1991.
5. Topazian R, Goldberg M (eds): Oral and Maxillofacial Infections. Philadelphia, W.B. Saunders, 1987.

IV. Central Nervous System

19. TRANSIENT ISCHEMIC ATTACK AND CEREBROVASCULAR ACCIDENT

Richard L. Hughes, M.D., and Michael Earnest, M.D.

1. We're number 3!

Despite the significant reduction in the morbidity and mortality from stroke in the past 30 years, stroke remains the third most common cause of death and the third most common diagnosis on admission to hospitals. Unfortunately, it is not always triaged and approached with the same aggressiveness as other life-threatening emergencies. The physician must quickly assess the stroke victim to ensure that the brain is receiving optimal supply of the three key metabolic substrates—glucose, oxygen, and blood flow. Severe hypoglycemia or hyperglycemia both are bad for ischemic brain. Hypoxemia is worse. Severe hypertension and hypotension likewise must be aggressively managed. The goal for acute treatment of severe hypertension should be about 150 systolic or 95 diastolic, as further drop in blood pressure may compromise collateral circulation and extend the ischemia.

2. What is the difference between a TIA and a CVA?

Let's face it. The nomenclature for stroke is less than ideal. Both cerebral vascular accident (CVA) and transient ischemic attack (TIA) refer to ischemia in the brain resulting in neurologic deficits. If the **clinical deficit** resolves by 24 hours, then the ischemia is referred to as a TIA. If the deficit is persistent at 24 hours, even if it resolves over a few days, then it is called a CVA or stroke. The nomenclature becomes more complicated because 30–50% of patients with **clinically** defined TIA actually have a permanent abnormality on their CT scan or in their brain at autopsy. Thus, TIAs can be the clinical expression of small areas of cell death in the brain, even though there is no permanent neurologic deficit.

3. You cannot do anything for a stroke, so what's the worry?

The highest risk for a recurrent stroke is in the first few days and weeks after an initial stroke or TIA. Therefore, it is crucial that patients have an appropriate evaluation to determine where their stroke came from so that a second ischemic event can be prevented. Because the exact mechanism of stroke is usually not apparent in the emergency department (ED), physicians will usually institute either aspirin therapy or anticoagulation (heparin) on a short-term basis during the hospital stay. Then, at discharge, a long-term plan can be devised to prevent another stroke from occurring.

Although we cannot resuscitate a stroke yet, a mistake in the ED or ICU can easily cause a stroke to extend or worsen. Mistakes include overtreating hypertension, ignoring dehydration, allowing aspiration, and neglecting treatment of concomitant coronary artery disease.

4. Why obtain a CT scan when somebody is stable and has an obvious stroke?

For the most part, a CT scan in a patient with "obvious" stroke adds very little. Unfortunately, in a small percentage (about 2%) of cases the deficit is caused by hemorrhage, tumor, or abscess. Even transient deficits can be caused by a small mass lesion. Because using anticoagulant or antiplatelet therapy in these patients can be catastrophic, it is advisable to obtain a CT scan in all patients with strokes and TIAs before such therapies are instituted.

5. Is MRI scanning useful in stroke?
In general, scanning is not indicated unless it will answer a specific question that CT cannot. Strokes usually will not show up on either CT *or* MRI scan in the first 24 hours. The role of scanning in this time frame is to exclude other processes (hemorrhage, tumor, abscess), something CT does as well as MRI. Both CT and MRI can adequately image a large stroke by 5–7 days. Smaller (i.e., milder) strokes may be better seen with MRI, but specificity is a problem (see below). MRI is clearly the test of choice to image a stroke (or anything else) in the posterior fossa (brain stem and cerebellum).

MRI has the advantage of imaging small vessel infarctions (e.g., lacunar infarcts) better. Unfortunately, MRI tends to have poor specificity because patients with typical vascular risk factors often have many high signal abnormalities in the white matter from stroke *or* age-related changes. A thorough knowledge of neuroanatomy can often identify the symptomatic abnormality from MRI scans with multiple abnormalities.

As MRI technology improves, we may be able to use MRI as a "single test" to look at the brain, intracranial vasculature, and the extracranial vasculature using magnetic resonance angiography (MRA). Protocols are being developed to use MRI to determine cerebral blood flow, too.

6. Does carotid surgery really work?
Yes, absolutely! Three prospective, randomized, multicenter carotid endarterectomy trials have recently reported their results in dealing with symptomatic patients. Patients with carotid stenosis of 70% or greater have a relative risk reduction of 71% at 24 months (North American Symptomatic Carotid Endarterectomy Trial, NASCET). These results have been confirmed by the European Carotid Surgery Trial and the Veterans' Administration Cooperative Study. The NASCET study is continuing to determine if there is a role for surgery and patients with moderate carotid stenosis (30–69%).

The answer in the asymptomatic carotid is not yet clear. Four major prospective trials are continuing, including the Asymptomatic Carotid Artherosclerosis Study (ACAS), the Veterans' Administration Cooperative Study, the Carotid Artery Surgery Asymptomatic Narrowing Operation vs. Aspirin (CASANOVA), and the Mayo Asymptomatic Carotid Endarterectomy Trial (MACE). At this time patients are encouraged to enroll in one of the ongoing trials of asymptomatic carotid stenosis.

There is strong feeling on both sides of the fence about the utility of carotid endarterectomy in asymptomatic carotid stenosis. Our personal approach is first to have a long discussion with the patient about the pros and cons of surgery and then to randomize the patient into ACAS or another study. Some patients understand the uncertainty but prefer to undergo a small operative risk for a better long-term outlook. Others would rather die than have a surgery (and some do die). Some die with surgery. Current acceptable levels of operative morbidity and mortality are less than 6%. Some institutions that do many endarterectomies have complication and death rates of less than 2%.

7. Do steroids help?
No. Despite the efficacy of steroids in cerebral edema associated with tumor and abscess, they do not work in ischemic stroke. The edema that is produced by stroke is more complicated than tumor edema. Because of anecdotal reports of success, they are sometimes used in large life-threatening strokes as an act of desperation. Similar attempts to use barbiturates, general anesthesia, naloxone, calcium channel blockers, or hemodilution to reduce the severity of the stroke have been disappointing.

8. Why isn't tissue plasminogen activator (TPA) or other lytic therapies used in stroke?

It is unclear how best to use them. The initial experience with urokinase, streptokinase, and TPA resulted in as many disasters as successes. The use of TPA is currently being evaluated by multiple trials that require its use within the first 90 minutes, 3 hours, or 6 hours of clinical symptoms. Because the average patient who sustains a stroke often does not even reach the ED for 6–8 hours, successful outcome of these trials will cause a tremendous change in the way strokes are handled in the field.

9. Which patients belong on a monitored bed?

In general, patients without a known etiology for their TIA or stroke or patients with uncertain cardiac risks can benefit from short-term (i.e., one day) monitoring. First, it increases the likelihood of identifying a cardiac arrhythmia or cardiac ischemia. Second, ICU monitoring allows close neurologic observation. Patients with a well-defined mechanism of stroke and a stable cardiac physiology do not usually require ICU or cardiac monitoring. Some institutions have dedicated stroke units, similar to step-down ICUs, to allow closer observation of stroke patients at less cost than a conventional ICU.

10. Do all stroke patients need a cardiac echo?

No, but all patients need to have the *mechanism* of their stroke defined. Cardiac ultrasound, either transthoracic or transesophageal, has demonstrated a larger number of potential cardiac sources for emboli. This includes the common sources such as atrial fibrillation, prosthetic valves, endocarditis, and mural thrombi as well as newer considerations such as paradoxical emboli through patent foramen ovale (PFO). Young stroke victims (less than 45 years old) have a two to three times greater prevalence of PFO than normal age-matched controls, suggesting that these abnormalities have an important role in causing strokes.

11. How can I prevent strokes from happening in my ED?

In-hospital strokes are a challenging problem to prevent. In the ED, two groups of patients are potentially identifiable before a stroke. The first group is patients with acute myocardial infarction (MI). Most emboli associated with MI occur early in their course. Patients with anterior wall MIs are at highest risk. Appropriate intervention with anticoagulation or antiplatelet therapy in the ED may prevent a stroke a few hours later. Patients with multiple traumatic injuries are notorious for having a stroke in the hospital after their "life has been saved." The highest risk of trauma-related stroke is in patients with direct trauma to the carotid or vertebral arteries that causes a penetrating injury or dissection. The vertebral artery is particularly prone to injury from rapid head motions. Facial fractures have been associated with a higher risk of carotid injury, leading to carotid occlusion, dissection, or artery-to-artery embolism. Recognition of high-risk patients and early angiography allows preventive measures to work.

12. Are stroke and TIA patients allowed to eat?

The majority of stroke and TIA patients are able to swallow without difficulty. Patients with obviously garbled speech, reduced alertness, or very large strokes should be NPO until tested. Neurologic dysphagia is better tested with liquids than solids. Although feeding can be deferred until patients reach the hospital floor, patients often need to take routine oral medications during the wait for a bed in the hospital.

13. How much aspirin is enough to prevent stroke?

Initially it was four a day, then three a day, and now evidence has demonstrated that one aspirin a day is as effective as the higher doses. It may be possible to reduce this dose further so that even lower doses of aspirin (80 mg a day, one aspirin 3 days a week, etc.) may eventually become the standard. Reducing the dose of aspirin can reduce the risk of gastro-intestinal hemorrhages and perhaps cerebral hemorrhages. A very small number of patients with hyperaggregable platelets will need higher doses of aspirin to effectively block platelet aggregation. At this time there are no specific guidelines on who might need platelet aggregation testing. The standard of care is to reserve it for patients who have failed aspirin, young patients, or patients without typical risk factors for stroke.

20. MENINGITIS

Andrew Ziller, M.D.

1. What is meningitis?
Meningitis is a disease of the central nervous system involving inflammation of the membranes surrounding the brain and spinal cord.

2. What are the causes of meningitis?
Causes of meningitis are divided into infectious (caused by bacteria, viruses, fungi, para-sites, and tuberculosis) and noninfectious causes (neoplastic, collagen-vascular).

3. Why is it important to know about meningitis?
Mortality from bacterial and fungal meningitis ranges from 10–50%. This is an important issue because prompt recognition and treatment of bacterial meningitis can lessen morbidity and mortality. In emergency departments (EDs), failure to diagnose meningitis ranks second in total malpractice dollars paid per case.

4. Which patients are at risk for meningitis?
Meningitis occurs most commonly in very young and older patients. Others at risk include immunocompromised patients (such as splenectomized patients), immunosuppressed patients, alcoholics, patients with recent neurosurgical procedures, and patients who have underlying infections such as endocarditis, pneumonia, sinusitis, or otitis media.

5. What are the common presenting symptoms?
Meningitis should be considered in any patient with a fever and change in mental status. Other symptoms that are not very specific include headache, photophobia, stiff neck, lethargy, irritability, malaise, confusion, and seizures.

6. What are the physical findings in meningitis?
Nuchal rigidity, Kernig's sign, and Brudzinski's sign are seen in some patients with menin-gitis. Kernig's sign is pain or resistance of the hamstrings when the knees are extended with the hips flexed at 90%. Brudzinski's sign is flexion of the hips caused by passive flexion of the neck. Unfortunately, these physical findings are often absent in the very young and older patients—the ones most likely to get meningitis. In infants, a tense or bulging fonta-nelle may be helpful but may not be manifest if there is associated dehydration.

7. If the symptoms are not specific and the physical findings are often absent, what are the indications for lumbar puncture (LP)?
LP should be performed whenever meningitis is suspected, because analyzing spinal fluid is the only way to diagnose meningitis. Many say, "If you think about the test, then you should do it."

8. What tests should be done before an LP?

When possible the patient should be checked for papilledema. A head CT scan should be done if papilledema is present, the patient has an altered mental status, a focal neurologic exam, new-onset seizure, or there is clinical suspicion for recent trauma or subarachnoid hemorrhage. If a bleeding disorder is suspected based on history or physical exam, coagulation studies and platelet count should be checked before performing an LP.

9. What is the most common error in the ED management of meningitis?

Delay in administering antibiotics until the LP is done. Antibiotics can and should be given in a patient who clinically has bacterial meningitis. Intravenous antibiotics given 2 hours or less before the LP (and ideally after blood and urine cultures are obtained) will not affect the results of the cerebrospinal fluid (CSF) analysis.

10. What are the risks of an LP?

Almost every physician has encountered patients who believe that an LP will cause paralysis. Paralysis is highly unlikely, because the needle is inserted below the level of the spinal cord at L4 or L5 in adults. This misconception probably arises from the fact that ocassionally patients experience transient leg paresthesias during LP from irritation of nerve roots by the needle. There are rare reports of cauda equina syndrome from hematoma formation, but only in patients with a coagulopathy. Headache is the most common sequelae, occurring in 5–30% of patients. Headache is believed to be minimized by using a small-gauge needle (for example a 20- or 22-gauge in adults) and having the patient lie flat for several hours after the LP. Most agree that tonsillar herniation is a potential complication following LP in a patient with increased intracranial pressure; however, this risk is eliminated if the patient has a normal head CT scan before the LP.

11. Which lab studies should I order for the CSF?

In an adult, 4 tubes are usually collected, each containing 1–1.5 ml. More CSF is needed if special tests are required.

Tube 1. Cell count and differential.
Tube 2. Gram stain and culture and sensitivity. Special tests in certain patients (such as immunocompromised patients) include viral cultures, tuberculosis cultures and acid-fast stain, fungal antigen studies and India ink stain (most commonly cryptococcosis), and serologic tests for neurosyphilis. Countercurrent immunoelectrophoresis (CIE) is occasionally used to detect specific bacterial antigens in the CSF.
Tube 3. Glucose and protein.
Tube 4. Cell count and differential.

In pediatric patients, three tubes are usually collected and the third is sent for cell count and differential.

12. What results from the CSF analysis indicate meningitis?

In adults a CSF white blood cell (WBC) count greater than 5 suggests meningitis. A WBC count of under 30 is considered normal in neonates. Polymorphonuclear leukocytes suggest a bacterial etiology. Elevated CSF protein is seen in meningitis. A CSF/serum glucose ratio of less than 0.5 occurs in patients with bacterial meningitis, and in patients with diabetes a CSF/serum ratio glucose of less than 0.6 is considered low. Gram stain is useful in diagnosing bacterial meningitis; up to 20% of the time, the etiologic organism can be identified. Finally, the CSF laboratory studies may be normal very early in meningitis, so if the clinical suspicion is high, a repeat tap may be indicated in 24 hours.

13. Which antibiotics should be prescribed when the causative organism is unknown?
For children, see chapter 66. For adults, see table below.

Antimicrobial Therapy for Meningitis When the Causative Organism Is Unknown*

PATIENTS	LIKELY PATHOGENS	RECOMMENDED TREATMENT
Otherwise healthy adult <40 yr of age	S. pneumoniae N. meningitidis	Penicillin G, 5 million IU IV at once, then 2 million IU IV q 2 hr, or ampicillin, 2 gm IV q 4 hr
Age >40 yr, otherwise healthy	S. pneumoniae N. meningitidis H. influenzae Gram-negative enteric bacilli	Cefotaxime,† 2 gm IV q 4 hr
Recent neurosurgery, traumatic dural defect, V/P shunt	Gram-negative enteric bacilli S. epidermidis S. aureus S. pneumoniae	Nafcillin, 50 mg/kg IV q 6 hr, plus cefotaxime,† 2 gm IV q 4 hr
Immunocompromised, IV drug abuser, alcoholic	S. pneumoniae N. meningitidis Gram-negative enteric bacilli L. monocytogenes H. influenzae S. aureus	Ampicillin‡ 2 gm IV q 4 hr plus cefotaxime† 2 gm IV q 4 hr plus nafcillin 50 mg/kg IV q 6 hr

* From Walls RM, Harrison DW: Adult meningitis, encephalitis, and intracranial abscess. In Rosen P, et al (eds): Emergency Medicine: Concepts and Clinical Practice. St. Louis, Mosby–Year Book, 1992, p 1853, with permission.
† Or equivalent third-generation cephalosporin.
‡ Coverage for L. monocytogenes may be discontinued when no longer indicated.

14. What additional pathogens should be considered in high-risk patients?

Additional Bacterial Pathogens in Meningitis in Patients at Increased Risk*†

RISK FACTOR	PATHOGEN
Age >60 yr	Gram-negative enterics, H. influenzae
Splenectomy	H. influenzae
Crowding	N. meningitidis
Sickle cell disease	Gram-negative enterics
Diabetes	Gram-negative enterics
Shunt, dural trauma, neurosurgery	S. aureus, S. epidermidis, Gram-negative enterics
Malignancy†	L. monocytogenes
Immunosuppression‡	Gram-negative enterics, S. aureus, S. epidermidis
Bacterial endocarditis	S. aureus

* From Walls RM, Harrison DW: Adult meningitis, encephalitis, and intracranial abscess. In Rosen P, et al (eds): Emergency Medicine: Concepts and Clinical Practice. St. Louis, Mosby–Year Book, 1992, p 1853, with permission.
† All patients in the above groups are still at highest risk for meningitis due to N. meningitidis and S. pneumoniae. Pathogens listed here are in addition to these.
‡ Patients also at increased risk for fungal meningitis.

15. What about steroids?
This is always a "good question" regardless of the disease or the rotation. Steroids (dexamethasone, 0.15 mg/kg) have been shown to reduce the incidence and severity of hearing loss in infants and children with meningitis caused by H. influenzae. To date, no study has shown a benefit from steroids in other pediatric or adult patients with bacterial meningitis.

BIBLIOGRAPHY

1. Keroack MA: The patient with suspected meningitis. Emerg Med Clin North Am 5:807–826, 1987.
2. Kooiker JC: Spinal puncture and cerebrospinal fluid examination. In Roberts JR, Hedges JR (eds): Clinical Procedures in Emergency Medicine, 2nd ed. Philadelphia, W.B. Saunders, 1991, pp 969–984.
3. Lebel MH, Freij BJ, Syrigiannopoulos GA, et al: Dexamethasone therapy for bacterial meningitis. N Engl J Med 319:964–971, 1988.
4. McGee ZA, Baringer JR: Acute meningitis. In Mandell GL, Douglas RG, Bennett JE (eds): Principle and Practice of Infectious Diseases, 3rd ed. New York, Churchill Livingstone, 1990, pp 741–755.
5. Talan DA, Hoffman JR, Yoshikawa TT, Overturf GD: Role of empiric parenteral antibiotics prior to lumbar puncture in suspected bacterial meningitis: State of the art. Rev Infect Dis 10:365–376, 1988.
6. Trunkel AR, Wispelwey B, Scheld WM: Bacterial meningitis: Recent advances in pathophysiology and treatment. Ann Intern Med 112:610–623, 1990.
7. Walls RW, Harrison DW: Adult meningitis. In Rosen P, et al (eds): Emergency Medicine: Concepts and Clinical Practice, 3rd ed. St. Louis, Mosby–Year Book, 1992, pp 1841–1859.

V. Respiratory System

21. BREATHING AND VENTILATION

Michael F. Murphy, M.D., FRCPC

1. What are the common breathing problems seen in the emergency department (ED)?
Naturally, the broad spectrum of medical and traumatic respiratory disorders present themselves to the ED. However, far and away the commonest problems are asthma, chronic obstructive pulmonary disease (COPD), and lower respiratory infections such as acute bronchitis and pneumonia.

2. How do I begin to sort these things out in the ED?
As for any other patient presentation to the ED, direct your attention to the presenting complaint and do a "directed" history and physical exam. However, because disorders of many systems can lead to respiratory symptoms, it is important not to be too narrow in your approach. Good examples include severe anemia presenting as fatigue and shortness of breath, or heart failure presenting as wheezing. Be complete in your assessment and do not jump to conclusions. Not all that wheezes is asthma!

3. List four categories of wheezing.
  1. Patients under 2 years of age in whom the diagnostic label is bronchiolitis.
  2. Asthmatics who experience punctuated episodes of dyspnea, cough, and wheezing interspersed with symptom-free periods.
  3. Patients with COPD in whom chronic obstruction to air flow secondary to chronic bronchitis, emphysema, or a mixture of the two leads to perpetual baseline respiratory symptoms, albeit with exacerbations and remissions back to baseline.
  4. Patients who wheeze because of nonintrinsic lung disease such as heart failure or foreign body aspiration.
These categories are by no means all-inclusive or mutually exclusive but merely represent a convenient means of classifying patients who present to the ED with a chief complaint of wheezing.

4. What is bronchiolitis?
Acute bronchiolitis is a viral disease that involves the small airways, leading to inflammation of these airways and signs of obstructive airways disease. Although it may occur in children up to 2 years of age, the majority of patients are less than 1. What starts as an upper respiratory infection progresses over 2–3 days to respiratory distress and wheezing. Many viruses have been implicated, although respiratory syncytial virus (RSV) is the causative agent more than 50% of the time.

5. Is it serious?
The most critical period is 48–72 hours after the onset of cough and dyspnea. The younger the infant, the greater the likelihood of serious illness. Apneic spells may occur in very small infants. Improvement tends to occur at a variable pace over the ensuing 1–3 days.

6. What do you see clinically?
The typical case is a 6-month-old infant with a runny nose and mild to moderate respiratory distress. Coughing, tachypnea, and wheezing are prominent. There is a low-grade fever. Chest auscultation reveals scattered rales, large airway sounds, and wheezing.

7. How should these infants be evaluated and managed?
It depends on how sick they look, but ordinarily you should start by determining room-air O_2 saturation. Saturations less than 95% indicate potentially severe illness. The next step is to administer supplemental oxygen, usually in a croupette. Once the infant stabilizes and the exam is completed, it is not unreasonable to try aerosolized bronchodilators, although only a small proportion (<20%) of infants tend to respond. Those who do respond may benefit from ongoing aerosolized or oral bronchodilators.

8. Should I do any tests?
A nasopharyngeal aspirate (NPA) for RSV culture or immunologic testing should be done. A chest x-ray will confirm air trapping and may be positive for more sinister findings such as atelectasis.

9. Which infants need to be admitted?
Several findings correlate with potentially severe disease and indicate admission: infants who appear toxic; room-air saturations <95%; premature infants <34 weeks at birth; respiratory rate >70/min; atelectasis on chest x-ray; and age <3 months. Infants who are feeding poorly because of respiratory distress should be carefully assessed for hydration status and considered for admission.

10. What about patients who do not require admission?
If a patient responded to bronchodilators, their use should be continued either orally or via aerosol. Nonresponders probably will not benefit from ongoing therapy. The most important thing to tell parents is to bring the child back for reevaluation if feeding tails off, as this may be a harbinger of serious disease.

11. How do you know these kids are not asthmatics?
The truth of the matter is you don't know for sure! Patients who have wheezing alone and no other stigmata of a viral illness seem to most closely resemble asthmatics. However, the diagnosis of asthma is uncommonly made with any degree of certainty before the age of 1 year. Some experts would say that the apparatus producing bronchospasm, namely bronchiolar smooth muscle, simply does not exist before 1 year of life, precluding a diagnosis of asthma. That subset of infants who have repeated attacks of respiratory distress and wheezing and respond to bronchodilators can probably be considered to be asthmatic and treated as such.

12. Define asthma.
Asthma is an inflammatory disorder of the airways triggered by a variety of intrinsic or extrinsic factors, leading to episodes of dyspnea, cough, and wheezing. Airway edema, mucous secretion, and bronchospasm are the culprits that produce the clinical picture of asthma.

13. Assuming other causes of wheezing have been ruled out, how is the asthmatic patient managed in the ED?
The asthmatic patient who presents to the ED is usually in status asthmaticus. The mainstays of therapy are oxygen, bronchodilators, and steroids. Use of 100% O_2 will ensure adequate hemoglobin saturation with oxygen and probably mitigate the pulmonary

hypertension that is associated with hypoxic pulmonary vasoconstriction accompanying the acute episode.

Beta$_2$ agonists (e.g., albuterol, fenoterol) and antimuscarinics (e.g., ipratropium) given as a combined aerosol should be administered on presentation. Adult aerosols should contain 5 mg of albuterol, 0.5 mg of ipratropium, and 2–3 ml of saline. These aerosols may be given virtually continuously in severely ill asthmatic patients until improvement occurs. Steroids should be given early and in moderate dosage (e.g., 2 mg/kg of methylprednisolone sodium succinate) because their effects are slow in onset and may take 8 hours or more until a clinically significant response occurs.

The more severe the asthmatic attack, the more aggressive the therapy and the more intensive the monitoring such as EKG and pulse oximetry.

14. How do you decide which asthmatic patients require admission?
There is no easy answer. An amalgamation of multiple bits of data tend to identify patients with moderate to severe asthma who will require admission, although consistency is not guaranteed. Some features include:
- Severe ongoing dyspnea despite therapy, irrespective of auscultatory chest findings
- Prolonged (>2 days) duration of symptoms
- Heart rate >120/min; respiratory rate >2 SD for age; pulsus paradoxus >18
- "Silent chest" on auscultation
- Oxygen saturation <91% on room air at presentation
- Forced expiratory volume in one second (FEV$_1$) and peak expiratory flow rate (PEFR) <50% of predicted at presentation, or <16% improvement with initial aerosol therapy

15. What is the approach to patients with chronic lung disease and other patients with wheezing?
The approach is no different from that described for asthma. The response to therapy is usually less dramatic in patients with COPD than in patients with asthma. In addition, you might want to be somewhat more conservative in the amount of supplemental oxygen you administer in case respiratory drive is hypoxically mediated. Arterial blood gases are rarely indicated in patients with asthma but are often indicated in patients with COPD as a measure of ventilatory status and to compare with previous results.

Other patients with wheezing who might be missed include those with cardiac asthma and children with foreign body aspiration. Consideration of these diagnoses will ordinarily suffice to exclude it in the majority of instances.

BIBLIOGRAPHY

1. Barnett PJ, Oberklaid F: Acute asthma in children: Evaluation of management in a hospital emergency department. Med J Aust 154:729–733, 1991.
2. Behrman RE, ct al (eds): Nelson Textbook of Pediatrics, 14th ed. Philadelphia, W.B. Saunders, 1992.
3. Fitzgerald JM, Hargreave FE: Acute asthma: Emergency department management and prospective evaluation of outcome. Can Med Assoc J 142:591–595, 1990.
4. Karem E, Tibshirani R, Canny G, et al: Predicting the need for hospitalization in children with acute asthma. Chest 98:1355–1361, 1990.
5. Rudolph AM (ed): Rudolph's Pediatrics. Norwalk, CT, Appleton & Lange, 1991.
6. Shaw KN, Bell LM, Sherman NH: Outpatient assessment of infants with bronchiolitis. Am J Dis Child 145:151–155, 1991.
7. Wilson JD, et al (eds): Harrison's Principles of Internal Medicine, 12th ed. New York, McGraw-Hill, 1987.

22. ASTHMA AND CHRONIC OBSTRUCTIVE PULMONARY DISEASE

Wayne Guerra, M.D.

ASTHMA

1. What is asthma?
Asthma is characterized by obstruction of the bronchi and bronchioles. The narrowing is caused by smooth muscle contraction and inflammation. The inflammatory component consists of leukocytic infiltrate and mucosal edema.

2. Describe the primary signs and symptoms of asthma.
The classic triad consists of cough, wheezing, and dyspnea. The degree of obstruction determines the severity of the symptoms.

3. Can an exacerbation of asthma occur without wheezing?
Yes. To exhibit wheezing a patient must have airway obstruction and enough airflow to produce turbulence. Patients with little air movement will not have wheezing. There is also a small subset of patients, mostly children, who present only with cough and shortness of breath.

4. What is the differential diagnosis of wheezing?
The major conditions to consider in the emergency department (ED) are asthma, chronic obstructive pulmonary disease (COPD), congestive heart failure, anaphylaxis, aspiration, foreign body bronchial obstruction, and tracheobronchitis.

5. What are the major factors that precipitate exacerbations of asthma?
The most common precipitant is a viral upper respiratory infection. Other considerations include dusts, pollens, dander, cold air, and exercise. Approximately 15% of asthmatics will suffer bronchoconstriction when exposed to aspirin, and cross-reactivity with the other nonsteroidal anti-inflammatory agents is common.

6. What elements of the history are important?
Vital information includes current medications, antecedent illnesses, allergies, how long the exacerbation has been occurring, and whether intubation was ever required in the past. In general, patients who have been wheezing for over 12–24 hours have a more inflammatory component to their bronchoconstriction and will require a longer treatment period to reverse the obstruction. Asthmatics who have required intubation in the past have a higher likelihood of subsequent respiratory failure.

7. What is the best clinical indicator of bronchoconstriction?
Auscultation, pulsus paradoxus, and vital signs are not very accurate in assessing airway obstruction, even by experienced clinicians. The most accurate measurement of broncho-constriction is use of spirometry to determine forced end-expiratory volume in one second (FEV_1) or peak expiratory flow rate (PEFR). These measurements can also be used to determine if a patient requires more aggressive treatment or admission. Patients who present with less than 20% of predicted air flow before treatment and only 60% after therapy have a high rate of outpatient failure.

Assessment of FEV₁ and PEFR with Clinical Outcome

	PEFR (L/MIN)		FEV₁ (L)	
	ABSOLUTE	% PREDICTED	ABSOLUTE	% PREDICTED
Probable Admission				
Before treatment	<100	$<20\%$	<0.7	$<20\%$
After treatment	<300	$<60\%$	<2.1	$<60\%$

8. Are laboratory data helpful in evaluating asthmatics?

In general they are not helpful. Arterial blood gases (ABGs) are usually unnecessary in most asthmatics because they are not predictive of who needs admission and will not be grossly abnormal if the patient's FEV₁/PEFR is greater than 25% of normal.

9. When should I order a chest x-ray?

Chest x-rays should be obtained only when there is clinical suspicion of pneumonia, foreign body aspiration, pneumothorax, or pneumomediastinum.

10. What is the first-line ED treatment?

Beta-agonist therapy is the mainstay of treatment. The aerosolized route is the most effective, and is usually delivered as a nebulizer. Albuterol (Proventil) and metaproterenol (Alupent) are the major agents, with albuterol being more beta-1-adrenergic selective. Initially treatments can be given back to back, with the rate-limiting factor being the side effects of tachycardia and tremors.

11. When should steroids be used?

Steroids are now the second line of therapy. Their primary mode of action is to inhibit the inflammatory component. Steroids should be instituted early in any asthmatic who does not experience clearing with the initial nebulizations. They are effective in intravenous and oral routes, but do not take effect for 6 hours after administration.

Patients requiring steroid therapy in the ED should be discharged with a 7-day course of corticosteroids to reduce the risk of failing outpatient treatment. A tapering dose is not required if the length of treatment is 7 days or less.

12. What are the indications for antibiotics?

Antibiotics should not be administered unless a bacterial infection is identified by chest x-ray or Gram stain. Many asthmatics will have productive purulent sputums. However, this finding alone should not prompt antibiotic administration since a Gram stain will reveal a predominance of eosinophils in the majority of patients.

13. When are anticholinergic agents indicated?

The results of aerosolized atropine have been conflicting. A trial is certainly indicated in a patient with significant bronchoconstriction, and should be continued if a clinical response is seen. Ipratropium bromide (Atrovent) is available only in the metered-dose inhaler form, but has been shown to produce increased bronchodilation when added to beta-agonists.

14. What is the role of xanthines?

Once a mainstay of therapy, xanthines have been relegated to a secondary role. In general, patients suffering from severe airway obstruction should probably be given aminophylline if they do not significantly clear with the initial therapy. If the patient is already taking theophylline, then maximizing treatment by ensuring a therapeutic level is warranted.

15. How does pregnancy change the treatment of asthma?
It does not. It is especially important to prevent maternal hypoxia, which could result in fetal demise. Aerosolized beta-agonists, steroids, and theophylline are all considered safe in pregnancy.

16. When does an asthmatic need intubation?
This can be a difficult clinical situation. Absolute indications for intubation include progressive exhaustion, altered mentation, and worsening hypoxia despite aggressive treatment.

17. What is the major complication of intubation?
Barotrauma resulting from too-vigorous bagging or excessively high peak airway pressures can result in pneumothorax or pneumomediastinum. Intubated patients who suffer barotrauma have been shown to have higher morbidity and mortality.

18. What are some other modalities that can be used for a patient in extremis?
Magnesium has been shown to have bronchodilating effects and should be given in critical situations. Other modalities such as helium/oxygen mixtures and inhaled anesthetics have been reported to have lifesaving results, although no well controlled studies have been performed.

CHRONIC OBSTRUCTIVE PULMONARY DISEASE (COPD)

19. What is COPD?
COPD is a disease process consisting of emphysema, chronic bronchitis, or varying combinations of both. Smoking is the major cause, and most patients have an element of reactive airways (i.e., asthma) as well.

20. What is emphysema?
Emphysema occurs from the gradual destruction of alveolar septi and interstitial capillary beds. This loss of the lung's infrastructure results in collapse of the bronchi and obstructive airflow.

21. What is chronic bronchitis?
Chronic bronchitis results from edema and inflammatory changes in the large and small bronchi, with superimposed bacterial infection. The airways become obstructed from edema, mucous secretion, and leukocytic infiltrate.

22. How do patients with COPD usually present?
Similar to asthmatics, most will have wheezing, although productive cough and progressive dyspnea play a more prominent role. In the end stages, respiratory failure and cor pulmonale are more common.

23. Are ABGs helpful in the evaluation of COPD?
ABGs are quite valuable in evaluating patients with COPD in respiratory distress. Although objective measurements such as FEV_1 and PEFR are helpful, they can be compared only with the patient's own baseline, which many times is not available to the emergency physician. In addition, patients with COPD frequently have chronically elevated PCO_2s and compensatory higher serum HCO_3s. Serial ABGs can identify a patient who is failing therapy by demonstrating hypoxia, hypercarbia, and respiratory acidosis.

24. What is the danger of high-flow O_2 therapy?
Patients with COPD lose their hypercarbic drive to breathe, allowing them to tolerate high PCO_2s. Their only stimulus to ventilate is hypoxemia. If these patients are placed

on excessively high O_2, they lose their only ventilatory drive and this can result in respiratory arrest.

25. How should patients with COPD be managed?
Beta-agonist bronchodilators, steroids, and theophylline are the mainstays of therapy. Parasympathetic agents such as atropine and ipratropium have also been shown to be effective and should be employed in moderate to severe disease.

26. What are the indications for intubation?
Patients with COPD with significant exacerbations usually take longer to recover and have less reserve to tolerate respiratory distress than those with pure asthma. Intubation should be performed sooner in this patient population. The patient with poor ventilatory effort and clouded consciousness requires immediate control of the airway. In less severe cases, serial ABGs and initial response to therapy can help determine if intubation is necessary.

27. What role do antibiotics play in the management of COPD?
Unlike asthma, in which antibiotics are rarely indicated, in COPD any patient with new or increased productive cough should be started on antibiotics. In the absence of pneumonia, sputum Gram stains and culture are not helpful, and a broad-spectrum agent covering *H. influenzae* (such as ampicillin) should be prescribed.

28. What are indications for chest x-rays?
Patients with COPD who have moderate to significant respiratory distress should have chest radiographs performed to rule out pneumonia, pneumothorax, or partial collapse.

23. PNEUMONIA

A. Roy Magnusson, M.D., FACEP

1. How common is pneumonia?
In the United States there are more than 500,000 hospital admissions each year for the diagnosis of pneumonia. It is currently the sixth overall cause of death and the leading infectious cause of death in the American adult.

2. By what mechanism does a pulmonary infection develop?
Pulmonary infections most often result from aspiration of oropharyngeal secretions. Aspiration of small amounts of oral secretions is common even in healthy patients. The development of pneumonia depends on the type of organisms aspirated, the number of organisms aspirated, and the underlying host defenses.

Pneumonia may develop when pathogens are spread hematogenously from another infected site such as the urinary tract or skin. For example, pneumonia is a common complication of intravenous drug use.

Finally, pathogens may be directly introduced into the lung during penetrating trauma or with insertion of a chest tube.

3. Who is at greatest risk for developing pneumonia?
The very old and the very young are at highest risk. Patients with an impaired gag reflex—from altered mental status caused by head injury, alcohol or drug intoxication, cerebrovascular accidents, or seizures—are also at higher risk.

Several underlying diseases are frequently complicated by pulmonary infection. These include pulmonary embolus, pulmonary contusion, bronchial foreign body or tumor, chronic obstructive pulmonary disease (COPD), and atelectasis. Patients with chest wall disorders such as rib fractures, surgical wounds, or myopathies are often unable to cough and clear secretions because of weakness or pain. Impaired function of the mucociliary clearance mechanisms from smoking, smog, alcohol, viral infections, or COPD increases the risk of infection. Impaired immune function from cancer and chemotherapy, malnutrition, immune deficiency syndrome, and sickle cell disease also predisposes patients to pulmonary infections.

Finally, patients with a history of diabetes, alcoholism, recent antibiotic therapy, or hospitalization may be colonized with more virulent organisms and therefore are at much higher risk for serious pulmonary infections. Colonization with gram-negative bacteria and *Pseudomonas aeruginosa* occurs in 35% of patients with diabetes and alcoholism compared with only 10% of normals.

4. Why is seasonal variation important to consider?

This information is helpful in guiding empirical therapy. Mycoplasma and streptococcal pneumonias are more common in the fall and winter. Legionella occurs in the summer and fall. The incidence of viral pneumonia and influenza peaks in the winter. These infections are often followed by superinfection with *Staphylococcus aureus*, *Hemophilus influenzae*, or *Streptococcus pneumoniae*.

5. Has the epidemiology of pneumonia changed in recent years?

Viral and mycoplasma pneumonias remain the leading causes of atypical pneumonia. However, *Moraxella catarrhalis* and the TWAR strain of Chlamydia have recently been recognized as important causes of atypical pneumonia. The AIDS epidemic has dramatically changed the epidemiology of pulmonary infections. *Pneumocystis carinii* pneumonia (PCP) is by far the most common cause of respiratory infection in AIDS patients; 80% of all AIDS patients have at least one episode of this type of pneumonia. AIDS patients are also predisposed to other unusual types of pneumonia, including infections due to atypical mycobacteria, fungi, and viruses.

6. Why is it important to ask about travel and hobbies?

Patients traveling to other parts of the world or who engage in certain activities may be at higher risk for unusual organisms. Those who travel to Southeast Asia, for example, may be exposed to tuberculosis. Histoplasmosis and blastomycosis are endemic in the Ohio and Mississippi River valleys. *Coccidioides immitis* is found in desert terrain such as the San Joaquin Valley in California. Patients exposed to parakeets, parrots, and turkeys may contract pneumonia caused by *Chlamydia psittaci*.

7. What physical findings should be expected in a patient with pneumonia?

The physical examination of patients with respiratory complaints begins with a review of the vital signs. Findings supporting the diagnosis of pneumonia include fever, tachypnea, and tachycardia. With severe infection, patients appear toxic and may have mental status changes due to hypoxia. Examination of the chest includes inspection, palpation, percussion, and auscultation. The respiratory pattern should be observed for evidence of pleuritic pain that prevents deep inspiration, use of accessory muscles, weak respiratory effort, or decreased respiratory drive.

When alveoli become filled with fluid (pus), the lung exam changes. Sound is transmitted more efficiently through consolidated areas of lung tissue. By palpating the chest while the patient speaks, the examiner will note an increase in vibration over the consolidated lobe, which is called vocal fremitus. By the same mechanism, whispered words will also be better transmitted. Whispered pectoriloquy is the term used to describe this finding. The chest should be percussed to identify areas of dullness due to consolidation or the development of an emphysema. Finally, the finding of localized rales on auscultation is suggestive of pneumonia.

8. What is the difference between typical and atypical pneumonia?
Pneumonias are often clinically characterized as typical or atypical. Typical pneumonia is caused by pyogenic organisms and the presentation is characterized by the abrupt onset of high fever, cough productive of purulent sputum, shortness of breath, and pleuritic chest pain. The atypical pattern is far more insidious. The onset may be over several days with mild respiratory symptoms and only moderate fever and sputum production. Pathogens that often present in this atypical manner include *Mycoplasma pneumoniae*, *Chlamydia pneumoniae* (TWAR strain), *Moraxella catarrhalis*, and *Coxiella burnetii* (Q fever).

9. How can I determine the most likely causative organism?
The appropriate treatment of pneumonia depends on establishing a specific etiologic diagnosis. A Gram stain of the sputum is the single most useful ED test in helping to identify the most likely causative organism. Unfortunately, treatment must be initiated before results of definitive microbiologic tests (sputum and blood cultures) are available. In addition to Gram stain interpretation (see question #13), the physician must make a "best guess" of the pathogen based on epidemiology. Four commonly used epidemiologic categories of pneumonia are community-acquired pneumonia, hospital-acquired pneumonia, pneumonia in the immunocompromised host, and aspiration pneumonia. Other clinical factors considered include age, typical vs. atypical presentations, the setting of acquisition, seasonal variation, travel and hobbies, use of intravenous drugs, and other host factors.

10. What are the most common etiologic agents in community-acquired pneumonia?
In the otherwise healthy patient, the vast majority of pulmonary infections are due to *Streptococcus pneumoniae* (pneumococci), *Mycoplasma pneumoniae*, or viruses. *Strep. pneumoniae* is responsible for 60–75% of bacterial pneumonias in most studies. Other bacteria that cause community-acquired pneumonia are the Legionella species (5–15%), *Moraxella pneumoniae* (5–18%), *Hemophilus influenzae* (2–5%), *Chlamydia pneumoniae* (2–3%), *Staphylococcus aureus* (1–5%), and *M. catarrhalis* (1–5%).

11. What are the most common etiologic agents in pneumonia in the hospitalized patient?
During hospitalization the oropharynx becomes colonized with much more virulent organisms and the pattern of pneumonia changes. Gram-negative bacilli, particularly the Klebsiella species, *Pseudomonas aeruginosa*, and *Escherichia coli*, are responsible for more than 50% of cases. *Staphylococcus aureus* accounts for 10–20% of hospital-acquired pneumonias. The balance are due to anaerobic oral flora (10%), *Strep. pneumoniae* (3–9%), the Legionella species (0–25%), and *M. catarrhalis* (1–5%).

12. What are the most common causes of aspiration pneumonia?
Patients who aspirate oral secretions may be infected with multiple anaerobic pathogens such as *Fusobacterium nucleatum*, Peptostreptococcus, and the Bacteroides species. Such mixed anaerobic infections occur after procedures such as upper gastrointestinal endoscopy or in patients who are debilitated to the point of not being able to protect their airway.

13. What is the role of a sputum Gram stain and cultures?
Careful examination of the patient's sputum is the most rapid method of determining bacterial cause. Unfortunately, it is only 40–60% sensitive. Specificity is compromised by contamination of the sputum by oral flora as it passes through the oral pharynx. Sputum

cultures are not very helpful, as more than 50% are contaminated with oral flora. However, a positive blood culture is usually diagnostic.

14. Is the white blood cell (WBC) count helpful?
Elevated WBC counts, especially when immature forms are present, support the diagnosis of severe infection. However, this finding is not specific for pneumonia and a normal WBC count does not rule out pneumonia. Therefore, it is of limited value.

15. Is oxygen saturation helpful?
Absolutely. This rapid noninvasive test should be done on all patients with suspected or documented pneumonia in order to ascertain whether supplemental O_2 is necessary.

16. What are the indications for an arterial blood gas (ABG) analysis?
ABGs may be helpful in patients who are significantly tachypneic, cyanotic, confused, or hypoxic (low O_2 saturation). Elderly patients may be particularly difficult to evaluate, and therefore ABGs should be considered whenever a significant pulmonary infection is present.

17. What are the x-ray findings?
Certain x-ray findings are suggestive of but not diagnostic for specific pathogens. X-ray findings fall into four major groups. (1) **Lobar infiltrates** suggest infection due to *Streptococcus pneumoniae*, the Klebsiella species, or pneumonia caused by obstruction of a bronchus by cancer or foreign body. (2) **Diffuse (patchy) infiltrates** involve multiple lobes of the lung and suggest infection with *Staphylococcus aureus*, *Hemophilus influenzae*, or gram-negative organisms. (3) When the supporting structures of the lung become involved in an inflammatory process, an **interstitial pattern** is seen on x-ray. This pattern occurs with Mycoplasma pneumonia, legionellosis, and viral infections., In HIV-positive patients, this pattern is consistent with PCP infection. (4) **Cavitary lesions** with air-fluid levels are seen with infection due to mixed anaerobes, *Staph. aureus*, the Klebsiella species, *Pseudomonas aeruginosa*, or *Mycobacterium tuberculosis*. Infiltrates and cavities in the upper lobes are very suggestive of tuberculosis.

The development and resolution of x-ray findings may lag behind clinical findings by several hours or even days. Therefore, treatment should be guided primarily by clinical findings.

18. What is the best way to diagnose PCP?
This diagnosis must be considered in any patient with risk factors for HIV-related disease. Physical exam may show other findings consistent with AIDS such as Kaposi's sarcoma, weight loss, diffuse adenopathy, and thrush. Induced sputum samples, examined with silver stain, have a sensitivity of 55–79%. Definitive diagnosis may require more aggressive sample collection using bronchoalveolar lavage or open lung biopsy.

19. Which patients with pneumonia need to be admitted to the hospital?
Not everyone with pneumonia needs to be admitted. Circumstances that influence the decision to hospitalize include:
    1. Age. The very old and the very young are at high risk for developing serious overwhelming infections.
    2. Failure of outpatient antibiotic therapy
    3. Immunocompromised host
    4. Inability to take oral antibiotics
    5. Significant clinical toxicity or significant abnormality of vital signs
    6. Poor underlying health, especially in patients with chronic lung disease
    7. Multilobar involvement

8. Possible empyema
9. Granulocytopenia
10. Infections most likely due to virulent organisms such as *Staphylococcus aureus* or gram-negative bacilli
11. Any patient who has a low O_2 saturation necessitating supplemental O_2 therapy.

20. What treatment should be initiated in the ED?
Supportive care, including oxygen and hydration, should be given as required. The antibiotic of choice varies with the clinical situation. Broad-spectrum empirical therapy for the most likely pathogens is begun, pending specific identification of the organism and its sensitivities.

BIBLIOGRAPHY

1. DeGowen EL, DeGowen RL: Bedside Diagnostic Examination, 3rd ed. New York, Macmillan, 1976, pp 284–308.
2. Goodman LR, Goren RA, Teplick SK: The radiographic evaluation of pulmonary infection. Med Clin North Am 64:553, 1980.
3. LaForce FM: Pneumonia 1987: New developments. Eur J Microbiol 6:613, 1987.
4. Levine SJ, White DA: *Pneumocystis carinii*. Clin Chest Med 9:395, 1988.
5. Levison ME, Kaye D: Pneumonia caused by gram-negative bacilli: An overview. Rev Infect Dis 7:656, 1985.
6. Marrie TJ, et al: Pneumonia associated with TWAR strain of chlamydia. Ann Intern Med 106:507, 1987.
7. Pennington JE: Community-acquired and hospital-acquired pneumonia in adults. Current Pulmonology, vol 7. Chicago, Year Book Medical Publishers, 1986.
8. Pennza PT: Aspiration pneumonia, necrotizing pneumonia and lung abscess. Emerg Med Clin North Am 7:279–307, 1989.
9. Rein MF, et al: Accuracy of Gram's stain in identifying pneumococci in sputum. JAMA 239:2671, 1978.
10. Rosen P, et al (eds): Emergency Medicine: Concepts and Clinical Practice, 3rd ed. St. Louis, Mosby–Year Book, 1992, pp 1162–1177.
11. Singal BM, Hedges JR, Radack KL: Decision rules and clinical prediction of pneumonia: Evaluation of low yield criteria. Ann Emerg Med 18:1, 1989.
12. Wilson JD, et al (eds): Harrison's Principles of Internal Medicine, 12th ed. New York, McGraw-Hill, 1991, pp 1064–1969.

24. DEEP VENOUS THROMBOSIS AND PULMONARY EMBOLISM

Polly E. Parsons, M.D.

1. What are some of the risk factors for the development of deep venous thrombosis (DVT)?
- Age >70
- Cancer
- Pelvic or lower extremity surgery or trauma
- Any surgery requiring general anesthesia for >30 minutes
- Prolonged immobility
- Estrogen/progesterone therapy
- Postpartum state
- "Hypercoagulable states," including circulating lupus anticoagulant, antithrombin III deficiency, and protein C or S deficiency

2. Are there classic symptoms and physical exam findings for a lower extremity DVT?
We are all taught that patients with DVT complain of leg swelling and pain and on physical exam have a swollen red leg, a palpable cord, and a positive Homan's sign. In reality, only half of patients have these complaints or findings on physical exam, so a high index of suspicion in patients at risk is paramount.

3. What other disease processes can present with similar signs and symptoms?
The differential diagnosis includes superficial thrombophlebitis, contusion, hematoma, Baker's cyst, and muscle strain.

4. What noninvasive methods are available for the diagnosis of DVT?
Radiofibrinogen leg scanning. Good for detecting distal clots, including those in the calf, popliteal ligament, and distal thigh vein, but relatively poor for more proximal clots.
Impedance plethysmography. The diagnostic sensitivity and specificity depend on the technical expertise of the person performing the study, but in many centers this test detects >95% of acute proximal lower extremity DVT.
Duplex ultrasound. Again, the sensitivity and specificity are operator dependent, but this test can also detect >95% of acute proximal DVT.

5. What is the gold standard test for the diagnosis of DVT?
Venogram.

6. How should DVT be treated?
Therapy depends on the location of the clot. Clots restricted to the distal (calf) veins can probably be treated symptomatically and do not require anticoagulation. However, clots extending into or starting in the proximal veins do require therapy. The treatment of choice currently is intravenous heparin followed by a 3- to 6-month course of warfarin or subcutaneous heparin. The use of thrombolytic agents for DVT is somewhat controversial because of conflicting data from clinical studies. There are, however, data that indicate that use of thrombolytic therapy in acute DVT may reduce venous valvular damage and decrease the incidence of postphlebitic syndrome. Therefore, many clinicians use thrombolytic therapy acutely for a DVT that is extensive and has been present for less than 5 days (based on symptoms).

7. Where do pulmonary emboli (PE) come from?
The majority (>90%) come from lower extremity DVT.

8. What percentage of patients with DVT have pulmonary emboli?
The incidence is higher than you think. In one study of 101 patients with proven DVT without pulmonary symptoms, 51% had a high-probability lung scan at the time of the diagnosis of DVT.

9. Are there any diagnostic signs or symptoms for PE?
No. The common clinical symptoms—shortness of breath and chest pain—and clinical signs—tachypnea and tachycardia—are nonspecific. Patient presentations can range from mild shortness of breath to cardiovascular collapse.

10. What studies should be considered if PE is suspected?
Although not diagnostic, an arterial blood gas (ABG), a chest x-ray, and an EKG may be helpful either in increasing the evidence for PE or in providing another explanation for the patient's symptoms. The following points should be noted, however.

ABGs. The most common findings are a mild acute respiratory alkalosis and hypoxemia (i.e., an abnormal AaO_2 gradient) although the ABG may be completely normal. Lack of hypoxemia does not rule out the diagnosis of PE.

Chest x-ray. The chest x-ray is often normal. Subtle abnormalities such as focal atelectasis, slight elevation of a hemidiaphragm, or focal hyperlucency of the lung parenchyma may be present.

EKG. The findings classically associated with PE (S_1, Q_3, T_3 pattern, new right bundle branch block) occur in less than 15% of patients. The more common findings are sinus tachycardia and nonspecific ST-segment and T-wave changes.

11. What studies are needed to make the diagnosis of PE?

Ventilation/perfusion scan. A normal lung scan essentially rules out a diagnosis of PE, although there are rare incidences of patients with a normal lung scan who subsequently had PE documented by pulmonary angiogram. A high-probability scan is diagnostic for PE. The problems arise when the lung scan is read as indeterminate, which is frequently the case when the chest x-ray is abnormal or the patient has underlying cardiopulmonary disease. An indeterminate scan should probably be followed up with a pulmonary angiogram. If a pulmonary angiogram cannot be performed the diagnosis of PE could be inferred if clinical suspicion for PE was high and the patient had documented DVT.

Pulmonary angiogram. The gold standard for the diagnosis.

12. What happens if the diagnosis of PE is missed?

PE is listed as one of the most common causes of death in the United States, and yet only about 25% of the cases are diagnosed. Of the undiagnosed 75%, a small number die within one hour of presentation, so it is unlikely that diagnosis and intervention could improve outcome in that group. In the rest, however, the mortality from untreated PE is approximately 30%.

13. What is a massive PE?

A massive PE can be either anatomically defined as the occlusion of greater than 50% of the pulmonary vasculature or physiologically defined as an embolus that is complicated by systemic hypotension and severe hypoxemia. These two definitions are not necessarily synonymous, as a normal individual can lose 50% of pulmonary circulation without significant hemodynamic compromise, whereas a patient with significant underlying cardiopulmonary disease could suffer major hemodynamic compromise with a much smaller clot.

14. What is the treatment for PE?

The best "treatment" is prevention. When PE does occur, the therapy of choice is generally anticoagulation with intravenous heparin followed acutely by oral warfarin or subcutaneous heparin therapy for 3–6 months.

15. When should inferior vena caval (IVC) filter placement be considered?

When a patient cannot be anticoagulated because of acute bleeding, recent trauma, and the like, or when a patient has a documented recurrent PE on a therapeutic anticoagulation regimen, IVC filter placement should be considered.

CONTROVERSY

16. Should thrombolytic therapy be used in patients with massive PE?

For: There are three major goals in the treatment of PE: (1) to prevent further thrombus formation, (2) to promote resolution of existing thrombus, and (3) to prevent the sequelae of PE, including recurrent emboli. The standard therapy, heparin, does prevent further thrombus formation but is not clearly effective in the other two areas. Thrombolytic therapy has been shown to increase the rate of resolution of PE, and some suggest in the literature that the long-term sequelae of PE may decrease slightly in patients who receive thrombolytic therapy.

Against: In large clinical trials, there were no differences in morbidity or mortality when heparin and thrombolytic therapy for PE were compared. Because thrombolytic therapy may be associated with a higher complication rate, heparin therapy may be preferred.

BIBLIOGRAPHY

1. Huisman MV, Buller HR, ten Cate JW, et al: Unexpected high prevalence of silent pulmonary embolism in patients with deep venous thrombosis. Chest 95:498–502, 1989.
2. Kelley MA, Carson JL, Palevsky HI, Schwartz JS: Diagnosing pulmonary embolism: New facts and strategies. Ann Intern Med 114:300–306, 1991.
3. Marder VJ, Sherry S: Thrombolytic therapy: Current status (second of two parts). N Engl J Med 318:1585–1595, 1988.
4. Moser KM: Venous thromboembolism. Am Rev Respir Dis 141:235–249, 1990.
5. Parsons PE, Neff TA: Pulmonary embolism. In Parsons PE, Wiener-Kronish J (eds): Critical Care Secrets. Philadelphia, Hanley & Belfus, 1992.
6. Rosenow ED, Osmundson PJ, Brown ML: Pulmonary embolism. Mayo Clin Proc 56:161–178, 1981.
7. Stein PD, Terrin ML, Hales CA, et al: Clinical, laboratory, roentgenographic, and electrocardiographic findings in patients with acute pulmonary embolism and no pre-existing cardiac or pulmonary disease. Chest 100:598–603, 1991.
8. The PIOPED Investigators: Value of the ventilation/perfusion scan in acute pulmonary embolism. Results of the Prospective Investigation of Pulmonary Embolism Diagnosis (PIOPED). JAMA 263:2753–2759, 1990.
9. White RH, McGahan JP, Daschbach MM, Hartling RP: Diagnosis of deep-vein thrombosis using duplex ultrasound. Ann Intern Med 111:297–304, 1989.

VI. Cardiovascular System

25. CONGESTIVE HEART FAILURE AND ACUTE PULMONARY EDEMA

Rodney W. Smith, M.D.

1. What is congestive heart failure (CHF)?

CHF refers to cardiac dysfunction that leads to an inability of the heart as a pump to meet the circulatory demands of the patient. As a result, pulmonary congestion occurs, and when the problem is severe enough, pulmonary edema results.

2. What causes CHF?

CHF is caused by myocardial disease, which may be primary (cardiomyopathies) or secondary (myocardial infarction due to coronary artery disease). Cardiac response to volume overload (as in mitral regurgitation) or pressure overload (as in hypertension or aortic stenosis) can also lead to CHF.

3. What are the symptoms of CHF?

Common symptoms are dyspnea (the subjective feeling of difficulty with breathing) and fatigue. Early in the course of CHF, the patient reports exertional dyspnea; the heart is able to supply enough cardiac output for sedentary activities, but does not have the reserve to increase cardiac output during exercise. As heart failure worsens, even minimal activity may be difficult. Patients also report orthopnea (dyspnea relieved by assuming an erect posture), paroxysmal nocturnal dyspnea (sudden onset of dyspnea at night), and nocturia.

4. What causes these symptoms?

When the patient with CHF assumes the supine posture, fluid is redistributed from the abdomen and lower extremities to the pulmonary vasculature, causing increased pulmonary hydrostatic pressure and increased ventricular filling pressures. The patient has difficulty lying flat, and will sleep with several pillows or even sitting in a chair to relieve these symptoms. Redistribution of fluid may also lead to increased urine output and thus nocturia. Finally, in severe CHF, volume redistribution may be sufficient to lead to acute pulmonary edema.

5. What are the four main determinants of cardiac function in CHF?

- Preload
- Afterload
- Myocardial contractility
- Heart rate

6. What is preload?

Preload refers to the fact that, within limits, the amount of work cardiac muscle can do is related to the length of the muscle at the beginning of its contraction.

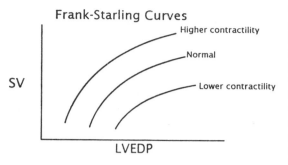

Frank-Starling Curves

Higher contractility

Normal

Lower contractility

SV

LVEDP

This relationship is shown graphically by the Frank-Starling curve, in which left ventricular end-diastolic volume (LVEDV) represents muscle length and the stroke volume (SV) represents cardiac work. (Actually, it is easier to measure pressure than volume, so we graph LVEDP vs. SV). Preload refers to LVEDP. As LVEDP increases, stroke volume increases. However, at higher LVEDP, the increase in stroke volume is less for a given increase in LVEDP. Note from the figure that the heart can function on different Frank-Starling curves, depending on the contractility.

7. What about afterload and heart rate?

Afterload refers to the pressure work the ventricle must do. The important components here are ventricular wall tension and systemic vascular resistance. Ventricular wall tension is directly related to intraventricular pressure and ventricular radius, and inversely related to ventricular wall thickness. Because cardiac output equals stroke volume times heart rate, the cardiac rate is an important determinant of cardiac output. At high heart rates, there may be insufficient time to fill the ventricle during diastole, leading to decreased LVEDP and SV, so that cardiac output may become compromised in spite of the fast heart rate.

8. How does this physiology relate to treatment?

The goal of treatment of CHF is to improve cardiac output. This can be accomplished by modifying each of these parameters. Diuretics and dietary salt and water restriction decrease preload and improve volume work. Digoxin improves contractility. Vasodilators are helpful in reducing afterload and thus the pressure work required of the heart.

9. What is acute pulmonary edema?

The most dramatic presentation of CHF is acute pulmonary edema. To understand pulmonary edema, we must go again to the physiologist Starling, who described the interaction of forces at the capillary membrane that lead to flow of fluid from capillaries to the interstitium. Simply put, there is a balance between hydrostatic pressure and osmotic pressure. Under normal circumstances, this leads to a small net movement of fluid from the capillaries into the lung interstitium. This fluid is then carried away by lymphatics. In CHF, the capillary hydrostatic pressure increases to the point that the lymphatics can no longer handle the fluid. Initially interstitial edema, and then alveolar edema, results.

10. What is the typical clinical presentation of acute pulmonary edema?

Patients develop acute shortness of breath and generally are fighting for air. These patients sit upright to decrease venous return (preload); they cough up frothy, red-tinged sputum. Auscultation of the lungs reveals wet rales throughout and often wheezes (due to bronchospasm). This presentation is a true emergency and requires immediate aggressive therapy.

11. What is the treatment of acute pulmonary edema?

First, follow the ABCs. In severe hypoxia, airway and breathing may be compromised and the patient will need to be intubated. Nasal intubation is often the best procedure, because it can be accomplished with the patient in an upright position. More often, intubation can be avoided with aggressive medical treatment. If you choose this route, however, constant attention to the patient is needed, and you need to set your decision point early. For example, you might decide, "I will intubate if the patient is not better in 15 minutes or worsens during that time." Administer oxygen to maintain sufficient oxygen saturation (>90%), either by nasal cannula or nonrebreather mask. Continuous positive airway pressure (CPAP) has also been used to avoid intubation. Continuously monitor oxygen saturation with pulse oximetry.

12. What about drug therapy?
Drug therapy is aimed at decreasing preload. Furosemide is given as a 40-mg IV bolus (larger amounts if the patient is on diuretics). Within 5–15 minutes of the injection, venodilation occurs and accounts for the rapid response to this drug. This action is followed within 30 minutes by diuresis. In addition to furosemide, morphine is given in a dose of 5–10 mg IV in order to decrease anxiety and thus the work of breathing. It is also a venodilator, decreasing preload. With decreased anxiety, there is decreased sympathetic response and thus decreased afterload. Finally, nitrates are useful in the form of sublingual nitroglycerin (NTG), topical NTG paste, or intravenous NTG drip. Nitroglycerin is predominantly a venodilator, reducing preload, but also dilates coronary arteries, so it may be especially helpful in the setting of coronary artery disease.

13. Are there other drugs that are useful in the treatment of acute pulmonary edema?
Yes: For the patient who is hypertensive, it is often helpful to lower the blood pressure (afterload). Remember that hypertension and tachycardia generally result from reflex mechanisms due to the acute decompensation, and often correct themselves with the initial treatment outlined above. With severe hypertension, nitroprusside is the treatment of choice. It is both a venodilator and arterial dilator, reducing both preload and afterload. Start the infusion at 10 μg/min and titrate upward every 5 minutes. It is important to monitor the blood pressure very closely. If the patient becomes hypotensive, stopping the infusion will cause a prompt increase in blood pressure, since nitroprusside has such a short half-life. Generally, doses of 0.5 to 2 μg/kg/min are sufficient.

14. What about giving positive inotropic drugs?
Digoxin, which is used in the treatment of chronic CHF, has little role in the treatment of acute pulmonary edema. Inotropic agents that are helpful include dobutamine, dopamine, and amrinone. Dobutamine and dopamine are both positive inotropic agents. Dopamine has more alpha effect, especially at higher doses, and thus should be reserved for the hypotensive patient. In cardiogenic shock that is refractory to these agents, amrinone infusion may be given. The ideal situation for administering these agents is in an intensive care unit with pulmonary artery monitoring to measure filling pressures, cardiac output, and other hemodynamic parameters.

15. Once the initial treatment has begun, what else needs to be done?
After the patient is stabilized, routine tests are performed, the most important being chest x-ray and EKG. Cardiac monitoring is begun, pulse oximetry is continuously monitored, and vital signs are recorded frequently. It is generally necessary to insert a Foley catheter for close monitoring of urine output. The search is on to try to discover the underlying reason for the acute decompensation.

16. What are the usual precipitating causes of acute pulmonary edema?
The most common cause of acute pulmonary edema is undermedication, either as a result of patient noncompliance with medication orders or dietary salt restrictions, or a change in medication under a physician's supervision. Other causes include pulmonary embolism, acute myocardial infarction, infection, anemia, arrhythmias, or severe hypertension. After precipitating factors are identified, specific therapy should be initiated.

17. What is the outpatient treatment of CHF?
Classically, the treatment has included diuretics and digoxin. More recently, vasodilators are playing an increasing role, especially angiotensin-converting enzyme (ACE) inhibitors.

18. How do ACE inhibitors work in CHF?
In response to cardiac decompensation, the renin-angiotensin system is activated. Angiotensin is a potent vasoconstrictor, leading to increased afterload. Stimulation of aldosterone leads to sodium retention and extracellular fluid volume expansion, and thus increased preload. ACE inhibitors help to decrease afterload by decreasing angiotensin II-mediated vasoconstriction, and decrease preload by blocking sodium retention and volume expansion. Placebo-controlled clinical trials have demonstrated significant improvement in survival of patients with CHF treated with ACE inhibitors.

19. What is the long-term prognosis for patients with CHF?
Prognosis depends on the etiology and severity of the heart failure. The prognosis is good when the underlying cause can be corrected, as in valvular heart disease. Patients with mild disease that can be controlled with low doses of diuretics or digoxin generally do well. Overall, however, patients who require hospitalization have an annual mortality of approximately 50%, and fewer than half of patients with CHF survive 5 years.

BIBLIOGRAPHY

1. Allison RC: Initial treatment of pulmonary edema: A physiologic approach. Am J Med Sci 302:385, 1991.
2. Bersten AD, Holt AW, Vedig AE, et al: Treatment of severe cardiogenic pulmonary edema with continuous positive airway pressure delivered by face mask. N Engl J Med 325:1825, 1991.
3. Braunwald E: Heart failure. In Wilson JD et al (eds): Harrison's Principles of Internal Medicine, 12th ed. New York, McGraw-Hill, 1991, pp 890–900.
4. Dzau VJ, Creager MA: Progress in angiotensin-converting enzyme inhibition in heart failure: Rationale, mechanisms, and clinical responses. Cardiol Clin 7:119, 1989.
5. McElroy PA, Shroff SG, Weber KT: Pathophysiology of the failing heart. Cardiol Clin 7:25, 1989.
6. Passmore JM, Jr, Goldstein RA: Acute recognition and management of congestive heart failure. Crit Care Clin 5:497, 1989.
7. Shesser R: Heart failure. In Rosen P, et al (eds): Emergency Medicine: Concepts and Clinical Practice, 3rd ed. St. Louis, Mosby–Year Book, 1992, pp 1266–1285.

26. ISCHEMIC HEART DISEASE

Edward P. Havranek, M.D., and Olivia Vynn Adair, M.D.

1. What presenting symptoms suggest acute ischemia or acute myocardial infarction (AMI)?
The most suggestive symptom of AMI is chest discomfort, typically retrosternal pressure, or a squeezing or heavy sensation. The discomfort often radiates to the left precordium, jaw, or medial aspect of the left arm. The pain usually increases over a few minutes and then plateaus until relief is obtained. Between 12 and 30% of AMIs go unrecognized because of the absence of typical symptoms, although less than 5% are actually "silent." Other symptoms include extreme fatigue, abdominal pain, nausea, vomiting, syncope, and respiratory difficulties. Duration of pain less than 30 minutes or greater than 18 hours rarely represents AMI. Elderly patients more frequently have atypical symptoms.

2. Who should be admitted when presenting with suspected angina?
Any patient presenting with suspected acute ischemia, AMI, or unstable angina should be admitted for evaluation and aggressive treatment. If the diagnosis of AMI is missed and the patient is sent home, the mortality during the next 72 hours is 25%, whereas in-hospital mortality is approximately 6%.

3. What questions should be asked to define the chest pain? How is the angina then classified?

First episode?	Intensity?
Location?	Frequency?
Radiation?	Precipitating factor(s)?
Duration?	Alleviating factor(s)?
Associated symptoms in last episode?	

The patient's chest pain, if defined as cardiac, can then be classified as (1) stable angina (angina for at least 60 days, with no change in frequency, precipitating causes, duration, ease of relief, or activity to avoid angina); (2) crescendo angina (increased frequency or diminished threshold of exertional angina); (3) unstable angina (provoked with less stimulation or at rest); (4) Prinzmetal's or variant angina (myocardial ischemia at rest with chest discomfort usually associated with EKG changes of ST elevation); or (5) angina equivalents (dyspnea and exhaustion due to left ventricular dysfunction secondary to ischemia).

4. What is the significance of abnormal ST-segment changes on an EKG?
The ST segment and the T-wave represent repolarization of the ventricles. Because repolarization is affected by many causes, both functional and organic, abnormal ST-segment changes may or may not represent ischemic cardiac injury. Ischemic current of injury is typically suggested by a convex-upward elevation of the ST segment; during early onset, it may simulate pericarditis or normal early repolarization. ST elevation may be due to normal repolarization (3–4 mm), acute pericarditis, acute cor pulmonale, hyperkalemia, hypothermia, cardiac tumor, or aneurysm. ST depression may represent cardiac ischemia, ventricular hypertrophy, drugs (e.g., digoxin), atrioventricular junctional rhythm with a retrograde P wave, or electrolyte abnormalities. If ST changes are ischemic in origin, they may be secondary to spasm, to obstruction of the coronary artery, or to both.

5. What are the typical EKG changes of ischemic cardiac injury?
The initial changes are T-wave prolongation and increased magnitude, either upright or inverted. Next the ST segment displays elevation and/or depression. A Q-wave may be seen in the initial EKG or may not develop for hours to days. As the ST segment returns to baseline, symmetrically inverted T-waves evolve. This classic evolution is documented in approximately 65% of patients with AMI.

6. Can the EKG be normal while a patient is having cardiac ischemia or an AMI?
Although serial EKGs show evolving changes diagnostic for AMI in over 90% of patients, 20–52% of initial EKGs will be normal or show only nonspecific abnormalities. Thus the initial EKG may be diagnostic for AMI in only half of the patients. An early repeat EKG may be helpful.

7. Are there any atypical features of the EKG that may indicate ischemia?
Atypical features are seen on about 40–50% of initial EKGs of patients later diagnosed with AMI. These include subtle ST-segment or T-wave changes, transient normalization of the ST segment or T-wave, or peaked T-waves. Between 20–30% of patients with AMI show

only T-wave abnormalities. An abnormal U-wave, negative or biphasic, is seen in 10–60% of patients with anterior infarctions and in up to 30% of patients with inferior myocardial infarction (this may precede other EKG changes). WPW, bundle branch blocks, and conduction defects may mask AMI EKG changes.

8. What other diagnoses should be differentiated in the patient with chest pain?
The history is paramount and helps to differentiate pleuritic chest pain associated with pleuritis, pericarditis, myocarditis, pneumothorax, or pulmonary embolism. Noncardiac chest pain may be found with local inflammation, such as onset of herpes zoster, or associated with neck, shoulder, or arm pain due to cervical or thoracic nerve-root compression. Gastritis, peptic ulcer, esophagitis, and esophageal spasm may also mimic angina. Patients with anxiety or depression syndromes often complain of chest pain. An important life-threatening condition, dissecting aortic aneurysm, may also cause sustained chest pain or typical angina.

9. What are the indications for thrombolytic therapy in AMI?
Thrombolytic therapy is of greatest benefit under the following conditions: (1) ST elevation greater than 1 mm in 2 leads, (2) pain not immediately responsive to nitroglycerin, and (3) pain lasting less than 6 hours.

10. What are the contraindications to thrombolytic therapy?
Risk for complications is excessive if patients have (1) active bleeding, (2) major surgery or trauma in the past 3 weeks, (3) neurosurgery or stroke in the past 3 months, or (4) prolonged (>10 min) or traumatic CPR. Relative contraindications include (1) major trauma or surgery >3 weeks ago, (2) neurosurgery or stroke >3 months ago, (3) active peptic ulcer, or (4) hemorrhagic ophthalmic condition, especially diabetic retinopathy.

In addition, patients with a known allergy to streptokinase or anisoylated plasminogen streptokinase activator complex (APSAC) should be treated with another agent. Exposure to streptokinase or APSAC in the previous 6 months or streptococcal infection in the previous 6 months are also reasons to use another agent.

11. What other diagnoses should be considered before giving thrombolytic therapy?
Aortic dissection and acute pericarditis can mimic AMI. Both have had fatal outcomes when thrombolytics were given. Dissection can be excluded with a careful history, examination of peripheral pulses, and chest x-ray. Pericarditis can be excluded by carefully listening for a rub and examining the EKG for widespread, concave-upward ST elevation.

12. What is the risk for fatal complications of thrombolytic therapy for AMI?
Mortality, which almost invariably results from intracranial hemorrhage, occurs in about 0.5% of treated patients.

13. Define reperfusion arrhythmias.
Approximately 45 minutes after initiation of a thrombolytic agent, blood flow is restored in most patients. This event may be accompanied by arrhythmias, especially ventricular tachycardia or accelerated idioventricular rhythm. In patients with inferior MI, sinus bradycardia or heart block may occur. These arrhythmias are transient, generally lasting less than 30 seconds. Reperfusion may be accompanied by a brief increase in pain.

14. What other medications are useful adjuvants to thrombolytic therapy?
    1. **Morphine.** Myocardial infarction can cause excruciating pain as well as severe fear and anxiety. Control of these symptoms with morphine is neglected too often.
    2. **Aspirin.** Should be given immediately.

3. **Beta blockers.** Given intravenously during thrombolytic therapy, they further reduce mortality and infarct size. They are better tolerated than one may think and are under-utilized.

4. **Heparin.** With tissue plasminogen activator (tPA), initiation of heparin is imperative at least 1 hour before the completion of the thrombolytic infusion. With streptokinase or APSAC, heparin should be started 4–6 hours later.

5. **Nitroglycerin.** If control of blood pressure is an issue, nitroglycerin is the preferred agent. Given routinely, it decreases mortality.

15. What is the role of lidocaine?

Prophylactic use of lidocaine infusion does not reduce mortality in AMI. It should be used in patients with frequent PVCs, ventricular tachycardia, or ventricular fibrillation. It must be monitored carefully because of the risk of seizures. It should not be used in patients who have had intermittent heart block because ventricular escape beats may be suppressed.

16. What other arrhythmias occur with AMI?

Ventricular irritability, with frequent PVCs, nonsustained ventricular tachycardia, and ventricular fibrillation, may occur and should be treated with lidocaine. Sustained ventricular tachycardia (lasting >30 seconds) is uncommon in AMI. Accelerated idioventricular rhythm (heart rate: 60–100) should not be treated.

Bradyarrhythmias may also occur. Second- or third-degree heart block that accompanies inferior MI is usually transient, and a temporary pacemaker is not required. When heart block accompanies an anterior MI, a temporary pacer *is* required. A prophylactic temporary pacer is probably indicated when severe conducting system disease (bifascicular block or left bundle branch block + first-degree block) accompanies an anterior AMI.

17. What is the role of emergency percutaneous transluminal coronary angioplasty (PTCA)?

In selected centers, personnel and facilities for performing PTCA may be readily available, and angioplasty may provide more rapid and more reliable reperfusion. It is emerging as the preferred treatment in AMI accompanied by cardiogenic shock. In patients who have received thrombolytic therapy, angioplasty appears to have no role unless recurrent ischemia is suspected.

CONTROVERSIES

18. What is the preferred agent for thrombolysis in AMI?

This issue is currently unresolved. Some cardiologists prefer tPA because in some studies it has produced higher rates of reperfusion than streptokinase (STK). Its major disadvantage is financial; it costs 8–10 times as much as STK. It also has a very short half-life (5–10 minutes), making reocclusion a significant problem if administration of the drug with adjuvant heparin is not carefully monitored.

Advocates of STK point out that large-scale studies of tPA vs. STK show no difference in mortality. Some concede that these studies are flawed by a failure to give adequate heparin after tPA, because adjuvant heparin has proved crucial to the success of tPA. The longer half-life and different effects on the coagulation system offered by STK may reduce the incidence of reocclusion after reperfusion.

APSAC is essentially a form of STK that requires biologic activation. It does not have the cost advantage of STK but is easier to administer. Evidence that it is more effective than either tPA or STK is lacking.

The definitive answer to this question awaits the results of large prospective multicenter trials currently under way.

19. How should unstable angina be managed in the emergency department (ED)?
Because unstable angina is associated with a high risk of AMI and sudden death, immediate intervention should include cardiac and hemodynamic monitoring, CCU admission, EKGs, intravenous nitroglycerin, intravenous morphine, intravenous infusion of heparin, and aspirin. Intravenous beta blockers and calcium-channel blockers may also be added for tachycardia, blood pressure, a history of rest angina, or continued/uncontrolled angina. Early coronary angiography is recommended immediately after stabilization or if pharmacologic therapy is not adequate. The use of thrombolytics in unstable angina is controversial. One study found higher mortality with their use in this group. However, adequate clinical trials are needed to evaluate their role in unstable angina.

20. If a cocaine user in the ED complains of chest pain, should there be true concern for ischemia or AMI? Do any EKG changes help in evaluation?
Chest pain in a cocaine user should be taken seriously, as sudden death and AMI associated with cocaine abuse are increasingly recognized. Acute coronary vasospasm and recurrent AMI are associated with prolonged use. Approximately one-third of these patients have preexisting atherosclerotic heart disease. Cocaine blocks the re-uptake of norepinephrine and dopamine, thus causing vasoconstriction, hypertension, tachycardia, and a predisposition to arrhythmias. Studies suggest various causes of cocaine-induced AMI: coronary spasm leading to thrombus formation; vasoconstriction and reduced coronary blood flow (possibly mediated by alpha-adrenergic stimulation); a direct effect on the myocardium; intimal proliferation; and increased platelet aggregation. Acute aortic rupture may also be associated with cocaine use secondary to acute increase in systemic arterial pressure.

21. What role does echocardiography play in evaluation of suspected cardiac ischemia or AMI in the ED?
Echocardiography is a powerful and sensitive diagnostic technique for evaluation of patients with chest pain, hypotension, or dyspnea in the ED. It provides immediate data to support AMI or ischemia; wall-motion abnormality has a reported sensitivity of 100% in transmural infarctions and an overall sensitivity of 90% in AMI. It is particularly useful when the EKG is negative or nondiagnostic, such as with bundle branch block. Other diagnoses are also easily investigated; i.e., valve dysfunction, endocarditis, cardiomyopathy, pericardial effusion or tamponade, and aortic dissection (which may require a transesophageal echocardiogram).

22. Do cardiac enzymes (CK-MB) have a role in evaluating chest pain in the ED?
If the patient presents with symptoms of chest discomfort and has a nondiagnostic EKG, the diagnosis is difficult. Studies show that a significant number of patients (5–15%) are inappropriately discharged or admitted to unmonitored beds with unrecognized AMI. Therefore, newer techniques that rapidly and sensitively indicate levels of CK-MB or serum myoglobin may be helpful and are expected to become more common in the ER evaluation of patients with chest discomfort and a nondiagnostic EKG. At present, the decision to admit or discharge should depend on the history, with supportive evidence supplied by the EKG.

23. Can lipoprotein analysis assist in the initial evaluation of patients with chest pain in the ED to predict patients with coronary artery disease?
Lipoprotein analysis has no predictive value and is not indicated in the initial evaluation of patients with chest pain.

24. What should be suspected if a patient with HIV disease presents with chest pain? Is there a suggested diagnostic aid?
The patient with HIV disease has the same risk for coronary artery disease as other patients presenting with chest pain. Recent studies have identified cardiac abnormalities in as many

as 70% of patients with HIV disease, more commonly in hospitalized patients. These abnormalities include cardiomyopathy, myocarditis, pericardial effusion and tamponade, pericardial and myocardial tumors, and valve disease. All of these may present as chest pain. Echocardiography is the recommended technique for early diagnosis and assistance in management decisions.

BIBLIOGRAPHY

1. Adair OV: Echocardiography in intensive care. In Parsons PE, Wiener-Kronish JP (eds): Critical Care Secrets. Philadelphia, Hanley & Belfus, 1992, pp 160–165.
2. Gay PC, Nishimura RA, Roth CS, et al: Lipoprotein analysis in the evaluation of chest pain in the emergency department. Mayo Clin Proc 66:885–891, 1991.
3. GISSI collaborators, GISSI-2: A factorial randomized trial of alteplase versus streptokinase and heparin versus no heparin among 12,490 patients with acute myocardial infarction. Lancet 336:65–71, 1990.
4. Green GB, Hansen KN, Chan DW, et al: The potential utility of a rapid CK-MB assay in evaluating emergency department patients with possible myocardial infarction. Ann Emerg Med 20:954–960, 1991.
5. Hauser AM: The emerging role of echocardiography in the emergency department. Ann Emerg Med 18:1298–1303, 1989.
6. Karlson BW, Herlitz J, Wiklund O, et al: Early prediction of acute myocardial infarction from clinical history, examination and electrocardiogram in the emergency room. Am J Cardiol 68:171–175, 1991.
7. Lamas GA, Muller JE, Turi ZG, et al: A simplified method to predict occurrence of complete heart block during myocardial infarction. Lancet 336:65–71, 1990.
8. Lau J, Antman EM, Jimenez-Silva J, et al: Cumulative meta-analysis of therapeutic trials for myocardial infarction. N Engl J Med 327:248–254, 1992.
9. Verstraete M, Bory M, Collen D, et al: Randomized trial of intravenous recombinant tissue-type plasminogen activator versus intravenous streptokinase in acute myocardial infarction. Lancet 336:65–71, 1990.

27. CARDIAC ARRHYTHMIAS

Elizabeth C. Brew, M.D., and Alden H. Harken, M.D.

1. Is it necessary to identify definitively a dysrhythmia in order to treat it?
No.

2. How do you know whether a patient's dysrhythmia is causing hemodynamic trouble?
Typically, if a patient's ventricular rate is between 60 and 100 beats per minute (bpm), then any hemodynmaic instability is caused by something else.

3. How much benefit is derived from atrial "kick"?
The standard answer is 10%, which is incorrect. The significance of atrial "kick" depends completely on ventricular function. Induced atrial fibrillation has absolutely no hemodynamic effect on a healthy medical student, whereas we have measured a 40% decrease in cardiac output in a patient with severe left ventricular dysfunction.

4. Is there a limit above which tachycardia does not further increase cardiac output?
A reasonable rule of thumb: You can increase cardiac output by increasing heart rate up to 200 bpm minus age.

5. What is a sinus beat?

At the end of each heart beat, all myocardial cells are depolarized and experience a refractory period. At this point, all cardiac cells float back up through phase IV depolarization toward "threshold potential." It is a race. Typically the sinoatrial (SA) nodal cells win this race, achieve threshold, fire, and assume pacemaker "sinus beat" function of the heart.

6. What is a premature ventricular contraction (PVC)?

A PVC occurs when a ventricular site wins the race and ventricular depolarization originates from an ectopic ventricular site.

7. What is a narrow-complex tachycardia?

The atrioventricular (AV) node attaches directly to the Purkinje system, which courses over the endocardial surface of the ventricles. An electrical impulse travels over the Purkinje very fast—2–3 m/sec. Thus, if an impulse enters the ventricles from the AV node, it can electrically activate the entire ventricular muscle mass very rapidly—in 0.12 sec or 120 ms or 3 little boxes on EKG paper. "Narrow complex" refers to the width of the QRS complex. Thus, a "narrow-complex" tachycardia must originate above the AV node and is therefore a supraventricular tachycardia.

8. What is the AV node?

The AV node is not simply a passive connection between the atria and ventricles. It is smart. With progressively rapid atrial impulse generation, all electrical impulses are conducted to the ventricles. When the ventricular rate becomes sufficiently rapid that cardiac output is compromised, conduction velocity begins to *slow* in the AV node. This progressive slowing filters the rapid atrial impulses so that serial atrial impulses are not conducted at all (Wenkebach). This progressive AV nodal conduction block is a protective mechanism to prevent dysfunctionally rapid ventricular rate.

9. What is a wide-complex tachycardia?

When an impulse originates from a typically damaged or ischemic bit of ventricular muscle, it takes a while to access the Purkinje superhighways, thus permitting electrical activation of the entire ventricular mass. The QRS is measured from its initial deflection (at the ectopic site) to the completion of all ventricular activity. When the major conduction pathways are not used primarily, it takes a long time (>0.12 sec or 120 ms or 3 little boxes on the EKG pager) to inscribe the QRS complex. This ectopic, ventricular origin complex is referred to as "wide."

10. What is a supraventricular rhythm with aberrancy?

Usually a supraventricular rhythm traverses the AV node and courses through the large endoventricular conduction fibers, activating the ventricles rapidly—narrow QRS complex <0.12 sec. If by virtue of major right or left conduction bundle damage a supraventricular impulse is forced to take a circuitous route through the ventricles, the activation time is longer and the QRS is wide. A "wide-complex" tachycardia represents a tachycardia of ventricular origin. A supraventricular rhythm with aberrancy is the infrequent exception. Of 100 patients presenting in the emergency department (ED) with a wide-complex tachycardia, 90% have ventricular tachycardia, and only 10% have a supraventricular tachycardia with aberrancy.

11. How do you treat bradyarrhythmias?

If the patient has a heart rate below 60 bpm and is hemodynamically unstable, (1) give 0.5 mg (.01 mg/kg in a child) atropine IV (may repeat); (2) begin intravenous isoproterenol (0.05 mg/kg/min); (3) initiate pacemaker (do not forget the external pacemaker). The transvenous pacemaker (especially without fluoroscopy) always takes much longer than you think it will.

12. How do you treat tachyarrhythmias?
If the rhythm is fast enough to cause hemodynamic instability (or to frighten the treating physician), proceed with cardioversion—for *all* tachyarrhythmias. You may start with 100–360 J (in the synchronous mode), depending on how frightened you are.

13. Does it make sense to cardiovert asystole?
Strictly speaking, no. But the answer is controversial. Theoretically, electrical cardioversion synchronously depolarizes all myocardial cells simultaneously. All cells then should repolarize synchronously and spontaneously reinitiate sinus rhythm. With asystole, there is nothing to depolarize and therefore nothing to cardiovert. Those in favor of attempting to cardiovert apparent asystole point out, however, that you have nothing to lose. Conceivably, the major QRS vector is perpendicular to the axis of the EKG lead, making ventricular fibrillation appear as asystole.

14. How do you treat wide-complex tachycardia?
With cardioversion. Although cardioversion is the mainstay of therapy, it is not wrong to give lidocaine (1 mg/kg IV bolus) to a patient with relatively slow, stable ventricular (wide-complex) tachycardia. If this patient becomes hemodynamically unstable, however, proceed directly to cardioversion.

15. How do you treat narrow-complex tachycardia?
A narrow-complex tachycardia must be supraventricular, originating above the AV node (see question 7). Thus, in order to control the ventricular rate, you need to block the AV node pharmacologically. Give adenosine, 6 mg IV bolus, followed by 12 mg *rapid* IV push, or verapamil, 1 mg/min IV × 10 min (to desired rate).

16. How do you treat a narrow-complex tachycardia in a hemodynamically unstable patient?
With synchronized cardioversion under adequate sedation.

17. Do you need to distinguish the multiple varieties of narrow-complex tachycardia (rapid atrial fibrillation, supraventricular tachycardia [SVT] atrial flutter) in order to treat effectively?
No.

18. What drug is contraindicated in the treatment of wide-complex tachycardia?
Verapamil. Since all wide-complex tachycardias must be considered to be of ventricular origin, verapamil is likely to cause hypotension and may cause degeneration of the rhythm to ventricular fibrillation or asystole.

CONTROVERSIES

There are none! In truth, the major controversy is whether the above material should be made more complex. We believe that effective therapy for all tachyarrhythmias can be summarized in three lines:

Diagnosis	*Treatment*
Unstable patient	Cardioversion
Wide-complex tachycardia	Cardioversion
Narrow-complex tachycardia	Verapamil or adenosine

BIBLIOGRAPHY

1. Harken AH: Cardiac arrhythmias. In Wilmore D, Brennan M, Harken AH, et al (eds): Care of the Surgical Patient, Vol. 1, Critical Care. New York, Scientific American, 1989.
2. Harken AH, Honigman B, Van Way C: Cardiac dysrhythmias in the acute setting: Recognition and treatment (or) anyone can treat cardiac dysrhythmias. J Emerg Med 5:129–134, 1987.
3. Lowenstein SR, Harken AH: A wide complex look at cardiac arrhythmias. J Emerg Med 5:519–531, 1987.

28. HYPERTENSION/HYPERTENSIVE EMERGENCIES

Alex M. Maslanka, M.D.

1. What is hypertension?
Blood pressure (BP) varies widely and no single BP value defines an emergency. Elevated values may be due to anxiety, pain, or drugs, and may resolve without treatment. Generally accepted guidelines regarding BP measurements are as follows: systolic values <140 mmHg and diastolic values <90 mmHg are considered normal. Diastolic pressures between 90 and 115 mmHg constitute mild to moderate hypertension, and values in excess of 115 mmHg constitute severe hypertension. Elevated systolic pressures (>160 mmHg) with normal diastolic pressures frequently are found in geriatric patients and are termed isolated systolic hypertension. Blood pressures must be elevated at least twice on two separate occasions with proper-sized cuffs in both arms before the diagnosis is made.

2. What causes hypertension?
In most cases (>90%) the cause is unknown and the disease is termed essential. Nervous, renal, hormonal, and vascular systems may all contribute. Secondary hypertension has an identifiable cause. Renal disease and endocrine abnormalities account for the majority of these cases.

3. What are the physiologic changes that occur in prolonged hypertension?
The contractile properties of smooth muscle in arterial walls are altered in hypertensive persons. It is not clear if this is the primary cause or a response to chronically elevated pressures from failure of normal autoregulatory mechanisms. **Cardiac response** to increased peripheral resistance results in left ventricular hypertrophy and dilatation. Congestive heart failure (CHF), angina pectoris, and myocardial infarction (MI) may follow. The **neurologic system** manifests both retinal and central nervous system changes. Narrowing of the retinal arterioles and focal spasm progress to hemorrhages, exudates, and papilledema. Funduscopic evaluation provides direct insight into the effect of hypertension on the arterial system. CNS dysfunction results from cerebral infarction, hemorrhage, and hypertensive encephalopathy. **Renal vascular lesions** result in decreased glomerular filtration and tubular dysfunction with ensuing renal failure.

4. What are the presenting symptoms in hypertensive patients?
Patients with mild to moderate hypertension are often asymptomatic. Symptoms of long-standing, severe, or accelerating hypertension include the following: **Cardiac decompensation** leads to dyspnea on exertion, nocturia, cough, weakness, and right upper quadrant pain

from passive hepatic congestion. **Retinal changes** may lead to scotoma, blurred vision, and even blindness. **CNS manifestations** include morning headaches (usually occipital), dizziness, light-headedness, vertigo, tinnitus, and syncope. **Renal failure** results in oliguria, hematuria, mental status changes, weight loss, and weakness.

5. What are some signs seen on physical exam?
Elevated serial measurements with a proper-sized cuff is the best initial screen. The **cardiopulmonary exam** may reveal cardiomegaly with a prominent left ventricular impulse, an S4, or an S3. Orthopnea, cyanosis, increased jugular venous distention, basilar rales, dependent edema, and hepatomegaly are also seen. **Funduscopic exam** shows evidence of retinal vessel spasm with arteriovenous nicking, copper-wiring and progression to hemorrhage, exudate, and papilledema. **CNS signs** resulting from decreased cerebral perfusion would depend on the vascular distribution. In cases of **renal artery stenosis**, abdominal bruits may be detected.

6. Is laboratory evaluation necessary?
Severe hypertension associated with end-organ damage requires hospitalization and extensive diagnostic testing. Less complicated patients may require only screening tests. The EKG may reveal left ventricular hypertrophy, ischemic changes, and possibly infarction patterns. Urinalysis may show proteinuria, microscopic hematuria, and glucosuria. Serologic studies include BUN and creatinine as indices of renal function. Electrolytes are studied for endocrine abnormalities and complications of diuretic therapy.

7. Discuss outpatient therapy.
Hypertensive patients may present to the ED under many circumstances not directly related to hypertension (e.g., trauma, toxicologic ingestion, noncompliance), and familiarity with conventional therapy is necessary. First, they should be referred for serial BP measurements in order to determine if they have hypertension. Nonpharmacologic treatment includes stress reduction, diet, regular exercise, and behavior modification. Pharmacologic intervention attacks the process at many sites. Diuretics, anti-adrenergics, vasodilators, calcium channel blockers, and ACE inhibitors are all used. Historically, therapy was begun with diuretics and/or beta blockers. Recently, ACE inhibitors and calcium channel blockers have become first-line drugs.

8. When is hypertension considered "urgent"?
Severe elevation of diastolic BP (>120–140 mmHg) without evidence of acute CNS, cardiac disease, or renal damage constitutes urgent hypertension. The patient may have minimal or no complaints and is often noncompliant with treatment. Therapeutic goals include gradual reduction of BP (diastolic BP 100–110 mmHg) within 24 hours. Oral agents are sufficient and hospitalization is unnecessary if close follow-up is available. The most frequently used agents are clonidine and nifedipine. **Clonidine** is a central alpha-adrenergic agonist that lowers blood pressure by decreasing sympathetic and peripheral vascular tone. **Nifedipine** is a calcium channel blocker that lowers systemic vascular resistance through arterial vasodilatation. It is capable of precipitous reduction of BP and resultant hypoperfusion. Myocardial infarction and stroke have been documented with its use.

9. What are hypertensive crises?
Acute syndromes that involve ongoing and life-threatening end-organ damage are considered hypertensive crises and require emergent therapy with prompt reduction in blood pressure. These include hypertensive encephalopathy, acute myocardial infarction, pulmonary edema, unstable angina, aortic dissection, or renal insufficiency.

10. What is the difference between accelerated and malignant hypertension?
Accelerated hypertension consists of elevated diastolic BP and funduscopic changes of flame hemorrhages and cotton wool exudates. Malignant hypertension has these factors along with papilledema.

11. What is hypertensive encephalopathy?
This is the classic neurologic hypertensive emergency, and it occurs when cerebral auto-regulation fails to control blood flow at markedly elevated mean arterial pressures, leading to ischemia, increased vascular permeability, and resultant intracerebral edema, petechial hemorrhages, and microinfarcts. Insidious (12–72 hr) onset of headache, vomiting, drowsiness, and confusion may be associated with seizures, visual changes, and focal neurologic changes. Papilledema and hypertensive retinopathy may be seen. The diagnosis is clinical and the process reverses with reduction of BP. Untreated, coma and death may result within hours.

12. What is the treatment for a hypertensive crisis?
Three treatment regimens are classically advocated for rapid reduction of BP. (1) The drug of choice is **nitroprusside**. Intravenous administration provides the rapid onset of powerful vasodilation that affects both resistance and capacitance vessels. Short half-life allows for dose titration. Use in the pregnant patient should be avoided. Intermediate metabolites include cyanide; however, toxicity is rare and not an issue in ED treatment. Light sensitivity requires that the solution be wrapped in an opaque material. (2) The second regimen involves the combination of **diazoxide and furosemide**. Diazoxide works primarily by vasodilatation of resistance vessels. It may exacerbate angina and is contraindicated in this setting. Because diazoxide causes sodium and water retention, administration of furosemide at doses of 20–40 mg IV is advocated. (3) **Labetalol** is the third choice. Its alpha₁ blocking effect in vascular smooth muscle decreases blood pressure while its beta effect prevents reflex tachycardia. Beta blockers should not be used in patients with CHF, heart block, severe tachycardia, and reactive airways disease. Neither diazoxide nor labetalol allows reduction of blood pressure as safely as nitroprusside.

13. What is the goal and rationale of this emergent therapy?
Gradual (2–3 hr) reduction of BP to levels of 140–160 mmHg systolic and 90 to 110 mmHg diastolic, but not more than a 25% reduction in the mean arterial pressure (MAP), which is the lower limit of cerebral autoregulation. Autoregulation (vasoactive response to changes in BP) keeps cerebral blood flow constant from a MAP of 60 mmHg to 150 mmHg. Chronic hypertension impairs normal autoregulation, so that rapid and profound reductions may result in cerebral hypoperfusion and ischemic insult.

14. What other neurologic syndromes are associated with hypertension?
Hypertension is associated with thromboembolic or hemorrhagic **stroke syndromes**. It is a predisposing factor for thromboembolic stroke and not the direct cause. A profound elevation in BP is not normally found. Rapid reduction of BP serves only to decrease cerebral blood flow and increase ischemia; therefore control patients with persistent and significant elevations (>130 mmHg diastolic). Patients may also present with **intracranial hemorrhage** as a result of hypertensive vascular disease or other factors (tumor, trauma, coagulopathy, aneurysm, or arteriovenous malformation). In patients who bleed for reasons other than hypertensive vascular disease, hypertension is often found, is transitory, and is secondary to increased intracranial pressure. Treatment is generally aimed at management of the underlying condition.

15. How are hypertension and pulmonary edema related?
Patients are hypertensive secondary to increased levels of catecholamine from the stress of hypoxia or as a reflex from myocardial ischemia. Severe hypertension and pulmonary

edema usually respond to standard treatment of pulmonary edema (morphine, nitrates, oxygen, furosemide). If the condition is refractory to this regimen, nitroprusside should be used to decrease the peripheral vascular resistance causing left ventricular failure and the resultant pulmonary edema.

16. What about the hypertensive patient with chest pain?

Acute ischemia of the left ventricle with **angina pectoris** is often accompanied by severe hypertension that may precede or appear in combination with infarction. Acute reduction of peripheral vascular resistance will decrease the work burden to the myocardium. Both **nitroglycerin and nitroprusside** have been used with success.

17. Is this the only cause of chest pain to worry about?

No. The patient may have **acute aortic dissection**. Dissection proximal to and involving the arch is treated surgically, whereas dissection distal to the arch is treated medically. In either case, immediate control of BP is necessary. Drugs that slow heart rate and lower pressure decrease the shearing force on the aortic intima. Current therapy advocates the coadministration of a beta blocker and nitroprusside. **Esmolol** is a short-acting beta blocker that can be administered initially in order to block the reflex tachycardia induced by **nitroprusside** therapy. Blood pressure should then be reduced within 15–30 minutes to maintain the systolic BP pressure between 100 and 120 mmHg, with the MAP no greater than 80 mmHg.

18. What renal emergencies result from hypertension?

Chronic renal failure exacerbates hypertension and vascular changes in the diseased kidneys, which can worsen the failure. If sodium retention and increased extracellular volume cannot be controlled by diuretics, then additional antihypertensives may be added. For patients who fail these regimens and present in renal failure with severe hypertension, **nitroprusside** therapy may be indicated.

19. Are there other causes of hypertensive emergencies in the ED?

Increased levels of catecholamines, seen in a number of conditions, can lead to hypertensive crises. **Pheochromocytoma** is uncommon and is treated with phentolamine, an alpha blocker. Abrupt **cessation of clonidine or beta blockers** may precipitate withdrawal and severe hypertension. For rapid reduction, labetalol, phentolamine, or nitroprusside may be needed prior to resumption of the original therapy. Patients taking **monoamine oxidase inhibitors** who ingest foods with tyramine or certain drugs may have severe and prolonged hypertension. Phentolamine is advocated. **Sympathomimetic ingestion** (cocaine, amphetamines, PCP, LSD, "diet pills") may also prompt a hypertensive response. Efficacious drug treatments include labetalol, esmolol, phentolamine, and nitroprusside.

BIBLIOGRAPHY

1. Calhoun DA, Oparil S: Treatment of hypertensive crisis. N Engl J Med 323:1177–1183, 1990.
2. Gifford RW Jr: Management of hypertensive crises. JAMA 266:829–835, 1991.
3. Mathews J: Hypertension. In Rosen P, et al (eds): Emergency Medicine, Concepts and Clinical Practice, 3rd ed. St. Louis, Mosby–Year Book, 1992, pp 1249–1265.
4. McDonald AJ: Hypertensive emergencies and urgencies. In Harwood-Nuss et al (eds): The Clinical Practice of Emergency Medicine. Philadelphia, J.B. Lippincott, 1991, pp 897–902.
5. Thacker HL, Jahnigen DW: Managing hypertensive emergencies and urgencies in the geriatric patient. Geriatrics 46:26–30, 35–37, 1991.
6. Williams GH: Hypertensive vascular disease. In Wilson JD, et al (eds): Harrison's Principles of Internal Medicine, 12th ed. New York: McGraw-Hill, 1991, pp 1001–1015.

29. PERICARDITIS AND MYOCARDITIS

Diana R. Williams, M.D.

PERICARDITIS

1. Describe a normal pericardium.

The pericardium is a 1–2 mm thick material that envelopes the heart. It has two layers, between which 25 to 50 ml of fluid are normally present, in the pericardial space.

2. What is pericarditis?

Pericarditis is inflammation of the pericardium.

3. What causes pericarditis?

Infectious agents such as viruses and bacteria can cause pericarditis as a result of direct spread of these infections to the pericardium. Viruses may also cause pericarditis 2–4 weeks after a viral illness as the result of an antibody-mediated autoimmune reaction. This post-viral pericarditis, termed idiopathic due to inability to isolate a viral source, is probably the most common form of pericarditis. Systemic illness may cause pericarditis, as may traumatic insults. Myocardial infarction, malignancy, drugs, and irradiation can also cause pericarditis.

Causes of Pericarditis

Infection	Systemic Illness	Myocardial Infarction
Viral	Rheumatic fever	Early
Coxsackie B	Lupus erythematosus	Late (Dressler's syndrome)
Echovirus	Sarcoidosis	
Adenovirus	Uremia	Drugs
AIDS		Procainamide
Bacterial	Trauma	Cromolyn sodium
Staphylococcus	Pericardiotomy	Hydralazine
Tuberculosis	Blunt	Radiation
Fungal	Penetrating	
Parasitic	Cardiac instrumentation	Neoplasm

4. Who is susceptible to infectious pericarditis?

Viral and idiopathic pericarditis occur most commonly in healthy persons 20–40 years of age. Bacterial pericarditis occurs in patients with a bacterial infection of the lungs, endocardium, blood, etc. Patients with acquired immunodeficiency syndrome (AIDS) are susceptible to pericarditis caused by opportunistic infections.

5. What is the clinical presentation of pericarditis?

The most common symptom is chest pain, described as midline and sharp. The pain is worse with movement and respiration, and relief is obtained from sitting up and leaning forward. It may radiate to the neck, back, or left shoulder. Dyspnea, malaise, and fever are other commonly associated symptoms.

A pericardial friction rub, a scratchy noise like creaking leather, is pathognomonic for pericarditis. The optimal patient position to hear a rub is sitting up and leaning forward, in full expiration. The diaphragm of the stethoscope should be pressed firmly to the chest at the lower left sternal border. A little luck may be needed to detect a rub, as it occurs intermittently.

6. How will the EKG appear in pericarditis?

The initial EKG abnormalities in pericarditis include ST-segment elevation in all leads except aVR and V_1, in which reciprocal depression occurs. The elevation is upwardly concave, and usually less than 5 mm above the baseline. In distinguishing pericarditis from early repolarization, the best discriminator is the ratio of the onset of the ST segment to the amplitude of the T wave in lead V_6. A ratio of 0.25 or more is indicative of pericarditis. A few days after the onset of pericarditis, the ST segments return to the baseline. PR depression may occur, followed by T-wave inversion, which may persist indefinitely or may normalize.

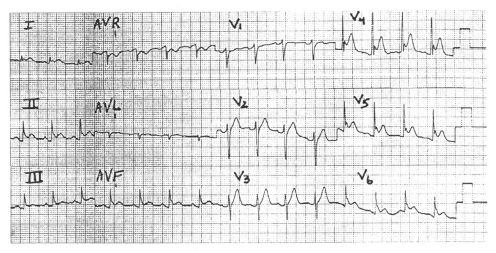

Example of an EKG consistent with acute pericarditis.

7. How can acute pericarditis be distinguished from acute myocardial infarction (AMI)?

Acute viral and idiopathic pericarditis typically occur in young, healthy patients without a cardiac history or risk factors for coronary artery disease. The pleuritic nature and sharp quality of the chest pain are distinct from ischemic chest pain, as is the relief obtained from sitting up and leaning forward. The pain of pericarditis is unresponsive to treatment with nitroglycerin.

Electrocardiographically, acute pericarditis contrasts with AMI in that the ST-segment elevations are diffuse and concave upward. The progression to T-wave inversion occurs after the ST segments have returned to the baseline, whereas in AMI it may accompany ST segment elevation.

8. How can acute pericarditis be distinguished from musculoskeletal chest pain?

Musculoskeletal chest pain generally is not relieved by sitting up, and the characteristic EKG abnormalities of pericarditis are not present.

9. Is pericardial effusion a concern in patients with pericarditis?

Yes. Pericardial effusion occurs most commonly in patients with acute viral or idiopathic, neoplastic, postradiation, or posttraumatic pericarditis. Its effects range from insignificant to life-threatening if tamponade occurs.

10. How much pericardial effusion is significant?

The normal pericardium can accommodate only 80–200 ml of fluid before intrapericardial pressure rises. A critical factor is the **rate** of accumulation of fluid—over 2000 ml may be tolerated, if it is accumulated slowly.

11. How can a pericardial effusion be diagnosed?
Echocardiography is the most sensitive test because it can detect as little as 15 ml of pericardial fluid. The cardiac silhouette will not be enlarged on chest x-ray until at least 250 ml of fluid has accumulated.

12. What is cardiac tamponade?
Cardiac tamponade exists when excess pericardial fluid prevents the atria and ventricles from filling adequately during diastole, decreasing the volume of blood available to be pumped during systole, and causing hemodynamic compromise. Although any form of pericarditis may lead to cardiac tamponade, acute tamponade is usually caused by trauma. Subacute tamponade occurs most commonly in neoplastic pericarditis.

13. How is cardiac tamponade diagnosed?
The diagnosis of this potentially life-threatening condition should be made clinically. Gradual accumulation of fluid will prompt patient complaints of dyspnea, with clinical findings of tachycardia, jugular venous distention, and pulsus paradoxus. **Rapid** accumulation of fluid producing tamponade, often due to penetrating cardiac injury, may cause decreased systemic arterial pressure, increased venous pressure, and muffled heart sounds, known as Beck's triad.

The chest x-ray usually demonstrates an enlarged cardiac silhouette with clear lung fields. The EKG may have low QRS voltage and T-wave flattening. An echocardiogram will quantitate the amount of pericardial fluid. The most accurate hemodynamic measurements are made by cardiac catheterization.

14. What is pulsus paradoxus?
Pulsus paradoxus is an abnormally large (more than 10 mmHg) drop in the systolic blood pressure with inspiration. Kussmaul termed this phenomenon "paradoxical" because of the disappearance of the pulse during inspiration when the heart was obviously still beating.

15. What is the appropriate ED management of pericarditis?
Anti-inflammatory agents such as indomethacin (Indocin), 25–75 mg four times a day, or aspirin, 650 mg every 3–4 hours, should be administered.

The use of corticosteroids is controversial. Although corticosteroids are effective anti-inflammatory agents, 10–20% of patients develop recurrent pericarditis as tapering occurs.

Echocardiography is indicated to rule out pericardial effusion.

If cardiac tamponade is present, percutaneous pericardiocentesis must be performed to relieve intracardiac pressure. Intravenous fluids should be infused rapidly to increase arterial pressure and cardiac output.

16. What is the prognosis for patients with pericarditis?
Most patients with pericarditis recover fully, although 15–20% will have a recurrence, probably due to an autoimmune mechanism. Nonsteroidal anti-inflammatory drugs (NSAIDs) are used for recurrences. If NSAIDs are ineffective, corticosteroid therapy is initiated. Colchicine holds promise as adjunctive therapy in recurrent pericarditis. Failure of medical therapy usually leads to pericardiectomy.

MYOCARDITIS

17. What is myocarditis?
Myocarditis is an inflammation of the myocardial wall.

18. What causes myocarditis?
Myocarditis is caused most commonly in the United States by viruses. Viruses can infiltrate the myocardium as they invade other body tissues. More commonly, a postviral myocarditis, which is a pathological autoimmune response to a recent infection, can occur. Protozoal (Chagas' disease), bacterial (diphtheria, tuberculosis), fungal, and spirochetal (Lyme disease) organisms can also infiltrate the myocardium. An autoimmune mechanism may cause myocarditis in systemic lupus erythematosus, Kawasaki disease, and the peripartum period.

19. When should a diagnosis of myocarditis be considered in the ED?
Diagnosing myocarditis in the ED is a challenge, as the symptoms and signs are non-specific. Myocarditis should be considered when a previously healthy person, usually young and often male, develops symptoms such as dyspnea, orthopnea, decreased exercise tolerance, palpitations, or syncope. Pericarditis frequently accompanies myocarditis, precipitating patient complaints of chest pain. Concomitant or recent upper respiratory or gastrointestinal illness may be elicited by history.

20. What clinical findings may be present?
The patient may be febrile. Sinus tachycardia is often present and may be out of proportion to the extent of temperature elevation. The specific clinical manifestations of myocarditis depend on the severity of the inflammatory process and the location of the lesions. A pericardial rub may be auscultated if myopericarditis is present. There may be conduction abnormalities, congestive heart failure, cardiogenic shock, or cardiac arrest.

21. Are there any chest x-ray or EKG abnormalities?
The chest x-ray may be abnormal, depending on the extent of disease. The cardiac silhouette may be enlarged due to ventricular cavity dilatation or pericardial effusion. The EKG most commonly shows sinus tachycardia. Other common and transitory abnormalities include rhythm disturbances, conduction defects, low voltage, and ST-T wave abnormalities. EKG abnormalities usually normalize within a few days to a few months.

22. How is myocarditis diagnosed?
The current definition is based on histopathologic examination of an endomyocardial biopsy rather than on clinical criteria. An inflammatory infiltrate and myocyte damage or necrosis are required to meet the "Dallas criteria." Failure to diagnose myocarditis in many clinical cases of myocarditis is believed to result from delay in obtaining the biopsy and from sampling errors.

Cardiac imaging with echocardiography may demonstrate ventricular wall motion abnormalities, dilated chambers, and depressed systolic function, but the etiology of heart failure is not revealed. Radionuclide scanning may identify areas of inflamed myocardium using gallium-67 and necrotic myocardium with indium 111-monoclonal antimyosin antibody imaging.

23. How can acute myocarditis be distinguished from AMI?
Myocarditis occurs primarily in young healthy patients without significant cardiac history or risk factors for coronary artery disease. Chest pain, dyspnea, EKG abnormalities, and cardiac enzyme elevation may occur in both conditions.

24. Is myocarditis a concern in acquired immunodeficiency syndrome (AIDS)?
Yes. The incidence of myocarditis found at autopsy of AIDS patients is as high as 52%, compared with 5% of the population as a whole. Their increased risk of myocarditis may be due to an abnormal autoimmune reaction, opportunistic infections, or the human immunodeficiency virus itself.

25. What is the appropriate ED management of a patient with myocarditis?
No specific drug has been found to be beneficial in the treatment of myocarditis. Therapy is based on bed rest and management of complications.

Specific treatment depends on the extent and location of myocardial dysfunction. Congestive heart failure is treated with conventional measures of oxygen and diuretics. Conduction abnormalities are managed with appropriate pharmacologic agents; a temporary transvenous pacer may need to be placed. The efficacy of immunosuppressive therapy has not been established. All patients with suspected acute myocarditis should be admitted to the hospital.

26. What is the prognosis for patients with acute myocarditis?
Most patients with myocarditis recover completely; dilated cardiomyopathy occurs uncommonly. Severe congestive cardiac failure may eventually require cardiac transplantation. Mural thromboses may develop due to reduced wall motion and blood flow, with the potential for thromboembolic complications.

27. Acute myocarditis is a disease of unknown incidence, with nonspecific symptoms and signs, imperfect diagnostic modalities, and no efficacious treatment. How can it possibly be appropriately diagnosed and managed in the ED?
As with any unusual but potentially life-threatening diseases, a high index of suspicion is necessary. Emergency medicine would not be fun and challenging if everything were easy!

BIBLIOGRAPHY

1. Ginzton LE, Laks MM: The differential diagnosis of acute pericarditis from the normal variant: New electrocardiographic criteria. Circulation 65:1004–1009, 1982.
2. Mizlozek CL, et al: Myocarditis presenting as acute myocardial infarction. Am Heart J 115:768–776, 1988.
3. Maze SS, Adolph RJ: Myocarditis: Unresolved issues in diagnosis and treatment. Clin Cardiol 13:69–79, 1990.
4. O'Connell JB, Mason JW: Diagnosing and treating active myocarditis. West J Med 150:431–435, 1989.
5. Peters NS, Poole-Wilson PA: Myocarditis: Continuing clinical and pathologic confusion (editorial). Am Heart J 121:942–947, 1991.
6. Shabetai R: Diseases of the pericardium. In Hurst JW (ed): The Heart: Arteries and Veins, 7th ed, vol. 2. New York, McGraw-Hill, 1990, pp 1348–1374.
7. Shabetai R: Acute pericarditis. Cardiol Clin 8:639–644, 1990.
8. Sternbach GL: Pericarditis. Ann Emerg Med 17:214–220, 1988.
9. Wenger NK, Abelmann WH, Roberts WC: Myocarditis. In Hurst JW (ed): The Heart: Arteries and Veins, 7th ed, vol. 2. New York, McGraw-Hill, 1990, pp 1256–1277.

30. AORTIC ANEURYSMS AND AORTIC DISSECTION

Thomas Drake, M.D.

1. Are aortic dissections and aortic aneurysms the same disease?
No. The processes occurring in the two diseases are different. Aortic dissection by definition involves intimal separation with formation of a pseudoaneurysm. A true aneurysm involves dilation of all layers of the arterial wall.

2. What are the risk factors for aortic aneurysms?

Hypertension is the most important predisposing factor for the development of aortic dissection. Atherosclerosis is thought to be another major predisposing factor. Others include diabetes, hyperlipidemia, smoking, hypertension, genetic predisposition and, more rarely, congenital defects. Other rare etiologies include syphilis, other infections, or aortitis. Males are ten times more likely to develop an aneurysm than females.

3. Describe the typical patient with an abdominal aneurysm.

An elderly male who has had manifestations of atherosclerosis, such as coronary artery disease or peripheral vascular disease.

4. What are the usual presenting signs and symptoms of abdominal aortic aneurysms?

Aortic aneurysms may often be found fortuitously on routine physical examination or via radiologic studies ordered for other reasons. The most common symptom with an acutely expanding or leaking aneurysm is constant abdominal pain, often localizing to the left middle or lower quadrant with radiation to the back. Depending on the degree of blood loss, the patient may have variable signs of hypovolemia, such as hypotension, syncope, or falling hematocrit.

5. Which studies should be ordered if an abdominal aneurysm is suspected?

No further studies should be performed in an unstable patient who has the clinical picture of a leaking aneurysm if performing the study delays operative intervention. If the patient is hemodynamically stable, the best screening exam is an ultrasound, which may be done quickly in the ED, where constant supervision of the patient is possible. If the aorta is normal, other potential conditions can be evaluated, such as biliary colic, nephrolithiasis, or pancreatitis. Disadvantages include potential obscuring of the aorta by bowel gas and the lack of demonstration of extravasation. Computed tomography (CT) is also an excellent way of visualizing the abdominal aorta and presence of retroperitoneal or free peritoneal blood. But it is time-consuming and requires moving the patient from the ED in most institutions. Angiography, considered the gold standard for evaluation of the aorta by many, gives excellent anatomic evaluation of the aorta and its branches but is invasive and time-consuming. Realistically, the study chosen is most often determined by judging the stability of the patient in relation to the specific anatomic questions to be answered.

6. What are the common reasons for missing this diagnosis?

Although physical examination is the best way of identifying an abdominal aneurysm (palpation possible in up to 80–90%), it may be difficult in the obese patient. Other more common and benign diagnoses that aortic aneurysm may mimic include pancreatitis, renal colic, biliary disease, or musculoskeletal back pain. Aneurysms may present atypically as gastrointestinal bleeding from a fistulous connection of the aorta with the small bowel. This most commonly occurs in patients with previous aortic surgery. A large aneurysm may cause unusual symptoms related to mass effect, such as bowel or ureteral obstruction. Radicular pain may occur if retroperitoneal bleeding causes a femoral or sciatic neuropathy. Peripheral embolization of mural plaque may cause peripheral ischemia as a presenting symptom.

7. What are the most common mistakes in the management of ruptured abdominal aneurysms in the ED?

1. Ascribing a patient's symptoms to a more benign condition.
2. Underaggressive fluid/blood volume resuscitation because of concerns about the patient's age or cardiac status.
3. Delay in operative intervention because of diagnostic studies.
4. Allowing hypothermia to occur from use of cold fluids and blood products. This causes many problems, most notably a significant coagulopathy.

8. Is the lateral abdominal x-ray useful?
The lateral abdominal x-ray may be useful if the aorta is calcified. A nonvisualized aorta has no diagnostic use.

9. What is the natural history of true aneurysms of the aorta?
Although smaller aneurysms fare better than larger ones, the natural history of this disease is progressive expansion and eventual rupture. The 1-year mortality rate of patients with initially asymptomatic abdominal aneurysm is about 50%. The elective operative mortality is 6% or less. The operative mortality for a ruptured abdominal aortic aneurysm is approximately 50%.

10. Do thoracic aortic dissections present in a different fashion?
Yes. Thoracic aortic dissections most commonly involve the proximal aorta and are more likely to cause chest and thoracic back pain that is typically excruciating. The patient usually looks acutely ill, requires large doses of narcotics to relieve pain, and is likely to be significantly hypertensive. Myocardial infarction may also be present if the dissecting process involves the coronary arteries.

11. Do all patients present with pain?
No. About 5–10% of patients with aortic dissection do not have pain as a major complaint. Indeed, aortic dissection may be painless in a minority of patients or, because of involvement of the carotids, may cause a stroke and render the patient incapable of communicating the pain. Unusual manifestations of dissection may relate to the process involving almost any peripheral artery. Thus the patient may present with abdominal pain from mesenteric artery involvement, renal failure from renal artery obstruction, or peripheral ischemia of an arm or leg. In addition, rupture of a bronchial artery may cause hemoptysis, or hoarseness may result from compression of the recurrent laryngeal nerve. Other mass effects may cause dysphagia or a chronic cough. Congestive heart failure may be caused by involvement of the aortic valve. Syncope and pericardial tamponade may be caused by rupture into the pericardial space.

12. What diagnostic studies prove thoracic aortic dissection?
Plain radiographs are abnormal in about 80% of patients. They may show dilation of the ascending aorta, mediastinal widening, loss of the aortic knob, left pleural effusion, deviation of the trachea or nasogastric tube, apical pleural "capping," or displacement of intimal calcium in the aorta. These signs are mostly indirect evidence and require confirmation by another study. CT is reported as the best noninvasive screening exam for dissection. It is sensitive and usually diagnostic, but it is now challenged by a relatively new mode of ultrasound called transesophageal echocardiography, which is performed by placing the transducer into the esophagus directly posterior to the heart and adjacent to the descending aorta. Because of proximity to these structures, it gives exceedingly detailed evaluation of the heart and aorta. Its advantages include availability in the ED, good sensitivity, and speed of evaluation. Disadvantages are its user-dependence, invasiveness, and need for sedation of the patient. Angiography remains useful in evaluation of aortic dissections because of its ability to evaluate the status of the coronary arteries and aortic valve.

13. What is the optimal ED treatment of aortic dissection?
Presumptive treatment of aortic dissection, which should be started before specific radiologic confirmation, includes aggressive control of blood pressure and pulse with nitroprusside and beta blockers. Some authorities now recommend using esmolol, a short-acting, intravenous beta blocker, because of its titratability. Narcotics should be used to relieve pain, but the goal of blood pressure/pulse control is to relieve pain by aborting or retarding the dissecting process.

14. Do all thoracic dissections require surgery?
Indications for surgery include all dissections involving the ascending aorta or aortic valve; rupture, enlargement, or progression in spite of medical therapy; or end-organ or limb ischemia. Medical treatment alone is indicated for patients not deemed surgical candidates or with isolated descending aortic involvement.

15. Where are true aneurysms most likely to occur?
They can occur in the thoracic aorta, but the abdominal aorta is more predisposed for several reasons. First, the abdominal aorta has higher systolic and larger pulse pressure than the thoracic aorta. This results from tapering of the aorta, smaller amounts of elastin in the infrarenal aorta, and turbulent flow from reflected pressure waves off the many branches of the abdominal aorta.

BIBLIOGRAPHY

1. Bergqvist D, Bengtsson H: Risk factors for rupture of abdominal aortic aneurysm. Acta Chir Scand 156:63–68, 1990.
2. Jehle D, Davis E, Evans T, et al: Emergency department sonography by emergency physicians. Am J Emerg Med 7:605–611, 1989.
3. Kronzon I, Demopoulos L, Schrem SS, et al: Pitfalls in the diagnosis of thoracic aortic aneurysm by transesophageal echocardiography. J Am Soc Echo 3:145–148, 1990.
4. Pierce GE: Abdominal aortic aneurysms. Surg Clin North Am 69(4):1989.
5. Rosen P, Baker FJ, Barkin RM, et al (eds): Emergency Medicine: Concepts and Clinical Practice, 3rd ed. St. Louis, Mosby–Year Book, 1992.
6. Swinton NW, Jewell ER, Tsapatsaris NP: Abdominal aortic aneurysms. Cardiol Clin 9:483–438, 1991.
7. Taams M, Gissemjpvem WK, Schippers LA, et al: The value of transesophageal echocardiography for diagnosis of thoracic aorta pathology. Eur Heart J 9:1308–1316, 1988.

31. PACEMAKERS IN EMERGENCY MEDICINE

Stanley J. Galle, Jr., M.D., FACEP

1. What is a pacemaker?
A pacemaker is an external source of energy used to stimulate the heart. It consists of a pulse generator (i.e., power source), head connections to the pulse generator, leads, and the myocardial-lead interface.

2. What is the difference between a fixed-rate mode and a demand mode?
In the fixed-rate mode, the pulse generator produces an electrical impulse at a fixed rate without influence from the patient's cardiac activity. In the demand mode, the pulse generator senses cardiac activity and fires only in the absence of cardiac depolarization.

3. What does a pacer setting of "DDD" mean?
The letters represent a pacing code. The code consists of 3 to 5 letters that describe the different types of pacer function. The first letter indicates the chamber paced, the second the chamber in which electrical activity is sensed, and the third the response to a sensed event. A fourth and fifth letter may be added to describe whether the pacemaker is programmable and whether special functions to protect against tachycardia are available. A DDD pacer is thus able to pace and sense both the atria and ventricle ((D)ual chambers)

and has a (D)ual response to the sensed ventricular and atrial activity, i.e., can pace either the atria or the ventricle. For example, spontaneous atrial and ventricular activity inhibits atrial and ventricular pacing; atrial activity without ventricular activity triggers only ventricular pacing.

Pacing Code

FIRST	SECOND	THIRD
A(trial	A(trial)	O(no response)
V(entricle)	V(entricle)	I(nhibition)
D(ual chamber)	D(ual chamber)	T(riggering)
		D(ual response)
Changer(s) paced	Chamber(s) sensed	Response of pacing function to a sensed event

4. What is the difference between temporary and permanent pacing?

In temporary pacing, the power source is external to the body. Temporary pacing is used to provide immediate stabilization when the indications for pacing are present (see question #5). Temporary pacing is generally accomplished with external cutaneous pacemakers and less commonly via the transvenous or transesophageal routes. In permanent pacing, the power source is placed subcutaneously. Permanent pacing is reserved for symptomatic bradycardia unrelated to self-limiting factors, or for documented persistent infranodal second- or third-degree blocks. Permanent pacemakers are implanted subcutaneously in the upper chest, with transvenous leads usually inserted via the subclavian vein to the endocardium of the right atrium or ventricle.

5. What are the indications for temporary pacing?

Sinus node dysfunction
  Symptomatic sinus bradycardia
  Sinus pauses >3 sec
AV nodal block
  Symptomatic second-degree AV block
    (Mobitz I)
  Symptomatic complete heart block

Infranodal block
  New bifascicular block associated
    with acute myocardial infarction
  Alternating bundle branch block
    with changing PR
  Second-degree AV block (Mobitz II)
  Complete heart block

6. Who should perform pacemaker placement in an emergency setting?

This depends on the patient's stability. If a condition exists that indicates pacing, and the patient has stable vital signs, placement should be performed in the best possible setting by the most experienced physician available. However, if the patient is hemodynamically compromised and cannot be stabilized with drug therapy, pacing should be performed by the emergency physician. Transthoracic external pacing should be attempted initially. If successful, a transvenous pacemaker should be inserted.

7. What is the best venous route for an emergency transvenous pacemaker?

Although all central venous routes (subclavian, internal jugular, femoral) may be used, emergency pacing is usually necessitated in the setting of low or absent forward flow. The straightest line from the insertion point to the tip of the right ventricle is the right internal jugular vein.

8. What is the most common cause of permanent pacemaker malfunction?

Because of greater technologic sophistication, patients with pacemaker problems present to the emergency department (ED) much less commonly now than in the past. Declining battery sources decay very slowly and are usually picked up by regular follow-up visits in pacemaker clinics. Today, most pacemaker failures are due to problems with the electrodes or the wires, not the battery or the pulse generator.

9. What complications typically occur in the month following pacemaker insertion?
Most of the early problems are related to implantation. A seroma or hematoma may occur at the pulse generator pocket. Of greater concern is infection of the pocket, which requires removal of the generator. Thrombosis may occur at the lead implant, the tricuspic valve, or the subclavian vein, and may even cause superior vena cava syndrome. Pacemaker syndrome is usually a late complication. Subacute bacterial endocarditis, lead infection, ventricular pacer failure, and "runaway pacemaker" are seen rarely.

10. What is pacemaker syndrome?
It is a clinical spectrum of lightheadedness, fatigue, palpitations, syncope, dyspnea on exertion, and hypotension that is usually attributed to asynchronous atrioventricular contraction.

11. Do patients with pacemaker syndrome require admission?
No. This complication occurs in 25% of patients with a pacemaker and, of those, no cause can be found in 25%. Before discharge, however, a careful exam should be done to rule out all potential causes.

12. What is "twiddler's syndrome"?
This is the most common cause of late lead dislodgement. It results from the twisting or "twiddling" of a pulse generator in its pouch to the point of twisting leads around the generator box, thus shortening and dislodging them from their proper position.

13. What is pacemaker-mediated tachycardia?
A normally functioning pacemaker may initiate a tachyrhythmia. Retrograde conduction of a ventricular beat may cause the atrium to trigger a second ventricular contraction that falls during the pacemaker's refractory period. Because this contraction is not sensed by the pacemaker, the pulse generator fires, initiating a reentrant tachycardia.

14. How is pacemaker-mediated tachycardia treated?
Treatment consists of lengthening the atrioventricular time by any of the following methods: (1) programming an increase in the atrial refractory time; (2) administering adenosine or verapamil; (3) increasing atrial sensory threshold; or (4) applying a magnet to stop atrial sensing by the pacemaker.

15. What is a runaway pacemaker?
It is malfunction of the pacemaker that is manifested by tachycardias secondary to rapid ventricular pacing. The problem is recognized when rates are greater than the upper rate limit settings of the pacemaker and may require drastic measures such as cutting the pacer leads.

16. What is the lifetime of a permanent pacemaker?
It varies depending on the amount of pacing, sensing, and thresholds for capture, but in general is 4–6 years.

17. What happens as pacemakers lose battery power?
Pacemakers usually show a decline in the rate of magnet-mediated pacing, usually to a predetermined manufacturer's rate. However, pacer response varies with manufacturer— some models may change pacer mode also (e.g., DDD to VVI).

18. How do I assess a patient with potential pacemaker malfunction?
First, take a careful history with regard to the perceived problem. The physical exam should include inspection of the neck for jugular venous distension and canon waves. An EKG should be obtained to evaluate pacemaker function, and anteroposterior and lateral chest x-rays obtained to ascertain pacemaker lead placement and connector integrity.

19. What is the most reliable indicator of pacer malfunction?
The most reliable indicator is rates that are usually inappropriate for paced hearts. A paced ventricular rate below 60 or above 100 is probably secondary to pacemaker malfunction.

20. What does a magnet do?
Placing a pacemaker magnet over the pulse generator stops the pacemaker from sensing or responding to a sensed event. The pacemaker thus reverts to a fixed rate mode: either the AOO (atrium paced) or the VOO (ventricle paced) mode. The purpose is to check the pacing rate, which should be done quickly, as the pulse generator is no longer prevented from firing during the T wave or from initiating serious arrhythmias.

21. Can a patient with a permanent pacemaker be defibrillated?
Yes, but it is important to place the paddles away from the pulse generator, preferably in the anterior-posterior position.

22. Can defibrillation damage the pulse generator when current passes through?
Yes. Temporary or even permanent loss of ventricular or atrial capture may occur secondary to elevation of the capture threshold of the pacer leads.

23. Can an external pacemaker be used if a permanent pacemaker malfunctions?
Yes, but be careful to place the external pacer on a PACE ONLY (fixed-rate) mode and not the sensing mode; otherwise it may sense spikes from the permanent pacer and not fire.

BIBLIOGRAPHY

1. Brinker JA: Pursuing the perfect pacemaker. Mayo Clin Proc 64:587, 1989.
2. Broka JJ: External transcutaneous pacemakers. Ann Emerg Med 18:1280, 1989.
3. Ellenbogan KA (ed): Cardiac Pacing. Boston, Blackwell Scientific Publications, 1992.
4. Ellenbogan KA, et al: New insights into pacemaker syndrome gained from hemodynamic, humoral, and vascular responses during ventriculoatrial pacing. Am J Cardiol 65:53, 1990.
5. Fujiki A, et al: Pacemaker syndrome evaluated by cardiopulmonary exercise testing. PACE 13:1236, 1990.
6. Furman S, Gross J: Dual chamber pacing and pacemakers. Curr Probl Cardiol 15:3, 1990.
7. Garson A: Stepwise approach to the unknown pacemaker ECG. Am Heart J 119:924, 1990.
8. Handley PC, et al: Two decades of cardiac pacing at the Mayo Clinic (1961 through 1981). Mayo Clin Proc 59:268, 1984.
9. Kissoon N, et al: Role of transcutaneous pacing in the setting of a failing permanent pacemaker. Pediatr Emerg Care 5:178, 1989.
10. Klottis TM, et al: Atrial pacing: Who do we pace and what do we expect? Experiences with 100 atrial pacemakers. PACE 13:625, 1990.
11. Lehman RB, et al: The potential utility of sensor-driven pacing in DDD pacemakers. Am Heart J 18:919, 1989.
12. Stapczynski JS: Disturbances of cardiac rhythm and conduction. In Tintinalli JE, Krome RL, Ruiz E (eds): Emergency Medicine: A Comprehensive Study Guide, 3rd ed. New York, McGraw-Hill, 1992.
13. Tilden SJ, et al: Runaway temporary pacemaker caused by a component defect. Crit Care Med 17:1231, 1989.
14. Zullo MA: Function of ventricular pacemakers during resuscitation. PACE 13:736, 1990.

VII. Gastrointestinal Tract

32. ESOPHAGUS AND STOMACH DISORDERS

Philip L. Henneman, M.D., FACEP

1. How are gastrointestinal (GI) problems differentiated from acute myocardial infarction?
Esophageal or gastric pain can present with visceral-type chest pain or upper abdominal pain and nausea that are difficult to differentiate from those related to myocardial ischemia or infarction. Description of the pain, determination of cardiac risk factors, and appropriate use of electrocardiography (EKG) in adult patients with visceral-type pain or cardiac risk factors will minimize clinical errors. It is important to remember that nitroglycerin, antacids, and GI cocktails are therapeutic interventions, not diagnostic tests. Patients with esophageal spasm may respond to nitroglycerin and antacids, or GI cocktails may provide a placebolike benefit to the patient with cardiac ischemia.

2. What is a GI cocktail?
The two most commonly used GI cocktails contain antacids (30 cc), viscous lidocaine (10 cc), and either Donnatal (10 cc) or dicyclomine (Bentyl) 20 mg. These cocktails may provide temporary symptomatic relief of minor esophageal and gastric irritation.

3. What is heartburn?
Heartburn is burning retrosternal discomfort that may radiate to the sides of the chest, neck, or jaw. It is characteristic of reflux esophagitis and is often made worse by bending forward or lying recumbent, or after meals. It may be relieved by upright posture, liquids (including saliva or water), or, more reliably, antacids. Heartburn is probably due to heightened mucosal sensitivity and can be reproduced by infusion of dilute hydrochloric acid (Bernstein test) into the esophagus.

4. How is reflux esophagitis treated?
In addition to antacids, general measures include elevation of the head of the bed (e.g., 4 inches), weight reduction, and elimination of factors that increase abdominal pressure. Patients should avoid alcohol, chocolate, coffee, fatty foods, mint, orange juice, smoking, ingestion of large quantities of food and drink, and certain medications (e.g., anticholinergics or calcium channel blockers). Antacids after meals and H_2 blockers (e.g., cimetidine) before bedtime are often helpful. Resistant cases may respond to sucralfate before meals and metoclopramide (10 mg q.i.d.). Treatment may need to be continued for as long as 6 months, and the disease may quickly recur.

5. What are the esophageal causes of odynophagia?
Odynophagia, or painful swallowing, is a characteristic of nonreflux esophagitis. Infectious esophagitis is a common cause and usually occurs in immunocompromised patients and can be due to fungal (e.g., monilial), viral (e.g., herpes, cytomegalovirus), bacterial (lactobacillus, beta-hemolytic streptococci), or parasitic organisms. Other types of nonreflux esophagitis include radiation, corrosive, pill-induced, and certain systemic diseases (e.g., Beçhet's,

Crohn's, pemphigus vulgaris, Stevens-Johnson syndrome). Odynophagia is unusual in reflux esophagitis but may occur with a peptic ulcer of the esophagus (Barrett's ulcer).

6. How does esophageal obstruction present?

Except in infants, there is usually a history of eating or swallowing something that is followed by the onset of chest pain, odynophagia, or inability to swallow. Foreign bodies usually lodge at one of four locations: cervical esophagus, upper esophageal sphincter, aortic arch, and lower esophageal sphincter. Obstruction by food may occur wherever there is narrowing of the lumen due to stricture, carcinoma, or a lower esophageal ring. Round, blunt objects may be removed using a Foley catheter that is inserted beyond the object; the balloon is inflated and then the catheter is gently withdrawn with the patient in a steep head-down position. This procedure is most often done under fluoroscopy. Foreign bodies, especially those that are sharp (e.g., needle), impacted food, or objects that cannot be removed with the Foley method are best removed endoscopically. Meat tenderizer should not be used to facilitate passage of obstructed meat. Glucagon (0.5–2 mg IV) may relieve distal esophageal food obstruction in about one-third of patients.

7. What is Mallory-Weiss syndrome?

Mallory-Weiss syndrome is a mucosal tear that usually involves the gastric mucosa near the squamocolumnar mucosal junction; it may also involve the esophageal mucosa. It is usually caused by vomiting and retching. Patients may present with upper GI bleeding.

8. What causes esophageal perforation? How is it diagnosed?

Esophageal perforation, a true emergency, is caused by iatrogenic damage during instrumentation, external trauma, increased intraesophageal pressure associated with forceful vomiting (Borhaave's syndrome), or diseases of the esophagus (e.g., corrosive esophagitis, ulceration, neoplasm). Esophageal perforation causes chest pain that is often severe and may be worsened by swallowing and breathing. Chest radiograph may reveal air within the mediastinum, pericardium, pleural space (pneumothorax), or subcutaneous tissue. Esophageal perforation may lead to leakage of gastric contents into the mediastinum and secondary infection (i.e., mediastinitis). The diagnosis is confirmed by swallow and leakage of radiopaque contrast material. Treatment includes broad-spectrum antibiotics, gastric suction, and surgical repair and drainage as soon as possible.

9. What causes abdominal pain of gastric or duodenal origin?

It is estimated that 10% of cases of abdominal pain seen in the emergency department (ED) are due to gastric or duodenal disease. Gastritis and peptic ulcer disease (PUD) (i.e., ulcer of the stomach or duodenum due to gastric acid) account for the majority of patients with abdominal pain due to gastric or duodenal disease. Perforated PUD and gastric volvulus are the two most serious conditions requiring immediate diagnosis and treatment.

10. What are the common causes of gastritis and PUD?

Exogenous causes of gastric mucosal damage include aspirin, alcohol, hemorrhagic shock, and indomethacin. Bile and pancreatic fluid may damage the gastric mucosal barrier. Cigarette smoking decreases pyloric sphincter tone and causes increased bile reflux. The importance of psychological factors in the development of PUD is controversial.

11. How does perforated peptic ulcer present?

Perforated peptic ulcer disease (and gastric volvulus) presents with sudden onset of abdominal pain that may or may not be related to eating. The pain is usually steady and refractory to antacids; it often radiates to the back but may also radiate to the chest or upper abdomen. Vomiting is present in approximately 50%.

On physical examination, patients appear in acute distress and often demonstrate tachycardia. Blood pressure may be elevated secondary to pain or decreased secondary to extensive fluid loss from generalized peritonitis. Patients usually lie still and avoid movement. Involuntary guarding, rebound tenderness, and abdominal rigidity are common. Bowel sounds are usually absent or significantly decreased.

Laboratory work may reveal nonspecific leukocytosis (40% have WBC >14,000). If vomiting has been significant, hypochloremic, hypokalemic, metabolic alkalosis may be seen. A small percentage of patients have mild hyperamylasemia. Free air will be present on upright chest x-ray or abdominal left lateral decubitus view in over 70%.

12. How should a patient suspected of having a perforated ulcer be managed?

Patients with severe abdominal pain should be undressed, placed on a cardiac monitor, and have a large-bore intravenous line placed for fluid resuscitation with crystalloid (normal saline or lactated Ringer's solution). Patients at risk for cardiac disease should be given supplemental oxygen. A prompt but thorough physical examination should be performed, including pelvic and rectal examinations. Blood should be drawn for complete blood count, electrolytes, blood urea nitrogen (BUN), creatinine, amylase, and type and screen. An EKG should be obtained on patients over the age of 40 years. A Foley catheter should be placed and urinalysis performed. A portable upright chest x-ray or abdominal left lateral decubitus view often helps to demonstrate free intraperitoneal air. A nasogastric tube should be placed and prompt surgical consultation obtained. Broad-spectrum antibiotics should be given and the patient prepared for emergency laparotomy. Once the decision has been made to operate on the patient, intravenous analgesics (opiates) should be administered for patient comfort.

13. What differentiates upper from lower GI hemorrhage?

Upper GI hemorrhage is bleeding that is proximal to the ligament of Treitz and lower GI bleeding is distal. In the ED, this is evaluated by placement of a nasogastric or orogastric tube and aspiration of gastric and proximal duodenal contents. Physical appearance of the aspirate (coffee grounds, red-tinged fluid or fresh blood) is the best way of determining the presence of significant upper GI bleeding; testing of gastric content for blood with various cards (e.g., Hemoccult, Gastroccult) is not reliable.

14. What are the causes of upper GI bleeding?

Etiology of Significant Upper GI Bleeding

ETIOLOGY	PERCENT
Peptic ulcer disease	45
Gastric erosions	23
Varices	10
Mallory-Weiss tear	7
Esophagitis	6
Duodenitis	6

Adapted from Henneman PL.[3]

15. What is the emergency management of upper GI bleeding?

Management of significant upper GI bleeding begins with a rapid assessment and management of the patient's airway, breathing, and cardiovascular status. Patients should be undressed, placed on a cardiac monitor, and given supplemental oxygen. Patients with compromised or unprotected airway should be promptly intubated. The history of GI bleeding (i.e., vomiting blood or passing black or blood stool) is sufficient to lead to the placement of a large-bore, peripheral intravenous catheter with infusion of either normal saline or lactated Ringer's solution. A focused physical examination should be performed, checking for signs of shock (altered mental status, tachycardia, hypotension, cool extremities, delayed capillary fill, etc.). The evaluation should include skin signs, pulmonary, cardiac and abdominal examination, and testing of stool for blood. Patients who demonstrate abnormal vital signs or signs of shock should have two or more intravenous lines placed and be given rapid infusion of crystalloid (5–30 cc/kg). During the initial examination and resuscitation, a history should be obtained. Patients with stable vital signs should be cautiously evaluated for postural changes in blood pressure or pulse. Blood should be drawn for type and cross-matching, hematocrit, platelet count, prothrombin time (PT), partial thromboplastin time (PTT), electrolytes, BUN, and creatinine. Elderly patients, patients with a history of cardiovascular disease, and patients who are severely anemic should have an EKG to evaluate for signs of cardiac eschemia (i.e., ST depression). A chest radiograph (portable, upright) should be taken to rule out subdiaphragmatic air or aspiration. A nasogastric (or orogastric) tube should be placed to determine the presence of blood in the stomach.

GI bleeding usually stops spontaneously and no further ED management is necessary other than admission and perhaps transfusion if there is significant anemia (i.e., Hct <25%). In 20% or less of patients, continued GI hemorrhage requires further management and treatment.

16. How should a patient with continued GI hemorrhage be managed?
Blood replacement should begin in patients who continue to demonstrate signs of shock or cardiovascular instability. Patients who do not respond promptly (i.e, remain hypotensive) to a 30 cc/kg infusion of crystalloid should be given O-negative blood if type-specific blood is not yet available. Cross-matched blood takes approximately 45–60 minutes to be available. If patients continue to demonstrate signs of shock or require more than 3 or 4 units of blood, a surgery and gastroenterology consult should be obtained. Upper GI bleeding may be stopped through the endoscope, but emergency operative repair is often required in patients with persistent GI bleeding.

17. Is placement of a nasogastric or orogastric tube contraindicated in someone with esophageal varices?
There is no evidence that a properly placed nasogastric or orogastric tube results in a significantly increased risk of tearing varices or increased size of a Mallory-Weiss tear. Nasogastric or orogastric tubes can perforate the esophagus or posterior pharynx if they are too aggressively placed. Diagnostic nasogastric or orogastric tubes are not necessary if the patient vomits gastric contents in the ED, as this may be inspected for the presence of blood.

18. Does iced saline lavage decrease gastric bleeding?
No, but it may result in hypothermia. The use of iced fluid to lavage patients with upper GI hemorrhage is no longer recommended. Gastric lavage is necessary only in patients who have no aspirate after the tube is placed. Lavage fluid need not be saline or sterile; regular tap water is fine. The only other indication for gastric lavage in patients with upper GI bleeding is immediately prior to endoscopy in order to improve visualization.

19. Should all patients with upper GI bleeding undergo endoscopy?
Endoscopy is the most accurate diagnostic tool available in the evaluation of patients with upper GI bleeding. Endoscopy identifies a lesion in 78–95% of patients with upper GI bleeding, if it is performed within 12–24 hours of hemorrhage. Endoscopy, however, has not been shown to affect hospital mortality, recurrence of bleeding, the number of transfusions required, or duration of hospital stay in such patients. Therefore, in most patients with upper GI bleeding, endoscopy is indicated for diagnostic purposes but not in the acute setting (i.e., during their stay in the ED). In patients with ongoing, persistent bleeding,

endoscopy may be acutely useful, especially if the active bleeding is due to an ulcer or varix that can be treated through the endoscope. Endoscopy also may identify the source of persistent bleeding and help the surgeon to decide on the proper operative approach.

20. Where should patients with upper GI hemorrhage be admitted?

Admission Guidelines for Upper GI Bleeding

ICU	WARD
Unstable vital signs	Stable* with melena
Persistent bleeding	Stable* with hematemesis that
Initial hypotension	quickly clears
Elderly (age >75 yrs)	History of bleeding, normal exam,
Severe anemia or large drop in Hct	comorbid disease
Significant complication(s)	
Unstable comorbid disease(s)	

Adapted from Henneman PL.[3]
*Stable means nonpostural vital signs, without signs of shock, significant anemia, or persistent bleeding.

21. Can I send someone home who reports a history of vomiting blood or passing a melenotic stool, but I find no objective evidence of significant blood loss?

Yes. Patients who report a history of GI bleeding but who have stable, nonpostural vital signs, a normal examination, a normal or near-normal hematocrit, stool that is negative or trace positive for blood, and no significant comorbid diseases can be discharged home from the ED with close (within 24 hours) follow-up. They should be instructed to return immediately to the ED if they become dizzy or lightheaded, vomit blood, or pass a black or bloody stool.

BIBLIOGRAPHY

1. Drugs for treatment of peptic ulcers. Med Letter 33:111–114, 1991.
2. Goyal RK: Diseases of the esophagus. In Wilson JD, et al (eds): Harrison's Principles of Internal Medicine, 12th ed. New York, McGraw-Hill, 1991, pp 1222–1229.
3. Henneman PL: Gastrointestinal bleeding. In Rosen P, et al (eds): Emergency Medicine: Concepts and Clinical Practice, 3rd ed. St. Louis, Mosby–Year Book, 1992, pp 1515–1532.
4. McGuigan JE: Peptic ulcer and gastritis. In Wilson JD, et al (eds): Harrison's Principles of Internal Medicine, 12th ed. New York, McGraw-Hill, 1991, pp 1229–1248.
5. Peterson WL, et al: Routine early endoscopy in upper gastrointestinal bleeding: A randomized, controlled trial. N Engl J Med 304:925, 1981.

33. APPENDICITIS

Denise Norton, M.D., and Charles Abernathy, M.D.

1. What is the most common cause of an acute abdomen?

Acute appendicitis.

2. Which patients should be suspected of having acute appendicitis?

The diagnosis of appendicitis must be considered in any patient presenting with abdominal pain who has not had an appendectomy.

3. What is the blood supply to the appendix?

Arterial blood is supplied by the appendicular branch of the ileocolic artery. Venous drainage occurs through the ileocolic vein, which empties into the superior mesenteric vein.

4. What causes appendicitis?

Most cases have no identifiable cause; however, an obstructive process (fecalith, foreign body, tumor, adhesion, or parasite) can occlude the lumen of the appendix and initiate an inflammatory response. The mucosa of the appendix continues to secrete behind the obstruction, increasing intraluminal pressure. This leads to edema and progressive vascular congestion, impeding arterial supply, and to eventual gangrene (after 24–36 hours) and perforation.

5. What is the classic sequence of symptoms for acute appendicitis?

Pain starts in the periumbilical region and moves to the right lower quadrant in 70% of cases. When the pain becomes severe, the patient may lie still with legs flexed. With appendiceal rupture the patient may experience temporary relief of pain; however, as peritonitis develops, the pain becomes diffuse and severe. The elderly and children are less likely to have this classic presentation.

6. Explain the sequence of physical findings.

Central, epigastric, colicky pain occurs secondary to stretching of the inflamed appendix wall. As intraluminal inflammation progresses, it involves the serosa and the parietal peritoneum, causing the sensation of pain to shift to the right lower quadrant. As serosal tension decreases with perforation, some patients experience a brief period of pain relief. Diffuse abdominal pain results from generalized peritonitis after perforation.

7. What physical signs may be associated with appendicitis?

- Tenderness may be experienced in the right lower quadrant.
- If the appendix is retrocecal, the patient may experience right flank pain.
- An appendix located low in the pelvis may be associated with tenderness on rectal or pelvic exam, but rectal tenderness is usually secondary to a concomitant pelvic abscess.
- Positive iliopsoas sign—tenderness is elicited with passive extension of the hip.
- Obturator sign is elicited by flexing the patient's right thigh at the hip with the knee bent and rotating the leg internally at the hip. Pain in the right lower quadrant with this maneuver may indicate appendicitis.

8. Which nonspecific symptoms may be associated with appendicitis?

Anorexia (90%), nausea and vomiting (75%), fever, malaise, diarrhea, and obstipation. However, patients may present with none of these symptoms. Infants with appendicitis are irritable, anorexic, and lethargic.

9. What laboratory tests might be helpful?

Leukocyte count—in approximately 90% of patients, it will be >10,000, but may be entirely normal.

Urinalysis—to rule out ureteral calculi or urinary tract infection.

Beta human chorionic gonadotropin (B-HCG)—to help rule out ectopic pregnancy.

Abdominal radiographs—nonspecific but may demonstrate a fecalith. These studies may also demonstrate some other cause of the abdominal pain (bowel obstruction, free air, etc.).

10. What is the role of ultrasound in diagnosing appendicitis?

In some studies ultrasound has decreased the negative laparotomy rate from as high as 20% to <10%. Sensitivities are reported to be as high as 96% and specificities as high as 94%

in the hands of some radiologists using graded compression ultrasound. Ultrasound criteria for appendicitis include: (1) any visualization of the appendix, (2) appendiceal diameter >6 mm, (3) muscular wall thickness ≥3 mm, and (4) presence of a complex mass indicating an appendiceal abscess.

11. What age group has the highest incidence of appendicitis?
Second and third decades of life.

12. In what group of patients is the incidence of perforation of the appendix greatest prior to operation?
Young children, particularly <5, and the elderly. The incidence of perforation in these groups is as high as 60–70% in some studies. Infants are more likely to have poor localization of an appendiceal abscess because the omentum, which functions to wall off infections, is thin and small. However, appendicitis is rare in infants since the appendix has a wide lumen, making the risk of luminal obstruction leading to acute inflammation unlikely.

13. What is the differential diagnosis for right lower quadrant pain in children?
Mesenteric adenitis, gastroenteritis, intussusception (<2 years old), and Meckel's diverticulum. Mesenteric adenitis, which is inflammation of the lymph nodes in the mesentery of the terminal ileum, is thought to be caused by ileal enteritis from *Yersinia enterocolitica*.

14. What might cause a mass and right lower quadrant tenderness in the elderly?
Acute diverticulitis in the cecum (rare) or redundant sigmoid colon. Cecal carcinoma must also be considered.

15. In which group of patients will the diagnosis of appendicitis have the highest false-positive rate?
Women of childbearing age, making a complete gynecologic and obstetric history essential.

16. What are the most common disorders confused with appendicitis in young women?
Acute salpingitis, in which pain begins in the lower abdomen, not the periumbilical region, is characterized by leukocytosis, high fevers, cervical motion tenderness (chandelier sign), and vaginal discharge. Other causes of right lower quadrant pain in young women are pelvic inflammatory disease, ruptured corpus luteum cysts, and ectopic pregnancy (always check a β-HCG on any female with lower abdominal pain). Mittelschmerz, the pain from the rupture of an ovarian follicle at the time of ovulation, may be differentiated from appendicitis by the characteristic of sudden lower abdominal pain at mid-menstrual cycle, rapid improvement in symptoms, and no gastrointestinal symptoms.

17. What clinical findings in pregnancy suggest appendicitis?
Because the location of the appendix changes in pregnancy, during the third trimester pain and tenderness tend to shift toward the right upper quadrant, right subcostal region, or right flank area. With a gravid uterus and accompanying laxity of the abdominal wall, pain may be difficult to localize, and guarding and rebound may be less obvious. With appendicitis, fetal mortality is estimated to be approximately 8%, and 30% when symptoms of peritonitis are present. Therefore, early operation is indicated for appendicitis during pregnancy.

18. How might appendicitis be confused with urologic disorders?
A retrocecal appendix or a gravid uterus may cause flank or costovertebral angle tenderness. Suprapubic pain may occur if the appendix irritates the bladder. In addition,

secondary to an inflammatory response from an adjacent appendicitis, patients may have sterile pyuria. However, the opposite is also true in that cystitis or the passage of a kidney stone may cause right lower quadrant pain.

19. How might the presentation of appendicitis differ in patients with AIDS/HIV infection or any other immunodeficiency?

Patients will present with the same signs and symptoms as immunocompetent patients; however, they are unlikely to demonstrate a leukocytosis. Patients with AIDS are prone to develop a number of gastrointestinal disorders such as gastroenteritis and typhlitis. The frequency of appendicitis has not been documented to be any different from that of the rest of the population.

20. What is the initial therapy for appendicitis?

Intravenous fluid hydration is immediately initiated to replace fluid deficits and to maintain hydration. A surgical consultation should be sought early, as the morbidity and mortality of appendicitis are directly related to progression to perforation and gangrene.

21. What is an acceptable rate for removal of normal appendices?

Figures as high as 15% have been quoted in the past. However, excluding females 12–25 years old, most surgeons' rate of removal of normal appendices will be less than 5%.

22. What are the complications of appendicitis?

Wound infection (most common), perforation, appendiceal abscess, and pylephlebitis.

23. What is pylephlebitis? What are its symptoms?

Portal vein pyemia leading to the development of hepatic abscesses. Symptoms include jaundice, high fevers, chills, and severe illness. The source is usually a perforated or gangrenous appendix, but with the use of antibiotics this is a rare complication.

24. Can antibiotics affect the rate of infectious complications?

Yes. Preoperative antibiotics have been demonstrated to decrease the rate of wound infections from 30% to 8% in patients with gangrenous appendicitis. They also decrease the rate of wound infections in acute appendicitis from 7% to 2%.

25. What are the most common organisms seen in early and late appendicitis?

Early appendicitis is associated with aerobic organisms: *Escherichia coli, Streptococcus viridans, Pseudomonas aeruginosa,* and group D Streptococcus. As appendicitis progresses, it becomes a mixed aerobic and anaerobic infection. A common anaerobic bacteria seen is *Bacteroides fragilis.* Antibiotics should cover both groups of organisms.

26. What are the operative options for appendectomy?

Open appendectomy and laparoscopic appendectomy. Laparoscopy has the advantage of allowing wide visualization of the abdomen and pelvis, which is particularly helpful in evaluating young women in that it allows differentiation of appendicitis from gynecologic disease with minimally invasive surgery. The laparoscopic procedure decreases irritation of patients' tissues in that they are not handled physically, resulting in decreased postoperative ileus and therefore shorter hospital stays. It should also result in decreased development of adhesions. In addition, the small incisions allow for earlier return to normal activity. In the larger studies of this procedure there were no mortalities; operating time was 15–20 minutes. Laparoscopy is not feasible in patients who may have had several previous operative procedures resulting in adhesions.

BIBLIOGRAPHY

1. Bennion et al: The bacteriology of gangrenous and perforated appendicitis. Ann Surg 211:165–171, 1990.
2. Binderow SR, Shaked AA: Acute appendicitis in patients with AIDS/HIV infection. Am J Surg 162:9–12, 1991.
3. Gamal R, Moore TC: Appendicitis in children aged 13 years and younger. Am J Surg 159:589–592, 1990.
4. Gotz et al: Modified laparoscopic appendectomy in surgery: A report of 388 operations. Surg Endosc 4, 1990.
5. Horattas MC, Guyton DP, Wu D: A reappraisal of appendicitis in the elderly. Am J Surg 160:291–293, 1990.
6. Tamir IL, Bongard FS, Klein SR: Acute appendicitis in the pregnant patient. Am J Surg 160:571–575, 1990.
7. Paulman AA, Huebner DM, Forrest TS: Sonography in the diagnosis of acute appendicitis. Am Fam Physician 44:465–468, 1991.
8. Pier A, Gotz F, Bacher C: Laparoscopic appendectomy in 625 cases: From innovation to routine. Surg Laparosc Endosc 1:8–13, 1991.
9. Ricci MA, Trevisani MF, Beck WC: Acute appendicitis: A 5-year review. Am Surg 57:301–305, 1991.
10. Rothrock SG, Skeoch G, Rush JJ, Johnson NE: Clinical features of misdiagnosed appendicitis in children. Ann Emerg Med 20:25–50, 1991.
11. Whitworth, et al: Value of diagnostic laparoscopy in young women with the possible diagnosis of appendicitis. Surg Gynecol Obstet 167:187–190, 1988.
12. Worrell JA, et al: Graded compression ultrasound in the diagnosis of appendicitis: A comparison of diagnostic criteria. J Ultrasound Med 9:145–150, 1990.

34. LIVER AND BILIARY TRACT DISEASE

Peter Moyer, M.D., FACEP

1. Why is it important to distinguish liver disease from biliary tract disease?
Biliary tract disease requires surgery. At times, the surgery must be immediate or the patient may die (e.g., cholecystitis in a diabetic, gallbladder empyema, cholangitis). In contrast, liver disease, whether viral, drug induced, or whatever, does not require surgery. In fact, surgery may increase morbidity or mortality.

2. What agents cause viral hepatitis?
Hepatitis A (fecal-oral transmission) and hepatitis B and C (sexual and parenteral transmission) are the usual agents. Hepatitis A and B can be diagnosed with readily available serologies. Cytomegalovirus (CMV) and herpes simplex also cause hepatitis.

3. Which patients with viral hepatitis should be admitted?
Those who are encephalopathic, bleeding, have an elevated prothrombin time (>4 sec beyond control), or who have intractable vomiting.

4. How should health care workers who have sustained a needlestick from a hepatitis-B-positive patient be treated?
The health care worker's own hepatitis B titer should be checked. Hyperimmune hepatitis B immune globulin (HBIG) should be administered as soon as possible and hepatitis B active immunization should be initiated. Consider HIV exposure and AZT prophylaxis in the same setting.

5. Which patients with alcoholic hepatitis should have ultrasound?

All. Those who appear acutely ill, especially those with fever and jaundice, should have ultrasound. In addition to liver disease, alcoholics commonly have gallstones. Fever and jaundice may indicate cholangitis, which requires immediate surgery.

6. Which patients with alcoholic hepatitis require admission?

Almost all of them. They need supportive care and hydration. Hospitalization also ensures abstinence.

7. What is cholestatic hepatitis? What causes it?

It is functional intrahepatic cholestasis with minimal other evidence of hepatocellular dysfunction and a normal biliary tract. It is typically caused by phenothiazines or androgens but may be seen in viral or alchoholic hepatitis and as an idiopathic condition in the third trimester of pregnancy. Cholestatic hepatitis must be distinguished from biliary tract disease by ultrasound.

8. What is the difference between biliary colic and cholecystitis?

Both entities are indicative of stones obstructing the cystic duct. Biliary colic suggests a bout of short duration (less than 6 hours) with a normal white blood cell count and no fever. The pain of cholecystitis lasts longer and may well be accompanied by leukocytosis and fever. Patients with biliary colic can usually be sent home. Those with cholecystitis require admission.

9. Are patients with cholecystitis typically jaundiced?

No, usually—only 10% are. Therefore, if a patient with suspected biliary tract disease is jaundiced, an ultrasound must be done emergently to rule out cholangitis.

10. Which patients with cholecystitis require emergency surgery?

Although most patients with cholecystitis may be operated on electively within the first 24 hours (before edema makes surgical dissection too difficult) or after a several-day defervescence, some patients require immediate surgery. For example, diabetics and patients with sickle cell disease are prone to empyema, perforation, and gangrene of the gallbladder, and require immediate surgery as do patients with cholecystitis who are clinically sick (febrile, jaundiced, hypotensive, etc.).

11. Which diagnostic tests confirm the diagnosis of cholecystitis?

The hepatoiminodiacetic acid (HIDA) scan is a functional radioisotope test in which failure to visualize the gallbladder suggests obstruction of the cystic duct and cholecystitis. Some advocate that the HIDA scan must be positive before operating for cholecystitis. Others believe that ultrasound is the diagnostic tool of choice, since it readily detects cystic duct stones. Additionally, it may show gallbladder wall thickening, pericholecystic fluid and a positive Murphy's sign on ultrasound. The combination of these findings is highly suggestive of cholecystitis.

12. When should cholangitis be suspected?

In patients with Charcot's triad (right upper quadrant tenderness, jaundice, and fever) should be suspected of having cholangitis. Shock and altered mental status may also be present (Reynold's pentad). Acute cholangitis and its systemic complications constitute a surgical emergency. Ultrasound is an excellent means (95% sensitivity) of detecting the common bile duct dilation seen in cholangitis. It may be negative in early cholangitis or in nongallstone cholangitis, such as sclerosing cholangitis and extraductal encasement by pancreatic cancer. In these cases, the diagnosis may be made by endoscopic retrograde cholangiopancreatography (ERCP) or percutaneous transhepatic cholangiogram.

13. Does cholelithiasis occur in children?
Yes. Its occurrence in infants is often associated with prematurity and manifested by jaundice, vomiting, and abdominal pain. It also occurs in adolescence when it is most commonly related to hemolytic disease or estrogen stimulation.

BIBLIOGRAPHY

1. Crossman SJ: Hepatobiliary imaging. Emerg Med Clin North Am 9:853–871, 1991.
2. Cunningham FG: Williams Obstetrics, 18th ed. Norwalk, CT, Appleton & Lange, 1989.
3. Heqarty J: Investigation of the jaundiced patient. The Practitioner 231:411–417, 1987.
4. Frank BB: Clinical evaluation of jaundice: A Guideline of the Patient Care Committee of the American Gastroenterological Association. JAMA 262:3031–3034, 1989.
5. Friesen CA, Roberts CC: Cholelithiasis: Clinical characteristics in children. Clin Pediatr 28:294–298, 1989.
6. Wolcott JK, Chen PS: Radiologic evaluation of the jaundiced patient. Postgrad Med 84:233–243, 1988.

35. BOWEL DISORDERS

Lisa S. Emmans, M.D.

1. What is the most common cause of small bowel obstruction (SBO)?
Postoperative adhesions are the most common cause of SBO, usually occurring long after surgery, although obstruction can be seen in the first few postoperative weeks. **Hernias** are the next most common cause, with incarcerated groin hernias the most frequent of these. Obturator hernias should be considered in elderly females presenting with SBO without a history of abdominal surgery and with pain in one knee or the thigh. Herniation may occur through mesentery defects. Other less common causes include **primary small bowel tumors, gallstones, inflammatory bowel disease, radiation enteritis, abscesses,** and **bezoars. Intussusception** and **congenital lesions** of the bowel wall should be considered in pediatric patients with SBO.

2. Why do patients with SBO die?
Even though the patient may not be eating, gastric pancreatic and biliary secretions continue. Most fluid resorption occurs distal to the obstruction in the large intestine, and the bowel loses the ability to resorb fluids and electrolytes. Vomiting or nasogastric suctioning can result in significant losses of fluids and electrolytes. Additional losses may occur into the bowel wall and peritoneal cavity. All this results in hypovolemia and hypotension, which progress to renal insufficiency, shock, and death. Strangulation occurs when the bowel becomes severely distended, resulting in gangrenous infarcted bowel. Bacteria pass into the lymphatics and bloodstream, leading to septic shock with a 70% mortality.

3. How do I differentiate radiographically between SBO and large bowel obstruction (LBO)?
Obstructed small bowel demonstrates a stepladder appearance of bowel gas (Fig. 1). There will still be gas and fecal matter in the large bowel in early SBO, but as obstruction progresses, the large bowel empties and the small bowel dilates out of proportion to the large bowel. Peristaltic activity causes fluid levels within "U loops" of bowel to lie at different levels within the limbs of the "U". Markedly distended small bowel may form a volvulus and become aperistaltic.

Large bowel gas is more round or square in shape, with haustral indentations every 3–4 mm (Fig. 2). Proximal large bowel has more haustra and is larger in diameter. Distally, gas is sausage-shaped. As the rectum becomes more dilated, it changes from diamond-shaped to circular.

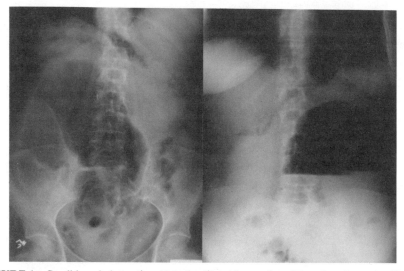

FIGURE 1.   Small bowel obstruction. Note the dilated loops of small bowel on the supine film (A). The upright view reveals multiple air-fluid interfaces at different levels (B).

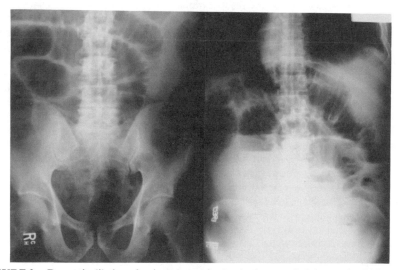

FIGURE 2.   Dramatic dilation of a single loop of colon in the central abdomen should immediately suggest the diagnosis of sigmoid volvulus. Both ends of the loop are located in the pelvis with the bow oriented superiorly. Also note that there is no rectal bubble and very little if any small bowel gas.

4. Can I differentiate clinically between SBO and LBO?

It is difficult to do so with great accuracy but there are some clues. The pain due to bowel obstruction is crampy or colicky and may be associated with high-pitched rushes on auscultation. In SBO pain tends to localize in the periumbilical region and occurs at intervals up to 5 minutes. Pain from LBO is usually less intense, localizes to the lower abdomen, and occurs at intervals up to 10 minutes. Vomiting is absent or develops later in LBO and is typically more feculent than that encountered in SBO.

5. What is the differential diagnosis for LBO?

LBO is most commonly due to fecal impaction, which is easily detected on physical examination. Carcinoma is the next most frequent cause. Tumors causing obstruction usually arise in the left colon or rectum, but it is important to consider gynecologic tumors in the differential. Diverticulitis may cause obstruction by acute swelling or chronic scarring. Volvulus should be considered in nursing home patients with chronic constipation (sigmoid volvulus) (Fig. 2) or in patients 25–35 years old (cecal volvulus).

6. When should strangulation be suspected?

Patients with strangulation are usually febrile and demonstrate persistent pain and abdominal mass after nasogastric decompression. Laboratory studies may show marked leukocytosis, metabolic acidosis, and elevated lactate dehydrogenase (LDH) and amylase. Radiographic studies are insensitive but may reveal the coffee-bean sign (single gas-distended loop with lumina separated by a broad dense band of edematous bowel), the pseudotumor sign (completely closed loop of bowel filled with fluid), or fixation of a single loop in three views.

7. Does the absence of vomiting or abdominal distention rule out obstruction?

No. In the early stages of obstruction, accumulation of gas and fluid is gradual, and pain may be the only symptom. Vomiting may be delayed 24–48 hours in low obstruction, and distention may be minimal in early high SBO.

8. How does ileus differ from obstruction?

There are no bowel sounds early in the course of ileus. Abdominal films in ileus show uniform distention throughout the entire GI tract. When barium studies are performed, barium will reach the colon within 1 hour in obstruction and may take up to 6 hours in paralytic ileus.

9. When should mesenteric vascular occlusion be suspected?

Patients at risk for mesenteric vascular occlusion are those with other manifestations of cardiovascular disease, including age >50 years, valvular or atherosclerotic heart disease, chronic congestive heart failure, recent myocardial infarction, dysrhythmias (atrial fibrillation), previous embolic events, hypovolemia, hypotension, and diuretics or vasoconstrictive drugs.

Initial presentation is frequently that of "pain out of proportion to the exam"—i.e., moderate to severe pain with minimal or no physical signs. Abdominal pain is encountered in 75–90% of patients and is typically dull, diffuse, and poorly localized. All patients eventually develop an acute abdomen. As the disease progresses, signs of systemic hypoperfusion, abdominal distention, and increased abdominal tenderness ensue. Death occurs as a result of hypovolemia and sepsis, and may occur over hours or days.

10. What is intestinal angina?

Intestinal angina is due to ischemia of the intestinal smooth muscle and manifests as postprandial abdominal discomfort lasting 1–3 hours.

11. What is the treatment of mesenteric vascular obstruction (MVO)?

The key to treating MVO is rapid diagnosis using abdominal angiography. Initial treatment focuses on resuscitation and correction of predisposing conditions with volume replacement, nasogastric suctioning, and parenteral antibiotics. Laparotomy for potential embolectomy and/or bowel resection is indicated in all patients with persistent peritoneal findings. Papaverine may be useful in patients with minor arterial occlusion, in those with major embolus but contraindications for surgery, and in those with splanchnic vasoconstriction but no occlusion.

12. Is intussusception seen only in children?
No. Ten percent of all intussusceptions occur in adults.

13. What causes intussusception in adults?
Intussusception, or invagination of a segment of bowel into itself, is associated with mass lesions in 90% of adult cases. Typical masses include tumors, Meckel's diverticulum, and inflammatory lesions. Malignancy is associated about 40% of the time. The remaining 10% of cases usually occur in the region of the terminal ileum and the ileocecal valve.

14. What are diverticula?
Diverticula are sac-like outpouchings of the colonic mucosa that occur through weakened areas of the muscularis.

15. In which portion of the bowel do diverticula occur most frequently?
Although diverticula may involve any or all of the colon, they form most frequently in the sigmoid colon and are typically limited to this region. Rectal diverticula are uncommon; however, persons of Chinese, Japanese or Hawaiian descent tend to have more cecal and ascending colon involvement.

16. Which patients develop diverticular disease?
Diverticulosis occurs in 50% of all persons by the age of 65 and 65% of persons reaching 85 years of age. Only 10–20% of individuals develop symptoms of the disease.

17. How do I differentiate clinically between diverticulosis and diverticulitis?
Patients with diverticulosis may describe intermittent left lower quadrant pain exacerbated by eating and relieved by defecation, with increased flatulence and diarrhea or constipation. Diverticulitis should be suspected when left lower quadrant pain becomes constant and is associated with malaise, altered bowel habits, anorexia, nausea, and vomiting. On exam, findings include a low-grade temperature and abdominal distention with typically localized tenderness. Occult bleeding is detected in >50% of patients on rectal exam but gross blood is rare.

18. What are the complications of diverticulitis?
Diverticulitis may result in obstruction, perforation, abscess, or fistula formation. Partial obstruction is fairly common during acute attacks, but complete obstruction occurs in less than 10% of patients. Fistula formation usually occurs only after repeated episodes; the most common is the colovesical fistula, which may cause pneumoturia. Abscess formation manifests with acute peritonitis. Immunocompromised and elderly patients may not develop fever, leukocytosis, and the clinical signs of peritonitis.

19. How are diverticulosis and diverticulitis treated?
Diverticulosis rarely requires hospitalization. Local heat and anticholinergics may help to relieve bowel spasm. A high-fiber diet, bulk laxatives, and stool softeners help decrease intraluminal pressure. Patients with a clear-cut diagnosis of diverticulitis and mild symptoms may be treated as outpatients and are given clear liquids and oral antibiotics. Any patient with evidence of perforation or abscess formation requires admission for surgical management. Even though bleeding from diverticula ceases spontaneously in 75–95% of patients, most require transfusion. Furthermore, patients without spontaneous cessation of hemorrhage will require definitive management. Finally, other etiologies such as carcinoma must be ruled out before lower GI hemorrhage can be attributed to diverticulosis.

20. Which patients with diverticulitis require surgery?
Patients with evidence of abscess formation (severe pain and local peritoneal signs) or diverticular perforation (severe pain, fever, and generalized peritoneal signs) require surgical drainage and bowel resection.

21. What causes volvulus?
In order for a volvulus to occur, a freely movable section of bowel must have its points of fixation in close proximity. The segment then rotates about its mesenteric axis, causing obstruction of the bowel.

22. Where does volvulus occur in the large intestine?
The sigmoid colon and cecum are affected in about 60% and 40% of cases of large bowel volvulus, respectively. Volvulus almost never occurs in the transverse colon or splenic flexure.

For nonstrangulated sigmoid volvulus, 85–90% of cases are detorsed and decompressed using a rectal tube and sigmoidoscope. Operative reduction of sigmoid volvulus is required only after failed tube decompression or when strangulation is suspected. Elective resection is sometimes recommended in eligible patients due to recurrence rates of almost 90% following nonsurgical decompression. In contrast, cecal volvulus almost always requires surgical reduction. Mortality rates range from 10–15%, increasing to 30–40% if gangrenous bowel is found at the time of surgery.

24. How do patients with Crohn's disease and ulcerative colitis initially present?
Although pathologically they are distinctly different entities, Crohn's disease and ulcerative colitis can be difficult to differentiate clinically. Both may present with chronic diarrhea, abdominal pain, fever, anorexia, and weight loss. Crohn's disease is associated more often with perianal manifestations and less often with bloody diarrhea than is ulcerative colitis. Both diseases have a peak incidence in the second and third decades of life. There is a family history or inflammatory bowel disease in 10–15% of patients with ulcerative colitis and whites are affected four times more frequently than nonwhites. Crohn's disease is more common in whites and four times more common in persons of Jewish descent. Because of the nonspecific nature of the symptoms, diagnosis of inflammatory bowel disease is often delayed months to years.

25. What is the difference between Crohn's disease and granulomatous ileocolitis?
There is no difference. Crohn's disease, granulomatous ileocolitis, and regional enteritis all refer to the same disease.

26. What are the common complications of regional enteritis?
Perianal complications include perianal or ischiorectal abscesses, fistulas (including recto-vaginal), fissures, and rectal prolapse. They occur in 50–80% of patients with Crohn's disease and are the initial presenting complaint in about half of all patients. Toxic mega-colon occurs less frequently than in ulcerative colitis (about 2–3% of cases). Strictures may form (less than 10% of patients) and, although rare (less than 1%), perforation or massive bowel hemorrhage has been associated with Crohn's disease. Risk of malignant neoplasm is three times greater in regional enteritis than in ulcerative colitis (which is about 1% per patient per year in patients with pancolitis: 10–30 times greater than in the general public).

27. What are the extraintestinal complications of regional enteritis?
Systemic manifestations have the same incidence (10–20%) in Crohn's disease and ulcerative colitis. These symptoms may actually precede intestinal symptoms (especially in children) and so may be the initial presenting complaint.

Extraintestinal Complications of Inflammatory Bowel Disease

HEPATOBILIARY DISEASE	OTHERS
Gallstones	Aphthous ulcers
Pericholangitis	Erythema nodosum
Chronic active hepatitis	Pyoderma gangrenosum
Primary sclerosing cholangitis	Nongranulomatous anterior uveitis
Cholangiocarcinoma	Polyarteritis
	Nephrolithiasis
	Pneumoturia

28. What are the indications for admission in a patient with inflammatory bowel disease?
Most patients with mild to moderate disease can be managed as outpatients and require admission only if they worsen or fail to improve. Admission is indicated in patients with severe disease (more than six bowel movements per day, severe abdominal pain, or grossly bloody stools), systemic toxicity (temperature greater than 38°, tachycardia, weight loss greater than 10% of premorbid weight, hematocrit less than 30%, albumin less than 3 gm/dl or sedimentation rate greater than 30 mm/hr) and those who are dehydrated or have metabolic disturbances. Admission with surgical consultation is indicated for patients with suspected toxic megacolon, perforation, massive lower GI bleed, obstruction, or possible colonic cancer.

29. What is toxic megacolon?
Toxic megacolon occurs in patients with advanced inflammatory bowel disease and has a 30% mortality rate. Involvement of all layers of the colon causes loss of muscular tone and colonic dilatation. Patients with toxic megacolon are ill-appearing with fever, tachycardia, evidence of hypotension, and a distended, tender tympanic abdomen. Laboratory data reveal leukocytosis, anemia, electrolyte abnormalities, and hypoalbuminemia. The colon will appear as a long, continuous segment of bowel dilated to >6 cm in diameter on plain film. Treatment consists of nasogastric suctioning and admission for observation. Steroid therapy should be avoided. Surgery is indicated in patients who fail to improve within 48–72 hours or in the approximately 25% in whom perforation occurs. This complication of inflammatory bowel disease carries a 30% mortality rate.

30. What is the differential diagnosis of abdominal pain in children?
Abdominal pain in children may be caused by many of the same disease processes encountered in adults. Certain causes, rare in adults, are seen more frequently in children.

Common Causes of Nontraumatic Abdominal Pain in Children

Infectious Conditions	Congenital Conditions	Masses
Gastroenteritis	Hirschsprung's disease	Ectopic pregnancy
Influenza	Sickle cell anemia	Incarcerated inguinal
Pneumonia	**Inflammatory Conditions**	hernia
Pyelonephritis or cystitis	Appendicitis	Tumor
Obstructive Conditions	Henoch-Schönlein	
Constipation	purpura	
Hirschsprung's disease	Meckel's diverticulitis	
Intussusception	Necrotizing enterocolitis	
Volvulus	Salpingitis	

Adapted from Diekman RA: Abdominal pain. In Grossman M, Dieckmann RA (eds): Pediatric Emergency Medicine: A Clinician's Reference. Philadelphia, J.B. Lippincott, 1991, p 199.

BIBLIOGRAPHY

1. Anderson GV, Woods JM: Intestinal obstruction. In Harwood-Nuss A, et al: The Clinical Practice of Emergency Medicine. Philadelphia, J.B. Lippincott, 1991, pp 138–141.
2. Bitterman RA: Disorders of the large intestine. In Rosen P, et al (eds): Emergency Medicine: Concepts and Clinical Practice, 3rd ed. St. Louis, Mosby–Year Book, 1992, pp 1644–1658.
3. Cayten CG: Colonic diverticular disease. In Harwood-Nuss A, et al (eds): The Clinical Practice of Emergency Medicine. Philadelphia, JB Lippincott, 1991, pp 144–146.
4. Diekman RA: Abdominal pain. In Grossman M, Dieckmann RA (eds): Pediatric Emergency Medicine: A Clinician's Reference. Philadelphia, J.B. Lippincott, 1991, pp 196–206.
5. Glover JL: Intestinal obstruction. In Tintinalli JE, Krome RL, Ruiz E (eds): Emergency Medicine: A Comprehensive Study Guide, 2nd ed. New York, McGraw-Hill, 1988, pp 319–321.
6. Hockberger RS, Henneman PL, Boniface K: Disorders of the small intestine. In Rosen P, et al (eds): Emergency Medicine: Concepts and Clinical Practice, 3rd ed. St. Louis, Mosby–Year Book, 1992, pp 1627–1644.
7. Krome RL: Colonic diverticular disease. In Tintinalli JE, Krome RL, Ruiz E (eds): Emergency Medicine: A Comprehensive Study Guide, 2nd ed. New York, McGraw-Hill, 1988, pp 328–329.
8. Preger L, Gronner AT, Glazer H, et al: Imaging of the nontraumatic acute abdomen. Emerg Med Clin North Am 7:453–496, 1989.
9. Werman HA: Inflammatory bowel disease. In Harwood-Nuss A, et al (eds): The Clinical Practice of Emergency Medicine. Philadelphia, J.B. Lippincott, 1991, pp 962–964.
10. Werman HA, Mekhjian HS, Rund DA: Ileitis and colitis. In Tintinalli JE, Krome RL, Ruiz E (eds): Emergency Medicine: A Comprehensive Study Guide, 2nd ed. New York, McGraw-Hill, 1988, pp 324–327.

36. ANORECTAL PROBLEMS

Mark Radlauer, M.D.

1. What are the causes of rectal bleeding?

In the vast majority of cases, rectal bleeding is from a benign cause—hemorrhoids, fissure, or infection—but an important minority have a more serious cause, such as carcinoma.

Causes of Rectal Bleeding

Hemorrhoids	Infection
Fissures	Colonic ulcers
Diverticulosis	Colonic varices
Polyps	Small bowel sources:
Cancer	Meckel's diverticulum
Inflammatory bowel disease	Tumors
Arteriovenous malformations	Ileitis
Ischemia	Varices
Radiation colitis	Upper GI source

From Lichtiger S, Kornbluth A, et al: Lower gastrointestinal bleeding. In Taylor MB (ed): Gastrointestinal Emergencies. Baltimore, Williams & Wilkins, 1992, with permission.

2. Differentiate between internal and external hemorrhoids.

The pectinate line, which separates the columnar epithelium of the GI tract from the squamous epithelium of the skin, differentiates internal from external hemorrhoids.

Internal hemorrhoids are mucosa-covered and are not visible externally. They are not palpable unless symptomatic. External hemorrhoids are skin-covered and are visible externally. Either type of hemorrhoid may bleed, become inflamed, or thrombose. External hemorrhoidal bleeding is visible, whereas internal hemorrhoidal bleeding may be seen on anoscopy. When inflammation or thrombosis occur, hemorrhoids are exquisitely tender. Thrombosed hemorrhoids appear dark blue and the clot is palpable.

3. How does hemorrhoidal bleeding generally present?
Patients notice drops of red blood in the toilet or on the toilet paper after a bowel movement. They may have constipation or have been straining excessively. Pain may or may not be present.

4. How are symptomatic external hemorrhoids treated?
Conservative therapy is usually adequate, with symptoms generally resolving in several days. Treatment centers on pain control, soothing with sitz baths, stool softeners, and a high-fiber diet. If an external hemorrhoid is acutely thrombosed and very painful, it can be excised.

5. How are symptomatic internal hemorrhoids treated?
In addition to inflammation and thrombosis, internal hemorrhoids are more prone to prolapse and significant bleeding than are external hemorrhoids. Internal hemorrhoids may prolapse below the pectinate line and be confused with external hemorrhoids. Reduction should be attempted if possible. If the prolapsed hemorrhoids are very inflamed, strangulated, or thrombosed, surgical consultation for hemorroidectomy is indicated. If bleeding is pronounced, cardiovascular assessment and IV access are indicated. Bleeding should be controlled if possible with suture ligation or cautery, and surgical consultation may be necessary. Inflamed internal hemorrhoids or nonprolapsed thrombosis may be handled conservatively, similar to external hemorrhoids, with appropriate referral.

6. What are common causes of rectal pain?
Anal fissures, abscesses, and thrombosed hemorrhoids are the most common causes. Malignancy, colitis, and foreign bodies are less common causes of rectal pain.

7. List some causes of anal pruritus.
Poor hygiene, hemorrhoids, prolapse, infections (including fungal and parasitic), and neoplasia.

8. Describe common types of abscesses encountered in the anorectal region.
Anorectal abscesses usually begin as infections at the glandular tissue between the internal and external sphincters (see figure on next page). An **intersphincteric abscess** is confined to the initial region of infection. A **submucosal abscess** results from proximal spread of the intersphincteric infection in the same tissue plane. A **perianal abscess**, the most common type, results from distal vertical spread of the intersphincteric infection and is localized to the subcutaneous space. **Ischiorectal or supralevator abscesses** and **perirectal abscesses** are more serious because of localization to deeper tissue planes.

Two other disorders may lead to abscess formation in this area. In the presacral region, cephalad to the anal opening, cysts may form secondary to ingrowth of hair follicles in the gluteal fold. These **pilonidal cysts** may become infected, forming abscesses or sinus tracts.

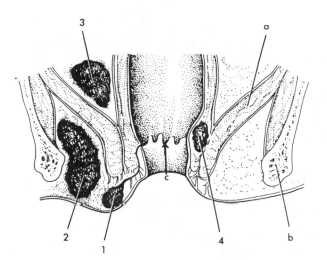

Perirectal abscesses. *a*, Levator ani. *b*, Ischeal tuberosity. *c*, Anal crypts. *1*, Perianal abscess with anal fistula; *2*, ischiorectal abscess; *3*, supralevator ani abscess; *4*, intersphincteric abscess. (From Meislin HW: Soft tissue infections. In Rosen P, et al (eds): Emergency Medicine: Concepts and Clinical Practice, 3rd ed. St. Louis, Mosby Year Book, 1992, p 857, with permission.)

9. How can these various abscesses be differentiated clinically?

Intersphincteric or submucosal abscesses present with dull pain within the rectum, worsened with bowel movements. Patients are usually not febrile. External exam of the anus is normal. Rectal exam reveals a localized tender mass at the level of the sphincter, often with purulent drainage.

Perianal abscesses present with moderate to severe pain in the anal region, worsened with sitting or defecation. Patients are usually not febrile, and external exam reveals a tender, fluctuant mass immediately adjacent to the anus.

Ischiorectal or supralevator abscesses are more severe and more difficult to diagnose. Patients often appear toxic and have fever and leukocytosis. They may report deep buttock or rectal pain, or pelvic or low abdominal pain. External skin exam is usually normal. Rectal exam, combined with external palpation, may reveal deep tenderness or an asymmetric fullness. Low ischiorectal abscesses tend to localize between the rectum and ischial tuberosity, resulting in a perirectal abscess that usually produces skin changes and points lateral to the anus.

10. Which of these abscesses can be treated in the emergency department (ED)?

Intersphincteric and perianal abscesses can be drained in the ED. Likewise, infected pilonidal cysts and hidradenitis cysts can be incised and drained in the ED, but surgical referral is indicated for definitive excision. Supralevator, ischiorectal, and perirectal space abscesses are surgical emergencies and usually require incision and drainage in the operating room.

11. What is an anal fissure?

Anal fissures, the most common cause of painful bowel movements, result from a tear in the anal mucosa, usually in the posterior midline. Passage of hard stool is the presumed initial injury, with secondary sphincter spasm leading to perpetuation of the fissure. Patients present with pain, generally acute and initiated by defecation, and rectal bleeding. Examination reveals a painful radial slit, usually posterior in the midline, that is often visible with traction of the anal skin.

12. What physical findings suggest that surgical treatment of a fissure may be necessary?
The presence of significant ulceration, hypertrophied tissue, or a skin tag (sentinel pile) suggests chronicity and necessitates surgical referral for operative treatment. Otherwise, simple fissures are treated with analgesics, stool softeners, and anal hygiene.

13. What other lesions resemble an anal fissure?
Chancres, inflammatory bowel disease, or anal cancer may present with fissure-like lesions. In each of these cases the lesions are often not midline and may be multiple. Chancres are painless, and associated lymphadenopathy is typically present. Chronic nonhealing lesions should raise the suspicion of neoplasm.

14. Who is susceptible to rectal prolapse? Why?
Rectal prolapse is most common in young children (usually less than 5) and in older female adults. Children's anal and rectal tissues are generally normal but immature. In adult females, the condition is related to loss of tissue integrity.

15. Is surgical referral for rectal prolapse necessary?
In children, the condition is generally self-limiting, possibly due to excessive straining with defecation. Manual reduction in the ED is indicated and generally successful. A high-fiber diet is recommended and parents are reassured that the child will outgrow the problem. Manual reduction in adults is reasonable, but recurrence is common, and surgical referral is appropriate.

16. Which sexually transmitted diseases are common in the anal region?
Condylomata acuminata (genital warts) and chancres from syphilis are seen in this region, usually secondary to anal intercourse.

17. What is Fournier's gangrene?
Fournier's gangrene is an acute and rapidly progressive infection of the scrotum that can quickly lead to sepsis and death. It is seen most commonly in diabetics. Gastrointestinal organisms are the usual cause, often secondary to a perirectal abscess or fistula. Scrotal infection is characteristic, but spread to the penis, abdominal wall, or perianal region is also seen, and patients generally have signs of systemic toxicity. This infection requires emergency surgical debridement and broad-spectrum antibiotics.

BIBLIOGRAPHY

1. Davis SM: Disorders of the anorectum. In Rosen P, et al (eds): Emergency Medicine: Concepts and Clinical Practice, 3rd ed. St. Louis, Mosby–Year Book, 1992.
2. Goligher J (ed): Surgery of the Anus, Rectum, and Colon. London, Balliere Tindall, 1984.
3. Halvorson GD, Halvorson JE, Iserson KV: Abscess incision and drainage in the emergency department. Am J Emerg Med 3:227, 1985.
4. Jones IT, Fazio VW: Anorectal diseases commonly encountered in clinical practice. In Kirsner JB, Shorter RG (eds): Diseases of the Colon, Rectum, and Anal Canal. Baltimore, Williams & Wilkins, 1988.
5. Kune GA: Anal symptoms. In Grant AK, Skyring A, Conn HO (eds): Clinical Diagnosis of Gastrointestinal Disease. Oxford, Blackwell Scientific Publishers, 1981.
6. Lichtiger S, Kornbluth A, et al: Lower gastrointestinal bleeding. In Taylor MB (ed): Gastrointestinal Emergencies. Baltimore, Williams & Wilkins, 1992.
7. Roberts JA: Infections of the genitourinary tract. In Howard RJ (ed): Surgical Infectious Diseases. Norwalk, Appleton & Lange, 1988.
8. Samuels L: Perianal, rectal, and anal diseases. In Harwood-Nuss A (ed): The Clinical Practice of Emergency Medicine. Philadelphia, J.B. Lippincott, 1991.
9. Smith LE: Hemorrhoids. Gastroenterol Clin North Am 16:79, 1987.
10. Thomson JPS: The rectum and anal canal. In Sabiston DC (ed): Textbook of Surgery, 13th ed. Philadelphia, W.B. Saunders, 1986.

VIII. Genitourinary Tract

37. RENAL COLIC

Grant Innes, M.D.

1. What are the most common forms of renal stone?
Calcium stones make up 80% of all renal stones—two thirds are calcium oxalate and the remainder calcium phosphate. Struvite (magnesium ammonium phosphate), uric acid, and cystine account for the remaining 20% of renal stones.

2. What factors predispose to stone formation?
Chronic dehydration, antacid use, hypercalciuria, hyperoxaluria, acid urine, and ingestion of vitamins A, C, and D predispose to calcium stones. Struvite stones are associated with chronic infection by urea-splitting organisms. Cystine stones are rare and occur in patients with cystinuria.

3. What lethal conditions are sometimes misdiagnosed as renal colic?
Aortic and iliac aneurysms. A careful search for bruits and pulsatile masses is mandatory when renal colic is suspected.

4. What clinical features help distinguish renal colic from other causes of abdominal pain?
Renal colic usually begins abruptly, causing terrible pain in the flank, costovertebral angle, lateral abdomen, and genitals. Patients are often profoundly distressed. Pallor, diaphoresis, restlessness, and nausea are prominent. Renal colic causes flank tenderness, but unlike other causes of lateralized abdominal pain (for example, appendicitis, diverticulitis, cholelithiasis, and ectopic pregnancy), it produces little or no abdominal tenderness.

5. What are the roles of the abdominal flat plate and the intravenous pyelogram (IVP)?
The abdominal flat plate, or KUB, is less sensitive and less specific than the clinical exam and has no role in the work-up of renal colic. The IVP is the gold standard diagnostic test for renal colic.

6. Name the two major contraindications to an IVP.
Allergy to contrast material and renal failure. Allergic reactions are uncommon. If a patient claims to be allergic to IVP dye, determine what the reaction was. Flushing and nausea often occur after injection and are not allergic reactions. Urticaria, stridor, wheezing, and syncope suggest a true allergy. If the patient has had a significant reaction in the past, there is a 15% chance of recurrence. Asthmatics are at higher risk for allergic reactions. In patients at risk for allergic reaction or contrast-mediated nephrotoxicity, nonionic contrast material is preferable.

7. In what other patients might an IVP be hazardous?
Patients over the age of 60 and those with underlying renal disease, diabetes, or myeloma are at high risk for contrast-mediated nephrotoxicity. Assess BUN and creatinine in all such

patients, and reconsider the need for IVP if serum creatinine is greater than 2.0. If IVP is deemed necessary in spite of risk factor, hydrate the patient adequately prior to infusion of contrast material.

8. Is pregnancy a contraindication to IVP?
Ultrasound is the investigation of choice in pregnant patients, but if ultrasound is non-diagnostic, a limited IVP (scout film and 20-minute postinjection film, preferably coned to the area of concern) is appropriate.

9. What IVP findings suggest a renal stone?
Typical findings include a delayed, intense, and often prolonged nephrogram on the involved side, delayed filling and dilatation of the affected collecting system (hydroureter and hydronephrosis), and an uninterrupted column of dye extending from the kidney to the calculus (an unobstructed ureter, being peristaltic, is not usually visualized in its entirety).

10. Why is the postvoid film important? What other "special" views are helpful?
The presence of contrast material in the bladder obscures the distal ureter. The postvoid film permits optimal visualization of the distal ureter and ureterovesical junction. The postvoid film also shows whether the bladder is emptying completely. Oblique views help to confirm that a visualized stone is in, rather than overlying, the ureter. Prone films often provide a better view of the ureter than standard supine films.

11. What if the ureter is not visualized on the standard IVP?
In high-grade ureteral obstruction, contrast material may not reach the distal ureter for many hours. If the ureter is not visualized at 1 hour, do a 2-hour film. If this fails, do a 4-hour film. The interval between films should be doubled until adequate visualization is achieved. It is important not to abandon the IVP until contrast material reaches the calculus.

12. What are the most common sites of stone impaction?
The ureteropelvic junction, the pelvic brim (where the ureter crosses the iliac vessels), and the ureterovesical junction—the narrowest point in the ureter—are the most common sites of impaction.

13. Can the likelihood of spontaneous passage be predicted based on the size and location of the stone?
Stones that reach the distal ureter are more likely to pass than those that impact proximally. Stones less than 4 mm will pass 90% of the time; stones from 4–6 mm will pass 50% of the time, and stones over 6 mm will pass 10% of the time. When estimating stone size, remember that the x-ray image is magnified—actual size will be 80% of what is measured on the films.

14. What if the IVP is normal but the patient still appears to have renal colic?
Reexamine the patient carefully to ensure that you have not missed some other abdominal disorder and to be sure that a surgical abdomen is not evolving. If the physical exam is still compatible with renal colic, treat the patient, not the test result. The IVP is falsely negative in about 10% of cases.

15. Isn't an ultrasound just as accurate as an IVP?
Ultrasound is safe and noninvasive, but is more prone to false negatives than IVP. Ultrasound is sensitive for detecting stones in the bladder and renal pelvis but often fails to reveal those in the mid and distal ureter—the most common sites for stone impaction. Even when ultrasound fails to identify a stone, it may demonstrate dilatation of the renal collecting system, providing evidence of ureteral obstruction.

16. What other tests are useful in the emergency department (ED)?
Urine dipsticks are sensitive for microscopic hematuria, which is present in 80% of patients with renal colic. Urinalysis is recommended to rule out pyuria and bacteriuria. Urine culture is indicated if there are symptoms, signs, or findings on urinalysis that suggest infection. Measurement of BUN, creatinine, and electrolytes is necessary if the patient has been vomiting or if presence of an underlying renal disease is suspected. A more extensive metabolic work-up in the ED is inappropriate.

17. Why is coexistent infection a major problem?
Bacteria in an obstructed collecting system can quickly cause abscess formation, renal destruction, and bacteremia. The presence of infection in an obstructed ureter mandates immediate surgical consultation and high-dose intravenous antibiotics.

18. Has lithotripsy supplanted percutaneous and open surgical methods of stone removal?
No. Optimal therapy depends on the size, type, and location of the stone. Ureteroscopic techniques are probably still preferable for lower ureteral stones. Extracorporeal shock wave lithotripsy (ESWL) is optimal for stones up to 2 cm, particularly those in the renal pelvis. Percutaneous stone removal techniques are indicated for larger stones, when there is obstructive uropathy, and when less invasive techniques have failed. For some stones, a combination of ESWL followed by percutaneous instrumentation is optimal. Some large stones will still require open surgery. The optimal method of removal is determined by a urologist.

19. What are the basics of ED treatment of renal colic?
Hydration, analgesics, and antiemetics. Unless the patient is elderly or has a history of renal or congestive heart failure, normal saline should be infused in volumes sufficient to produce a urine output of at least 100 cc/hr. Various analgesics and antiemetics are available for rapid control of symptoms. Although nonsteroidal anti-inflammatory drugs (NSAIDs) have been studied in patients with renal colic, intravenous narcotics remain the analgesics of choice for reasons of cost, efficacy, and ease of administration.

Analgesics and Antiemetics for Renal Colic

Narcotic analgesics			
Meperidine (Demerol)	IV	25–50 mg	q 5–10 min prn
	IM	1–2 mg/kg	q 2–3 hr prn
Morphine sulfate	IV	3–5 mg	q 5–10 min prn
	IM	.1–.2 mg/kg	q 3–4 hr prn
Oxycodone and aspirin (Percodan)	PO	1–2 tabs	q 4 hr prn
Oxycodone and acetaminophen (Percocet)	PO	1–2 tabs	q 4 hr prn
Antiemetics			
Metoclopramide (Reglan)	IV	10–30 mg	q 30 min prn
Perphenazine (Trilafon)	IM	5 mg	q 6 hr prn
	PO	4 mg	q 6 hr prn
Prochlorperazine (Compazine)	IM	5–10 mg	q 4–6 hr prn
	PO	5–10 mg	q 4–6 hr prn
Droperidol (Inapsine)	IV	2.5–5 mg	q 2–4 hr prn
	IM	2.5–5 mg	q 2–4 hr prn
Nonsteroidal Analgesics			
Indomethacin	50- or 100-mg suppositories, 200 mg/day		
Diclofenac (Voltaren)	50- or 100-mg suppositories, 150 mg/day		
Ketorolac* (Toradol)	IM 30–60 mg	q 6	hr*

*Not to exceed 150 mg/day.

20. Who requires hospitalization?

Patients with high-grade obstruction, intractable pain or vomiting, associated urinary tract infection, or a solitary or transplanted kidney, and those in whom the diagnosis is uncertain should be hospitalized. Obtain urologic consultation for patients with stones greater than 6 mm in diameter, irrespective of symptoms.

21. What advice should be given to patients being discharged from the ED?

Patients are advised to drink plenty of fluids, strain their urine, follow up with their family doctor in 3 days, and return to the ED if symptoms of infection or recurrent severe pain develop.

22. Which analgesics are recommended for outpatient pain control?

GI irritation limits the usefulness of oral NSAIDs in patients with renal colic; however, rectal NSAIDs (diclofenac, indomethacin) may provide adequate analgesia. If necessary, oral narcotics are appropriate for patients with documented ureteral calculi.

23. How should I counsel patients about the long-term prevention of renal stones?

Stone formers should hydrate themselves to the point that they are passing dilute urine. Elimination of rhubarb, beets, spinach, beer, cola, coffee, citrus fruit, and vitamin C may reduce the risk of calcium oxalate stones. A variety of specific treatment regimens exist, depending on the type of stone produced by the patient. Given the uncertainty of recurrence—only 50–70% of patients will have recurrent stones—and the fact that lifetime compliance with dietary modification and drugs is poor, prophylactic measures for renal colic may not be reasonable.

BIBLIOGRAPHY

1. Fontanarosa PB: Radiologic contrast induced renal failure. Emerg Med Clin North Am 3:601–613, 1988.
2. Hendricks SK, Ross SO, Krieger JN: An algorithm for diagnosis and therapy of management and complications of urolithiasis during pregnancy. Surg Gynecol Obstet 172:49–54, 1991.
3. Hetherington JW, Philp NH: Diclofenac sodium versus pethidine in acute renal colic. BMJ 292:237–238, 1986.
4. Juul N, Brns J, Torp-Pedersen S, Fredfeldt KE: Ultrasound versus intravenous urography in the initial evaluation of patients with suspected obstructing urinary calculi. Scand J Urol Nephrol Suppl 137:45–47, 1991.
5. Kraebber DM, Torres SA: Extracorporeal shock wave lithotripsy. South Med J 81:48–51, 1988.
6. Loberant N: Emergency imaging of the urinary tract. Emerg Med Clin North Am 10:59–92, 1992.
7. Marthak KV, Gokarn AM, Rao AV, Sane SP, et al: Comparative study of diclofenac sodium and pethidine in renal colic patients in India. Curr Med Res Opin 12:366–373, 1991.
8. Mutgi A, Williams JW, Nettleman M: Renal colic—utility of the plain abdominal roentgenogram. Arch Intern Med 151:1589–1592, 1991.
9. Rosen P, et al (eds): Stone disease. Emergency Medicine: Concepts and Clinical Practice, 3rd ed. St. Louis, Mosby–Year Book, 1992, pp 1902–1908.
10. Segura JW: Current surgical approaches to nephrolithiasis. Endocrinol Metab Clin North Am 19:919–935, 1990.
11. Segura JW: Role of percutaneous procedures in the management of renal calculi. Urol Clin North Am 17:207–216, 1990.
12. Sinclair D, Wilson S, Toi A, Greenspan L: The evaluation of suspected renal colic: Ultrasound scan versus excretory urography. Ann Emerg Med 18:556–559, 1989.
13. Stewart C: Nephrolithiasis. Emerg Med Clin North Am 6:617–629, 1988.
14. Sutton RA: Causes and prevention of calcium-containing renal calculi. West J Med 155:249–252, 1991.
15. Thompson JF, Pike JM, Chumas PD, Rundle JSH: Rectal diclofenac compared with pethidine injection in acute renal colic. BMJ 299:1140–1141, 1989.
16. Uribarri J, Oh MS, Carroll HJ: The first kidney stone. Ann Intern Med 111:1006–1009, 1989.
17. Van Arsdalen KN, Banner MP, Pollack HM: Radiologic imaging and urologic decision making in the management of renal and ureteral calculi. Urol Clin North Am 17:171–190, 1990.

38. SCROTAL PAIN

Robert E. Schneider, M.D., FACEP, FACS

1. What is the differential diagnosis in a patient with acute scrotal pain?
Testicular torsion must always be considered in any patient with a history of acute scrotal pain. The differential diagnosis is somewhat age dependent. In the patient 15 years of age or younger, the differential diagnosis includes testicular torsion, torsion of a testicular or epididymal appendix, epididymitis, and rarely, orchitis, acute hematocele, or idiopathic scrotal edema. In patients older than 15, the differential includes testicular torsion, epididymitis, torsion of a testicular or epididymal appendix, and testicular tumor.

2. What is testicular torsion?
Testicular torsion is the result of a congenital developmental abnormality that involves the testicle and the tunica vaginalis. In the normal state, the visceral tunica vaginalis covers the anterolateral portion of the testis and the lateral portion of the epididymis, while the parietal tunica vaginalis acts as an envelope and fixes both the testis and epididymis to the posterior scrotal wall. This fixation eliminates the freedom for rotation and subsequent torsion. In the abnormal state, both layers of the tunica vaginalis totally encircle the testis and epididymis (similar to a clapper in a bell, hence bell-clapper deformity), so that these structures are free to rotate on their cord secondary to any stimulus that may promote cremaster muscle contraction. This can lead to varying degrees of testicular torsion.

3. How is testicular torsion diagnosed?
Surgical exploration is the only definitive diagnostic method. For complete torsion, the window of warm ischemia is 4–6 hours. Unfortunately, no clinical findings. laboratory tests or radiographic studies can approach the sensitivity of surgical exploration. Adjunctive studies used in the diagnosis include the following: (1) physical exam to document the presence or absence of the cremasteric reflex; (2) attempted manual detorsion with or without the aid of a Doppler stethoscope; (3) radionuclide testicular scan; (4) duplex color Doppler ultrasonography; and (5) magnetic resonance imaging (MRI).

4. What is the significance of cremasteric reflex?
The cremasteric reflex is a spinal cord reflex encompassing T12–L2 nerve roots and is elicited by stroking the inner aspect of the involved thigh. In a normal state, the ipsilateral testis will retract in a superior fashion as the cremaster muscle contracts. Any inflammatory process that fixes the testis to the surrounding scrotal wall or inhibits contraction of the cremaster muscle will prevent elicitation of this reflex. A torsed testis may lose its cremasteric reflex due to twisting of the spermatic cord.

5. What is manual detorsion?
Manual detorsion is a maneuver used to untwist the spermatic cord in order to reestablish blood flow to the testis. This procedure should be done in any patient with suspected testicular torsion while the patient is being readied for the operating room. Since most testes torse lateral to medial, the procedure is done as follows. If you were to stand at the foot of the patient's bed, you would perform the detorsion maneuver for either testis just as you would open a book, rotating each testicle in a medial to lateral direction. If testicular torsion has progressed to the point where there is fixation of the scrotal contents to the overlying scrotal skin, testicular detorsion will not be possible. Successful detorsion results in immediate reduction of pain or complete pain relief and allows an emergent operative

procedure to be done electively within 24–48 hours. However, in many cases it will not be successful or the testis will twist again. Therefore, surgical fixation is still indicated.

6. What is Doppler evaluation of the spermatic cord?

Doppler evaluation of the cord is done by placing a Doppler stethoscope over the superior portion of the at-risk spermatic cord and attempting to measure arterial flow to the involved testis. Unfortunately, the interpretation of this examination is subjective and by itself is not diagnostic. Absent or diminished arterial flow strongly supports the diagnosis of torsion. However, the presence of flow **does not exclude** this diagnosis. The use of this technique in conjunction with manual detorsion to confirm an increase in blood flow following the detorsion maneuver has some merit.

7. What is the utility of radionuclide scans and Doppler ultrasound?

Following the injection of a radionuclide substance into a peripheral vein, a scanner is used to document the presence of the radionuclide substance in the testis, thus demonstrating arterial inflow. This examination is invasive, time-consuming, and reader dependent, and has no place in the time-sensitive diagnostic armamentarium of testicular torsion. Duplex color Doppler ultrasonography is noninvasive, can be done much faster, and has a specificity of 100%. However, it also is reader dependent and should not delay surgical exploration.

8. How are these tests helpful in the management of testicular torsion?

These studies are truly adjunctive and in no way should preclude or delay surgical exploration once the diagnosis of testicular torsion is suspected.

9. What is the treatment of choice for testicular torsion?

Unequivocally, the treatment of choice is surgical exploration. The involved testis must be surgically detorsed and then evaluated for viability. If the testis is deemed to be salvageable, it is fixed (pexed) to the medial and lateral scrotal wall with nonabsorbable suture material. If it is deemed unsalvageable, the testis is removed. Because testicular torsion is a bilateral phenomenon, the uninvolved testis must always be prophylactically pexed to prevent subsequent development of torsion.

10. What is torsion of the appendix testis and appendix epididymis?

The testicular and epididymal appendices are mullerian and wolfian duct remnants that have no physiologic function. They are subject to torsion because of their anatomic stalk. Unlike torsion of the testis, physical examination of a torsed appendix early in its course will disclose point tenderness over the involved appendix. Late in its course, generalized scrotal tenderness may be encountered, making differentiation from testicular torsion impossible and necessitating scrotal exploration. In an unequivocal case of appendiceal torsion, ice, bed rest, NSAIDs, and pain medication are the treatment modalities. The affected appendix will subsequently necrose over 10–14 days and become asymptomatic.

11. What is orchitis? How common is it?

Orchitis is inflammation of the testis. It occurs most commonly in association with mumps. Its relatively infrequent occurrence should prompt reconsideration of the history and physical findings to be certain not to miss a more serious diagnosis, such as testicular torsion, epididymitis, or testicular tumor.

12. What is epididymitis? What are the physical findings?

Epididymitis is inflammation of the epididymis, the tubular structure that lies on the posterolateral portion of the testis. Epididymitis begins in the area of the ejaculatory ducts found in the prostatic urethra. Infected and occasionally sterile urine refluxes in a retrograde fashion down the vas deferens to the globus minor or tail of the epididymis, initiating the inflammatory response. When evaluated at this stage, the examiner will feel an isolated mass at the inferiormost portion of the epididymis adjacent to the testis. The remainder of the testis and scrotal contents will be normal. With inflammation confined solely to the epididymis, the sulcus or groove that separates the epididymis from the testis is uninvolved and easily identifiable during examination. If the process is allowed to progress, inflammation will spread to the body of the epididymis and subsequently to the superiormost portion of the epididymis known as the globus major or head of the epididymis.

13. What is epididymo-orchitis?
It is severe inflammation of the epididymis that has progressed onto the contiguous testis. The normally palpable sulcus between the epididymis and testis is obliterated, and a large tender scrotal mass results. This severe form of epididymitis must be treated aggressively.

14. List the most common cause(s) of epididymitis in a 20-year-old male; a 50-year-old male.
In a 20-year-old male, the most common cause of epididymitis is related to sexually transmitted diseases (STDs). The most common organisms are *Chlamydia trachomatis*, followed by *Neisseria gonorrhoeae* and *Ureaplasma urealyticum*. In contrast, the most common cause of epididymitis in a 50-year-old male is gram-negative rods such as *E. coli*, Klebsiella, and rarely Pseudomonas. The older patient with epididymitis presents an additional diagnostic challenge, as the physician must discover why the patient's urine is infected, e.g., is it outlet obstruction or a urethral stricture?

15. What is the treatment for epididymitis or epididymo-orchitis?
A patient who is febrile and toxic must be admitted to the hospital for intravenous anti-biotics and possible diagnostic studies to exclude a scrotal or testicular abscess (testicular ultrasound). Otherwise, outpatient therapy includes bed rest with placement of a folded towel between the legs to elevate the affected hemiscrotum. Ice is placed on the affected testis/epididymis for 10 minutes at a time, 3 or 4 times a day. The patient may get up to eat or to go to the bathroom. Once he is pain-free at rest, he may begin to ambulate with some type of scrotal supporter. If pain recurs, the patient should resume absolute bed rest and begin the process again.

When STD is suspected to be the cause of the epididymitis, the patient should be cultured for chlamydia and gonorrhea, and then treated empirically with ceftriaxone, 250 mg IM, and doxycycline, 100 mg b.i.d., for 7–10 days. The patient's sexual partner should be referred for evaluation and treatment. When gram-negative organisms are thought to be the cause of the epididymitis, treatment is based on the suspected organism.

All patients should be treated with antiinflammatory agents. If it becomes necessary to prescribe narcotics, it is prudent to place the patient on stool softeners to avoid straining to have a bowel movement, as this may exacerbate the inflammatory process.

All patients should be referred to a urologist within 1 week of initiation of outpatient therapy. If a large inflammatory mass is present, the urologist will need to proceed with testicular ultrasound to be certain the patient does not have a testicular abscess or testicular tumor.

BIBLIOGRAPHY

1. Cattolica EV: Preoperative manual detorsion of the torsed spermatic cord. J Urol 133:803–805, 1985.
2. Chen DCP, Holder LE, Melloul M: Radionuclide scrotal imaging: Further experience with 210 patients. II. Results and discussion. J Nucl Med 24:841, 1983.
3. Edelsberg JS, Surh YS: The acute scrotum. Emerg Med Clin North Am 6:521, 1988.

4. Kaver I, Matzkin H, Braf ZF: Epididymo-orchitis: A retrospective study of 122 patients. J Fam Pract 30:548, 1990.
5. Lindsey D, Stanisic TH: Diagnosis and management of testicular torsion: Pitfalls and perils. Am J Emerg Med 6:42, 1988.
6. Melekos MD, Asbach HW, Markou SA: Etiology of acute scrotum in 100 boys with regard to age distribution. J Urol 139:1023, 1988.
7. Middleton WD, Siegel BA, Melson GL, et al: Acute scrotal disorders: Prospective comparison of color Doppler US and testicular scintigraphy. Radiology 177:177, 1990.
8. Rabinowitz RL: The importance of the cremasteric reflex in acute scrotal swelling in children. J Urol 132:89–90, 1984.
9. Smith GI: Cellular changes for graded testicular ischemia. J Urol 73:355, 1955.

39. ACUTE URINARY RETENTION

Elizabeth L. Mitchell, M.D.

1. What is acute urinary retention (AUR)?

It is an uncomfortable inability to urinate that is precipitated by obstructive, neurogenic, pharmacologic, and psychogenic, or other causes. Urine is produced normally but is retained in the bladder.

2. What is the most common cause of AUR?

Obstruction is the most common cause of AUR seen in the emergency department (ED), with benign prostatic hypertrophy (BPH) being the most common.

3. How does BPH cause AUR? What do I do about it?

Urine outflow is obstructed by enlargement of the median lobe of the prostate, impinging on the internal urethral lumen. A careful history will elicit symptoms of heistancy, nocturia, dribbling, and diminished stream. The acute obstruction is usually precipitated by increased fluid load, infection, or medications. Physical exam may reveal a palpable enlarged bladder and rectal exam reveals an enlarged prostate. The immediate therapy is relief of the obstruction to urine flow usually accomplished by catheterization and bladder decompression. Chronically distended bladders should be decompressed slowly in order to avoid precipitating mucosal hemorrhage.

4. What if I can't pass a Foley catheter?

One trick that often helps is to fill a 30-cc syringe (Toomey-tipped) with xylocaine jelly and inject it into the urethral meatus. If that does not work, the next step is to try a Coude catheter. This catheter has a curved tip designed to slip over an enlarged prostate. If there is resistance proximally (<16 cm from the external meatus), a stricture may be present. Use of special dilators called filiforms and followers, under the strict supervision of a urologist, or suprapubic catheterization may be necessary.

5. What is suprapubic catheterization? How is it performed?

Suprapubic catheterization is a procedure used to pass a urinary catheter directly into the bladder through the lower anterior midline abdominal wall. It is indicated when bladder drainage is necessary and (1) other methods have failed or (2) in the face of suspected urethral damage from trauma. The procedure is performed under sterile conditions and with local anesthesia. The bladder is percussed and a small incision is made 2 cm above the symphysis pubis midline. Depending on technique, either a needle or a trochar is then used to penetrate the bladder through the incision. When urine is aspirated, a catheter is advanced over the cannula.

6. I'm sure there must be some studies or x-rays that I should order. What are they?
You probably won't need any x-ray studies. You should, however, always do a urinalysis, microscopic exam, and culture. Check BUN and creatinine to evaluate renal function and electrolytes to look for abnormalities sometimes found in AUR.

7. Are there any other obstructing lesions that cause AUR?
Absolutely. In men there are prostatitis, phimosis, and paraphimosis. In both sexes, etiologies include urethritis, urethral strictures, urethral calculi, tumor, clot, and foreign bodies.

8. I have heard that women have only psychogenic AUR. True?
No. Women may also have neurogenic and pharmacologic AUR. Psychogenic urinary retention is a diagnosis of exclusion and has been inappropriately overdiagnosed in the past.

9. Which medications cause AUR?
Anticholinergics are commonly associated with the problem; however, a variety of medications may cause AUR. Some are listed below.

Medications That May Cause Acute Urinary Retention

Sympathomimetics (alpha-adrenergic)	**Hormonal agents**
Ephedrine	Progesterone
Phenylephrine hydrochloride (Neo-Synephrine)	Estrogen
Phenylpropanolamine hydrochloride (Contac)	Testosterone
Pseudoephedrine (Sudafed, Actifed)	**Antipsychotics**
Sympathomimetics (beta-adrenergic)	Haloperidol
Isoproterenol	Chlorpromazine (Thorazine)
Terbutaline	**Antihypertensives**
Antidepressants	Hydralazine
Tricyclics	**Muscle Relaxants**
Antiarrhythmics	Diazepam (Valium)
Quinidine	Cyclobenzaprine (Flexeril)
Procainamide	**Miscellaneous**
Anticholinergics	Nifedipine (Procardia)
Antihistamines	Indomethacin
	Carbamazepine (Tegretol)
Antiparkinsonian agents	Amphetamines
Trihexyphenidyl (Artane)	Mercurial diuretics
Benztropine (Cogentin)	Dopamine
Amantadine (Symmetrel)	Vincristine
Levodopa (Sinemet)	Morphine sulfate

10. Can you help me sort out the neurogenic etiologies of AUR?
Neurogenic causes of AUR can be loosely divided into three categories.
    1. **Upper motor neuron lesions.** Lesions above the sacral micturition center (L2 vertebral level, S2–4 spinal segments) in the spinal cord lead to spastic or reflex bladder. The most common causes are spinal cord trauma, tumor, and multiple sclerosis (MS). Lesions in the cerebral cortex (e.g., acute stroke, bleed) usually cause loss of bladder control and incontinence, except in an acute phase.

2. **Lower motor neuron lesions.** Lesions at the micturition center in the cauda equina produce loss of sensation of bladder fullness, leading to overstretch, muscle atony, and poor contraction, and resulting in increased capacity and large residuals. Spinal trauma, tumor, metastases, herniated intervertebral discs, and MS are the most common causes.

3. **Bladder afferent and efferent nerve dysfunction.** Dysfunction in this pathway disrupts the micturition reflex arc, causing AUR. Causes include diabetes mellitus, herpes simplex infection, and postoperative state.

11. Are any complications associated with AUR?

Yes. The most common are infection, hemorrhage, and postobstructive diuresis.

12. What is postobstructive diuresis? How is it managed?

Persons with chronic urinary retention may develop postobstructive diuresis, which is an inappropriate excretion of salt and water after relief of urinary obstruction. A physiologic diuresis is normal, as the kidneys excrete the overload of solute and volume retained while obstructed. However, if urine output persists at high levels, significant fluid and electrolyte derangements will develop. Therefore, such patients should be observed closely following bladder decompression. Any patient who exhibits a continuous diuresis after clinical euvolemia is reached requires hospitalization for hemodynamic monitoring and fluid and electrolyte repletion.

13. Which patients with AUR should be admitted?

Good question! Patients with chronic obstructive urinary retention secondary to anatomic lesions such as BPH usually require continuous catheterization. Patients in good health, with no sign of infection, normal vital signs, uncomplicated relief of obstruction, and relatively timely follow-up can usually go home with a Foley catheter and leg bag. The use of prophylactic antibiotics in these patients is controversial. Patients with neurogenic AUR usually require hospital admission. Younger patients with pharmacologic urinary retention should have the catheter removed after relief of obstruction. The causative medication should be discontinued and the patient discharged with instructions to return if symptoms recur.

BIBLIOGRAPHY

1. Fontanarosa PB, Roush WR: Acute urinary retention. Emerg Med Clin North Amer 6:419–437, 1988.
2. Hastie KJ, et al: Acute retention of urine: Is trial without catheter justified? J R Coll Surg Edinb 35:225–227, 1990.
3. Higgins PM, et al: Management of acute retention of urine: A reappraisal. Br J Urol 67:365–368, 1991.
4. Koch MO: Fluid and electrolyte abnormalities in urologic practice. AUA Update Series, Lesson 12, Vol XI, pp 90–95.
5. O'Reilly PH, et al: High-pressure chronic retention: Incidence, aetiology and sinister implications. Br J Urol 58:644–666, 1986.
6. Purkerson ML, et al: Role of atrial peptide in the natriuresis and diuresis that follows relief of obstruction in rats. Am J Physiol 256(4 Pt 2):F583–589, 1989.
7. Seeley EC, et al: Diagnostic skills for primary care physicians. Prim Care 16:875–877, 1989.
8. Sophasan S, Sorrasuchart S: Factors inducing post-obstructive diuresis in rats. Nephron 38:125–133, 1984.
9. Stine RJ, et al: Diagnostic and therapeutic urologic procedures. Emerg Med Clin North Am 6:547–577, 1988.

40. URINARY TRACT INFECTION: CYSTITIS, PYELONEPHRITIS, PROSTATITIS

Marc A. Davis, M.D.

1. What is the spectrum of urinary tract infection (UTI)?
Bacteriuria is the presence of bacteria anywhere in the urinary tract. **Cystitis** refers to bacteriuria with bladder mucosal invasion. **Pyelonephritis** is a clinical syndrome of fever, flank pain, and tenderness associated with nausea and vomiting, leukocytosis, pyuria, and bacteriuria. **Acute urethral syndrome** or **urethritis** is the clinical syndrome of dysuria and frequency with less than 100,000 bacterial colonies per ml on urine culture. **Prostatitis** (chronic or acute) is a syndrome of prostatic inflammation that presents with a wide range of symptoms.

2. Describe the pathogenesis of UTIs.
The perineum and periurethral area are colonized by fecal bacteria that gain access to the urinary tract by retrograde movement through the urethra. Hematogenous seeding occurs much less commonly from systemic illness, such as staphylococcal sepsis and disseminated tuberculosis.

3. Why is the incidence of UTI much lower in males than in females?
The increased length of the urethra and antibacterial substances in prostatic fluid help to prevent infections in males. Females have more frequent colonization of the urethral meatus because the vagina serves as a bacterial reservoir. Because cystitis and pyelonephritis are uncommon in normal males, a search for underlying anatomic abnormalities should be initiated when these conditions are diagnosed.

4. What are the most common causes of UTI?
The Enterobacteriaceae family, particularly *E. coli*, are the most common. Klebsiella, Proteus, and Enterobacter are less commonly involved. In immunocompromised and chronically ill patients, Pseudomonas, *Staphylococcus aureus*, and Candida account for a small percentage of infections. *Staph. saprophyticus* and Enterococcus also cause infections. In the acute urethral syndrome, *Chlamydia trachomatis* is often isolated.

5. Why is a pelvic examination helpful in a female with dysuria?
Often dysuria is described as an external sensation associated with vulvovaginitis. Herpes genitalis may also present with dysuria and severe genital pain. Pelvic inflammatory disease (PID) may present similarly to pyelonephritis. The pelvic exam is invaluable in helping to distinguish between these entities.

6. What is the role of the urine dipstick in the diagnosis of UTI?
The nitrite test is based upon the ability of most urinary pathogens (with the exception of enterococcus) to reduce urine nitrates to nitrite. In order to be positive, the bacteria must act on the urine nitrate for 6 hours, requiring a first-voided morning specimen. This limits the test's utility in the emergency department. The leukocyte esterase test depends upon the ability of leukocytes to convert indoxyl carboxylic acid to an indoxyl moiety. The test is highly specific for detecting pyuria. False positives can result from vaginitis. A positive leukocyte esterase test combined with microscopic bacteriuria is most predictive of a UTI.

7. Does the presence of pyuria on microscopic examination confirm UTI?
Not always. Although pyuria, which is defined as >5 WBCs per high power field (HPF), is often present, false positives occur when pyuria is found in the absence of bacteriuria. Other inflammatory conditions such as appendicitis and PID cause pyuria without bacteriuria. The presence of both pyuria and bacteriuria on microscopic analysis is about 80% accurate for UTI.

8. Is microscopic bacteriuria predictive of a positive urine culture?
In an unspun urine specimen, one bacteria per HPF correlates with a urine culture >100,000 colony-forming units (CFUs) per ml. Examination of the urine sediment after centrifuge may be more sensitive in diagnosing patients with low-bacterial-count UTI (less than 100,000 CFUs). Ten or more bacteria per HPF in urine sediment usually predicts infection.

9. When should I order a urine culture?
Clearly, a urine culture is not required to presumptively treat the patient who presents with frequency, dysuria, and suprapubic pain. Most would recommend a culture in children, males, pregnant patients, immunocompromised patients, and patients with known anatomic abnormalities of the urinary tract, as well as in instances of suspected pyelonephritis, relapse in recently treated patients, and suspected sepsis or fever with neutropenia.

10. Can upper tract infection be clinically differentiated from lower tract infection?
Not by clinical exam, since 30–50% of patients with symptoms restricted to the lower urinary tract may have subclinical pyelonephritis. Several techniques, including bladder washout, antibody-coated bacteria, and ureteral catheterization, may be helpful in localizing the site of infection. These tests are not available. Symptoms such as frequency, dysuria, and suprapubic pain are found in a large percentage of both upper and lower tract infection. Fever, CVA tenderness, and white blood cell casts are more specific for pyelonephritis but are not 100% sensitive.

11. Which patients with pyelonephritis can be treated as outpatients?
Nonpregnant, nonimmunocompromised females who are not toxic appearing, who are able to take oral fluids and antibiotics without vomiting, and who have access to good follow-up care are candidates. Observation for 6–8 hours with treatment of 1–2 doses of IV antibiotics may help clarify who will do well with outpatient treatment of 10 days of oral antibiotics.

12. Which patients with pyelonephritis should be admitted?
Admission should be strongly considered for all pregnant patients, males, and patients with serious medical illnesses such as diabetes or an immunocompromised state. Of course, any patient who appears septic should be aggressively treated. Patients with anatomic abnormalities of the urinary tract or with urinary obstruction are at high risk for urosepsis and should be treated as inpatients.

13. What is the duration of treatment?
It depends. Single-dose therapy is now acceptable treatment for uncomplicated UTI. It is well tolerated, ensures compliance, is less expensive, and may be a good way to screen for subclinical pyelonephritis. Patients with recurrent symptoms after single-dose therapy, symptoms longer than 48 hours, symptoms suggestive of upper tract disease, hemorrhagic cystitis, or indwelling catheters should be treated with the traditional 7–10-day course of antibiotics.

14. Is it important to treat asymptomatic bacteriuria?
Certainly in pregnant patients (2–10% of all pregnant patients have asymptomatic bacteriuria; if left untreated, up to 30% will develop pyelonephritis) and probably in patients who are immunosuppressed. Patients with indwelling catheters should be treated only if symptomatic, as treatment may result in development of resistant bacteria and yeast.

15. How do I choose the proper antibiotic?
Many antibiotics are useful in treating UTI because of high concentrations achieved in the urine. Allergies, frequency of administration, most likely causative organism, and cost should be taken into account when prescribing antibiotics.

Oral Antibiotics for UTI

MEDICATION	DOSE	COST (10-DAY COURSE)*	SINGLE DOSE
TMP/SMX ds†	1 b.i.d.	$ 2.40	3 tabs
Ampicillin	500 mg q.i.d.	$ 3.45	3.5 gm
Amoxacillin	500 mg t.i.d.	$ 4.62	3 gm
Cephalexin	500 mg q.i.d.	$11.37	2 gm
Sulfasoxazole	500 mg q.i.d.	$ 6.45	2 gm
Nitrofurantoin	100 mg q.i.d.	$ 1.04	N/A
Norfloxacin	400 mg b.i.d.	$44.98	N/A
Ciprofloxacin	250 mg b.i.d.	$46.78	N/A
Doxycycline	100 mg b.i.d.	$ 2.39	N/A

* 1992 Red Book wholesale lowest generic price.
† Trimethoprim-sulfamethoxazole double strength.

16. What are the signs and symptoms of acute prostatitis?
Fever, chills, malaise, arthralgias, and myalgias may be present. Pain in the low back, perineal, or rectal area may be accompanied by dysuria, urgency, and frequency. Urinary retention may result from the acutely swollen prostate. The prostate is difficult to examine because of extreme tenderness.

17. How is acute prostatitis managed?
Antibiotics such as trimethoprim-sulfamethoxazole (TMP/SMX) and the newer quinolones (ciprofloxacin) are used to treat acute prostatitis. Prostatic massage and urethral catheterization should be avoided, as they may lead to hematogenous spread of bacteria and are painful. If urinary retention is a problem, suprapubic aspiration may be used initially. Toxicity with fever, chills, and urinary retention requires parenteral antibiotics and hospitalization. Outpatient treatment consists of antibiotics, bed rest, analgesics, and stool softeners.

18. What is the most common cause of recurrent urinary tract infection in males?
Chronic prostatitis.

19. List the potential complications of pyelonephritis.
Bacteremia, renal or perinephric abscess, papillary necrosis, and recurrent UTIs.

20. Infection with which organism produces alkalotic urine?
Proteus contains ureases, which lead to the formation of ammonia and alkalinization of the urine.

BIBLIOGRAPHY

1. Israel RS, Lowenstein SR, Marx JA, et al: Management of acute pyelonephritis in an emergency department observation unit. Ann Emerg Med 20:253–257, 1991.
2. Latham R: Urinary tract infections and the urethral syndrome in adult women: Pathogenesis, diagnosis and therapy. Emerg Med Clin North Am 3:75, 1985.
3. McCabe JB: Cystitis and pyelonephritis. In Callaham ML (ed): Current Therapy in Emergency Medicine. Philadelphia, B.C. Decker, 1987.
4. Meares EM Jr: Urinary tract infection in men. In Harrison JH, et al (eds): Campbell's Urology, 4th ed. Philadelphia, W.B. Saunders, 1978.
5. Stamm WE, Running K, Mckevitt M, et al: Treatment of the acute urethral syndrome. N Engl J Med 16:956, 1981.
6. Terndrup TE, McCabe JB: Urinary tract infection in women. In Harwood-Nuss (ed): The Clinical Practice of Emergency Medicine, Philadelphia, J.B. Lippincott, 1991.

41. CHRONIC RENAL FAILURE AND DIALYSIS

Allan B. Wolfson, M.D., FACEP, FACP

1. Isn't renal failure just another genitourinary disorder?

No. End-stage renal disease (ESRD) is a complex multisystem disorder. The absence of renal function has obvious consequences for the regulation of total body fluid and electrolyte balance, limiting the ability of dialysis patients to handle fluid and electrolyte loads. Chronic renal failure results in subtle metabolic abnormalities such as glucose intolerance and lipid disturbances. Renal failure is associated with numerous end-organ effects, ranging from pericarditis to renal osteodystrophy, that compromise comfort and normal function.

2. What are the special concerns in patients with renal failure?

Iatrogenic illness is the most important consideration, whether through overadministration of fluids or drug toxicity. Because the effects of renal failure on drug metabolism and disposition are often complex, it is always advisable to check recommended dosage adjustments for patients with ESRD before administering or prescribing medications. Even apparently innocuous drugs such as antacids and cathartics may cause morbidity and mortality if used improperly. Patients with ESRD also have complications from underlying disease that may have caused renal failure, as well as complications from dialysis therapy. They also have a limited capacity to respond to infection, trauma, or other intercurrent illnesses.

3. How is hemodialysis performed?

In hemodialysis, the patient's blood is brought into contact with a semipermeable artificial membrane, on the other side of which is a chemically balanced aqueous dialysis solution. Metabolic waste and electrolytes flow from the patient's blood into the dialysate, and other substances (e.g., calcium) may flow from the dialysate into the blood, acting to normalize blood chemistries. In order to achieve adequate total body clearances over the time available for hemodialysis, a high blood flow rate is necessary. This requires the cannulation of large vessels or, for chronic dialysis, the creation of an artificial vascular access that can be used repeatedly. Hemodialysis is typically performed for 4–5 hours, 3 times per week.

4. How is peritoneal dialysis performed?

The patient's peritoneal membrane serves as the semipermeable barrier between the blood (in the peritoneal capillaries) and a balanced dialysate solution, which is introduced into the patient's peritoneal cavity and allowed to dwell for a period of hours before being drained and replaced. An osmolar gradient is created by using a dialysate with high concentrations of glucose that, through osmosis, pulls water from the intravascular space into the dialysate, acting to correct volume overload. For patients with ESRD on chronic ambulatory peritoneal dialysis (CAPD), about 2 liters of dialysate dwells continuously within the peritoneal cavity. It is exchanged for fresh dialysate in a sterile fashion by the patient 4 times a day. Special peritoneal access is required in the form of a surgically implanted Teflon catheter (Tenkhoff catheter), through which dialysate is infused and drained.

5. What is the most common problem relating to the vascular access device in the emergency department (ED)?
Thrombosis should be suspected when patients report loss of thrill in the vascular device. The only intervention necessary is a prompt call to a vascular surgeon. An angiogram will define the nature and extent of the obstruction and delineate anatomic lesions, allowing the surgeon to revise or replace the access.

6. How do I diagnose and treat a vascular access infection?
Such infection is obvious when the patient presents with signs of inflammation localized to the access area. The difficulty is that many patients present only with fever and without specific localizing signs. A useful rule of thumb in such instances is to assume that an endovascular access infection is present and to treat accordingly. Patients can typically be sent home after one dose of an appropriate antibiotic, provided they look well and are reliable for follow-up. Vancomycin, 1 gm IV, is the treatment of choice because the vast majority of infections are staphylococcal and the duration of action is 5–7 days in ESRD. The drug is not hemodialyzable, and its major toxicity is to the kidneys. If gram-negative infection is suspected, a loading dose of tobramycin may be added to the regimen, with reloading after each of the next several dialysis treatments. Careful follow-up should be arranged with the patient's dialysis nurse or physician. Blood cultures should be obtained before treatment is initiated.

7. When can the vascular access device be used for giving IV infusions or for drawing blood?
Hemodialysis patients are instructed never to allow anyone to take the blood pressure in the arm with the vascular access or to allow drawing blood or giving IV infusions. This is to protect the access device, which is truly the patient's lifeline. However, occasionally there is no reasonable alternative but to use the access device for blood drawing or IV lines. In these situations, very cautious use of the vascular access device is permissible, provided certain guidelines are followed.

When using the access to draw blood, a tourniquet should not be used. At most, one finger can be used to lightly tourniquet the vein. The presence of a thrill should be documented both before and after the procedure. The area should be cleaned thoroughly with povidone-iodine or another antiseptic, and sterile technique should be observed. Care should be taken not to puncture the back wall of the vessel, and after the puncture firm but nonocclusive pressure should be applied to the site for several minutes to ensure that extravasation does not occur. Obvious aneurysms should not be punctured.

When using the vascular access for an IV line, similar precautions should be observed. Because the vessel is under arterial pressure, a pressure bag or, preferably, an automated infusion device is an absolute requirement (certainly when infusing medications).

8. How is CAPD-associated peritonitis diagnosed?
Peritonitis associated with CAPD occurs about once per year in even the most fastidious and well-motivated patients. In contrast to other types of peritonitis, it tends to be quite

mild clinically, and most patients can be managed without hospital admission. CAPD-associated peritonitis is most commonly caused by gram-positive organisms, which are thought to have been introduced during the exchange procedure. The diagnosis is suspected by the patient on the basis of the new development of a cloudy appearance of the dialysis effluent. Patients are instructed to seek medical attention promptly when this occurs, and for this reason most episodes of peritonitis are relatively mild. If, however, the patient delays seeking attention, the symptoms tend to become progressively more severe. Most patients have abdominal pain and tenderness, but a minority have fever, nausea, vomiting or even (at least early on) an elevated peripheral white count. Localized peritoneal findings are suggestive of an acute surgical abdomen rather than CAPD-induced peritonitis.

9. How is CAPD-associated peritonitis treated?

Once fluid has been obtained through the effluent bag and laboratory studies have confirmed the presence of a significant number of white cells ($>100/mm^3$ with $>50\%$ polymorphonuclear leukocytes) or a positive Gram stain, treatment is initiated with a loading dose of a first-generation cephalosporin such as cefazolin. Gram-negative coverage, usually tobramycin, can be added if felt appropriate. After this loading dose, if the patient is otherwise suitable for outpatient management, a 10-day regimen of self-administered intraperitoneal antibiotics is prescribed. A typical regimen is cefazolin, 250 mg/2-liter bag of dialysate. Follow-up should be in 48 hours, at which time cultures and clinical findings are rechecked and therapy adjusted as necessary.

Admission criteria include severe pain, nausea and vomiting, a toxic appearance, or the inability for the patient to comply with outpatient therapy and follow-up.

10. What are the indications for emergency dialysis?

Emergency dialysis is indicated for patients with ESRD who present with acute pulmonary edema, life-threatening hyperkalemia, or life-threatening intoxication or overdose secondary to dialyzable toxins that ordinarily are excreted by the kidneys.

11. What is unique about a dialysis patient with cardiac arrest?

Two potentially reversible entities should always be considered in an ESRD patient with cardiac arrest.

1. **Severe hyperkalemia** may cause severe rhythm disturbances and ultimately cardiac arrest without any other warning or clinical signs. Once a patient suffers an arrest from whatever cause, respiratory and metabolic acidosis and the efflux of potassium from cells can be expected to produce hyperkalemia secondarily. In the patient who may already have a tendency toward hyperkalemia, this further increase could cause the patient to be refractory to standard advanced cardiac life support (ACLS) interventions. Thus, ESRD patients in cardiac arrest should always be given intravenous calcium if they do not respond immediately to the first round of ACLS measures.

2. **Acute pericardial tamponade** may result from accumulation of pericardial fluid or spontaneous bleeding into the pericardial sac. Patients with tamponade tend to display refractory hypotension and/or electromechanical dissociation (EMD). Although less likely than other entities to be the cause of refractoriness to resuscitation measures, the possibility of pericardial tamponade should always be considered in patients in whom other measures have failed. Emergency pericardiocentesis may be life-saving.

12. What are the treatment options for acute pulmonary edema in patients with ESRD?

ESRD patients with pulmonary edema do not have the ability to rid themselves of excess fluids through the kidneys, and therefore ultimately require dialysis to correct volume overload. Interventions that are useful in patients with functioning kidneys are also useful in patients with ESRD before dialysis can be initiated. The patient should be given oxygen and placed in a sitting position. Nitrates administered sublingually or intravenously are the mainstay of temporizing therapy. Sublingual nitroglycerin can be given every 3 minutes to decrease preload and afterload as blood pressure permits. Intravenous nitroglycerin is a useful alternative. Intravenous morphine, although less popular in recent years, may also be helpful in decreasing pulmonary venous hypertension, although patients may be more likely to require intubation and mechanical ventilation because of its sedative action. Intravenous furosemide, although it cannot act as a diuretic, has some action in decreasing pulmonary venous pressure.

Dialysis, however, is the definitive therapy and should usually be instituted as early as possible. The CAPD patient with acute pulmonary edema presents a slightly different problem, because intensified dialysis, even with 4.25% glucose solution, is a slow means of removing fluid and because the presence of 2 L of dialysate in the peritoneal cavity tends to have an adverse affect on diaphragmatic excursion and pulmonary mechanics. Therefore intubation and mechanical ventilation may be necessary while continuing hourly exchanges of high-concentration dialysate.

In the past, it has been recommended that patients without immediate access to dialysis be given oral sorbitol in order to produce a "gastrointestinal dialysis." This modality should rarely, if ever, be used because of its rather slow action, the almost universal availability of conventional dialysis modalities, and the clinician's desire to work harmoniously with the ED nursing staff in the future.

13. What about air embolism?

Air embolism is an uncommon but well-reported complication of hemodialysis. Although it has become rare in recent years with the advent of sophisticated monitoring and alarm systems on hemodialysis machines, when air embolism does occur it is often a devastating event and one for which the patient will almost surely be brought to the nearest ED.

Air embolism should be suspected when a patient experiences a sudden acute decompensation during the course of hemodialysis treatment. Several immediate measures are thought to be helpful. Any IV lines should be clamped. The patient should be given 100% oxygen and laid on the left side with the head down, in an attempt to cause the air to collect at the apex of the right ventricle. At this point, if the patient is reasonably stable, an interventional radiologist can be consulted for consideration of passage of a central venous catheter into the right ventricular apex, through which the air can be directly aspirated out of the heart. For patients who are in close proximity to a hyperbaric chamber, treatment with 100% oxygen at several atmospheres can directly shrink the size of the bubbles and enhance resorption of the gas. One should be certain before embarking on this course, however, that the patient's symptoms are indeed due to air embolism rather than, for example, a sudden spontaneous pneumothorax.

14. How should a patient with acute shortness of breath be evaluated?

The rule of thumb is: if they are short of breath, dialyze them, because it is most commonly volume overload. It is sometimes very difficult to make the diagnosis of volume overload. The patient's weight may be the best guide. Physical examination is not always helpful and even chest x-ray may be misleading.

15. What are the main differential diagnostic elements of chest pain in ESRD?

One should always think first of either angina or pericarditis. Some patients with ESRD, particularly those who are anemic, may have angina and cardiac ischemia even if a previous cardiac catheterization has shown a "noncritical" coronary obstruction. This is because there are increased cardiac oxygen demands and decreased oxygen delivery to the heart. Although cardiac enzyme levels may be altered somewhat in ESRD, renal failure does not obscure the usual EKG and enzyme changes of acute myocardial infarction.

16. What is the differential diagnosis of hypotension in a patient with ESRD?
Always consider hypovolemia after dialysis, hemorrhage, acute pericardial tamponade, and sepsis.

17. What are the major causes of altered mental status in patients with ESRD?
"Disequilibrium syndrome," caused by rapid solute shifts during hemodialysis, is a common consideration, but a major pitfall is to attribute every change in mental status to this entity. Drug effects are a major cause, as is spontaneous intracranial hemorrhage. Any patient with localizing signs should certainly have a CT scan of the head; those without localizing signs probably should as well, since subdural hematoma may not cause focal findings.

BIBLIOGRAPHY

1. Anderson CC, Shahvari MBG, Zimmerman JE: The treatment of pulmonary edema in the absence of renal function. JAMA 241:1008, 1979.
2. Bennett WM, Aronoff GR, Golper TA, et al: Drug Prescribing in Renal Failure: Dosing Guidelines for Adults. Philadelphia, American College of Physicians, 1987.
3. Kohen JA, Opsahl JA, Kjellstrand CM: Deceptive patterns of uremic pulmonary edema. Am J Kidney Dis 7:456, 1986.
4. Wolfson AB: End-stage renal disease: Emergencies related to dialysis and transplantation. In Wolfson AB, Harwood-Nuss A (eds): Renal and Urologic Emergencies. New York, Churchill Livingstone, 1986.
5. Wolfson AB: Dialysis-related emergencies. In Harwood-Nuss A, Linden CH, Luten RC, et al (eds): The Clinical Practice of Emergency Medicine. Philadelphia, J.B. Lippincott, 1991, pp 1010–1014.
6. Wolfson AB: Chronic renal failure and dialysis. In Rosen P, et al (eds): Emergency Medicine: Concepts and Clinical Practice, 3rd ed. Philadelphia, Mosby–Year Book, 1992, pp 1928–1944.
7. Wolfson AB, Singer I: Hemodialysis-related emergencies (Part I). J Emerg Med 5:553, 1987.
8. Wolfson AB, Singer I: Hemodialysis-related emergencies (Part II). J Emerg Med 6:61, 1988.

IX. Hematology/Oncology

42. HEMOSTASIS AND COAGULOPATHIES

Andrew M. Johanos, M.D.

1. I'm an emergency physician, not a hematologist. Why do I need to know about coagulopathies?
Patients with coagulopathies cannot schedule their crises to fall during their hematologist's office hours. You need not recall that the gene for von Willebrand factor is on band 21 of chromosome 12, but you must know that a hemophiliac with an intracerebral bleed needs 50 U/kg of factor VIII concentrate.

2. But hemostasis and coagulation are complicated. How can I remember all the steps?
Simply recall the three phases of hemostasis: (1) vasoconstriction, (2) platelet adhesion and aggregation, and (3) fibrin clot formation. Coagulation occurs via intrinsic (factors VIII and IX) and extrinsic (factor VII) pathways, each of which activates factor X in the common pathway; factor X converts prothrombin to thrombin, which cleaves fibrinogen into fibrin.

3. What clinical findings suggest platelet versus coagulation factor disorders?
Patients with platelet defects cannot efficiently initiate hemostasis. They present with bruising, epistaxis, and gingival and mucosal bleeding; bleeding may be prolonged. Once bleeding stops, fibrin clot formation usually prevents recurrence. Patients with coagulation factor defects cannot effectively reinforce platelet-induced hemostasis. They present with hematomas, hemarthroses, and deep space bleeds; presentation may be delayed and recurrent.

4. When and how should I give platelets to a patient with thrombocytopenia?
A platelet count of 10–20,000 in a nonbleeding medical patient is cited as the threshold for transfusion; in reality, spontaneous hemorrhage is rare above 5,000. In the surgical patient, the threshold rises to 50–60,000. For adults, each unit of platelets raises the platelet count by 5–10,000 in the absence of peripheral destruction. The hemorrhaging patient with thrombocytopenia needs 8–10 units of platelets, regardless of the count.

5. Why do alcoholics have bleeding diatheses?
Alcoholics have decreased hepatic synthesis of clotting factors and decreased marrow production of platelets. Splenic sequestration reduces the number of circulating platelets, and alcohol induces a toxic effect on platelet function.

6. Why do patients with renal failure have prolonged bleeding times despite normal platelet counts?
As uremia progresses, unspecified uremic toxins in the plasma interfere with platelet function. Platelet transfusions are of little benefit, for the metabolic disorder persists; dialysis is the definitive treatment. Short of this, DDAVP (1-desamino-8-D-arginine-vasopressin) can help; the dose is 0.3 μg/kg IV.

7. What is von Willebrand's disease (VWD)?

VWD is the most common congenital hemostatic disorder. Unlike the X-linked hemophilias, the vast majority of VWD is autosomal dominant, affecting males and females alike. The disease involves decreased levels of von Willebrand factor (VWF), a protein produced by endothelial cells. VWF enhances platelet–platelet and platelet–endothelial adhesion and stabilizes factor VIII in plasma.

8. How is VWD treated?

Mild bleeding often responds to DDAVP, 0.3 μg/kg IV. DDAVP increases the release of VWF and factor VIII from endothelial cells. If this fails to control bleeding, the treatment of choice is cryoprecipitate. Cryoprecipitate is concentrated from fresh frozen plasma (FFP) and contains large amounts of VWF, factor VIII, and fibrinogen. Dosing is in "bags" of cryoprecipitate per 10 kg of body weight and is based on severity of injury; epistaxis and superficial trauma = 0.5–1.0 bags/10 kg; GI bleeding and menorrhagia = 1.0–1.5 bags/10 kg; head injury or intracranial bleed = 2.0 bags/10 kg.

9. What is classic hemophilia?

Classic hemophilia (hemophilia A) is an X-linked recessive disorder characterized by deficient activity of factor VIII; symptomatology varies from mild, with bleeding following trauma or surgery, to severe, with recurrent spontaneous bleeding. The most common presentations include hemarthrosis, hematuria, gastrointestinal bleeding, and dental-related bleeding. Screening tests reveal a prolonged partial thromboplastin time (PTT) and a normal prothrombin time (PT), along with a normal platelet count and bleeding time.

10. What is Christmas disease?

Hemophilia B, also known as Christmas disease, is one-seventh as common as hemophilia A; it is an X-linked recessive disorder characterized by deficient activity of factor IX. Clinical symptoms and screening tests are identical to those for hemophilia A; the distinction is made by specific factor assays. The disease shows no seasonal predilection; the name stems from its first report in the Christmas 1952 issue of the *British Medical Journal.*

11. How do I treat hemophilia A?

The approach is based on the source and severity of bleeding. Mild epistaxis, hemarthrosis, or hematoma may respond to DDAVP, 0.3 μg/kg IV, or 8–10 bags of cryoprecipitate (10 U/kg; 80–100 U/bag). If these treatments are unsuccessful, use 10–15 U/kg of factor VIII concentrate. Moderate-to-severe hemarthroses and hematomas require 20–30 U/kg; intracranial hemorrhages and major trauma require 50 U/kg of factor VIII concentrate.

12. How do I treat hemophila B?

Mild bleeding may respond to FFP alone, 5–6 units, because FFP retains significant factor IX activity. Authorities differ as to empirical dosing with factor IX concentrate, but a good approximation is to use the same guidelines as with factor VIII concentrate in hemophila A. Intracranial hemorrhages and major trauma require 50 U/kg of factor IX concentrate.

13. What anatomic sites of bleeding pose immediate life threats for hemophiliacs?

Central nervous system, retroperitoneal, and retropharyngeal bleeds are true emergencies with the potential for neurologic deterioration, uncontrolled hemorrhage, and airway obstruction. Patients should receive 50 U/kg of the appropriate factor concentrate in the emergency department (ED) and be admitted to the hospital.

14. What if the patient has a factor inhibitor?

Of patients with severe hemophilia A, 5–10% develop antibodies to factor VIII, foiling any efforts at correction with factor VIII concentrate. First-line treatment is to use factor IX concentrate, 100 U/kg IV; a fraction of the factor IX is activated and bypasses the factor VIII-dependent step of the intrinsic pathway. If this fails, use activated IX complex. Management must be coordinated with a hematologist and the blood bank.

15. What are the most common causes of prolonged PT and PTT in the hospitalized or chronically ill patient?

Aside from anticoagulant therapy, the common culprits include vitamin K deficiency (nutritional or secondary to broad-spectrum antibiotics and depletion of bowel flora), liver disease (predominantly alcoholic), and disseminated intravascular coagulation (DIC).

16. How is heparin-induced bleeding treated?

Minor bleeding is treated with simple cessation of heparin therapy; the half-life of heparin is only 1 hr. Hemorrhage or intracerebral bleeds require immediate inactivation of heparin with protamine sulfate; the dose is 1 mg of protamine sulfate for every 100 units of heparin in circulation, given at a maximum rate of 50 mg over 10 min.

17. What about bleeding induced by warfarin (Coumadin)?

Bleeding can be controlled with 4–5 units of FFP. Vitamin K, 5–10 mg, given IV or SQ, partially reverses the effect of warfarin; 20–30 mg completely reverses the effect and causes refractoriness to therapy for several weeks.

18. How is the cirrhotic patient with bleeding varices treated?

Above all, wear a mask, goggles, and gloves; in fact, put on a second pair of gloves! In addition to red blood cell transfusion, these patients deserve treatment with 6–10 units of FFP. If the platelet count is <70,000, give 8–10 units of platelets. Vitamin K should be given once the patient is stable.

19. How do I diagnose and treat DIC?

In the appropriate clinical setting (retained fetus, amniotic fluid embolism, shock, sepsis, widespread malignancy, major trauma, or burns), with prolonged PT and PTT and falling platelet counts, the diagnosis is confirmed by decreased fibrinogen levels and elevated fibrin split products. The easy answer to the second part of this question is treat the underlying condition. But the hemorrhaging patient needs red blood cell transfusions; FFP and platelets are needed to replace consumed factors and platelets, despite the unsubstantiated theoretical fear of "feeding the fire." Paradoxically, some authorities advocate the use of heparin to inhibit thrombin and break the consumptive cycle; this approach calls for a higher sphincter tone than most physicians can tolerate.

BIBLIOGRAPHY

1. Burns ER: Clinical Management of Bleeding and Thrombosis. Boston, Blackwell, 1987.
2. Carr ME Jr: Disseminated intravascular coagulation: Pathogenesis, diagnosis, and therapy. J Emerg Med 5:311, 1987.
3. Harwood-Nuss A, et al (eds): The Clinical Practice of Emergency Medicine. Philadelphia, J.B. Lippincott, 1991.
4. Hilgartner MW, Pochedly C (eds): Hemophilia in the Child and Adult, 3rd ed. New York, Raven Press, 1989.
5. Ratnoff OD, Forbes CD (eds): Disorders of Hemostasis, 2nd ed. Philadelphia, W.B. Saunders, 1991.
6. Rosen P, et al (eds): Emergency Medicine Concepts and Clinical Practice, 3rd ed. St. Louis, Mosby–Year Book, 1992.

43. SICKLE CELL ANEMIA

Linda L. Hanson, M.D.

1. What causes sickle cell anemia?
Sickle cell anemia is an autosomal dominant disease that results from substitution of valine for glutamine at the sixth position on both chains of the beta-globulin chain in a hemoglobin molecule.

2. What factors promote sickling?
Sickling is promoted by low pH independent of oxygen tension by shifting the oxygen dissociation curve to the right. Low oxygen tension from whatever cause induces sickling. Causes include cardiovascular disease, circulatory stasis that results in local tissue hypoxia, high altitude, or breathing through special devices as when SCUBA diving or during anesthesia. A high intracellular concentration of sickle hemoglobin from dehydration promotes sickling. Low temperature promotes sickling through vasoconstriction.

3. Why do patients with sickle cell anemia develop clinical problems?
Sickled cells and chronic hemolysis produce sludging in the microcirculation, with obstruction of flow causing regional hypoxia and acidosis, further increasing sickling and obstruction of flow. Ischemic injury and infarcts occur, resulting in a propensity for infection and chronic organ damage.

4. What are the various types of sickle cell crises?
Vaso-occlusive crisis is caused by ischemic tissue injury. The presenting complaint is usually pain, which may affect any organ, but common sites include bone, abdomen, and chest. **Hemolytic crisis** usually occurs in response to infection, resulting in a more rapid rate of hemolysis. A rapidly falling hematocrit, an elevated reticulocyte count, pallor, and jaundice are usually observed. **Aplastic crisis** is often induced by infection and rarely folic acid deficiency. Patients present with a decreased hematocrit, depressed reticulocyte count, fatigue, dyspnea, or pallor. **Sequestration crisis** occurs when large numbers of red blood cells pool in the spleen. The inciting event is thought to be infection. Patients present with splenic enlargement, abdominal pain, a falling hematocrit, pallor, tachycardia and dyspnea. Pooling can be so massive that hypovolemic shock and death can ensue. It usually occurs between the ages of 5 months and 2 years and is the most dangerous crisis for the young child.

5. Why is sequestration crisis more common in very young children?
Fetal hemoglobin inhibits sickling and has a protective effect until about 4 months of age, when it declines. Therefore, splenic sequestration is unusual until after 4 months of age, when the spleen may undergo repeated infarcts that result in autosplenectomy (usually before the age of 2).

6. Why do patients with sickle cell anemia have an increased risk of infection?
Patients with sickle cell anemia experience repeated splenic infarctions that lead to functional asplenia. In addition, ischemia produced by sludging in the microcirculation by sickled cells serves as a nidus for infection. Phagocytic activity is depressed because of blockage of sinusoids in the liver and spleen. Decreased nonantibody opsonic activity and decreased IgM antibody production also contribute to infection.

7. Why should I worry about a child with sickle cell anemia who presents with fever?
Fever in children, especially those under 5 years of age, may indicate life-threatening infection. Severe overwhelming sepsis secondary to *Streptococcus pneumoniae* is still the

most common cause of death during early childhood. In addition, a twofold increase in the incidence of *Hemophilus influenzae* is seen. Appropriate cultures should be done and antibiotics should be used liberally.

8. What is the "acute chest syndrome"?
It is an acute pulmonary process that occurs in patients with sickle cell anemia. Typical findings include fever, pleuritic chest pain, and radiographic evidence of an acute pulmonary process. Hypoxemia and leukocytosis may be present. The differential diagnosis includes viral, bacterial, or mycoplasmal infections or pulmonary infarcts. It may be difficult to determine whether infection or infarction is responsible for the condition.

9. Which diagnostic studies are indicated in acute chest syndrome?
In general, diagnostic studies are indicated only when deep venous thrombosis is suspected, in which case a venous Doppler study should be performed. Because the hypertonicity of contrast agents may produce cellular dehydration (resulting in more sickling), pulmonary angiograms and venograms are contraindicated. Ventilation-perfusion scans can safely be done in patients with sickle cell anemia; however, interpretation is often difficult, owing to repeated pulmonary insults, unless baseline ventilation-perfusion scans are available.

10. How is acute chest syndrome treated?
Patients should be admitted to the hospital. Analgesics, IV hydration, and oxygen for hypoxemia are the basic treatment strategies. Early treatment with broad-spectrum antibiotics and oral erythromycin is instituted until culture results are available. In severe, rapidly progressive cases with marked hypoxemia, exchange transfusion is indicated to acutely lower the concentration of HgS.

11. Is heparin beneficial in the treatment of acute chest syndrome?
No. In fact, it is dangerous. Patients with sickle cell anemia and pulmonary infarcts have not been shown to benefit from heparin, and it imposes the risk of bleeding. Again, severe cases should be treated with exchange transfusion to acutely lower the concentration of HgS, which retards sickling.

12. Are neurologic complications a predominant feature in patients with sickle cell disease?
Yes! They occur in 26% of all patients with sickle cell anemia. Most such complications result from vascular occlusion and embolic events. Possible complications include transient ischemic attacks (TIAs), cerebrovascular accidents (CVAs), meningitis, seizures, coma, and subarachnoid and intracerebral hemorrhage.

13. Which neurologic complications occur more frequently in young patients?
Children and young adults are more susceptible to CVAs and are more likely to have recurrent CVAs. The mean age at onset of CVA is 10. The youngest patient reported to have a CVA was 6. CVAs account for 16% of deaths in children. Up to 67% of patients who have one stroke will suffer another, usually within 36 months, presumably secondary to stasis.

14. What steady-state laboratory abnormalities are present in sickle cell anemia?
Patients with sickle cell anemia at steady state have underlying hemolytic anemia. Hemoglobin levels are generally between 5 and 10 gm/dl. Reticulocyte counts are in the range of 5–30%. Polymorphonuclear leukocytosis is common from demargination. Increased indirect bilirubin and lactate dehydrogenase (LDH) result from hemolysis. Increased alkaline phosphatase results from increased bone metabolism.

15. Which screening tests are helpful?

The diagnostic work-up is guided by the presentation of the patient. Minimum screening tests are complete blood count, reticulocyte count, and oxygenation, which are compared to the patient's baseline values to determine severity and type of crisis. Severely ill patients with toxemia or hypoxemia require screening of all systems and panculture because of the potential for multiple organ failure.

16. What is the fluid of choice and rate for IV hydration?

Aggressive rehydration is one of the mainstays of therapy. D5 ½ normal saline is the fluid of choice because it is relatively hypotonic and will restore intracellular volume, thereby reducing the intracellular concentration of sickle hemoglobin, and in turn retarding sickling. Severely ill patients with hypovolemia should be given normal saline, then switched to D5 ½ normal saline as intravascular volume is repleted. Adults should be given 200–300 cc/hr, children 100 cc/kg/day.

17. What is the rationale for the use of rapid partial exchange transfusion (RPET)?

RPET is used to decrease the sickle hemoglobin concentration rapidly to less than 30%, which decreases sludging in the microcirculation and thereby increases tissue perfusion and limits infarct size.

18. What are some indications for RPET?

RPET is indicated for life-threatening events, including acute impending or suspected CVA or TIA, acute hepatic or splenic sequestration in the face of a falling hematocrit, acute priapism unresponsive to medical management after 6 hours, acute progressive lung disease, fat embolization, prior to surgery, and prior to administration of IV contrast material or other hypertonic fluids.

BIBLIOGRAPHY

1. Alavi J: Sickle cell anemia. Med Clin North Am 68:545, 1984.
2. Bromberg P: Pulmonary aspects of sickle cell disease. Arch Intern Med 133:652, 1974.
3. Charache S, Lubin B, Reid C: Management and therapy of sickle cell disease. National Institutes of Health Publication No. 85-2117. Bethesda, MD, U.S. Department of Health and Human Services, 1985, p 485.
4. Charache S, Scott J, Charache P: Acute chest syndrome in adults with sickle cell anemia. Arch Intern Med 139:67, 1979.
5. Galloway S, Harwood-Nuss A: Sickle cell anemia: A review. Am J Emerg Med 6:213, 1988.
6. Lukens J: Sickle cell disease. Disease a Month 27:1, 1981.
7. Mozzarelli A, Hofricter J, Eaton W: Delay time of hemoglobin S polymerization prevents most cells from sickling in vivo. Science 237:500, 1987.
8. Poncz M, Kane E, Gill F: Acute chest syndrome in sickle cell disease: Etiology and clinical correlates. J Pediatr 107:861, 1985.
9. Serjeant G: What's new in sickle cell. Trans Roy Soc Trop Med 82:177, 1988.
10. Shapiro B: The management of pain in sickle cell disease. Pediatr Clin North Am 36:1029, 1989.
11. Vichinsky EL, Lubin B: Sickle cell anemia and related hemoglobinopathies. Pediatr Clin North Am 27:429, 1980.

44. ONCOLOGIC EMERGENCIES

Nicholas J. Jouriles, M.D.

1. What is an oncologic emergency?

An oncologic emergency is a life- or limb-threatening problem in a patient with an underlying neoplastic disease. These problems may be caused directly by the cancer or its systemic effects, or by therapeutic maneuvers used in treatment.

2. Is this important?

Yes. Cancer is the second leading cause of death in the United States. It is also second only to trauma in years of potential life loss.

3. Name several oncologic emergencies.

Emergencies in Patients with Underlying Neoplastic Diseases (Partial List)

Airway Compromise	Emotional Stress
Head and neck mass	Death and dying
Tracheal compression	DNR orders
Adrenal Crisis	Family issues
Primary tumor	Graft vs. Host Disease
Metastatic lesion	Hyperviscosity Syndrome
Anemia	Infection
Bone marrow replacement	With neutropenia
with tumor	Postobstructive pneumonia
Chemotherapy effects	Intestinal Obstruction
Bleeding	Intestinal Perforation
Primary mass	Malignant Pericardial Effusion
Low platelet count	With tamponade
Abnormal clotting factors	Metabolic Abnormalities
secondary to liver metastases	Hypercalcemia
Carcinoid Syndrome	Acute tumor lysis syndrome
Complications of Chemotherapy	Hyponatremia/SIADH
Bone marrow suppression	Obstructive Jaundice
Cardiac toxicity	Pain
GI toxicity	Peptic Ulcer Disease
Pulmonary toxicity	Seizures
Renal toxicity	Spinal Cord Compression
Complications of Radiotherapy	Motor/sensory loss
Dermatitis	Incontinence
GI toxicity	Back pain
	Superior Vena Cava Syndrome
	Tinnitus

4. Which on this list are life or limb threatening?

The life-threatening diseases are those that can lead to shock or death. They can be divided into the standard categories of shock: volume loss (bleeding) or impaired vascular return (superior vena cava syndrome); pump impairment (cardiac tamponade); and derangement of systemic vascular resistance or afterload (infection/sepsis). In addition to life-threatening problems, there are diseases that can cause serious metabolic derangements (hypercalcemia) and those that can lead to neurologic impairment (spinal cord compression).

5. Tell me about these.

Superior vena cava syndrome is caused by obstruction of the superior vena cava. Although it may be caused by such relatively benign processes as mediastinitis or aortic aneurysms, it is most often caused by a neoplastic process. Lung cancer is the most common cause, usually the small cell or squamous cell types. Adenocarcinoma of the breast, lymphoma, and thymus neoplasms are also common. Superior vena cava syndrome may also occur secondary to metastatic lesions from distant primary sites. Treatment usually involves radiation therapy.

Pericardial tamponade occurs secondary to metastatic disease to the pericardium, and has been found in 2–21% of patients dying of cancer. Even with proper treatment, patients with pericardial tamponade usually have a large tumor burden and poor 6-month survival. The diagnosis of a malignant pericardial tamponade is made in the hypotensive patient with muffled heart sounds, elevated neck veins, and an enlarged cardiac silhouette on chest x-ray. It is most commonly seen in lung and breast carcinomas as well as lymphoma. Treatment involves pericardial drainage.

Infections. Because all patients with tumors are by definition immunocompromised, the variety of infections is unlimited. Immune status may be further compromised by chemotherapeutic agents. When patients become neutropenic secondary to treatment, any types of infection may occur (bacterial, viral, or fungal), potentially leading to septic shock, adult respiratory distress syndrome, and death. The neutropenic febrile patient should immediately be treated with prophylactic broad-spectrum antibiotics.

Hypercalcemia occurs in approximately 5% of patients followed in a hospital-based oncology practice. Neoplasms that lead to metastatic involvement of the skeletal system are commonly associated with hypercalcemia. Common presenting signs are lethargy, constipation, and altered mental status. Treatment involves hydration with normal saline followed by forced calcium excretion.

Spinal cord compression occurs in up to 5% of all patients with metastatic disease. The spinal cord or nerve root is directly compressed by an extradural mass, causing secondary neurologic dysfunction. The most common causes of spinal cord compression are lung cancer, breast cancer, prostate cancer, and multiple myeloma. The most common presenting symptom is back pain. Any patient with an underlying malignancy who presents with back pain, motor or sensory losses, or incontinence should be considered as having spinal cord compression until proved otherwise. Prompt diagnosis can save neurologic function. All patients who fit the clinical criteria should undergo either myelography or MRI. Treatment is emergent surgical decompression or radiation therapy. Steroids can be used in the ED.

6. Are these common problems?
Of the life-threatening problems, spinal cord compression, infection, and hypercalcemia are common.

7. Which problems are common in patients with an underlying malignancy?
The most common problems are complications of cancer treatment. Each chemotherapeutic agent has side effects, including nausea and vomiting, renal involvement (e.g., cis-platinum), pulmonary toxicity (e.g., bleomycin), cardiac toxicity (e.g., adriamycin), and diarrhea/enteritis secondary to radiation. These problems are usually treated by the oncologist before the patient leaves the clinic or office. However, onset of symptoms may be delayed and the patient may present to the ED for treatment.

Other problems associated with neoplasms are pain, death, and dying.

8. How is a patient with a terminal neoplastic disease treated?
Often the best treatment for a patient with a terminal malignancy is adequate analgesia, comfort measures, and supportive care. Patients with terminal neoplastic disease should

be given analgesics, narcotics, or other medication as needed. The emergency physician must also deal with problems related to "do not resuscitate" orders in the ED and the pre-hospital arena.

9. How is an oncologic emergency diagnosed?

The most important element is clinical suspicion. In any patient with an underlying neoplastic process (not only patients with an ongoing process but patients who had a "cure" in the remote past), a complication related to that process should be suspected.

After concentrating on *A*irway, *B*reathing, *C*irculation, and vital signs, an extensive history should be taken, followed by a complete physical examination. A presumptive diagnosis should be made and appropriate data obtained. (See table.)

Management of Selected Oncologic Emergencies

CLINICAL PROBLEM	PRESENTING SYMPTOMS	ED DATA BASE	ED PRIORITIES
Superior vena cava syndrome	Plethora Cyanosis Dyspnea Dilated head/arm veins Jugular venous distention Cough Chest pain	Mediastinal mass on CXR	Emergency radiotherapy Consider tissue biopsy Consider chemotherapy Consider surgical debulking
Infection	Fever Varies with source	CBC with differential Urinalysis CXR Blood cultures Wound culture(s) Catheter culture(s) LP if not contra-indicated	Complete physical exam to locate source Culture all possible sources Protective isolation if neutropenic Begin broad-spectrum anti-biotics (varies with known community antibiotic resistance patterns)
Malignant pericardial effusion	Chest pain Cardiac rub Jugular venous distention Distant heart sounds Hypotension	Elevated CVP Low-voltage EKG Cardiomegaly on CXR Pericardial fluid on echocardiogram CVP/PCWP pressure equalization	IV fluid challenge (NS or LR) Drainage Pericardial window (preferred) Pericardiocentesis
Hypercalcemia	Dehydration Constipation Lethargy Altered mental status	Elevated free calcium Abnormal EKG	IV fluid rehydration (NS) Furosemide Consider calcitonin Consider prednisone, mithramycin
Spinal cord compression	Back pain Motor/sensory deficits Incontinence	Spinal x-ray abnormality Image spinal cord (CT vs. myelogram vs. MRI)	Initiate high-dose steroids Analgesics Emergent surgical decompression Emergent radiotherapy

CXR = chest x-ray, CBC = complete blood count, LP = lumbar puncture, CVP = central venous pressure, EKG = electrocardiogram, IV = intravenous, NS = normal saline, LR = lactated Ringer's, PCWP = pulmonary capillary wedge pressure, CT = computed tomography, MRI = magnetic resonance imaging.

10. Which neoplastic processes are the most worrisome?

Those that occur most commonly are lung, breast and colon cancer. All may have complications. In addition, leukemias, lymphomas, and prostate cancer also commonly lead to complications. Because of their common nature and high propensity for complications, these are the most worrisome neoplastic processes.

11. What common symptoms can be related to an underlying neoplastic emergency?

Any presenting symptom can be caused by a neoplastic process. For example, a neoplastic process should be considered in any patient who presents with weakness, dizziness, altered mental status, headache, or seizure. The common symptoms of back pain or abdominal pain can be the initial presentation for an oncologic process that has led to spinal cord compression (back pain) or intestinal obstruction or perforation (abdominal pain).

12. What treatment is used for patients with oncologic emergencies?

Treatment is identical to that for patients without an underlying neoplastic process and should be initiated early. Treatment of selected life-threatening problems is provided in the table on the previous page.

13. When should the patient be admitted?

All patients with life- or limb-threatening disease must be admitted. Patients in whom the diagnosis of an oncologic process is first made in the ED are usually admitted. A special group of patients who need to be admitted are those who lack the resources at home to care for themselves. It is not uncommon for families to give so much of themselves that they need a break, and an admission for respite care is indicated.

For all other patients, it is probably best to discuss the matter with the patient and the primary physician. Most patients with neoplastic processes have a primary oncologist who knows the patient and his or her situation in detail. One needs to balance the medical risks of the current problem with the patient's psychological needs. Many patients have already spent much time at the hospital and want to spend as much time at home as possible.

BIBLIOGRAPHY

1. Bockman RS, Delaney TF, Fair WR, et al: Oncologic emergencies. In DeVita VT, Hellman S, Rosenberg SA: Cancer: Principles and Practice of Oncology, 3rd ed. Philadelphia, J.B. Lippincott, 1989.
2. Davis KD, Ahie MF: Management of severe hypercalcemia. Crit Care Clin 7:175–190, 1991.
3. Health D: The treatment of hypercalcemia in malignancy. Clin Endocrinol 34:155–157, 1991.
4. Lange B, D'Angio G, Ross AJ: Oncologic emergencies. In Pizzo PA, Poplack DG (eds): Principles and Practice of Pediatric Oncology. Philadelphia, J.B. Lippincott, 1989.
5. Mosekilde L, Eriksen EF, Charles P: Hypercalcemia of malignancy: Pathophysiology, diagnosis and treatment. Crit Rev Oncol/Hematol 11:1–27, 1991.
6. Parish JM, Marschke RF, Dines DE, Lee RD: Etiologic considerations in superior vena cava syndrome. Mayo Clin Proc 56:407–413, 1981.
7. Pizzo PA, Rubin M, Freifield A, Walsh TJ: The child with cancer and infection. I. Empiric therapy for fever and neutropenia, and preventive strategies. J Pediatr 119:679–694, 1991. II. Nonbacterial infections. J Pediatr 119:845–857, 1991.
8. Ratanatharathorn V, Powers WE: Epidural spinal cord compression from metastatic tumor, diagnosis and guidelines for management. Cancer Treat Rev 18:55–71, 1991.
9. Rinkevich D, Borovik R, Bendett M, Markiewicz W: Malignant pericardial tamponade. Med Pediatr Oncol 18:287–291, 1990.
10. Siegal T, Siegal T: Current considerations in the management of neoplastic spinal cord compression. Spine 14:223–228, 1989.

X. Metabolism and Endocrinology

45. FLUIDS AND ELECTROLYTES

Corey M. Slovis, M.D., FACP, FACEP

1. Why is the study of fluid and electrolytes so difficult?
Most people who teach fluid and electrolytes are very smart and talk about things like "the negative log of the hydrogen ion concentration," "idiogenic osmols," and "pseudo-pseudo triple acid base disturbances." Luckily this chapter won't be written by a person who believes in, or understands, negative logarithms.

2. What is the anion gap?
The anion gap (AG) measures the amount of negatively charged ions in the serum (unmeasured anions) that are not bicarbonate (HCO_3^-) or chloride (Cl^-). The AG is calculated by subtracting the sum of HCO_3^- and Cl^- values from the sodium (Na^+) value, the major positive charge in the serum. Potassium (K^+) values are not generally used in the calculation because of the huge amount of intracellular potassium (155 mEq) and the relatively low amount of K in the serum (only about 4 mEq). The formula for determining AG is as follows:

$$AG = Na^+ - (Cl + HCO_3^-)$$

The normal value of the AG is 10–15.

3. Why do you have to calculate AG every time you evaluate an electrolyte panel?
Elevated AG means there is some unmeasured anion, toxin, or organic acid in the blood. If you do not calculate the gap, you could miss one of the only clues to a potentially life-ending disease or overdose. The AG also allows acidosis to be divided into two types: wide gap (gap above 10–15), and normal gap (gap below 10–15).

4. Okay. There are two types of acidosis: wide gap and normal gap. What's all this about hyperchloremic metabolic acidosis?
Hyperchloremic acidosis is just another name for a normal gap acidosis. Just think: if the AG is going to be normal, and the formula for AG = $Na^+ - (HCO_3^- + Cl^-)$, then if HCO_3^- goes down, Cl^- has to rise—or more simply, you become hyperchloremic—hence the name hyperchloremic metabolic acidosis.

5. Is there any easy way to remember the differential diagnosis for wide gap metabolic acidosis?
Of course. My favorite is taken from Dr. Louis Goldfrank and is called MUDPILES.

M	=	Methanol	P	=	Paraldehyde
U	=	Uremia	I	=	INH (Isoniazid) and Iron
D	=	DKA and AKA	L	=	Lactic acidosis
			E	=	Ethylene glycol
			S	=	Salicylates

6. What are three clues to each of the entities in MUDPILES?

DISEASE	CLUES
Methanol	Alcoholism, blindness or papilledema, profound acidosis
Uremia	Chronically ill-appearing, history of chronic renal failure, BUN above 100, and Cr above 5 mg/dl
DKA	History of diabetes mellitus, polyuria, and polydipsia, glucose above 500
AKA	ETOH, glucose <250, nausea and vomiting
Paraldehyde	Alcoholism, distinctive breath, access to this now-hard-to-find drug
INH	TB, suicide-prone, refractory status seizures
Iron	Pregnant or postpartum, hematemesis, radiopaque tablets on abdominal film (unreliable finding!!)
Lactic acidosis	Hypoxia, hypotension, sepsis
Ethylene glycol	Alcoholism, oxalate crystals in urine with/without renal failure, fluorescent mouth (from drinking antifreeze)
Salicylates	History of chronic disease requiring aspirin use (i.e., rheumatoid arthritis); mixed acid-base disturbance (primary metabolic acidosis plus primary respiratory alkalosis); aspirin level above 20–40 units

7. What are the causes of narrow gap acidosis?
Just memorize HARDUP.

H	=	Hyperalimentation/hyperventilation (chronic)
A	=	Acetazolamide, acids like hydrochloric, lysine hydrochloride, etc.
R	=	Renal tubular acidosis (RTA)
D	=	Diarrhea
U	=	Uterosigmoidostomy
P	=	Pancreatic fistulas, drainage and also parenteral saline in 1 gm amounts

If you don't want to memorize anything, then it is important to know that diarrhea, especially in children, and RTA, especially in adults, are by far the two most common causes of narrow gap acidosis.

Enough acid-base, let's do some fluids.

8. Why should normal saline (NS) or lactated Ringer's (LR) solution rather than ½ normal saline or D₅W be given to someone who needs volume replacement?
Things would be pretty simple if you could just give fluid and it would stay in the vasculature. Fluid goes into three different body compartments: (1) inside blood vessels (intravascular); (2) into cells (intracellular); and (3) in-between the two (interstitial). Normal saline (NS) and lactated Ringer's (LR) solution go into all three compartments, and only 25–33% stays in the intravascular compartment. A person who lost 2 units of blood (1000 cc) would need 3–4 liters of crystalloid for volume resuscitation. One-half NS (0.45 NS) obviously provides only half of what NS or LR provide; thus, each liter of 0.45 NS provides just 125–175 cc to blood vessels (versus the 250–333 cc for NS and LR). D₅W is the worst for trying to give intravascular volume; it puts only about 80 cc per 1000 cc D₅W into the vasculature. The rest goes into cells and the interstitium.

9. Which solution is better, NS or LR?
Both fluids are "good" and both are excellent for early volume replacement. NS has a pH of 4.5–5.5 and has a sodium *and* chloride content of 155 mEq/L each. Thus it is acidotic,

has an osmolarity of 310, and has a little more sodium than serum does and a lot more chloride than serum (155 mEq/L of Cl⁻ vs. about 100 mEq/L of Cl⁻ in serum). Too much NS too quickly may cause hyperchloremic metabolic acidosis.

LR is considered more physiologic in that it is much closer to serum in its content. Its sodium content is lower than NS at 130 mEq/L and its chloride is only 109 mEq/L (vs. the 155 mEq/L of NS). The solution is called lactated because it has 28 mEq/L of bicarbonate in the form of lactate, which becomes bicarbonate once it is in the body. LR has 4 mEq of potassium (none in NS) and also has 3 mEq/L of calcium. Critics of LR do not like all the bicarb in it and believe that potassium therapy should be individualized. The bottom line is that neither is better; both are equal in quantities of 2–4 L. When large quantities of volume are required rapidly (i.e., trauma), LR is the preferred fluid. Patients with protracted vomiting should get NS, which is higher in chloride.

10. What is the most dangerous electrolyte abnormality? What are its five most common causes?

Hyperkalemia. It may result in sudden arrhythmogenic death because of its effect on the cells' resting membrane potential. By far the most common cause of hyperkalemia is "lab error." Actually, the lab does a perfect analysis, but the serum sample has hemolyzed after or while it is being drawn. Other common causes are (1) chronic renal failure (the #1 cause of true hyperkalemia), (2) acidosis (K moves out of the cell during acidosis), (3) iatrogenic (from giving too much KCl in an IV), (4) drug induced (including NSAIDs, K-sparing diuretics, digoxin, and captopril), and (5) burn or crush injuries (where K comes out of injured muscle and red cells). Less common causes include hemolysis, tumor lysis syndrome, adrenal insufficiency, and hematologic illnesses.

11. What EKG changes are associated with hyperkalemia?

The first EKG change seen in hyperkalemia is usually a tall, peaked T-wave that may occur as potassium values rise to 5.5–6.5 mEq/dl. Loss of the P-wave may follow as potassium levels rise to 7.0 mEq/dl. The most dangerous EKG finding associated with levels of 7.0–8.0 mEq/dl or higher is widening of the QRS, which may merge with the abnormal T-wave and create a sine-wave-appearing ventricular tachycardia.

12. What is the best treatment for hyperkalemia?

Treatment is based on: (1) the patient's serum levels, (2) the presence or absence of EKG changes, and (3) underlying renal function. If the patient has life-threatening EKG changes of hyperkalemia (widening QRS or a sine wave-like rhythm), 10% calcium chloride should be given in an initial dose of 5–10 cc to temporarily reverse potassium's deleterious electrical effects. Most patients with hyperkalemia usually require (1) moving potassium intracellularly, and then (2) removing potassium from the body, rather than receiving a potentially dangerous calcium infusion.

13. How can potassium be moved intracellularly?

The two most effective ways are by giving either bicarbonate or glucose and insulin. Bicarbonate will drive potassium into the cell as the patient's pH rises. Usually 1–2 ampules of bicarbonate (44.6–50 mEq of bicarbonate per ampule) are given over 1–20 minutes, depending on how sick and/or acidotic the patient is. Glucose and insulin work by activating the glucose transport system into the cell. As glucose is carried intracellularly, potassium is carried along. The usual dose of glucose is 2 ampules of D_{50} (100 cc) and 10 units of insulin. Other, less common methods of driving potassium into the cell include inhalation of bronchodilators—a good approach in a renal failure patient with fluid overload, as it may also help treat the bronchospasm of pulmonary edema, and intravenous magnesium—a great maneuver if the patient is having ventricular ectopy, but potentially dangerous if the patient has hypermagnesemia in association with chronic renal failure. Magnesium in a dose of 1–2 gm may, like beta agonists, lowers serum potassium by 0.5 mEq.

14. After potassium's electrical effects have been counteracted (if indicated) and potassium has been driven intracellularly, how do you remove it from the body?
Potassium can be removed from the body by (1) diuresis, (2) potassium-binding resins, and (3) hemodialysis. Diuresis with saline, supplemented by furosemide, is an excellent way to lower total body potassium. Unfortunately, most patients have renal failure and cannot make much urine—that's how they got hyperkalemic in the first place! Kayexalate is a sodium-containing resin that exchanges its sodium content for the patient's potassium. Each gram of Kayexalate can remove about 1 mEq of potassium from the patient's body. The best method of lowering potassium is by hemodialysis and it is the method of choice for any severely ill, acidotic or profoundly hyperkalemic patient.

15. What are the most common etiologies of hyponatremia?
Hyponatremia is defined as a serum sodium of less than 135 mEq/dl. Most patients with mild hyponatremia (levels of above 125–130 mEq/dl) are either on diuretics and/or have some degree of fluid overload due to congestive heart failure (renal failure or liver disease). Diuretic-induced hyponatremia is most common in the elderly. Patients with congestive heart failure, liver failure and renal failure develop hyponatremia due to secondary hyperaldosteronism. Aldosterone is released because of renal hypoperfusion and volume overload with subsequent hyponatremia that occurs even in the face of total body sodium excess. Moderate to severe hyponatremia (levels below 125) are most commonly due to the syndrome of inappropriate secretion of antidiuretic hormone and psychogenic polydipsia (compulsive water drinking).

16. What is SIADH?
The syndrome of inappropriate secretion of antidiuretic hormone is abnormally high levels of hormone from the posterior pituitary gland, which blocks free water excretion. Normally, when sodium levels fall, levels of this hormone also decrease, resulting in urinary losses of water (diuresis). Unfortunately, in this syndrome, ADH is released inappropriately and serum sodium levels fall as more and more excess free water is retained (antidiuresis). The hallmark of this syndrome is relatively concentrated urine, rather than the maximally dilute urine one sees in a water-overloaded patient. Patients cannot be labeled with this diagnosis if they are on diuretics, or have a reason to be water overloaded, i.e., congestive heart failure, chronic renal failure, or liver failure.

17. What are the classic neurologic signs of hyperkalemia? What are the classic EKG signs of hyponatremia?
No, not a misprint, just a trick to wake you up after antidiuresing. Potassium causes cardiovascular symptoms via its effects on the EKG (see question 11). Sodium causes no EKG changes, but does affect the brain because of its effects on osmolality—symptoms include dizziness, confusion, coma, and seizures.

18. How fast should hyponatremia be corrected?
There has been much debate over how rapidly (about 2 mEq/hr) or how slowly (about 0.5 mEq/hr) sodium should be corrected. It appears that patients should be corrected slowly over 1–2 days and serum sodium should be allowed to rise by only about 0.5 mEq/hr. This will avoid the possible development of central pontine myelinosis, a catastrophic neurologic illness of coma and paralysis, seen with too rapid correction.

19. Should sodium levels *ever* be treated quickly?
There are some very specific indications for raising someone's sodium rapidly by infusing 3% saline at 100 cc/hr. Patients who have serum sodium levels of less than 110 *and* who have acute alterations in mental status, seizures, or focal findings should have their levels raised about 4–6 mEq/dl over a few hours. Other than these rare patients with profound hyponatremia, slow correction by water restriction, slow infusion of saline, and judicious use of furosemide should be employed.

20. What is osmolality? What is the osmolal gap?
Osmolality is calculated by multiplying the serum sodium by 2 and adding the glucose (GLU) divided by 18, plus the blood urea nitrogen (BUN) divided by 2.8. Normal is approximately 280–290 mOsm.

$$\text{Osmolarity} = 2 \times NA + GLU/18 + BUN/2.8$$

The osmolal gap is determined by using the above formula and then asking the lab to determine it by the molal freezing point depression. The difference should only be about 10; if it is more, something else is in the serum, e.g., an alcohol or IVP dye.

$$\text{Osmolal Gap} = \text{Lab-determined Osmolarity} - \text{Calculated Osmolarity}$$

21. How do you use the osmolal gap in figuring out if someone has ingested methanol or ethylene glycol?
If osmolal gap is elevated, you should immediately measure the patient's serum ethanol level. Because of ethanol's molecular weight, every 4.2 mg/dl of alcohol "weighs" 1 milliosmol (mOsm). Thus, if the alcohol level is 100 mg/dl, then the patient's osmolal gap should be about 30–35 (about 25 from alcohol, added to the normal osmolal gap, which is about 5–10).

If there is a higher gap, these unaccounted osmols may represent methanol, ethylene glycol, or isopropyl alcohol. Because isopropyl alcohol causes ketosis without acidosis, acidosis plus an unexplained osmolal gap may mean a life-threatening overdose. Hints to methanol and ethylene glycol overdose appear in answer 6.

22. What are the most common causes of hypercalcemia? How do they present?
Mild hypercalcemia is usually due to dehydration, thiazide diuretics, or hyperparathyroidism. It is often asymptomatic, but mild fatigue, renal stones or nonspecific GI symptoms may be present. Severe hypercalcemia, with levels more than 2–3 mg/dl above normal, presents as alteration in mental status with the signs and symptoms of profound dehydration.

23. What is the emergency treatment of hypercalcemia?
Hypercalcemia is treated symptomatically by aggressive volume resuscitation with saline supplemented by furosemide once intravascular volume has been normalized. Hypercalcemia is one of the only true indications left for forced diuresis (rhabdomyolysis may be the other). Patients should receive 300–500 cc of NS plus enough furosemide to keep urine flow high. Saline will block the proximal tubules from absorbing calcium and furosemide will block distal tubular absorption.

BIBLIOGRAPHY

1. Blumberg A, et al: Effect of various therapeutic approaches on plasma potassium and major regulating factors in terminal renal failure. Am J Med 85:507–512, 1988.
2. Campbell WH, Marx JA: Disorders of water metabolism. In Wolfson AB (ed): Endocrine and Metabolic Emergencies. New York, Churchill Livingstone, 1990, pp 1–17.
3. Goldfrank LR, Starke CL: Metabolic acidosis in the alcoholic. In Goldfrank's Toxicologic Emergencies, 3rd ed. Norwalk, CT, Appleton Century Crofts, 1986, pp 435–444.

4. Narins RG, et al: Diagnostic strategies in disorders of fluid, electrolyte and acid-base homeostasis. Am J Med 77:496–519, 1982.
5. Narins RG, Emmett M: Simple and mixed acid-base disorders—a practical approach. Medicine 59:161–187, 1980.
6. Sterns RH: The treatment of hyponatremia: First, do no harm (editorial): Am J Med 88:557–560, 1990.
7. Wrenn K, Slovis C, Slovis BS: The ability of physicians to predict hyperkalemia from ECG. Ann Emerg Med 20:1229, 1991.

46. ACID-BASE DISORDERS

Stephen L. Adams, M.D., FACP, FACEP, and John Longano, M.D., FACEP

1. What are the four types of acid-base disorders seen in the emergency department (ED)? Give a common example of each.

Actually, there are five: metabolic acidosis (cardiac arrest), respiratory acidosis (COPD with CO_2 retention), metabolic alkalosis (protracted vomiting), respiratory alkalosis (hyperventilation syndrome), and a mixed acid-base disorder (e.g., salicylate intoxication in the adult: respiratory alkalosis and metabolic acidosis; metabolic acidosis with respiratory compensation). We will not "Hasselbalch" the reader by reviewing basic physiology, since an understanding of basic acid-base physiology is assumed.

2. What does pulse oximetry contribute to the understanding of the patient's acid-base status?

Nothing. Pulse oximetry measures oxygen saturation and does not provide a measurement of acid-base or ventilatory status. Arterial blood gas (ABG) analysis is necessary to determine acid-base status.

3. What are the most commonly cited causes of an elevated anion gap?

An elevated anion gap, usually indicating a low bicarbonate level, should give the clinician cause to consider the presence of a metabolic acidosis. The differential diagnoses may be remembered by the mnemonic "DR. MAPLES":

D	=	Diabetic ketoacidosis
R	=	Renal failure
M	=	Methanol
A	=	Alcoholic ketoacidosis
P	=	Paraldehyde
L	=	Lactic acidosis
E	=	Ethylene glycol
S	=	Salicylate intoxication

These are only some of the causes of a metabolic acidosis.

4. Name some obscure causes of an elevated anion gap metabolic acidosis.

Sulfuric acidosis, short bowel syndrome (D-lactic acidosis), nalidixic acid, methenamine, mandelate, hippuric acid salt, rhubarb (oxalic acid) ingestion, and inborn errors of metabolism such as the methylmalonic acidemias and isovaleric acidemia have all been associated with a metabolic acidosis with an elevated anion gap. Toluene intoxication can cause either an elevated anion gap metabolic acidosis or a hyperchloremic metabolic acidosis (no anion gap).

5. Is the size of the anion gap clinically useful?

In one study, an anion gap of greater than 30 mEq/L was usually due to an identifiable organic acidosis (i.e., lactic acidosis or ketoacidosis). However, almost 30% of patients with an anion gap of 20–29 mEq/L had neither a lactic acidosis nor a ketoacidosis.

6. What are some causes of lactic acidosis?

Shock, seizure, hypoxemia, isoniazid (INH) toxicity, cyanide poisoning, ritodrine, inhaled industrial acetylene, phenformin ingestion, iron intoxication, ethanol abuse, and carbon monoxide poisoning are some causes to consider. Sodium nitroprusside, povidone-iodine ointment, sorbitol, xylitol, and streptozocin are other drugs that have been listed as causing increased lactic acid formation.

7. How severe is the acid-base disturbance that results from a grand mal seizure? How long does it take to resolve the acidosis?

A grand mal seizure can result in a profound lactic acidosis. The pH levels may plummet to 6.9 or lower. The acidosis in an uncomplicated seizure usually resolves spontaneously within an hour.

8. Can one have a metabolic acidosis without evidence of an elevated anion gap?

Absolutely. A patient with a hyperchloremic metabolic acidosis may have no evidence of an elevated anion gap. This condition is caused, in effect, by adding hydrogen chloride (HCl) to the serum. The fall in serum bicarbonate is offset by the addition of Cl^-; consequently, there will be no increased anion gap.

9. How can I remember some of the causes of normal anion gap metabolic acidosis?

Use the mnemonic "USED CARP":

U	=	Ureteroenterostomy	C	=	Carbonic anhydrase inhibitors
S	=	Small bowel fistula	A	=	Adrenal insufficiency
E	=	Extra chloride	R	=	Renal tubular acidosis
D	=	Diarrhea	P	=	Pancreatic fistula

10. In a patient with diabetic ketoacidosis (DKA) who is improving with appropriate therapy, why might the measurement of serum ketones actually show an increase?

There are three ketone bodies that exist: beta-hydroxybutyrate (BHB), acetoacetate (AcAc), and acetone. BHB and AcAc are acids; acetone is not. The proportion of BHB to AcAc depends on the oxidation/reduction status of the patient. A patient who is in DKA upon presentation is often severely dehydrated, and the preponderance of ketone bodies may be in the form of BHB. The test by which ketones are noted is the nitroprusside reaction test (Acetest, Ketostix), which measures AcAc and acetone, but is not sensitive to BHB. In the patient with DKA, as fluids and insulin therapy are instituted, the amount of BHB converted to AcAc increases, and the nitroprusside reaction, which initially may have been weakly positive or even negative, becomes increasingly positive.

11. Name nine disorders that can cause a hyperketonemic state.

Isopropyl alcohol intoxication, DKA, alcoholic ketoacidosis, starvation, stress hormone excess, cyanide intoxication, industrial acetylene inhalation, hyperemesis gravidarum, and bovine ketosis. Paraldehyde intoxication may cause pseudoketosis.

12. Name four acids that may contribute to metabolic acidosis in an abuser of alcohol.

Ketoacidosis has been well documented in the chronic alcoholic who binges and then presents with nausea, vomiting, abdominal pain, and poor caloric intake. Lactic acid, acetic acid, and indirect loss of bicarbonate in the urine (nonanion gap metabolic acidosis) may also contribute to an alcoholic acidosis.

13. Which electrolyte is most commonly affected by a change in acid-base status?

Serum potassium. Patients with severe acidosis tend to have elevated serum potassium levels, whereas patients with severe alkalosis tend to have low serum potassium levels. A change of pH of 0.10 is consistent with a corresponding change in serum K^+ of about 0.5 (0.3–0.8) mEq/L. If the pH is elevated by 0.10, then the serum K^+ will fall by about 0.5 mEq/L. If the pH is diminished by 0.10, then the serum K^+ will rise by about 0.5 mEq/L. This concept is well known to those who treat patients who present in DKA. Although the patient's total body potassium may be severely depleted, initial serum potassium levels may actually be elevated in the severely acidotic patient. As the patient is appropriately treated and acidosis resolves, potassium supplementation is indicated, as serum levels may fall precipitously.

14. What is a pseudometabolic acidosis?

Underfilling of Vacutainer tubes can cause a significant decline in bicarbonate and an increase in anion gap that may be mistaken for metabolic acidosis. It is theorized that because atmospheric pressure contains less than 5% carbon dioxide (CO_2), the lower partial pressure of CO_2 over the blood in an underfilled tube causes CO_2 to diffuse out of the venous solution, decreasing the bicarbonate with which it is in equilibrium. Therefore, tubes should be completely filled to prevent creating a pseudometabolic acidosis.

15. Are there any potential ill effects of using paper bag rebreathing in the treatment of hyperventilation syndrome?

Yes. When normal volunteers hyperventilated into a brown paper bag, inspired oxygen was sufficiently decreased so as to endanger hypoxic patients. Paper bag rebreathing therapy should probably not be used unless myocardial ischemia can be ruled out and arterial blood gas analysis or pulse oximetry excludes hypoxia.

16. How does core temperature affect ABGs?

Uncorrected ABGs will yield a falsely elevated pH as well as a falsely decreased pO_2 and pCO_2 in hypothermia. For every $1°C$ decrease in body temperature, the pH will be elevated 0.015, pCO_2 (mmHg) will decrease 4.4%, and pO_2 will decrease 7.2% ($37°C$ reference). Hyperthermia will decrease the pH and increase the pCO_2 and pO_2 by an equivalent amount. The clinical use of corrected versus uncorrected pH determinations in hypothermia remains controversial.

BIBLIOGRAPHY

1. Adams SL: Alcoholic ketoacidosis. Emerg Med Clin North Am 8:749–760, 1990.
2. Callaham M: Hypoxic hazards of traditional paper bag rebreathing in hyperventilating patients. Ann Emerg Med 18:622–628, 1989.
3. Emmet M, Narins RG: Clinical use of the anion gap. Medicine 56:38–54, 1977.
4. Gabow PA, Kaehny WD, Fennessey PV, et al: Diagnostic importance of an increased serum anion gap. N Engl J Med 303:854–858, 1980.
5. Halperin ML, Hammeke M, Josse RG, Jungas RL: Metabolic acidosis in the alcoholic: A pathophysiologic approach. Metabolism 32:308–315, 1983.
6. Herr RD, Swanson T: Pseudometabolic acidosis caused by underfill of Vacutainer tubes. Ann Emerg Med 21:177–180, 1992.
7. Orringer CE, Eustace JC, Wunsch CD, Gardner LB: Natural history of lactic acidosis after grand-mal seizures. N Engl J Med 297:796–799, 1977.
8. Reuler JB: Hypothermia: Pathophysiology, clinical settings, and management. Ann Intern Med 89:519–527, 1978.
9. Schade DS, Eaton RP: Differential diagnosis and therapy of hyperketonemic state. JAMA 241:2064–2065, 1979.
10. Shapiro BA, Harrison RA, Cane RD, Kozlowski-Templin R: Clinical Application of Blood Gases, 4th ed. Chicago, Year Book Medical Publishers, 1989.
11. Wilson RF: Acid-base problems. In Tintinalli JE (ed): Emergency Medicine: A Comprehensive Study Guide, 4th ed. New York, McGraw-Hill, Inc., 1992, pp 35–50.

47. DIABETIC DISORDERS

R. Scott Israel, M.D.

HYPERGLYCEMIC HYPEROSMOLAR NONKETOTIC COMA

1. What is hyperglycemic hyperosmolar nonketotic coma (HHNK)? How does it differ from diabetic ketoacidosis (DKA)?
HHNK is characterized by elevated serum glucose levels, increased osmolality, and absence of ketoacidosis. Insulin levels are lower than would be appropriate for the degree of hyperglycemia seen but are higher than those in patients with DKA. There is enough insulin to suppress ketoacid production in the liver but not enough to maintain euglycemia.

2. Who is at risk for HHNK?
Patients with HHNK tend to be elderly and 30–90% have a history of diabetes. Precipitating events can be identified in approximately 50% of patients and include acute infections, particularly pneumonia or urinary tract infections, stroke, pancreatitis, gastrointestinal bleed, myocardial infarction, or burns. Drugs associated with HHNK include diuretics, beta blockers, corticosteroids, psychotropic drugs, and diphenylhydantoin.

3. What is the typical clinical presentation of HHNK?
Patients report polyuria, polydipsia, nocturia, and weakness. They may also present with nausea, vomiting, or dizziness. Physical examination generally shows dehydration secondary to polyuria. Half of patients with HHNK present comatose, with the remainder exhibiting some signs of confusion. The degree of mental status alteration corresponds mostly closely to serum osmolality. Focal neurologic findings such as aphasia, hemianopsia, hemiparesis, ataxia, nystagmus, or seizures may be seen and lead to a mistaken diagnosis of stroke. Seizures are typically focal and motor in nature. Most neurologic findings disappear when hyperosmolality normalizes.

4. What are the laboratory findings in HHNK?
Glucose levels range from 350–3000 mg/dl. Spurious hyponatremia commonly occurs. Corrected serum sodium levels are normal or high (for each 100 mg/dl increase in serum glucose, the serum sodium will decrease 1.6 mEq/L). Serum potassium levels may be normal initially but there is always a significant total body potassium deficit. BUN and creatinine may be increased, reflecting dehydration. Bicarbonate will be normal or slightly diminished, but qualitative tests for ketoacids will be negative or only trace positive. There may be an anion gap acidosis, but this is related to accumulation of lactate or renal failure rather than to ketoacid production.

5. How should HHNK be treated?
Patients with HHNK may have lost 25% of their total body water. Initial replacement therapy should begin with normal saline until the patient no longer appears grossly dehydrated, after which ½ normal saline can be used. An initial rate of rehydration of 1 L/hr should be adequate. When ½ normal saline is initiated, the rate may be decreased to 250–500 cc/hr.

6. Should patients with HHNK receive insulin?
Most patients with HHNK require insulin. An initial infusion of 3–5 units/hr should be adequate. There is some concern that early insulin therapy may lead to hypovolemic shock

as glucose moves from the extracellular to the intracellular compartment. This facet, however, has not been well studied and early insulin treatment has been used safely in many patients.

7. Do patients with HHNK require potassium (K⁺) replacement?

Because insulin causes a rapid shift of K⁺ into cells and drop in serum K⁺ levels, it may be prudent to withhold insulin until K⁺ replacement has been initiated in patients who are initially hypokalemic.

8. What are the complications of HHNK?

The overall mortality associated with HHNK is related most closely to underlying diseases and precipitating factors rather than to hyperglycemia or hyperosmolality. It is important to search carefully for infection, primary neurologic events, and myocardial infarction. Another source of morbidity is vascular thrombosis related to dehydration, hemoconcentration, and hyperviscosity. Arterial or venous thrombosis may occur in the cerebral, pulmonary, mesenteric, or portal vasculature.

HYPOGLYCEMIA

9. How is glucose metabolism normally regulated?

Five to six hours after a meal, insulin levels decrease and energy stores are utilized. Glucose is initially supplied by the breakdown of liver glycogen which, in the average adult, supports normal glucose levels for 8–10 hours of fasting. Liver disease, starvation, recent illness, or exercise may shorten the period during which glycogen stores maintain euglycemia. After that, gluconeogenesis occurs in the liver from lactate, pyruvate, and amino acids. The hormones responsible for converting metabolism from an energy storage mode to one of substrate liberation are collectively referred to as counterregulatory hormones. They include glucagon, epinephrine, cortisol, and growth hormone. Glucagon and epinephrine are responsible for acute glucose mobilization. Hypoglycemia results from deficiencies in counterregulatory hormones or when excessive insulin levels overcome the counterregulatory response.

10. What are the signs and symptoms of hypoglycemia?

Hypoglycemic symptoms fall into two major groups. Symptoms that result from the effects of counterregulatory hormones include sweating, tachycardia, hunger, and other adrenergic symptoms. These are most prominent when serum glucose levels fall rapidly. The second group, neuroglycopenic symptoms, include headache, confusion, coma, seizures, and focal neurologic findings. These follow a gradual decline in plasma glucose and may be present without adrenergic symptoms if the drop in serum glucose levels has been slowly progressive.

11. What is a normal serum glucose level? How is the diagnosis of hypoglycemia made?

A normal blood sugar is generally considered to be between 80 and 110 mg/dl, depending on the laboratory. Healthy adults may have fasting serum glucose levels of 25 mg/dl without symptoms. On the other hand, diabetics in poor control may have symptoms when their serum glucose drops to 80 mg/dl. The diagnosis of hypoglycemia requires demonstration of (1) neuroglycopenic symptoms, (2) laboratory evidence of hypoglycemia, and (3) clearing of symptoms following glucose administration.

12. What are the two broad categories of hypoglycemia?

Fasting hypoglycemia (symptoms begin 4 hours or longer after a meal) and **reactive hypoglycemia** (onset of symptoms shortly after a meal).

13. What are the primary causes of fasting hypoglycemia?
Fasting hypoglycemia may be caused by increased peripheral use of glucose or by under-production of glucose. When overutilization of glucose is the cause, hypoglycemia may be associated with either increased or normal insulin levels. In the ED, hypoglycemia is most commonly associated with increased insulin levels as the result of an accidental or intentional overdose of insulin, oral hypoglycemic agents, or sepsis. Insulinoma is a rare cause of hypoglycemia. Patients with fasting hypoglycemia and normal insulin levels include those in a starvation state, those subjected to strenuous activity, and those with tumors that secrete insulinlike substances. Underproduction of glucose is associated with drugs (particularly alcohol, salicylates, and beta blockers), counterregulatory hormone deficiencies (e.g., adrenal insufficiency), liver disease, or limited substrate due to malnutrition.

14. What is reactive hypoglycemia?
Reactive hypoglycemia is seen in patients with symptoms of anxiety and sweating beginning within 1–2 hours of a meal. However, these symptoms are nonspecific and the syndrome is still controversial. The presumed mechanism is rapid gastric emptying followed by excessive insulin release.

15. How should hypoglycemia be treated?
Patients with mild hypoglycemia who are able to take oral solutions may be managed with fruit juices or oral administration of 50% dextrose. These patients should receive more complex carbohydrates as their symptoms resolve. Alcoholics at risk for malnutrition should receive thiamine. Unresponsive patients may be given 50% dextrose intravenously. One 50-cc ampule raises the serum glucose an average of 150 mg/dl, although patients exhibit a broad range of responses. In some patients a second or third ampule may be necessary. Side effects include volume overload, congestive heart failure, and hypokalemia due to the movement of potassium into cells along with glucose. D25 is preferred in children; D10 is most commonly given in neonates. For patients at risk for recurrent hypoglycemia, such as overdose of insulin, a continuous infusion of D5 or D10 is indicated. If intravenous access is delayed, glucagon (1 mg for adults, 0.5 mg for children under 1 year of age) may be given IM. Patients respond clinically within 20 minutes. Side effects include nausea and vomiting. Hydrocortisone, 120 mg IV, should be given if adrenal insufficiency is suspected.

16. How quickly do patients improve?
Adrenergic symptoms generally respond within minutes; however, neuroglycopenic symptoms may require longer to resolve, as glucose must cross the blood-brain barrier. Failure of neurologic symptoms to improve after an hour suggests neurologic injury, a preexisting neurologic condition, or another cause of the patient's symptoms.

17. What is an appropriate disposition for patients presenting with a hypoglycemic episode?
If the cause of the hypoglycemic episode is not clear, admission for observation and evaluation is warranted. Patients with episodes of hypoglycemia resulting from unintentional mild insulin overdose may be discharged if symptoms have resolved, oral intake has been reestablished, and a reliable person will be available to assist them. Patients with intentional overdoses of hypoglycemic agents should be admitted because late hypoglycemia is not unusual, given the kinetics of insulin elimination in overdose and for psychiatric evaluation.

BIBLIOGRAPHY

1. Addler PM: Serum glucose changes after administration of 50% dextrose solutions: Pre- and in-hospital calculations. Am J Emerg Med 4:504, 1986.
2. Arem R: Insulin overdose in eight patients: Insulin pharmokinetics and a review of the literature. Medicine 64:323, 1985.

3. Arieff A, Carroll H: Cerebral edema and depression of sensorium in nonketotic hyperosmolar coma. J Diabetes 23:525–531, 1974.
4. Chardori R, Soler N: Hyperosmolar hyperglycemic nonketotic syndrome. Am J Med 77:809–904, 1984.
5. Ellis E: Concepts of fluid therapy in diabetic ketoacidosis in hyperosmolar hyperglycemic nonketotic coma. Pediatr Clin North Am 37:313–321, 1990.
6. Fajans SS: Fasting hypoglycemia in adults. N Engl J Med 294:766–772, 1976.
7. Hare J, Rossini A: Diabetic comas: The overlap concept. Hosp Pract 95–108, 1975.
8. Malouf R, Brust JCM: Hypoglycemia: Causes, neurologic manifestations, and outcome. Ann Neurol 17:421–425, 1985.
9. McCurdy D: Hyperosmolar hyperglycemic nonketotic diabetic coma. Med Clin North Am 54:683–699, 1970.
10. Service FJ: Hypoglycemias. West J Med 154:442–454, 1991.
11. Tchertkiff V, Nyak S, Camath C, et al: Hyperosmolar nonketotic diabetic coma: Vascular complications. J Am Geriatr Soc 22:462–466, 1974.

48. THYROID DISORDERS

Sarah K. Scott, M.D.

1. Which thyroid related conditions are considered emergencies?

True emergencies are represented by the life-threatening extremes of myxedema coma and thyroid storm. Thyroid disease is common. The frequency of hypothyroidism in adults in the United States is 1 in 20. However, myxedema coma is rare, accounting for significantly less than 1% of hypothyroid cases. Thyroid storm occurs in 1–2% of thyrotoxic patients. The mortality of thyroid storm and myxedema coma *without* treatment ranges from 80–100%, and *with* treatment, from 15–50%.

2. Are "thyrotoxicosis" and "hyperthyroidism" interchangeable terms?

Not exactly. **Thyrotoxicosis** refers to hypermetabolic states that occur in response to excess circulating thyroid hormone originating from multiple etiologies (e.g., thyroid hormone overdose, thyroid inflammation, or thyroid hyperfunction). **Hyperthyroidism** refers to excess circulating hormone resulting only from thyroid hyperfunction.

3. What are the most common etiologies of thryotoxicosis? How do they present?

• **Excess thyroid hormone production:** (1) Graves' disease accounts for up to 85% of all cases of thyrotoxicosis. Typically, patients are females between 20 and 40 years of age who variably have a goiter, exophthalmos, and smooth, moist skin. (2) Toxic multinodular goiter is the second most common cause of thyrotoxicosis. The usual patient is elderly and has cardiovascular abnormalities, with congestive heart failure and tachydysrhythmias predominating. (3) Exposure to iodine can precipitate thyrotoxicosis in patients with toxic nodular goiter or Graves' disease. Agents include radiographic contrast material, potassium iodine solution, amiodarone, and large doses of topical providone-iodine.

• **Leakage of thyroid hormone:** (1) Subacute thyroiditis is an inflammatory condition commonly seen in young women. Typically, a painful or painless goiter is present and is most common in postpartum thyrotoxicosis. (2) Radiation-induced thyroid inflammation.

• **Exogenous thyroid hormone administration:** (1) Thyrotoxicosis factitia is a Munchausen-type syndrome in which thyroid hormone is taken to cause illness. (2) Thyroid hormone overdose or ingestion of meat containing beef thyroid tissue can cause thyrotoxicosis.

4. What are the main manifestations of thyrotoxic states?
Essentially all organ systems are affected. Symptoms and physical findings can include tremor, fatigue, weakness, hyperreflexia, apathy or anxiety, emotional lability, psychosis, heat intolerance, diaphoresis, fever, goiter, eye dryness, exophthalmos, lid lag, palpitations, tachycardia, congestive heart failure, weight and hair loss, diarrhea, onycholysis, edema, and multiple laboratory abnormalities such as anemia, leukocytosis, and electrolyte disorders.

5. Is goiter always associated with thyrotoxicosis?
No. A goiter is often not present in a patient with thyrotoxicosis. Thyroid disease is a spectrum of physical findings dependent on the disease state. Two thyrotoxic states without goiter are exogenous administration of thyroid hormone and apathetic thyrotoxicosis. To make it even more confusing, a goiter may be present in hypothyroidism. The latter case is seen in goiterous forms of thyroditis where, in advanced stages, the gland is "burned out" and scar tissue causes gland enlargement.

6. What is apathetic thyrotoxicosis?
It is an atypical and frequently missed presentation of hyperthyroidism seen commonly in the elderly. The typical patient is 70–80 years old with a small or no palpable thyroid gland. Few exhibit ophthalmologic findings characteristic of hypothyroidism. The diagnosis should be considered in the elderly with chronic weight loss, proximal muscle weakness, depressed affect, new-onset atrial fibrillation, or congestive heart failure.

7. How does thyroid storm differ from thyrotoxicosis?
Thyroid storm is a medical emergency. While no absolute criteria exist, the most suggestive of thyroid storm include (1) exaggerated manifestations of thyrotoxicosis, (2) temperature higher than 100° F, (3) tachycardia out of proportion to fever, and (4) dysfunction of the central nervous system, cardiovascular system, or gastrointestinal system.

8. What other conditions may mimic thyroid storm?
Similar presentations may be seen with toxicity caused by cocaine, amphetamines, and other sympathomimetics as well as alcohol withdrawal syndromes, anticholinergics, and infections, including encephalitis, meningitis, and sepsis. A history of thyroid disease or previous thyroid treatment or surgery may be helpful in distinguishing thyroid storm from these other conditions.

9. Are thyroid function studies helpful in confirming the diagnosis of thyroid storm?
Although they will be abnormal, thyroid function tests in the patient with thyroid storm may not be appreciably different from those with thyrotoxicosis and will not differentiate between the two.

10. What is the role of thyroid function tests in the ED?
Thyroid function tests are not helpful for ED diagnosis and management because laboratory turnaround is prolonged. However, TSH, free T_3 (FT_3), and free T_4 (FT_4) levels should be measured to confirm the diagnosis of thyroid disease. "Sensitive" thyroid-stimulating hormone (TSH) (sTSH) assays should be used, as they are 10–100 times more sensitive than routine TSH assays at discriminating between very low TSH levels seen in patients with thyrotoxicosis and those in normal individuals. In hypothyroid patients, measurement of T_3 is not useful, as up to 30% may have normal levels.

11. What precipitates thyroid storm?
Possible triggers include emotional stress, infection or serious illness, surgery, trauma, childbirth, and withdrawal of antithyroid therapy.

12. How is thyroid storm treated?

ED management of thyroid storm is essentially the same as for thyrotoxicosis, only more urgent:

Step Therapy of Decompensated Thyrotoxicosis

1. Supportive Care

General: Oxygen, cardiac monitor

Fever: External cooling, acetaminophen (aspirin is contraindicated since it may increase free T_4)

Dehydration: Intravenous fluids

Nutrition: Glucose, multivitamins, including folate (deficient secondary to hypermetabolism)

Adrenal replacement (depletion secondary to hypermetabolism):
Hydrocortisone, 200 mg IV initially, then 100 mg TID until stable

Cardiac decompensation (atrial fibrillation, congestive heart failure):
Digoxin (increased requirements), diuretics, sympatholytics as required

2. Inhibition of hormone biosynthesis—thionamides:

Propylthiouracil (PTU),* 1200–1500 mg/day given as 200–250 mg q 4 hr PO, by nasogastric (NG) tube or rectally (also blocks peripheral conversion of T_4 to T_3)

or

Methimazole (MMI), 120 mg/day given as 20 mg PO q 4 hr (or 40 mg crushed in an aqueous solution rectally)

3. Blockade of hormone release—iodides* (after step 2):

Lugol's solution, 30–60 drops/day orally

or

Saturated solution potassium iodide (SSKI), 8 drops q 6 h PO

or

Sodium iodide, 0.5–1 gm IV q 12 h

or

Lithium carbonate (if allergic to iodine or agranulocytosis occurs with thionamides), 300 mg orally q 6 h and subsequently to maintain serum lithium at 1 mEq/L

4. Antagonism of peripheral hormone effects—sympatholytics:

Propranolol,* 2–5 mg IV q 4 hr or IV infusion at 5–10 mg/hr. For less toxic patients use PO at 20–200 mg q 4 h (contraindicated in bronchospastic disease† and congestive heart failure; digitalize patients with congestive heart failure before starting propranolol)

or

Reserpine, 2.5–5 mg IM q 4 h, preceded by 1-mg test dose while monitoring blood pressure (use if beta blocker contraindicated and congestive heart failure and hypotension and cardiac shock not present)

or

Guanethidine, 30–40 mg PO q 6 h

---

* Preferred medication.
† Consider esmolol if history of pulmonary disease. Effective dose may be higher than recommended. Begin with 500 mg/kg load over one minute, followed by 50 mg/kg/min IV. Repeat load and double infusion as necessary.

13. Are there special considerations when treating thyrotoxicosis during pregnancy and lactation?

Propylthiouracil (PTU) is preferable to methimazole (MMI). Both drugs cross the placenta and can block fetal thyroid function, but PTU crosses less readily. PTU is transferred in breast milk, but less so than MMI. Breastfeeding while on PTU may be continued, as long as neonatal thyroid function is monitored. Beta blockers may be used as clinically indicated.

14. How is thyroid hormone overdose treated?

Thyroid hormone overdose presents as thyrotoxicosis and is most common after chronic ingestions. Fatalities are rare with acute ingestion. Toxicity following massive acute overdose may occur within 4–12 hours or may be delayed as long as 5–11 days, particularly with T_4 (levothyroxine) ingestion. Overdose management is as usual, including charcoal and cathartic. The acute treatment of symptomatic patients is the same as that of thyrotoxicosis.

15. What causes hypothyroidism?

Hypothyroidism is caused by a deficiency of thyroid hormone. The major mechanisms include (1) primary—dysfunction of the gland; (2) secondary—deficiency of TSH from the pituitary; (3) and tertiary—deficiency of TRH from the hypothalamus. Primary hypothyroidism is the most common, and causes include autoimmune and subacute thyroiditis, end-stage Graves' disease, post thyroidectomy or irradiation drug induced (iodides, lithium, thionamides), congenital, and tumor.

16. What are the common signs and symptoms of hypothyroidism?

Signs and symptoms are myriad and nonspecific, including cold intolerance, weight gain, hypothermia, joint pain, muscle cramps, weakness, delayed deep tendon reflexes, lethargy, dementia, psychosis, cool, dry skin, hair loss, nonpitting edema, angina, bradycardia, hoarse, deep voice, slow speech, dyspnea, hypoventilation, and pleural effusion, among others. More age-sex specific findings include menorrhagia in child-bearing women and dementia in the elderly.

17. If the presentation of hypothyroidism is so nonspecific, how is myxedema coma diagnosed?

There may be a history of thyroid disease, thyroid replacement therapy, previous thyroid surgery, or scan. Classic physical findings of hypothyroidism may be present. Hallmark clinical features of myxedema coma are hypothermia (75%) and coma. Laboratory evaluation may reveal anemia, electrolyte abnormalities, hypercarbia, respiratory acidosis, or respiratory failure. EKG and chest radiograph may show bradycardia and pleural effusion or frank congestive heart failure.

18. What is the treatment of hypothyroidism and myxedema coma?

General treatment is supportive with intravenous access, oxygen, and cardiac monitor. Glucose, naloxone, and thiamine are to be administered as necessary. Other immediate life threats are assessed and treated. In severe hypothyroidism or myxedema coma, after thyroid function studies are done, an initial dose of 4 μg/kg lean body weight of T_4 (levothyroxine or thyroxine) should be administered. An alternative treatment is to administer T_4 as a single dose of 500 μg IV, regardless of weight. Because of the risk of decreased T_3 generation from T_4 in severely hypothyroid patients, a simultaneous dose of T_3 (liothyronine) at 10 μg PO q 8 h or 15–30 μg IV should be administered. Intravenous T_3 is approved for commercial use and may become the preferred mode of therapy for myxedema. Hydrocortisone, 100–200 mg IV, is indicated because of the metabolic stress associated with hypothyroidism.

An evaluation for intercurrent illness should be performed. Hypothermia is treated with passive rewarming. Patients should be intubated and hyperventilated for respiratory failure. Hypotension is treated with crystalloids. Patients may be refractory to vasopressors without thyroid hormone replacement. Hyponatremia is managed by free water restriction or infusion of saline and furosemide. Hypertonic saline is rarely indicated.

BIBLIOGRAPHY

1. Bayer MF: Effective laboratory evaluation of thyroid status. Med Clin North Am 75:1–26, 1991.
2. Becks GP, Burrow GN: Thyroid disease and pregnancy. Med Clin North Am 75:121–150, 1991.

3. Braverman LE, Utiger RD (eds): Werner and Ingbar's The Thyroid: A Fundamental and Clinical Text, 6th ed. Philadelphia, J.B. Lippincott, 1991.
4. Brunette DD, Rothong C: Emergency department management of thyrotoxic crisis with esmolol. Am J Emerg Med 9:232–234, 1991.
5. Gavin LA: Thyroid crises. Med Clin North Am 75:179–193, 1991.
6. Levy EG: Thyroid disease in the elderly. Med Clin North Am 75:151–167, 1991.
7. MacKerrow SC, Osborn LA, Lev et al: Myxedema-associated cardiogenic shock treated with intravenous triiodothyronine. Ann Intern Med 117:1014, 1992.
8. Mitchell JM: Thyroid disease in the emergency department—thyroid function tests and hypothyroidism and myxedema coma. Emerg Med Clin North Am 7:885–902, 1989.
9. Roth RN, McAuliffe MJ: Hyperthyroidism and thyroid storm. Emerg Med Clin North Am 7:873–883, 1989.
10. Wilson JD, Foster DW (eds): William's Textbook of Endocrinology, 8th ed. Philadelphia, W.B. Saunders, 1992.

49. ADRENAL DISORDERS

Michael W. Brunko, M.D., FACEP

1. Since adrenal emergencies are rare, why should I spend time learning about them?
Adrenal emergencies are rare, but if you are confronted with one and do not recognize it, the results can be devastating. Overall, the treatment is simple, but you must understand some adrenal physiology to recognize a problem and know how to treat it.

2. What are the adrenal emergencies that I need to worry about?
The most serious adrenal emergency is acute adrenal insufficiency. Hypercortisolemia or Cushing's disease is rare and it is unlikely you will make that diagnosis in the emergency department (ED).

3. Will I ever need to worry about hypercortisolemia in the ED?
Cortisol excess can lead to psycho-emotional disturbances such as insomnia, mood disorders, mania, depression, and psychosis. If a woman presents with signs of masculinization, or a man presents with signs of feminization, and the above-mentioned symptoms, think of hypercortisolemia.

4. What adrenal physiology do I need to know?
You must know the primary functions of the glucocorticoid cortisol and the mineralocorticoid aldosterone.

5. What are the primary effects of cortisol?
Cortisol has essential effects on all organ systems. It influences fat, protein, and carbohydrate metabolism. It affects immunologic and inflammatory responses, bone and calcium metabolism, growth and development, the GI tract, and the central nervous system. It is a major mediator of the stress response—affecting the heart, the vascular bed, water excretion, and electrolyte balance.

6. What are the primary effects of aldosterone?
To maintain sodium and potassium concentrations and to regulate extracellular volume.

7. How is normal secretion of cortisol controlled?
Cortisol is secreted from the cortex of the adrenal gland in response to direct stimulation by adrenocorticotropic hormone (ACTH). ACTH secretion is stimulated by the hormone

corticotropin-releasing factor (CRF) from the hypothalamus. This occurs in a diurnal rhythm, with higher levels secreted in the morning and lower levels in the evening. By negative feedback inhibition, plasma cortisol levels act to suppress release of ACTH.

8. How is secretion of aldosterone controlled?

Aldosterone secretion is controlled primarily by the renin-angiotensin system and the serum potassium concentration. The renin-angiotensin system controls aldosterone levels in response to changes in volume, posture, and sodium intake. Potassium influences the adrenal cortex directly to increase secretion of aldosterone.

9. What causes acute adrenal insufficiency?

Adrenal insufficiency may be due to either destruction of adrenal gland (primary adrenal insufficiency) or inadequate production of ACTH (secondary adrenal insufficiency). Adrenal crisis will often present in a patient with chronic adrenal insufficiency who undergoes some form of stress such as an acute myocardial infarction, surgery, or trauma, enabling the patient to be unable to mount a stress response by increasing circulating cortisol levels.

10. What are the main causes of primary adrenal insufficiency?

Tuberculosis and autoimmune destruction account for 90% of the cases of primary adrenal insufficiency.

Causes of Adrenal Insufficiency

Primary adrenal insufficiency
  Idiopathic (autoimmune)
  Tuberculosis
  Miscellaneous
    Bilateral adrenal hemorrhage or infarction
    AIDS
    Drugs: adrenolytic agents (metyrapone, aminoglutethimide, mitotane),
      ketoconazole
    Infections: fungal, bacterial sepsis
    Infiltrative disorders: sarcoidosis, hemochromatosis, amyloidosis, lymphoma,
      metastatic cancer
    Bilateral surgical adrenalectomy
    Hereditary: adrenal hypoplasia, congenital adrenal hyperplasia, adreno-
      leukodystrophy, familial glucocorticoid deficiency

Secondary adrenal insufficiency
  Exogenous glucocorticoid administration
  Pituitary or suprasellar tumor
  Pituitary irradiation or surgery
  Head trauma
  Infiltrative disorders of the pituitary or hypothalamus: sarcoidosis, hemo-
    chromatosis, histiocytosis X, metastatic cancer, or lymphoma
  Infectious diseases: tuberculosis, meningitis, fungal
  Isolated ACTH deficiency

---

11. Has primary adrenal insufficiency increased since there has been an increased incidence of tuberculosis?

This has yet to be documented in the literature, but with the increasing spread of acquired immunodeficiency syndrome (AIDS), more cases of primary adrenal insufficiency are being reported.

12. How can AIDS cause primary adrenal insufficiency?
The human immunodeficiency virus (HIV) has been found in the adrenal gland, where it may cause impaired function of the gland. Opportunistic infections may cause adrenal insufficiency; cytomegalovirus, Cryptococcus and Mycobacterium species, and Kaposi's sarcoma have been found in the glands of patients with AIDS. Some drugs used to treat AIDS can cause adrenal insufficiency. For example, ketoconazole is an inhibitor of steroid hormone synthesis, and rifampin alters cortisol metabolism and decreases cortisol bioavailability.

13. What is the most common cause of secondary adrenal insufficiency?
Chronic therapy with pharmacologic doses of glucocorticoid is the most common cause of secondary adrenal insufficiency. These drugs are used to treat a wide variety of medical problems, and if they are used for any significant time, some degree of suppression of the hypothalamic-pituitary-adrenal (HPA) axis will occur.

Diseases in Which Glucocorticoids Are Therapeutically Effective

1. Rheumatoid arthritis	21. Idiopathic thrombocytopenic purpura
2. Psoriatic arthritis	22. Autoimmune hemolytic anemia
3. Gouty arthritis	23. Lymphomas
4. Bursitis and tenosynovitis	24. Immune nephritis
5. Systemic lumpus erythematosus	25. Tuberculous meningitis
6. Acute rheumatic carditis	26. Urticaria
7. Pemphigus	27. Chronic active hepatitis
8. Erythema multiforme	28. Ulcerative hepatitis
9. Exfoliative dermatitis	29. Regional enteritis
10. Mycosis fungoides	30. Nontropical sprue
11. Allergic rhinitis	31. Dental postoperative inflammation
12. Bronchial asthma	32. Cerebral edema
13. Atopic dermatitis	33. Subacute nonsuppurative
14. Serum sickness	thyroiditis
15. Allergic conjunctivitis	34. Malignant exophthalmos
16. Uveitis	35. Hypercalcemia
17. Retrobulbar neuritis	36. Trichinosis
18. Sarcoidosis	37. Myasthenia gravis
19. Loffler's syndrome	38. Organ transplantation
20. Berylliosis	39. Alopecia areata

14. What period of time is required to cause suppression of the HPA axis?
Any patient who is on larger doses of steroids (e.g., >20 mg/day of prednisone) for 2 weeks or more has the potential for long-term suppression of the HPA axis. It depends on the dose and potency of the glucocorticoid, the time of day the drug was taken (suppression is greater when taken in the evening), and the potency of the drug. Recovery of the HPA axis may take from a few months up to a year.

15. What are some signs and symptoms of primary adrenal insufficiency?
Fatigue, weakness, weight loss, anorexia, hyperpigmentation, GI symptoms (nausea, vomiting, abdominal pain, and diarrhea), and hypotension (usually with orthostatic changes) are seen with primary adrenal insufficiency.

16. What are the characteristic laboratory findings?
Hyperkalemia, hyponatremia, and hypoglycemia are usually present with primary adrenal insufficiency. If the patient is dehydrated, volume depletion may lead to azotemia. A mild metabolic acidosis is often present.

17. How is the presentation of secondary adrenal insufficiency different from that of primary adrenal insufficiency?

In secondary adrenal insufficiency there is no deficiency of aldosterone secretion. Thus, the volume depletion and hypotension are not as severe (unless crisis is present), hyperkalemia is absent, and hyponatremia, if present, is due to water retention and not salt wasting, as in primary adrenal insufficiency. Patients usually have a cushingoid appearance because of chronic glucocorticoid use. If the patient has a pituitary or hypothalamic cause for the adrenal insufficiency, findings may include symptoms of other pituitary hormone deficiencies such as hypothyroidism and amenorrhea.

18. When does acute adrenal crisis usually occur?

It usually occurs in response to a major stress such as acute myocardial infarction, surgery, major injury, or other illness in any patient with primary or secondary adrenal insufficiency.

19. What is the most frequent iatrogenic cause of acute adrenal crisis?

Rapid withdrawal of steroids in patients with adrenal atrophy secondary to chronic steroid administration.

20. What are the most common clinical features of acute adrenal crisis?

Patients appear to be profoundly ill. They are significantly volume-depleted with hypotension and shock. Nausea, vomiting, and severe abdominal pain, many times mimicking an acute abdomen, are present. Fever may occur as a result of infection or the adrenal insufficiency itself. Central nervous system symptoms of confusion, disorientation, and lethargy may be present.

21. Will these patients always be hyponatremic and hyperkalemic?

No. If a patient has been taking mineralocorticoid replacement, such as fludrocortisone, these laboratory findings may be near normal.

22. Why do patients have a metabolic acidosis?

There are multiple reasons. Volume depletion and shock lead to increased lactate production. If aldosterone deficiency is present, decreased renal acid secretion will be present, contributing to a metabolic acidosis.

23. How is adrenal crisis diagnosed in the ED?

First and foremost, you must suspect it if a patient has been taking high-dose steroids and presents with the symptoms mentioned. The most useful and practical laboratory test in the ED is the **rapid ACTH stimulation test.**

24. How is the rapid ACTH stimulation test performed?

A baseline sample of blood is drawn at time zero for a cortisol level. Then, 0.25 mg of Cosyntropin (synthetic ACTH) is given intravenously. Cortisol levels are checked at 30 minutes, 1 hour, and 6 hours.

25. Does performance of the rapid ACTH stimulation test delay treatment of the patient with glucocorticoids?

No. You can begin treatment using a glucocorticoid that will not cause an increase in measurable cortisol levels. Dexamethasone, 6–10 mg, is generally recommended.

26. How is acute adrenal insufficiency treated?

Intravenous hydrocortisone (100 mg minimum) and crystalloid IV fluids containing dextrose must be initiated early. A detailed history and examination should be performed to attempt to elicit what may have instigated the stress that caused the acute adrenal insufficiency. If a cause is found, supportive and definitive measures need to be instituted in the ED. Mineralocorticoid replacement is usually not necessary if salt and water replacement is adequate and if the patient receives hydrocortisone—100 mg of hydrocortisone has the salt-retaining effect of 0.1 mg of fludrocortisone.

27. What about the patient with chronic adrenal insufficiency who presents to the ED with a minor illness or injury? Should I treat this patient any differently?
Yes. These patients usually require 20–30 mg/day of hydrocortisone. Some also require mineralocorticoid replacement. If these patients experience a minor illness or injury, they should be told to double their daily cortisol dose for 24–48 hours until symptoms improve. Increasing the mineralocorticoid dose is usually not necessary. Follow-up care should be coordinated closely with their private physician or endocrinologist. Patients should be told that if nausea or vomiting develops and they are unable to keep down the medication, they should seek immediate medical care.

BIBLIOGRAPHY

1. Aron DC: Endocrine complications of the acquired immunodeficiency syndrome. Arch Intern Med 149:330–333, 1989.
2. Bondy PK: Disorders of the adrenal cortex. In Wilson JD, Foster DW (eds): Williams' Textbook of Endocrinology, 7th ed. Philadelphia, W.B. Saunders, 1985, pp 816–871.
3. Brunko MW, Wolfe R: An unusual cause of an acute surgical abdomen. J Emerg Med 6:411–416, 1988.
4. Loriaux DL: Tests of adrenocortical function, Cushing's syndrome, adrenocortical insufficiency. In Becker KL (ed): Principles and Practice of Endocrinology and Metabolism. Philadelphia, J.B. Lippincott, 1990, pp 591–604.
5. Nelson DH: Diagnosis and treatment of Addison's disease. In DeGroot LJ (ed): Endocrinology, Vol 2. New York, Grune & Stratton Co., 1985, pp 1193–1201.
6. Tuck ML: Complications of corticosteroid therapy. In Hershman JM (ed): Practical Endocrinology. New York, John Wiley & Sons, 1981, pp 31–51.
7. Wogan JM: Endocrine disorders. In Rosen P, et al (eds): Emergency Medicine: Concepts and Clinical Practice, 3rd ed. St. Louis, Mosby–Year Book, 1992, pp 2242–2259.

XI. Infectious Disease

50. CELLULITIS/ABSCESS

Harvey Meislin, M.D., FACEP

1. How do you differentiate cellulitis from an abscess?
Cellulitis is a soft tissue infection of the skin and subcutaneous tissue usually characterized by blanching erythema, swelling, tenderness, and local warmth. A cutaneous abscess is a localized collection of pus resulting in a painful soft tissue mass that is often fluctuant but surrounded by firm granulation tissue and erythema.

2. What are the causes of cellulitis/abscess? How do they progress?
Cellulitis, although most often acute, may be subacute or chronic. Minor trauma is often the predisposing cause, but hematogenous and lymphatic dissemination may account for its appearance in previously normal skin. Cellulitis that is caused from bacterial infection tends to spread radially both proximately and distally with associated swelling. Nonbacterial or inflammatory cellulitis tends to stay localized. Although abscesses occur on all areas of the body, they have a predominance for the head and neck, upper extremities, and torso. Abscesses are usually caused by interruptions of the integrity of the protective epithelium but may be associated with obstruction of apocrine glands or spread via mucosal involvement in the oral and anorectal area. Superficial abscesses tend to stay localized and often will rupture through the skin if not incised and drained. Cellulitis may progress to ascending lymphangitis and septicemia.

3. What is the significance of the presence of pus?
Abscesses contain pus; cellulitis does not. Although soft tissue infections tend to spread, and both abscess and cellulitis may be present in the same anatomic area, the presence of pus defines the presence of the abscess and therefore the need for incision and drainage.

4. How can one determine if pus is present?
In cutaneous abscesses, the presence of a raised painful mass with a fluctuant center surrounded by erythematous tissue signifies the presence of pus. Adjunctive techniques such as ultrasound or CT scanning may be useful for deeper soft-tissue infections but are rarely indicated in superficial abscesses. The use of a "localizer" needle is often helpful, especially in wounds in which the purulence is loculated. Needle aspiration(s) of the involved area with a needle large enough to withdraw thick pus often helps to define the location of purulence for incision and drainage and makes the process more comfortable by decreasing the pressure and pain in the area.

5. What is the differential diagnosis of cellulitis/abscess?
The differential is one of bacterial versus nonbacterial infection. Nonbacterial cellulitis includes arthropod envenomation, chemical or thermal burns, inflammatory joints, and healing wounds. Nonbacterial cellulitis is usually localized and often does not have the presence of lymphangitic streaking. The differential diagnosis of abscesses includes sterile

abscesses, cutaneously borne bacterial abscesses, and mucous membrane abscesses. Abscesses of the oral and anorectal area usually originate from flora of the oral or rectal cavity, respectively. Sterile abscesses, which occur approximately 5% of the time, tend to be associated with drug abuse and subcutaneous injections.

6. Is it useful to culture cellulitis/abscesses?

Culturing cellulitis is often futile, with only 10–50% of such efforts yielding successful results. Often there is secondary skin contamination. Culturing is useful in patients who do not respond to initial management or patients with recurrent disease. Culturing the portal of entry may be useful, even if distal to the site of the cellulitis. Culturing of cutaneous abscesses is seldom clinically indicated. Because normal host defenses tend to contain and localize the process, culturing is not necessary for management. In recurrent abscess or failure of initial therapy, culture and Gram stain may be indicated.

7. Is there any role for routine laboratory studies?

Laboratory studies are generally not helpful in the treatment of superficial soft-tissue infections. These patients are often not systemically ill, and even an elevated white count does not necessarily differentiate bacterial from nonbacterial infection, identify the presence of abscess or cellulitis, or demonstrate systemic involvement. An exception may be *Hemophilus influenzae* cellulitis, in which white counts often exceed 15,000 with a left shift, usually in the pediatric population. Laboratory analysis may be useful in the immunocompromised host or in patients who appear to be septic or systemically ill.

8. What is the most appropriate treatment?

The time-honored treatment for cellulitis is immobilization, elevation, heat or warm moist packs, analgesics, and antibiotics. The treatment for cutaneous abscesses is incision and drainage. Antibiotics are not indicated in the patient with a cutaneous abscess and with normal host defenses. If antibiotics are used for soft-tissue infections, the selection of antimicrobial agents can be facilitated by knowing the flora associated with the anatomic area involved, and whether the abscess is from a cutaneous or mucosal process. Abscesses of the face and neck that originate in the oral cavity may contain aerobes, anaerobes, and other facultative organisms. Abscesses in the anorectal usually reflect fecal flora.

Oral Therapy of Superficial Soft Tissue Infections

Streptococcus—Group A	
Penicillin V (phenoxymethylpenicillin)	250–500 mg qid
Erythromyicn	250 mg–1 gm q6h
Staphylococcus aureus	
Cloxacillin	250–500 mg q8h
Dicloxacillin	125–500 mg q6h
Erythromycin	250 mg–1 gm q6h
Clindamycin	150–450 mg q6h
Cephradine	250–500 mg q6h
Cephalexin	250–500 mg q6h
Amoxicillin/clavulanate	250–500 mg q8h
Hemophilus influenzae	
Cefaclor	250–500 mg q8h
Cephradine	250–500 mg q6h
Cephalexin	250–500 mg q6h
Amoxicillin/clavulanate	250–500 mg q8h
Trimethoprim/sulfamethoxazole	160 mg TMP
	800 mg SMX bid

9. Are there anatomic areas of significance in a patient with an abscess/cellulitis?
Cellulitis of the mid face, especially in the area of the orbits, must be treated aggressively. The venous drainage of these infections is through the cavernous sinus of the brain, with the potential for causing cavernous sinus thrombosis. In true orbital cellulitis, there must be aggressive intravenous antibiotic therapy. Often a CT scan is performed to detect abscess formation. *Hemophilus influenzae* cellulitis usually occurs in children, resulting in high fevers, high white cell counts, and bacteremia. Perirectal/perianal abscesses that are large or extend into the supralevator or ischiorectal space often need management in the operating room, removing not only the abscess but the fistulas that are often associated with it. Deep-space abscesses of the groin and head and neck region often must be drained in the operating room because of their proximity to major neurovascular structures.

10. When are antibiotics always indicated for cellulitis/abscesses?
Antibiotics are indicated for cellulitis along with other supportive therapies such as immobilization, elevation, and heat. Cutaneous cellulitis occurs most often in the upper or lower extremities, and so initial therapy to cover common skin organisms such as *Staphylococcus aureus* and streptococcus can be achieved with the use of oral cephalosporins, erythromycin and/or dicloxacillin. If there is no response to such therapy, one must search aggressively for an etiologic factor and attempt to culture the cellulitis. A broader spectrum antibiotic or multiple antibiotics may be indicated. The treatment for the majority of abscesses is incision and drainage, and neither antibiotics nor cultures are indicated in patients with normal host defenses as long as the abscess is localized. For abscesses associated with immunocompromise or progressing cellulitis, as well as for those that may be penetrating into deeper soft tissues, incision and drainage, antibiotic therapy, culture, and Gram stain constitute a reasonable initial approach. The choice of antibiotics depends on the location and most likely cause of the infection.

11. What is appropriate follow-up care?
Most patients with simple cellulitis and localized abscesses need to be seen only once or twice in the ED. The packing can usually be removed after 48–72 hours and the patient can irrigate the cavity by bathing or showering at home. It is important to be sure that the cellulitis is responding to therapy and, with abscesses, to make sure that all pus has been drained and evacuated. Further follow-up is indicated only when the processes are recurrrent, there is no response to therapy, or in the immunocompromised patient.

12. Who should be admitted to the hospital?
Patients who appear septic, are immunocompromised, and are not responding to treatment, patients who appear toxic, and patients with soft-tissue infections in certain anatomic sites such as the central area of the face should be admitted for close observation and treatment. Patients with infections that have the potential for causing airway closure, such as sublingual abscesses, Ludwig's angina, and retropharyngeal abscesses should also be admitted for observation. Close attention must be paid to immunosuppressed patients, who may develop abscesses or cellulitis as secondary infections from gram-negative or anaerobic gas-forming organisms. Abscesses in the perineal area may spread quickly through the fascial planes, resulting in Fournier syndrome.

13. Is there an association between abscesses or cellulitis and systemic disease?
Patients who are immunocompromised or have peripheral vascular disease have a tendency to develop superficial soft-tissue infections. Recurrent abscesses in the head and neck and/ or groin regions may be associated with hydradenitis suppurativa, which is a disease of chronic suppurative abscesses of the apocrine sweat glands. Inflammatory bowel disease, diabetes, malignancies, and pregnancy have been associated with a higher incidence of

perirectal abscesses. Recurrent abscesses in the perineal and lower abdominal area may signify the presence of associated inflammatory bowel disease. All patients with recurrent soft-tissue infections, whether superficial or deep, should be evaluated for underlying systemic disease.

14. What is the best advice overall?
Cellulitis usually responds to antibiotic therapy and immobilization. Cutaneous abscesses respond to incision and drainage; antibiotics are not indicated. All soft-tissue infections should be observed to ascertain that healing is occurring. Selection of antibiotics, when indicated, is guided by location and cause of the infection.

BIBLIOGRAPHY

1. Fleisher G, Ludwig S, Henretig F, et al: Cellulitis: Initial management. Ann Emerg Med 10:356, 1981.
2. Ginsberg MB: Cellulitis: Analysis of 101 cases and review of the literature. South Med J 74:530, 1981.
3. Goligher JC, Ellis M, Pissidis AG: Critique of anal glandular infection in the etiology and treatment of idiopathic anorectal abscesses and fistulas. Br J Surg 54:977, 1967.
4. Llera TL, Levy RC: Treatment of cutaneous abscess: A double-blind clinical study. Ann Emerg Med 14:15, 1985.
5. Meislin HW, McGehee MD, Rosen P: Management and microbiology of cutaneous abscesses. JACEP 7:186, 1978.
6. Meislin HW, Lerner SA, Graves MH, et al: Cutaneous abscesses: Anaerobic and aerobic bacteriology and outpatient management. Ann Intern Med 87:145, 1977.
7. Spencer LV, Callen JP: Cutaneous manifestations of bacterial infections. Dermatol Clin 7:579, 1989.

51. ACQUIRED IMMUNODEFICIENCY SYNDROME (AIDS)

Catherine A. Marco, M.D.

1. What is the significance of AIDS in the emergency department (ED)?
Disease caused by human immunodeficiency virus (HIV) infection, ranging from asymptomatic infection to AIDS, with serious, possibly life-threatening complications, is commonly encountered in the practice of emergency medicine. As of 1991, over 206,000 cases of AIDS had been reported in the United States. The yearly incidence continues to grow. Seroprevalence among ED patients varies greatly depending on the location and type of hospital. Among inner-city ED patients, it ranges from 4.2 to 8.9%. Knowledge of HIV infection and related disease is essential to diagnose and treat disease, as well as to ensure adequate protection of health care workers.

2. How is the diagnosis of AIDS made?
The diagnosis of AIDS is most commonly made with laboratory evidence of HIV infection and the presence of one of the indicator diseases, some of which are listed in the table on the next page. HIV infection should be suspected in all patients with known risk factors or with presenting symptoms suggestive of opportunistic infection. Questioning the patient

directly about risk factors may be crucial to diagnosing HIV-related disease. Risk factors that are commonly associated with HIV infection include homosexuality or bisexuality, intravenous drug use, heterosexual exposure, blood recipients prior to 1985, and maternal-neonatal transmission.

Testing for HIV is rarely indicated in the ED because of difficulty in maintaining confidentiality and assuring appropriate reporting and counseling. However, referral for testing and counseling can be initiated in the ED.

AIDS-Defining Conditions

Laboratory evidence of HIV infection and any of the following:

Esophageal candidiasis	Brain lymphoma	HIV wasting syndrome
Cryptococcosis	*Mycobacterium avium* complex	Disseminated histoplasmosis
Cryptosporidiosis	*Pneumocystis carinii* pneumonia	Isosporiasis
Cytomegalovirus retinitis	Progressive multifocal leukoencephalopathy	Disseminated *Mycobacterium tuberculosis* disease
Herpes simplex virus	Brain toxoplasmosis	Recurrent Salmonella septicemia
Kaposi's sarcoma	HIV encephalopathy	CD4 lymphocyte count $<200/\mu l$

3. How do patients with HIV infection present to the ED?

Patients may present with involvement of virtually any organ system. HIV infection should be suspected in any patient who presents with abnormally severe symptoms of a common disease or with symptoms of opportunistic infection or other debilitating HIV-related disease, such as AIDS wasting syndrome or AIDS dementia. Among AIDS patients, systemic infection or malignancy must always be considered and may present with malaise, anorexia, fever, weight loss, GI complaints, or other symptoms. Because of the wide spectrum of disease related to HIV infection, many specific diagnoses cannot be definitively made in the ED; therefore, treatment focuses on recognition of disease, institution of initial therapy, and admission or outpatient follow-up.

4. How is the HIV-positive patient with systemic symptoms evaluated in the ED?

In addition to a complete history and physical examination, appropriate laboratory investigation may include electrolytes, complete blood count, blood cultures (aerobic, anaerobic, and fungal), urinalysis and culture, liver function tests, chest radiography, serologic testing for syphilis, blood tests for cryptococcal antigen, and Toxoplasma and Coccidioides serologies. Lumbar puncture may also be appropriate if no other source of fever is identified.

5. What is the significance of fever in these patients?

Fever may indicate bacterial, fungal, viral, or protozoal infection. The most common etiologies of fever include HIV-related fever, systemic infections such as *Mycobacterium avium-intracellulare* (MAI), cytomegalovirus (CMV), Hodgkin's disease, and non-Hodgkin's lymphoma.

Many HIV-infected patients with fever may be managed as outpatients. Outpatient management may be attempted if the source of the fever does not dictate admission, if appropriate laboratory studies have been initiated, if the patient is able to function adequately at home (able to ambulate and tolerate oral intake), and if appropriate medical follow-up can be arranged.

6. What are the common neurologic complications of AIDS?

The most common acute symptoms are seizures, altered mental status, headache, and meningismus. ED evaluation should include a complete neurologic examination, and, when appropriate, computed tomography and lumbar puncture. Specific cerebrospinal fluid

(CSF) studies that may be of value include opening and closing pressures, cell count, glucose, protein, Gram stain, India ink stain, bacterial culture, viral culture, fungal culture, toxoplasma and cryptococcal antigen, and coccidioidomycosis titer. The most common etiologies of neurologic symptoms include *Toxoplasma gondii*, AIDS dementia, *Cryptococcus neoformans, Mycobacterium tuberculosis,* and Herpes simplex virus (HSV).

7. What is AIDS dementia?

Manifested by decline in attention, cognitive reasoning, speech, motor function, and motivation, AIDS dementia is the most common neurologic problem and affects 40–60% of patients. It may be the presenting sign of overt AIDS in up to 25% of patients. Other causes of dementia must be ruled out.

8. What are the pulmonary complications of HIV infection? How are they managed?

Common presenting pulmonary complaints are cough, hemoptysis, shortness of breath, or chest pain. After history and lung exam, arterial blood gases, chest radiography, sputum culture, Gram stain, acid-fast stain, and blood cultures should be obtained if clinically indicated.

The most common pulmonary complication is *Pneumocystis carinii* pneumonia (PCP), which occurs in 70–80% of seropositive patients and typically presents with dyspnea, nonproductive cough, fever, and weight loss. Rapid institution of therapy with trimethoprim/ sulfamethoxazole may prevent excessive morbidity and mortality. Other etiologies include *Mycobacterium tuberculosis* pneumonia, CMV, *Cryptococcus neoformans, Histoplasma capsulatum,* and neoplasm.

ED management includes supplemental oxygen, volume repletion if indicated, and, when appropriate, antibiotic therapy. Admission should be considered for patients with new-onset pulmonary symptoms or those with a significant deterioration in respiratory status.

9. How should GI complaints be managed?

Approximately 50% of AIDS patients will present with GI complaints at some time during their illness. The most common presenting symptoms are abdominal pain, bleeding, and diarrhea. Diarrhea is the most common GI complaint and is estimated to occur in 50–90% of AIDS patients. Helpful laboratory studies include microscopic examination of stool for leukocytes, acid-fast stain, examination for ova and parasites, and bacterial culture of stool and blood. Cryptosporidium and Isospora infections in particular are common etiologies and are associated with prolonged watery diarrhea. Other common infectious agents include Candida, Kaposi's sarcoma, MAI, HSV, CMV, *Campylobacter jejuni, Entamoeba histolytica,* Shigella, Salmonella, Giardia, Cryptosporidium, and Isospora species. Management should be directed at repletion of fluid and electrolytes and appropriate antibiotic coverage.

10. What are the common cutaneous presentations of AIDS? How are they treated?

Kaposi's sarcoma (KS) is the most common cutaneous manifestation of AIDS. It is usually widely disseminated and may involve mucous membranes. Complaints such as xerosis (dry skin) and pruritus are common and may be manifested prior to development of opportunistic infections. Traditional therapy is employed. Xerosis may be treated with emollients, and, if necessary, with mild topical steroids. Pruritus may respond to oatmeal baths, and, if necessary, antihistamines. Exacerbation of any underlying dermatologic condition in the HIV-infected patient is common.

Infections, including *Staphylococcus aureus* (presenting as bullous impetigo, ecthyma, or folliculitis), *Pseudomonas aeruginosa* (which may present with chronic ulcerations and macerations), herpes simplex, herpes zoster, syphilis, and scabies, are common and should be treated with standard therapies.

Other dermatologic conditions that occur with increased frequency in HIV-infected patients include seborrheic dermatitis, psoriasis, atopic dermatitis, and alopecia. Dermatologic consultation is generally indicated. Admission may be indicated for patients with any disseminated cutaneous infection requiring intravenous antibiotics.

11. What ophthalmologic emergencies occur in AIDS patients?
Eye complaints such as change in visual acuity, photophobia, redness, or pain are common and may represent retinitis or invasion of eye or periorbital tissues with a malignant process. CMV retinitis occurs in 10–15% of AIDS patients and accounts for the majority of retinitis among AIDS patients. It has a characteristic appearance of fluffy white retinal lesions, often perivascular (sometimes referred to as "tomato and cheese pizza" appearance). Ophthalmology consultation is indicated followed by treatment with ganciclovir (5 mg/kg/day) for 2 weeks and long-term maintenance therapy.

12. Should HIV-infected patients receive tetanus immunization?
According to the U.S. Public Health Service Immunizations Practices Advisory Committee (ACIP), routine immunization recommendations for diphtheria (DPT), tetanus (Td), and measles, mumps and rubella (MMR) are unchanged for HIV-infected patients.

13. How should symptoms of side effects from drugs be managed?
Reactions to pharmacologic therapy are common in HIV-infected patients and must always be considered as the cause of new symptomatology. In a recent series, 5% of ED visits by symptomatic HIV-positive patients were related to complications of pharmacologic therapy. A decision about discontinuing therapy depends on balance between the benefit of the drug and the severity of side effects.

Common Drug Reactions in HIV-Infected Persons

	FEVER	RASH	N/V	DIARRHEA	HEAD-ACHE	CON-FUSION	PHLE-BITIS	DYS-RHYTHMIA
Antibiotics								
TMP-SMX	x	x	x					
Pentamidine		x						x
Isoniazid	x	x	x					
Clindamycin		x						
Dapsone	x	x	x		x			
Antifungals								
Amphotericin	x		x		x		x	x
5-Fluorouracil			x	x			x	
Ganciclovir			x	x				
Clotrimazole			x	x				
Nystatin			x	x				
Ketoconazole			x	x				
Antivirals								
Zidovudine (AZT)			x		x	x		
Acyclovir			x	x	x			
Dideoxyinosine (DDI)								x
Pain medications								
Ibuprofen	x	x	x					
Narcotics			x					

Laboratory Abnormalities in HIV-infected Persons

	↑LFTs	↑GLUC	↓GLUC	↓K	↓Mg	↓WBC	↓PLTS	↓HCT	↑AMYLASE
Antibiotics									
TMP-SMX	x					x	x		
Pentamidine		x	x			x		x	
Isoniazid	x					x	x	x	
Clindamycin									
Dapsone	x					x		x	
Antifungals									
Amphotericin				x	x			x	
5-Fluorouracil	x					x			
Ganciclovir						x			
Clotrimazole									
Nystatin									
Ketoconazole	x								
Antivirals									
Zidovudine (AZT)						x		x	
Acyclovir									
Dideoxyinosine (DDI)	x				x				x
Pain medications									
Ibuprofen	x					x		x	
Narcotics									

14. What are the common ethical problems?

Several important ethical considerations are HIV testing of patients and physicians, confidentiality, and resuscitation efforts.

At this time, testing for HIV is generally not indicated in the ED, and many departments have adopted strict policies against HIV testing because of difficulties in ensuring adequate confidentiality and availability of counseling. This may change as the need for early identification and treatment of patients is demonstrated. Initiation of counseling and referral for testing are recommended for patients at high risk.

Confidentiality regarding HIV-related diagnoses is paramount to providing appropriate patient care. Discretion when discussing the patient's diagnosis and condition with staff members, as well as with the patient's family and friends, will help to maintain confidentiality.

Resuscitation of patients with advanced AIDS is controversial. Decisions about life-support measures are best made prior to the need for their institution. Discussions with the family and the primary care physician may aid in making appropriate decisions. Because ED physicians may not have sufficient information about individual patients, their wishes, and the state of their disease, it is recommended that appropriate therapy and resuscitative measures be undertaken unless specifically otherwise stated.

15. How can physicians protect themselves from acquiring HIV?

Health care workers are often exposed to HIV-infected patients and their body fluids. Precautions in handling potentially infectious fluids are crucial. Because HIV infection is often undiagnosed at the time of the ED encounter, the use of universal precautions is strongly recommended, including the appropriate use of gown, gloves, mask, and goggles for procedures in all patients.

16. Should zidovudine (AZT) prophylaxis be administered following HIV exposure?
There is no clearcut nationwide recommendation regarding this issue. Although AZT may provide some decreased risk of HIV seroconversion, its efficacy has not been established and potential risks (the most serious of which are neutropenia and anemia) must also be considered. Some centers now advocate its use for prophylaxis after a high-risk exposure. Local policies should be instituted and followed until further data regarding its efficacy are available.

17. Should health care workers be tested for HIV?
Routine testing for HIV in health care workers is not currently recommended. There are several controversial issues, such as cost, confidentiality, and the potentially needless removal of skilled health care workers from practice. To date there have been no documented cases of direct physician-to-patient transmission of HIV. Currently the Centers for Disease Control recommends that health care workers who perform invasive procedures should know their HIV antibody status, and that expert review panels determine whether HIV-positive health care workers should continue to perform invasive procedures on a case-by-case basis.

BIBLIOGRAPHY

1. Callahan ML: Prophylaxis with zidovudine (AZT) after exposure to human immunodeficiency virus: A brief discussion of the issues for emergency physicians. Ann Emerg Med 20:1351–1354, 1991.
2. Centers for Disease Control: HIV/AIDS Surveillance Report. Jan 1992, pp 1–22.
3. Centers for Disease Control: Review of draft for revision of HIV infection classification system and expansion of AIDS surveillance case definition. MMWR 40:787, 1991.
4. Centers for Disease Control: The HIV/AIDS epidemic: The first 10 years. MMWR 40:357–369, 1991.
5. Cohen PT, Sande MA, Volberding PA (eds): The AIDS Knowledge Base. Waltham, MA, Massachusetts Medical Society, 1990.
6. Go GW, Baraff LJ, Schriger DL: Management guidelines for health care workers exposed to blood and body fluids. Ann Emerg Med 20:1341–1350, 1991.
7. Kelen GD: Human immunodeficiency virus and the emergency department: Risks and risk protection for health care providers. Ann Emerg Med 19:242–248, 1990.
8. Lo B, Steinbrook R: Health care workers infected with the human immunodeficiency virus. JAMA 267:1100–1106, 1992.
9. Marco CA: HIV infection and AIDS. In Tintinalli JE, Krome RL, Ruiz E (eds): Emergency Medicine: A Comprehensive Study Guide, 3rd ed. New York, McGraw-Hill, 1991, pp 519–524.
10. Talan DA, Kennedy CA: The management of HIV-related illness in the emergency department. Ann Emerg Med 20:1355–1365, 1991.

52. TOXIC SHOCK SYNDROME

Steven M. Chernow, M.D., FACEP

1. What is toxic shock syndrome (TSS)?
TSS is a toxin-mediated multisystem disease associated with *Staphylococcus aureus* colonization or infection.

2. When was TSS first described?
In 1978 Todd described a new shock syndrome in seven children. An exotoxin producing *S. aureus* was isolated from 5 of these patients.

3. Describe the epidemiology of TSS.

The number of new cases increased until it reached epidemic proportions in 1980 and 1981. The majority of cases occurred in menstruating females using tampons, although cases not related to menstruation also occurred. Procter and Gamble's super-absorbent Rely tampon was found to have a sevenfold greater risk over other tampons and was removed from the market. During the last decade the incidence and mortality of menstruation-related TSS has decreased from 812 cases and a 13% mortality in 1980 to 53 cases and a 2.5–5.0% mortality in 1988. Nonmenstrual TSS may occur in almost any clinical setting where *S. aureus* exists. These cases account for about one-third of TSS cases and are associated with a significant mortality of 10–15%.

4. How does *S. aureus* cause TSS?

An *S. aureus* exotoxin, TSS toxin-1 (TSST-1), has been isolated and genetically sequenced. This exotoxin is produced by 90–100% of *S. aureus* strains associated with menstrual TSS and 60–75% of strains associated with nonmenstrual TSS. In contrast, only 20% of random samples of *S. aureus* produce TSST-1. Because not all *S. aureus* strains associated with TSS produce TSST-1, other staphylococcal toxins may also cause the syndrome.

5. What is the Centers for Disease Control (CDC) case definition of TSS?

In July 1980, the CDC published their case definition of TSS.

CDC Case Definition of TSS

Fever: Temperature $\geq 38.9°$ C ($102°$ F)
Rash: Diffuse macular erythroderma
Desquamation: 1–2 weeks after illness, particularly of palms and soles
Hypotension: Systolic blood pressure ≤ 90 mmHg (adults), <5th percentile
   (children) or orthostatic dizziness, syncope, or diastolic decrease ≥ 15 mmHg
Multisystem Involvement (3 or more of the following):
   Gastrointestinal: vomiting or diarrhea at onset of illness
   Muscular: myalgia or elevated CPK (twice normal)
   Mucous membranes: vaginal, oropharyngeal, or conjunctival hyperemia
   Renal: twice-normal BUN or creatinine or pyuria (>5 WBC/hpf)
   Hepatic: twice-normal bilirubin or transaminases
   Hematologic: platelets $\leq 100,000/mm^3$
   Central nervous system: disorientation or alteration in consciousness without
      focal neurologic signs when fever and hypotension are absent
Negative Results (if obtained):
   Cultures: Blood, throat, CSF (blood cultures may be positive for *S. aureus*)
   Serology: Rocky Mountain spotted fever, leptospirosis, or measles

6. What are the clinical manifestations of TSS?

The syndrome may have an early prodrome with malaise, myalgias, low-grade fever, vomiting, or diarrhea. Symptoms may rapidly progress to become a multisystem disease with a wide range of severity.

Clinical Manifestations of TSS

Cardiovascular
   Hypotension
   Syncope or near-syncope
   Decreased systemic vascular resistance
   Decreased myocardial function
   EKG abnormalities and heart blocks
   Hypovolemia from loss of body fluids due to fever, vomiting, and diarrhea

Table continued on next page.

Clinical Manifestations of TSS (Continued)

Pulmonary
  Increased alveolar-arterial gradient
  Noncardiac pulmonary edema, i.e., adult respiratory distress syndrome
  Pleural effusions
Dermatologic
  Macular erythroderma (a flat, sunburnlike blanching rash)
  Desquamation of the rash 1–2 weeks after the illness
  Hyperemia of the mucous membranes (look for subconjunctival hemorrhages
      and hyperemia of the vagina and oropharynx)
Gastrointestinal
  Vomiting and/or watery diarrhea (usually early in the disease)
  Abdominal pain
  Hepatomegaly with abnormal liver function tests
Musculoskeletal
  Myalgias and arthralgias
  Nonpitting edema, especially of the hands and feet
Neurologic
  Headache
  Altered mental status
  Seizures
Renal
  Decreased urine output (possible acute tubular necrosis)
  Sterile pyuria, hematuria, elevated BUN, creatinine
Hematologic
  Possible disseminated intravascular coagulation (DIC)
  Thrombocytopenia, mild anemia, leukocytosis

---

7. What host or other factors increase susceptibility to TSS?
Patients with TSS demonstrate low antibody levels to TSST-1, whereas most controls have high levels. Frequently, convalescent titers of anti-TSST-1 antibodies do not rise and many patients may go on to have recurrent episodes of TSS. Local factors such as the absorbency and chemical composition of tampons are also important.

8. Are there any laboratory tests that definitively make the diagnosis of TSS?
No. The diagnosis is a clinical one with fulfillment of the CDC case definition.

9. Are there cases of TSS that do not meet the CDC case definition?
Probably. The original case definition was deliberately designed to ensure that only true cases of TSS were included. Milder cases do occur that do not fulfill all the requirements of the case definition and are considered to be probable TSS.

10. What is the differential diagnosis of TSS?
All the exclusions listed by the CDC case definition should be considered, including Rocky Mountain spotted fever, leptospirosis, and measles. In addition, other sources of shock such as meningococcemia, typhus, Lyme disease, tularemia, staphylococcal scalded skin syndrome, Stevens-Johnson syndrome, toxic epidermal neurolysis, Kawakaki disease, and, most recently, toxic streptococcal syndrome, may mimic TSS.

11. What is toxic streptococcal syndrome?
In the late 1980s a syndrome similar to TSS was recognized to be associated with a variety of a group A streptococcus that produced toxins with biologic activity similar to that of TSST-1.

12. What is the treatment for TSS?

The first priority is to recognize the syndrome early and remove any possible source of staphylococcal organisms such as vaginal tampons, nasal or surgical packs, or wound abscesses. Aggressive support to obviate multiple organ system failure is the cornerstone of successful management. Hypotension should be aggressively treated initially with crystalloid. Patients with decreased systemic vascular resistance or myocardial dysfunction may have hypotension refractory to fluid resuscitation and require pressors such as dopamine and admission to an intensive care unit for arterial and pulmonary wedge pressure monitoring. Complications include heart failure, noncardiac pulmonary edema, renal failure, and electrolyte abnormalities. Whether antibiotics alter the acute disease is controversial; however, they do reduce the likelihood of recurrent TSS. Therefore a beta-lactamase-resistant antistaphylococcal antibiotic should be administered. The use of corticosteroids may be useful if given early, although this is controversial and no prospective study supports their use. The efficiency of intravenous immune globulin and specific antitoxin antibody is not yet proved but may play an important role in the future.

BIBLIOGRAPHY

1. Bonventure PF, Linnemann C, Lana S, et al: Antibody responses to toxic-shock syndrome toxin by patients with TSS and by healthy staphylococcal carriers. J Infect Dis 150:662–666, 1984.
2. Freedman JD, Beer DJ: Expanding perspectives on the toxic shock syndrome. Adv Intern Med 36:363–397, 1991.
3. Hirsch MD, Kass EH: An annotated bibliography of toxic shock syndrome. Rev Infect Dis 8(Suppl 1):S1–S104, 1986.
4. Stevens DL, Tanner MH, Winship J, et al: Severe group A streptococcal infections associated with a toxic shock-like syndrome and scarlet fever toxin A. N Engl J Med 321:1–7, 1989.
5. The Toxic Shock Syndrome: Ann Intern Med 96 (Part 2):831–996, 1982.
6. Todd J, Fishaut M: Toxic-shock syndrome associated with phage-group-I staphylococci. Lancet 2:1116–1118, 1978.
7. Torres-Martinez C, Mehta D, Butt A, Levin M: Streptococcus associated toxic shock. Arch Dis Child 67:126–130, 1992.
8. Wright S, Trott A: Toxic shock syndrome: A review. Ann Emerg Med 17:268–273, 1988.

53. FOOD POISONING

Kim M. Feldhaus, M.D.

1. What causes food poisoning?

- Exotoxins produced by microorganisms
- Microorganisms, e.g., bacteria, fungi, viruses, parasites (these may be further classified as invasive, noninvasive, or toxin-producing organisms)
- Toxic substances present in the food naturally, e.g., mushrooms, dinoflagellates, or thallophytes

2. What are the common symptoms of food poisoning?

Nausea, vomiting, diarrhea, low-grade fever, and crampy abdominal pain.

3. What history is suggestive of food poisoning?

Presence of similar symptoms in other family members or others who ingested the same food or water, presence of blood in stools, and recent travel to underdeveloped countries or to mountainous regions are suggestive of food poisoning. Other historical points include course of disease (acute vs. subacute vs. chronic), recent food ingested, other medical problems (HIV status, hypertension), previous abdominal surgeries, sexual history, and pets at home.

4. What are the usual physical findings?
Generally, the abdomen is soft and minimally tender without peritoneal signs and with hyperactive or normal bowel sounds. Blood may be present in the stool. The physical exam is generally nonspecific.

5. Which physical findings are atypical in food poisoning?
Discrete areas of abdominal tenderness, peritoneal signs, and grossly bloody stools or melena should be warning signs that further investigations, including surgical consultation or GI consultation, may be warranted. High fever is not a common feature of bacterial diarrhea with the exception of shigellosis.

6. Differentiate diarrhea caused by invasive versus noninvasive organisms.
Organisms that invade the mucosa (Salmonella, Shigella, Campylobacter, *E. coli,* and Yersinia) cause bloody mucoid stools. Enterotoxins produced by other organisms (viruses, *Vibrio cholerae, E. coli, Staphylococcus aureus, Clostridium perfringens, Clostridium difficile,* and *Bacillus cereus*) affect the cyclic adenosine monophosphate pump on the gut mucosa and produce watery diarrhea.

7. What is the initial ED treatment of food poisoning?
Once a history and physical exam have been obtained and the working diagnosis is that of gastroenteritis (regardless of cause), the degree of dehydration **must** be assessed and treated. Intravenous hydration with crystalloids may be required. Oral rehydration is accomplished with isotonic glucose-containing fluids (which will help to facilitate sodium and therefore water absorption). Antiemetics may be administered. The patient should be able to tolerate fluids in the ED before being discharged.

8. What is the best test for diagnosing invasive diarrhea?
The best test is examination of the stool for fecal leukocytes. A thin smear of stool should be placed on a microscope slide and examined for the presence of leukocytes. Some recommend staining with methylene blue, Wright's stain, or Gram's stain, but an unstained specimen may work as well. The presence of numerous leukocytes indicates an invasive cause of the diarrhea.

9. What is "Montezuma's revenge"?
Traveler's diarrhea, or Montezuma's revenge, is caused by *E. coli. E. coli* can produce diarrhea by three mechanisms: (1) Enterotoxigenic strains produce a toxin that causes watery diarrhea (traveler's diarrhea) similar to that which occurs in cholera. (2) Entero-pathogenic strains colonize the bowel, causing outbreaks of diarrhea in hospital nurseries. (3) Enteroinvasive strains may cause a shigellalike illness with bloody mucoid stools.

10. What is the treatment for traveler's diarrhea?
Double-strength trimethoprim-sulfamethoxazole (160 mg of TMP and 800 mg SMZ), one tablet twice daily, is recommended. If the patient is allergic to sulfa drugs, ciprofloxacin (500 mg BID), norfloxin (400 mg BID), or ofloxin (300 mg BID) may be used. Treatment is continued until symptoms resolve, up to 4 days.

11. Is there any role for prophylaxis against traveler's diarrhea?
Prophylactic antibiotics are generally not advocated; however, Pepto-Bismol (bismuth subsalicylate) has been shown to prevent the onset of diarrhea in travelers who take 2 tablets

4 times daily. This product should not be used by patients on anticoagulants or salicylates, or who are allergic to salicylates.

12. Which diarrhea-producing agent is associated with febrile seizures in children?
Shigella infections in young children often cause high fevers with febrile seizures before the onset of diarrheal illness. The disease can be quite severe, and death has been known to occur within 8 hours of the onset of diarrhea secondary to dehydration. Abdominal pain and fever usually precede the diarrhea. Stools are typically bloody, mucoid, and explosive. Elevated white blood counts may be seen and a marked leftward shift is typical.

13. When are antibiotics indicated for invasive diarrhea?
Antibiotics are recommended only for severe cases of shigellosis or for outbreaks of *Shigella flexneri*. Bactrim is the drug of choice; most strains are also sensitive to ampicillin.

14. Describe a patient with Salmonella food poisoning.
Typically, patients have watery diarrhea, with abdominal cramping about 12–36 hours after ingestion of contaminated foods. Vomiting is rare. If septicemia is present, systemic symptoms of fever, cough, headache, and meningismus occur. Enteric fever should be treated with hospitalization and antibiotics.

15. Name the frequent food and pet sources of salmonella poisoning.
Eggs, egg products such as yogurt, egg nog, and hollandaise sauce, chicken, and turkey are commonly discovered to be the source of outbreaks of salmonella food poisoning. Pet turtles frequently are the source of salmonella gastroenteritis.

16. Which bacterial organism typically causes abdominal cramps and diarrhea 12 hours after eating contaminated food?
Clostridium perfringens. Time of onset is longer than that of salmonella poisoning. It is frequently associated with food-service establishments where food is prepared in advance. Usual symptoms include diarrhea, abdominal pain, and occasionally nausea. Fever and vomiting are unlikely.

17. What is the most common food-borne disease in the U.S.?
Staphylococcus aureus food poisoning. Cooled meat, fish, poultry, and bakery goods, especially those with cream or custard fillings, are common sources. Vomiting, cramping, and watery diarrhea without fecal leukocytes occur within 1–6 hours of ingestion of contaminated foods.

18. Which parasite should be highly suspected in a camper with chronic abdominal bloating and intermittent diarrhea with constipation?
Giardia lamblia is endemic to many areas of the country and is the most common parasite in the U.S. Infection is acquired through drinking contaminated water. Up to 5% of the population harbors the parasite in the cyst stage. Treatment with metronidazole has frequently been used effectively, although its use for this infection is not approved.

19. Should antibiotics be used for invasive causes of bacterial diarrhea?
Older studies have indicated that the use of antibiotics in salmonella gastroenteritis prolongs the shedding of the organism and may give rise to carrier states. Antibiotics *do* hasten the recovery of patients with infection by *other* invasive organisms. Trimethoprim-sulfamethoxazole (one double-strength tablet 2 times daily) is effective against most organisms. The quinolones are also active against the most common bacterial agents. In general, antibiotics are reserved for severe cases of food poisoning.

20. What about symptomatic relief? Should this be offered to patients?
Historically, symptomatic relief was offered only to those with noninvasive diarrhea (no fecal leukocytes in stool smears). Those with invasive diarrhea can develop toxic megacolon and have continued shedding of the organism if they are placed on antimotility drugs. Recently, however, loperamide (Imodium) has been used safely for all forms of gastroenteritis, but diphenoxylate (Lomotil) should be avoided in invasive diarrhea.

21. What is an appropriate disposition for the patient with food poisoning?
Most patients can be discharged to home with instructions to avoid lactose-containing foods until the diarrhea stops. They should receive instructions on proper use of clear liquids and how to advance their diet. Follow-up should be arranged if the symptoms persist for 1 week. Be sure to rule out other causes of vomiting and diarrhea in the elderly. Close follow-up to assess for dehydration is crucial in young infants.

BIBLIOGRAPHY

1. Baird-Parker AC: Foodborne salmonellosis. Lancet 336:1231–1235, 1990.
2. Doyle MP: Pathogenic *Escherichia coli, Yersinia enterocolitica,* and *Vibrio parahaemolyticus.* Lancet 336:1111–1115, 1990.
3. Fang G, Araujo V, Guerrant RL: Enteric infections associated with exposure to animals or animal products. Infect Dis Clin North Am 5:681–701, 1991.
4. Heller M: Diarrhea and proctitis. In Harwood-Nuss A (ed): The Clinical Practice of Emergency Medicine. Philadelphia, J.B. Lippincott, 1991, pp 964–966.
5. Levine MM: Antimicrobial therapy for infectious diarrhea. Rev Infect Dis 8(Suppl 2):S207–S215, 1986.
6. Lund BM: Foodborne disease due to *Bacillus* and *Clostridium* species. Lancet 336:982–986, 1990.
7. Seidel JS: Diarrhea and food poisoning. In Tintinalli J (ed): Emergency Medicine: A Comprehensive Study Guide. New York, McGraw-Hill, 1988, pp 333–337.
8. Todd E: Epidemiology of foodborne illness: North America. Lancet 336:788–790, 1990.
9. Tranker HS: Foodborne staphylococcal illness. Lancet 336:1044–1046, 1990.

54. BOTULISM

Mark Langdorf, M.D., FACEP, and Lisa Josephson, M.D.

1. What is the causative agent of botulism? How does it cause disease?
Botulism is caused by the toxin produced by *Clostridium botulinum*. This toxin binds to peripheral presynaptic cholinergic membranes, preventing the release of acetylcholine and thereby producing a life-threatening paralytic illness. Adrenergic synapses are unaffected. By weight, botulism toxin is the most potent toxin known.

2. What are the three circumstances by which a patient can contract botulism?
    1. Botulism is most commonly contracted by ingesting food that contains the preformed toxin. Most cases are due to home-canned or prepared foods and occur in isolation or in small clusters.
    2. Wound botulism occurs when *C. botulinum* organisms contaminate traumatic wounds. These occur most often in IV drug users and wounds grossly contaminated by soil. Children are at risk because they so often sustain extremity injuries while playing in the dirt. The incubation period for development of wound botulism is 4–14 days, and the wound may appear "clean" at the time of initial medical evaluation.

3. Infant botulism occurs when *C. botulinum* infects the infant gastrointestinal tract, most commonly from contaminated raw honey. This is the most common form of botulism in the United States, usually occurring in infants 3–20 weeks of age.

3. How does infant botulism present?

Often the first sign is constipation. This is followed by a feeble cry, floppy or weak neck, pooling of oral secretions or food in the oropharynx, decreased gag reflex, hypotonia, and areflexia. Cranial nerve deficits also occur, including flaccid facial expression, ptosis, and ophthalmoplegia. Respiratory arrest occurs in up to half of babies affected. Infants with botulism are afebrile and have normal cerebral spinal fluid.

4. What is the treatment for infant botulism?

Supportive care, including respiratory support, is the mainstay of treatment. Antitoxin is not recommended, as infants recover without it. The organism and toxin may remain in the bowel for up to 8 weeks after recovery. It has been suggested that infant botulism accounts for some cases of sudden infant death syndrome.

5. How can we prevent food-borne botulism?

Foods contaminated with botulism may have a normal appearance and taste, and only a small amount of it is necessary to cause disease. Appropriate processing of foods is vital to preventing illness. Botulism spores are heat resistant. Therefore, even when home-prepared food is cooked prior to canning, the spores can still produce toxin. Proper methods of cooking canned foods prior to eating, either by boiling for 10 minutes or heating at 80°C (176°F) for 30 minutes, destroy botulism toxin.

6. How does a patient with adult botulism present?

Early symptoms are nonspecific and usually begin 12–36 hours (range, 6 hours to 8 days) after ingestion. They include nausea, vomiting, weakness, lassitude, and dizziness. The patient then develops anticholinergic symptoms, including extreme dry mouth unrelieved by fluids, decreased lacrimation, constipation, and urinary retention. Neurologic symptoms, which may be delayed up to 3 days after the appearance of anticholinergic symptoms, most often first involve cranial nerves. The patient develops diplopia, blurred vision, photophobia, dysphonia, and dysphagia—all ocular and bulbar symptoms. In addition, the patients develop symmetric descending weakness of the extremities. Ominously, the weakness may progress to involve respiratory muscles.

7. What are the characteristic physical findings?

The most characteristic findings are postural hypotension, ptosis, extraocular palsies, and dilated, fixed pupils. Deep tendon reflexes may be normal, increased, or absent. Sensory exam is normal, as is temperature in the absence of wound infection. The patient may have decreased bowel sounds and abdominal distention from ileus. Pulmonary function tests may reveal decreased vital capacity.

Therefore, the constellation of postural hypotension, dilated and unreactive pupils, dry mucous membranes, descending paralysis with progressive respiratory weakness, and absence of fever strongly suggests the diagnosis.

8. What is the differential diagnosis of botulism?

There are many causes of acute weakness, such as disorders of nerves, muscles, or the neuromuscular junction. Myasthenia gravis, Guillain-Barré syndrome, multiple sclerosis, tick paralysis, Eaton-Lambert syndrome, periodic paralysis, paralytic shellfish poisoning, coral snake envenomation, and drug-induced disorders of neuromuscular transmission caused by aminoglycosides, phenytoin, lithium, organophosphate, and carbamate insecticide poisonings may all present similarly to botulism.

9. How can you confirm your clinical suspicion that a patient has botulism?
You must isolate either the organism itself or the toxin from suspect food or the patient. Examine the patient's stool, blood, wound, and, in the case of infant botulism, gastric contents. Other lab studies are not helpful. Solicit help from a poison center such as the Centers for Disease Control and local health department, as this is a reportable condition.

10. How do you treat adult botulism? Which organ system requires the most intensive monitoring?
Treatment is largely supportive. The most life-threatening effect of botulism is respiratory failure. Therefore, intensive monitoring of vital capacity and negative inspiratory force, preferably in an intensive care unit, is mandatory. Early and controlled intubation is preferable to crash intubation, because patients can deteriorate within minutes. Nasogastric suction and total parenteral nutrition are necessary for profound ileus. Urinary catheterization avoids retention. Penicillin may eradicate colonization of the intestine but is of unproven value. Botulism antitoxin, available through state health departments, should be given as soon as possible. Even if diagnosis is delayed, antitoxin should still be used, as toxin has been demonstrated in the blood for as long as 30 days. It is an equine antitoxin, effective against toxin types A, B, and E. Patients must be tested for hypersensitivity to horse serum prior to administration, as described on the antitoxin package insert.

11. What is the prognosis of a patient with botulism?
With the use of antitoxin and respiratory support, adult mortality has decreased from 60% to 25% over the past 30 years. Recovery is very gradual over weeks to months.

BIBLIOGRAPHY

1. Barrett DH: Endemic food-borne botulism: Clinical experience 1973–1986 at the Alaska Native Medical Center. Alaska Med 33:101–108, 1991.
2. Cherington M: Botulism. Semin Neurol 10:27–31, 1990.
3. Critchley EM, Mitchell JD: Human botulism. Br J Hosp Med 43:290–292, 1990.
4. Dunbar EM: Botulism (published erratum appears in J Infect 20:273, 1990). J Infect 20:1–3, 1990.
5. Frankovich TL, Arnon SS: Clinical trial of botulism immune globulin for infant botulism. West J Med 154:103, 1991.
6. Jagoda A, Renner G: Infant botulism: Case report and clinical update. Am J Emerg Med 8:318–320, 1990.
7. Kudrow DB, Henry DA, Haake DA, et al: Botulism associated with *Clostridium botulinum* sinusitis after intranasal cocaine abuse. Ann Intern Med 109:984–985, 1988.
8. Lecour H, Ramos H, Almeida B, Barbosa R: Food-borne botulism: A review of 13 outbreaks. Arch Intern Med 148:578–580, 1988.
9. McCarthy JD, Fleischmann J, George WL: Fever, dyspnea, and slurred speech following lower extremity trauma (clinical conference). Rev Infect Dis 13:172–176, 1991.
10. Mills DC, Arnon SS: The large intestine as the site of *Clostridium botulinum* colonization in human infant botulism. J Infect Dis 156:997–998, 1987.
11. Oh SJ, Cho HK: Edrophonium responsiveness not necessarily diagnostic of myasthenia gravis. Muscle Nerve 13:187–191, 1990.
12. Schaffner W: *Clostridium botulinum* (botulism). In Mandell GL, Douglas RG, Bennett JE (eds): Principles and Practice of Infectious Diseases. New York, Churchill Livingstone, 1990.
13. Spika JS, Shaffer N, Hargrett-Bean N, Collin S, et al: Risk factors for infant botulism in the United States (published erratum appears in Am J Dis Child 144:60, 1990). Am J Dis Child 143:828–832, 1989.
14. Suen JC, Hatheway CL, Steigerwalt AG, Brenner DJ: Genetic confirmation of identities of neurotoxigenic *Clostridium baratii* and *Clostridium butyricum* implicated as agents of infant botulism. J Clin Microbiol 26:2191–2192, 1988.
15. Swedberg J, Wendel TH, Deiss F: Wound botulism. West J Med 147:335–338, 1987.

55. TETANUS

James Mathews, M.D.

1. No one I know has seen a clinical case of tetanus. Why should I worry about it?
It is true that because of mandated immunization in the U.S., the incidence of tetanus is less than one case per million per year. However, many people are at risk. This group includes immigrants from countries in which tetanus prophylaxis is not mandated, and elderly persons who have lost their immunity.

2. Worldwide, what is the most common cause of death from tetanus?
The neonatal form, arising from poor hygiene of the umbilical stump and from circumcision practices, is the most common cause of death.

3. What are "tetanus-prone" wounds?
Wounds that produce anaerobic conditions are the most worrisome. These include puncture wounds, crush injuries, and burns (even superficial ones). Any wound heavily contaminated with debris such as soil or feces is at high risk.

4. Are there other problems that may lead to tetanus?
Yes. Otitis media, tonsillar crypt infection, septic abortion, and problems with the lower GI tract have all been implicated.

5. What bacteria causes tetanus?
The causative bacterium, *Clostridium tetani*, is an obligate anaerobe. It is shaped like a drumstick and produces spores. This organism is ubiquitous in soil and feces, and occurs worldwide. The organism itself is easily killed by heat and antiseptics, but the spores are extremely tough. Disease occurs when the spores germinate, multiply in tissue under anaerobic conditions, and produce the toxin.

6. How can I diagnose tetanus?
The most common presenting symptom is trismus, possibly associated with dysphagia, excessive pain in the area of injury, and a painful stiff neck. This usually begins within 10–15 days of injury, and onset is over a 2–5-day period. Onset is the period between earliest symptoms and the first generalized spasm. Onset over less than 48 hours is associated with severe disease. Progression of the disease involves increasing numbers of spastic muscle groups and increasing pain during spasm.

7. Which muscle group is often profoundly affected?
The muscles of the neck and back. Severe spasm of these muscles may produce opisthotonos to the extent that only the heels and the back of the head are touching the bed. In the worst cases, these spasms have caused rupture of the rectus abdominis muscles and fractured vertebrae.

8. Are there systemic symptoms?
Yes, but these may be minimal. In severe cases, wide swings in blood pressure and heart rate, and high fever may be seen. These signs seem to be due to excessive catecholamines.

9. What usually causes death?
In modern developed countries, the most common causes of death are the autonomic problems, especially fatal arrhythmias and hyperpyrexia. In the past and in underdeveloped countries, the most common cause of death was and is respiratory failure secondary to spasm of the muscles of respiration.

10. What diseases may mimic tetanus?

In the established case it can be confused only with strychnine poisoning. In strychnine poisoning, the jaw muscles are usually involved late or not at all, and between spasms there is no rigidity. Early tetanus may be confused with dental infections that produce trismus and with dystonic reactions. Observation will reveal that trismus secondary to dental infection does not progress, and the patient with a dystonic reaction can open the mouth, which does not occur with true trismus.

11. Which laboratory studies are helpful?

There are no diagnostic laboratory studies. Routine testing includes EKG, arterial blood gases (ABGs), and vital capacity (VC). These last two should be followed closely to recognize early respiratory failure. The site of infection should be identified.

12. What do I do in the emergency department (ED)?

An IV should be started and human tetanus immunoglobulin given, 1000 units IV and 2000 units IM. This must be done prior to surgical wound debridement in order to bind any released toxin. Penicillin is the drug of choice in a dose of 1 million units IV every 6 hours. Penicillin-allergic patients are treated with erythromycin, 500 mg IV every 6 hours.

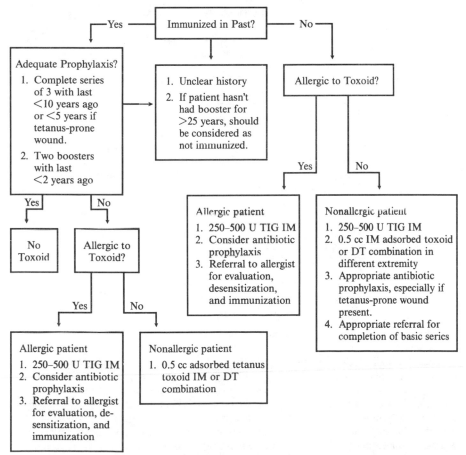

Guidelines for Tetanus Immunization

13. What about supportive measures?
If the vital capacity (VC) is <50% predicted, the patient must be paralyzed with long-acting agents, such as curare or pancuronium, and placed on a ventilator. If VC is >50% but trismus is severe with compromise of the airway, either an endotrachael tube or tracheostomy is indicated. Mild disease may be controlled with sedatives such as diazepam. A nasogastric tube should be placed.

14. How can tetanus be prevented?
Mandatory immunization. Proper wound care and good hygiene are important components of prevention. Proper cleansing irrigation and debridement must be done on all wounds and appropriate immunization is mandatory (see figure). Tetanus immunization must always be confirmed and documented. If there is any doubt regarding earlier immunizations, both toxoid and tetanus immune globulin (TIG) should be given.

15. What are the pitfalls?
The early symptoms of tetanus are easy to ascribe to psychoneurotic disorders. A dystonic reaction should respond immediately to 50 mg of intravenous diphrenhydramine. The careful observer will not make this error.

BIBLIOGRAPHY

1. Adams EB, Laurence DR, Smith DWG: Tetanus. Oxford, Blackwell Scientific Publications, 1969.
2. Bartlett JG: Tetanus. In Wyngaarden JB, et al (eds): Cecil Textbook of Medicine, 19th ed. Philadelphia, W.B. Saunders, 1992.
3. Dowell VR Jr: Botulism and tetanus, selected epidemiological and microbiologic aspects. Rev Infect Dis 6(Suppl 1):S202, 1984.
4. Edmondson RS, Flowers MW: Intensive care in tetanus management, complications, and mortality in 100 cases. Br Med J 1:1404, 1979.
5. Mathews JJ: Tetanus. In Harwood-Nuss A (ed): The Clinical Practice of Emergency Medicine. Philadelphia, J.B. Lippincott, 1991.
6. Patel JC, Mehta BC: Tetanus. Study of 8,697 cases. In Proceedings of the Fourth International Conference on Tetanus, April 6–12, 1975, Dekar, Senegal. Lyon, France, Foundation Merieuz.
7. Trujillo MJ, Castillo A, Espana J, Guevara P, Eganex H: Tetanus in the adult: Intensive care and management experience with 233 cases. Crit Care Med 8:419, 1980.

56. SEXUALLY TRANSMITTED DISEASES

David S. Howes, M.D., FACEP

1. What are the more common sexually transmitted diseases (STDs) and their annual frequency?
Overall STDs affect about 12 million people annually in the U.S. **Chlamydial infection** is estimated to infect 4 million people annually and is a major health risk for young women, as it may be associated with minimal symptoms, yet cause serious infertility from chronic infection. Cases of **gonorrhea** appeared to be on the decline through the mid-1980s, only to surge since that time, especially in nonwhite, urban settings; 1.4 million cases were identified in 1990. Approximately 1 million annual cases of **genital warts** are found. They are more unpleasant than dangerous clinically, but there are links to genital neoplasms, making this a tremendous health care problem. Each year, 500,000 new cases of **genital**

herpes are identified, and asymptomatic shedding of the virus remains a problem for sexual partners. **Pelvic inflammatory disease** will complicate the lives of over 400,000 women this year. **Sexually transmitted hepatitis** infects about 300,000 persons annually. New cases of **syphilis**, after four successive decades of declining incidence, are very much on the rise and will be diagnosed in over 150,000 patients this year. Despite intensive public education, **HIV acquisition** due to sexual activity, especially heterosexual transmission, is increasing and will account for a tremendous health care burden in the years to come. Over a million Americans are now HIV infected and 200,000 cases of AIDS were identified in 1991.

2. Explain the significance of finding mucopurulent cervicitis in a woman with lower abdominal pain.

The normal endometrial secretion, as noted on exit from the endocervical canal, should be transparent and have the consistency of viscous styling gel. The presence of a mucopurulent secretion from the endocervix, which may appear yellow when viewed on a white cotton-tipped swab (positive Q-tip sign), suggests mucopurulent cervicitis (MPC). MPC, most commonly due to gonorrhea or chlamydia, is a likely precursor to most cases of ascending pelvic infection in young, sexually active women, and should be carefully sought in all women with lower abdominal pain.

3. How does one suspect on epidemiologic and clinical grounds that chlamydial infection may be responsible for symptoms of a urinary tract infection (UTI)?

Epidemiologic evidence for chlamydial infection includes younger women, women with a new or multiple sexual partner(s), a partner with symptoms of urethritis, or a past history of STD. Pyuria without bacteriuria is a typical finding. The presence of MPC is supportive, as is cervical motion and tubal tenderness, of an alternative diagnosis to simple UTI. Therefore, lower abdominal pain and dysuria should prompt strong consideration of a speculum and bimanual pelvic examination in most sexually active women.

4. A young, sexually active male presents with dysuria. How likely is it due to UTI?

About as likely as getting gonorrhea from sitting on a toilet seat. Dysuria in young men is almost always due to STD-related urethritis. The likely pathogens include gonorrhea, chlamydia, ureaplasma, trichomonas, and herpes simplex virus. Ironically, a large study of adolescent males with dysuria revealed that a urinary specimen demonstrating pyuria was as effective as a urethral swab in identifying which patients had an active STD-related urethritis; no patient was felt to have true UTI in this study.

5. Are there suitable oral alternatives to parenteral therapy for gonorrhea?

Uncomplicated urethral, endocervical, or rectal gonorrheal infections can be suitably treated with a single intramuscular injection of ceftriaxone, 250 mg, or equivalent cephalosporin antibiotic. Though clinical experience is less extensive, alternative single-dose oral regimens have been recommended: ciprofloxacin, 500 mg; norfloxacin, 800 mg; and cefuroxime axetil, 1 gm (the latter with probenecid, 1 gm). The incidence of coexistent chlamydial infection in a patient with suspected or proven gonorrhea is as high as 50%. Therefore, all patients being treated for gonorrhea should also be treated for chlamydia. In an uncomplicated case, the preferred regimen is doxycycline, 100 mg BID for 7 days.

6. A young, sexually active female presents with an acutely swollen, warm, painful right knee. What are your concerns and therapeutic plans?

The patient should be presumed to have disseminated gonococcal infection (DGI), in this instance acute gonococcal arthritis. A pelvic examination must be performed, even if the patient is asymptomatic from a gynecologic standpoint, to assess for MPC and to obtain cultures from the cervix, the most common primary infection site. An arthrocentesis for cell count, a Gram stain, and culture must be performed and the patient should be considered for admission and given intravenous antibiotics. A suitable regimen includes intravenous ceftriaxone, 1 gm q 12 hr, or equivalent cephalosporin and treatment for coexistent chlamydia.

7. Are there any single-dose regimens for the treatment of uncomplicated chlamydial infection?

Until recently, there were no recommended single-dose regimens for the treatment of uncomplicated chlamydial infection. The availability of azithromycin, a macrolide antibiotic with an unusually long duration of action, may substantially cut down on compliance problems in difficult-to-treat patient populations. A single oral dose of 1 gm was as effective as a conventional course of doxycycline given for 7 days. However, it does not effectively treat gonorrhea or syphilis.

8. Which factors are associated with an enhanced risk of acquiring syphilis?

The incidence of syphilis in the U.S. had declined over the last four decades and was primarily a problem in the homosexual population. However, during the 1980s, syphilis reached epidemic proportions in inner-city, primarily black, heterosexual populations. Epidemiologic factors that enhance risk include multiple sexual partners, prostitution, cocaine or crack cocaine use, intravenous drug abuse, HIV-positive status, or a history of STD, especially gonorrhea or herpes. Findings of cervicitis, generalized or groin rash, groin or rectal lesions, or active herpes have been associated with an increased risk of syphilis. It is clear that selected ED screening of patient populations at risk who do not seek out primary health providers will be increasingly important in order to effectively address this problem.

9. What are four STD-related causes of groin adenopathy? How are they treated?

1. The most common cause of groin adenopathy is active, **primary herpes simplex virus** (HSV) infection. It may also be seen with severe recurrences. Oral acyclovir, 200 mg 5 times a day for 7–10 days, is recommended to provide partial control of symptoms and accelerate healing. Unfortunately, use of acyclovir neither eradicates the infection nor decreases the subsequent risk, frequency, or severity of recurrences.

2. **Chancroid**, due to *Hemophilus ducreyi*, has become an important STD in the U.S. It remains sensitive to oral erythromycin base, 500 mg QID for 7 days, or a single intramuscular dose of ceftriaxone, 250 mg.

3. **Syphilis** must always be considered in the differential of groin adenopathy and a VDRL or similar screening test for syphilis must be obtained in all patients who present with groin adenopathy. In this stage, a single intramuscular injection of benzathine penicillin G, 2.4 million units, is the treatment of choice.

4. **Lymphogranuloma venereum** (LGV) is caused by *Chlamydia trachomatis*. It may be confused with chancroid. It is uncommon in the U.S. Treatment of LGV requires a prolonged course of oral doxycycline, 100 mg BID for 21 days.

10. Proctitis is a problem primarily seen in the homosexual community. Discuss the approach and treatment.

Any individual, male or female, with onset of acute proctitis symptoms who has recently practiced unprotected receptive anal intercourse is at risk for an STD-related problem. Such patients should be examined by anoscopy (go easy on this) and be evaluated for infection with gonorrhea, chlamydia, HSV, and syphilis. All patients should undergo serologic testing for syphilis. As with genital herpes, HSV proctitis is treated with oral acyclovir but at a higher dose, 400 mg 5 times a day for 10 days. Most patients should be empirically treated for gonorrhea with a single dose of intramuscular ceftriaxone, 250 mg, and be given treatment for chlamydia with oral doxycycline, 100 mg BID for 7 days.

11. Vaginitis is a common problem in young, sexually active women. Discuss the approach to this problem.

The problem is easier if you have a female with a long-standing single sexual partner and she has recently received a course of antibiotics. This infection is likely due to Candida, and the findings of vulvar erythema and a cheesy, non-foul-smelling vaginal discharge confirm the diagnosis. Treatment with a 3–7 day course of miconazole vaginal suppository (or cream), 200 mg at bedtime, should take care of the problem.

Anything else is more complicated. A recent study showed that it was difficult to distinguish clinically between candidal vulvovaginitis, *Trichomonas vaginalis* infection, and bacterial vaginosis. Of interest, symptoms did not differ significantly between patients with different causes, and a lack of vaginal odor in yeast infections was the only significantly different physical sign. This has led some to recommend that most young women who are sexually active and present with vaginitis be treated comprehensively with a 3-day regimen of intravaginal miconazole and a 7-day course of oral metronidazole, 500 mg BID.

BIBLIOGRAPHY

1. Abramowicz M (ed): Drugs for sexually transmitted diseases. Med Letter 33:119, 1991.
2. Brandt AM: Sexually transmitted diseases: Shadow on the land, revisited. Ann Intern Med 112:481, 1990.
3. Brunham RC, Paavonen J, Stevens CE, et al: Mucopurulent cervicitis: The ignored counterpart in women of urethritis in men. N Engl J Med 311:1, 1984.
4. Centers for Disease Control: Sexually transmitted diseases: Treatment guidelines. MMWR 38:S-8, 1989.
5. Handsfield HH, McCormack WM, Hook EW, et al: A comparison of single-dose cefixime with ceftriaxone as treatment for uncomplicated gonorrhea. N Engl J Med 325:1337, 1991.
6. Koutsky LA, Stevens CE, Holmes KK, et al: Underdiagnosis of genital herpes by current clinical and viral-isolation procedures. N Engl J Med 326:1533, 1992.
7. Rolfs RT, Nakashima AK: Epidemiology of primary and secondary syphilis in the United States, 1981 thorugh 1989. JAMA 264:1432, 1990.
8. Sadof MD, Woods ER, Emans SJ: Dipstick leukocyte esterase activity in first-catch urine specimens: A useful screening test for detecting sexually transmitted disease in the adolecent male. JAMA 258:1932, 1987.
9. Schaaf VM, Perez-Stable EJ, Borchardt K: The limited value of symptoms and signs in the diagnosis of vaginal infections. Arch Intern Med 150:1929, 1990.
10. Stamm WE: A comparison of single-dose azithromycin with doxycycline for uncomplicated genital Chlamydia infection. Am J Med 91(3A):19S, 1991.
11. Stone KM, Whittington WL: Treatment of genital herpes. Rev Infect Dis 12:610, 1990.

57. TICK-BORNE ILLNESSES OF NORTH AMERICA

Cheryl Melick-Casanova, M.D.

1. Are tick-related illnesses of medical importance?

The answer is a resounding *yes*. They transmit a greater variety of infectious agents than any other arthropod and are second in importance only to the mosquito as a vector for human illness.

2. How many illnesses are transmitted by ticks in North America?

Ten different illnesses are currently identified as being transmitted by a tick vector. They range from protozoan, bacterial, viral, spirochetal, and rickettsial to toxic in origin.

3. Classify ticks.

Ticks are from the class Arachnida, which includes spiders, mites, and scorpions. There are two major families of ticks. The Ixodidae, or hard tick, and the Argasidae, or soft tick. All major tick-borne illnesses are transmitted by hard ticks except for relapsing fever.

4. What time of year do tick-related illnesses occur?

The peak incidence is late spring and early summer, with 64% of illnesses presenting May through July. Illness is seen, however, through the month of October in most regions.

5. In which age groups are the majority of tick-related illnesses seen?

Most cases of tick-borne illness occur in children under 15, probably due to lack of recognition of tick attachment while playing outdoors. Another peak occurs in the 25–44 age group, possibly related to increased outdoor recreational activities in this group.

6. Name the vector and infectious agent for each tick-borne illness.

Tick-borne Illnesses

DISEASE	VECTOR	AGENT	ORGANISM
Lyme disease	*Ixodes dammini*	Spirochete	*Borrelia burgdorferi*
Relapsing fever	Ornithodoros	Spirochete	*Borrelia hermsii*
			Borrelia turicatae
			Borrelia parkeri
Rocky Mountain spotted fever	*Dermacentor andersoni* *Dermacentor variabilis*	Rickettsia	*Rickettsia rickettsii*
Ehrlichiosis	Unknown	Rickettsia	*Ehrlichia canis*
Q fever	Unknown	Rickettsia	*Coxiella burnetii*
Colorado tick fever	*Dermacentor andersoni*	RNA virus	Orbivirus
Encephalitis	Multiple	Viral	Arbovirus
Babesiosis	*Ixodes dammini*	Protozoan	*Babesia microti*
Tularemia	*Dermacentor andersoni* *Dermacentor variabilis* *Amblyomma americanum*	Bacterial	*Francisella tularensis*
Tick paralysis	Multiple	Toxin	None

7. Describe the classic initial presentation of Lyme disease.

A pathognomonic rash, erythema chronica migrans (ECM), develops at the site of inoculation of the spirochete in 60–80% of infected individuals. Initially a small red papule forms which expands peripherally over the ensuing 3 days to weeks, creating a characteristic lesion consisting of a bright red outer border with partial central clearing. Lesions enlarge to 15 cm or greater. In 50% of patients, multiple secondary annular lesions develop. Untreated, the rash resolves in 4 weeks; with treatment, resolution occurs in 5 days. Constitutional symptoms include headache, stiff neck, fever, lethargy, malaise, and anorexia.

8. Describe the later stages of untreated Lyme disease.

The heart, central nervous system, joints, and eyes may be affected. Lyme carditis, seen in 8% of cases, consists of fluctuating degrees of atrioventricular block, including complete heart block. Temporary pacing may be necessary, but complete resolution occurs with time. Neurologic complications occur in 15% and include headache, meningitis, cranial neuritis with bilateral facial palsies, and peripheral radiculoneuritis. Encephalopathy with progression and neuropsychiatric syndromes may occur over years. In 60% of patients, asymmetric monoarticular arthritis affects the large joints, primarily the knee, with increasingly longer periods between attacks. Chronic degeneration develops in 10% of patients.

9. What is the geographic distribution of Lyme disease?

Most cases of Lyme disease occur along the coastal regions of the Northeast, upper Midwest, and Pacific regions, and 97% of cases occur in nine states: Connecticut, Massachusetts, Rhode Island, New York, New Jersey, Pennsylvania, Wisconsin, Minnesota, and California.

10. What is relapsing fever?

Relapsing fever is caused by a spirochete and is the only tick-borne illness transmitted by the Argasidae, or soft-bodied tick. Outbreaks usually occur in backpackers from the western mountains who stay in old cabins infested by rodents. The tick is harbored in the rodent's nest and feeds on the unwary for brief periods at night. The 4–18 day incubation period is followed by the abrupt onset of a high fever associated with chills, severe headache, myalgia, weakness, and occasional GI complaints. Symptoms last 3 days and then resolve. If the condition is not treated, multiple relapses ensue at weekly intervals. In 25% of patients an erythematous macular rash may develop. Diagnosis is by identifying spirochetes on a peripheral blood smear using a Giemsa stain.

11. What is Rocky Mountain spotted fever?

Infection by this rickettsial organism causes an overwhelming vasculitis. Organisms multiply within the vascular endothelium with development of increased vascular permeability and microinfarction of organs. Onset is abrupt, with initial complaints of high fever, headache, and myalgia. The classic rash, which is initially macular, becomes petechial over several days. It begins on the palms and soles then spreads centripitally to involve the trunk. It does not appear until the fourth day of illness but is absent in 15%. The classic triad of fever, rash, and tick exposure is present in less than half of patients. Meningismus, focal neurologic signs, myocarditis, pneumonitis, and GI symptoms may occur. Death is due to multi-system organ failure with intracerebral hemorrhage, DIC, and vascular collapse. Diagnosis is entirely clinical; serologic evidence is helpful only for confirmation following recovery.

12. What is the mortality rate for Rocky Mountain spotted fever?

The case fatality rate has remained constant at 4%, with mortality highest in the elderly (>8%) and those whose treatment is begun after the third day of symptoms. In regions with endemic Rocky Mountain spotted fever, a trial of doxycycline is recommended for anyone who presents with fever, headache, and myalgia from May through September.

13. What is the geographic distribution of Rocky Mountain spotted fever?

Initially the condition was isolated and diagnosed in the Rocky Mountains, but a change in the epidemiology of the illness occurred around 1931. The illness is now seen almost exclusively in the southern Atlantic and western south-central parts of the United States. The states with the highest incidence are Oklahoma, Kansas, and the Carolinas.

14. What is human ehrlichiosis?

First described in humans in 1986 but known as a veterinary pathogen since 1935, ehrlichia is characterized by the ability of the rickettsial organism to parasitize white blood cells. After an incubation period of 10–14 days, an acute febrile illness associated with myalgia, headache, nausea, and other GI symptoms develops. A rash, if present, is rare and fleeting. Laboratory results are noteworthy for leukopenia, thrombocytopenia, and a mild elevation of liver enzymes. Its geographic distribution is the south-central and southern Atlantic states. Serologic testing has shown it to be misdiagnosed as Rocky Mountain spotted fever in these regions.

15. What is Q fever?

It is a highly infectious rickettsial infection in which a single inhaled organism is sufficient to initiate infection. The infection, although carried by and transmitted to animals by ticks, is rarely transmitted to humans by this route. Most human infection follows exposure during parturition of livestock, especially sheep. Following an incubation period of 14–39 days, an acute febrile illness associated with rigors, severe headache, malaise, myalgia, and chest pain develops. Pneumonia and hepatitis may be the primary manifestations. The most serious and often fatal complication of unrecognized and untreated Q fever is the development of endocarditis 1–20 years later. Most patients recover without treatment.

16. What is Colorado tick fever?
Following infection with this RNA virus, the incubation period averages 4 days (range 1–14 days). Onset is sudden with high fever, chills, headache, myalgia, fatigue, retro-orbital pain, and GI symptoms occurring. Meningeal or encephalitic symptoms are common in children. Rash is fleeting if present. The characteristic biphasic or "saddleback" fever lasts 2–3 days and abates for 1–2 days before returning. A marked leukopenia (1000–3000 range) develops, reaching its lowest point during the second fever spike. The diagnosis is made by identifying the virus in blood specimens. An erythrocyte viremia persists for 120 days, so blood donations should be avoided in this period. Recovery is complete after 3 weeks, with only supportive care required. Lifelong immunity develops. As the name implies, this illness is found in the Rocky Mountain states.

17. What is babesiosis?
Babesiosis is a rare protozoan parasite of red blood cells. The illness is characterized by a mild febrile illness with headache, fatigue, weakness, and anemia. The illness is most severe in the elderly, immunocompromised, or asplenic patients. Diagnosis is by identifying parasitized red blood cells on peripheral blood smears. It is endemic to Nantucket, Martha's Vineyard, Shelter Island, and parts of Long Island in the northeastern United States. The major concern is that the same tick that transmits this illness also transmits Lyme disease, and coinfection with both organisms, causing a more severe illness, has been documented.

18. What is tularemia?
Prior to 1950, most cases of tularemia were seen in hunters exposed to rabbits. Since then, most cases are secondary to tick transmission, with an average of 250–300 cases per year, most occurring in the Midwest. The ulceroglandular variety accounts for 85% of cases. About 48 hours after skin exposure, a firm erythematous papule develops. Ulceration develops within 2 days, whereas regional lymph nodes enlarge and form suppurating buboes. Constitutional symptoms of fever, myalgia, headache, and cough are present. Mortality from untreated ulceroglandular tularemia is 5–7%. The disseminated typhoidal variety develops in 10% of cases and is characterized by severe disabling fatigue, weight loss, and pulmonary involvement. The pneumonic variety is associated with nonproductive cough, diffuse patchy infiltrates on chest x-ray, and a mortality approaching 30%.

19. What is tick paralysis?
It is a rare toxin-mediated illness seen following prolonged attachment (4–7 days) and feeding of a female tick. The toxin is secreted in the saliva and affects central and peripheral nerves. Victims are usually children. Initially they are irritable, restless, and may complain of paresthesia of extremities but will have a normal neurosensory exam. Over the subsequent 24–48 hours, an ascending symmetric flaccid paralysis develops. Eventually respiratory paralysis, stupor, myocarditis, and death result. Recovery is usually rapid once the tick is removed.

20. What it the proper method for tick removal?
Extensive folklore and home remedies exist. Most are ineffective or dangerous to the victim and increase the risk of transmission of infectious agents to the person involved in the removal. The best method for removal is to use a gloved hand to grasp the tick as close to the head or mouth as possible with forceps and to pull upward with steady traction. If parts remain embedded, excision with a scalpel should be performed.

21. What are the best methods for prevention of tick-borne disease?
The best methods of prevention are appropriate awareness and use of precautions while enjoying the outdoors. Long-sleeved shirts should be worn and pants should be tucked into socks or boots. Light clothing allows identification of crawling ticks. Twice-daily "tick checks" aid early removal and prevention of transmission of illness. DEET repellents repel ticks but in toxic amounts may cause seizures in children. Permethrin that is made for clothing only kills ticks on contact but is not readily available.

22. Are prophylactic antibiotics indicated for tick bites?
The current recommendation generally is "no." Most tick illnesses require prolonged attachment for transmission of the infectious agent. In Lyme disease attachment of 24–48 hours may be necessary. Many tick-transmitted diseases are not responsive to antibiotics. In rickettsial infections, prophylaxis with doxycycline, which is a bacteriostatic agent, requires a host immune response to aid clearance of the infectious agent, making prophylaxis ineffective. The exception to this recommendation occurs in regions with high endemic rates of Lyme disease. A recent study shows that prophylactic treatment of documented tick bites in these regions may be cost effective, as 20–25% of patients do not develop the classic ECM rash.

23. What is the treatment for each tick-borne illness?

Treatment of Tick-borne Illnesses

	DRUG	ADULT DOSAGE
SPIROCHETES		
Lyme Disease (*Borrelia burgdorferi*)		
Acute Phase		
Drug of choice:	Doxycycline[1]	100 mg PO BID 10–21 days
Alternate:	Amoxicillin	500 mg PO TID 10–21 days
	Erythromycin	250 mg PO QID 10–21 days
	Cefuroxime axetil	500 mg PO BID 10–21 days
Late Phase		
Drug of choice:	Ceftriaxone	2 gm IV qd 14–21 days
Alternate:	Penicillin G	20 million U IV 14–21 days
Relapsing Fever (Borrelia)		
Drug of choice:	Doxycycline[1]	100 mg PO BID 10–14 days
Alternate:	Amoxicillin	500 mg PO TID 10–14 days
	Erythromycin	250 mg PO QID 10–14 days
RICKETTSIAE		
Rocky Mountain Spotted Fever (*Rickettsia rickettsii*)		
Drug of choice:	Doxycycline[1]	100 mg PO BID 10–14 days
Alternate:	Chloramphenicol[2]	
	Fluoroquinolone[3]	
Ehrlichiosis (*Ehrlichia canis*)		
Drug of choice:	Doxycycline[1]	100 mg PO BID 10–14 days
Alternate:	Fluoroquinolone[3]	
Q Fever (*Coxiella burnetii*)		
Drug of choice:	Doxycycline[1]	100 mg PO BID 10–14 days
Alternate:	Chloramphenicol[2]	
	Fluoroquinolone[3]	
Endocarditis		
Drug of choice:	Doxycycline[1]	100 mg PO BID for 1 year
Plus:	Septra or Lincomycin or Rifampin	

Table continued on next page.

Treatment of Tick-borne Illnesses (Continued)

	DRUG	ADULT DOSAGE
PROTOZOA		
Babesiosis (*Babesia microti*)		
Drug of choice:	Clindamycin	1.2 gm IV BID or
		600 mg PO TID for 7 days
Plus:	Quinine	650 mg PO TID for 7 days
BACTERIA		
Tularemia (*Francisella tularensis*)		
Drug of choice:	Streptomycin	30–40 mg/kg/day IM divided
		BID for 3 days, then half this
		dose PO for 4–7 days
Alternate:	Gentamicin	1–1.5 mg/kg/dose IM for 5 days
	Doxycycline[4]	
	Chloramphenicol[4]	
TOXIN		
Tick paralysis		
Drug of choice:	None	
VIRUS		
Colorado tick fever		
Drug of choice:	None	

[1] Tetracyclines are generally not recommended for pregnant women or children less than 8 years.

[2] This is the drug of choice in pregnant females and children less than the age of 8 years. The penicillins, cephalosporins, aminoglycosides, sulfonamides, and erythromycins are not effective against rickettsial infections.

[3] Ciprofloxacin or ofloxacin. Neither of these agents is recommended for children.

[4] Doxycycline and chloramphenicol will control the acute phase but their bacteriostatic nature prevents eradication, and therefore relapses may occur.

BIBLIOGRAPHY

1. Centers for Disease Control: Babesiosis—Connecticut. MMWR 38:649–650, 1989.
2. Centers for Disease Control: Outbreak of relapsing fever—Grand Canyon National Park, Arizona, 1990. MMWR 40:296–297, 1991.
3. Doan-Wiggins L: Tick-borne diseases. Emerg Med Clin North Am 9:303–325, 1991.
4. Goodpasture HC, Poland JD, Francy DB, et al: Colorado tick fever: Clinical, epidemiologic and laboratory aspects of 228 cases in Colorado in 1973–1974. Ann Intern Med 88:303–310, 1978.
5. Kamper CA, Chessman KH, Phelps SJ: Therapy reviews: Rocky Mountain spotted fever. Clin Pharmacol 7:109–116, 1988.
6. Magid D, et al: Prevention of Lyme disease after tick bites: A cost effectiveness analysis. N Engl J Med 327:534, 1992.
7. McDade JE: Ehrlichiosis: A disease of animals and humans. J Infect Dis 161:609–617, 1990.
8. Needham GR: Evaluation of five popular methods for tick removal. Pediatrics 75:997–1002, 1985.
9. Rahn DW, Malawista SE: Lyme disease: Recommendations for diagnosis and treatment. Ann Intern Med 114:472–481, 1991.
10. Sawyer LA, Fishbein DB, McDade JE: Q fever: Current concepts. Rev Infect Dis 9:935–946, 1987.
11. Wright SW, Trott AT: North American tick-borne diseases. Ann Emerg Med 17:964–972, 1988.

58. ARTHRITIS

Carl M. Ferraro, M.D., FACEP

1. What is arthritis?
Arthritis is any inflammatory process that involves a joint. It may involve a single joint (monoarticular) or many joints (polyarticular), and may be acute or chronic.

2. What are common signs and symptoms of acute arthritis?
Patients typically report pain, swelling, loss of motion, and redness about the involved joint. There may be tenderness to palpation, swelling or effusion, erythema, and painful, decreased range of motion on exam. Children may present because of a limp or not using an extremity.

3. What are the common causes of acute arthritis?
Common causes in order of importance and treatability are:

1. Infection
   Bacterial
   Granulomatous
   Viral
2. Crystal-induced
   Gout
   Pseudogout
3. Trauma
   Traumatic hemarthrosis
   Traumatic synovitis
4. Nontraumatic hemarthrosis
   Inherited coagulopathy
   Anticoagulant induced
   Spontaneous
5. Inflammatory
   Small joint ("rheumatoid arthritis") pattern
   Large joint or axial skeleton
      ("rheumatoid variant") pattern
6. Degenerative
   Primary degenerative joint disease
   Secondary degenerative joint disease

4. What are the most serious causes of arthritis?
Acute bacterial arthritis is by far the most serious cause of acute monoarticular arthritis. It carries a risk of permanent joint damage that may occur in as little as 7–10 days, causing chronic disability. There may be associated sepsis as well.

5. What other diseases should be considered when arthritis is suspected?
In addition to the various causes of arthritis listed above, diseases that may mimic arthritis include tendinitis, bursitis, cellulitis, and other soft-tissue infections.

6. How do you differentiate an intraarticular process from a periarticular process?
Diseases that involve the synovial cavity of a joint cause tenderness and swelling about the entire joint, whereas with diseases near joints, the tenderness and swelling are localized to a small area. Active and passive range of motion is painful in all directions in intraarticular processes, whereas in periarticular diseases there may be little pain with passive motion and only in limited planes.

7. What other physical findings may be helpful?
Besides examining the involved joint, looking elsewhere may be helpful in determining the etiology of the underlying process. Other findings may include evidence of sepsis (such as fever, rash, or genital lesions), gouty tophi, or other findings of metabolic or endocrine disorders.

215

8. Which diagnostic studies are useful?

X-rays of the affected joint should be obtained; however, the most common finding in acute monoarticular arthritis is a normal film except for presence of soft-tissue swelling.

Synovial fluid should be collected by arthrocentesis, inspected for its general appearance, and sent for Gram stain and culture. Cell counts may give additional information but absolute numbers are not diagnostic in any individual disease. The finding of crystals under polarized light suggests gout or pseudogout in the absence of evidence of infection.

Blood tests such as white cell counts, sedimentation rate, or uric acid are usually of little help in the acute setting.

9. When should arthrocentesis be performed?

Indications for arthrocentesis include obtaining synovial fluid for diagnosing nontraumatic joint diseases and for diagnosing ligamentous or bony injury when not readily evident, and for effecting pain relief by instillation of medications or relief of a tense effusion. Contraindications to arthrocentesis are overlying infections and prosthetic joints (left for the orthopedist), and care should be taken in the face of a bleeding diathesis.

10. How is acute bacterial arthritis treated?

Appropriate parenteral antibiotics should be administered based on specific Gram stain findings or empirically based on the history, physical, and statistical data. The most common organism causing monoarticular infectious arthritis in adults is gonococcus followed by staphylococcus and streptococcus. In children, Hemophilus has predominated, followed again by staphylococcus and streptococcus. When an organism is not identified on Gram stain, empirical therapy should be based on these findings.

In addition to use of antibiotics, the involved joint must be drained either by repeated needle aspirations, open arthrotomy, or continuous irrigation.

11. Who should be admitted?

All patients with confirmed or suspected acute bacterial arthritis should be admitted. In all other acute processes, the need for admission must be based on clinical grounds, such as intractable pain or inability to ambulate.

12. How do I interpret the results of the arthrocentesis?

Normal findings and those of various rheumatic disease states are shown in the following table:

Synovial Fluid Analysis

DIAGNOSIS	APPEARANCE	TOTAL WBC COUNT (Per Cubic mm)	PMN %	MUCIN CLOT TEST	FLUID/BLOOD GLUCOSE DIFF. (mm/dl)	MISCELLANEOUS (CRYSTALS/ ORGANISMS)
Normal	Clear, pale	0–200 (200)	<10%	Good	NS	—
Group I (noninflammatory; degenerative joint disease, traumatic arthritis)	Clear to slightly turbid	50–4000 (600)	<30%	Good	NS	—
Group II (noninfectious, mildly inflammatory: SLE, scleroderma)	Clear to slightly turbid	0–9000 (3000)	<20%	Good (occ. fair)	NS	Occ. LE cell, decreased complement

Table continued on next page.

Synovial Fluid Analysis (Continued)

DIAGNOSIS	APPEARANCE	TOTAL WBC COUNT (Per Cubic mm)	PMN %	MUCIN CLOT TEST	FLUID/BLOOD GLUCOSE DIFF. (mm/dl)	MISCELLANEOUS (CRYSTALS/ ORGANISMS)
Group III (noninfectious, severely inflammatory)						
Gout	Turbid	100–160,000 (21,000)	70%	Poor	10	Uric acid crystals
Pseudogout	Turbid	50–75,000 (14,000)	70%	Fair– poor	Insuff. data	Calcium pyro-phosphate
Rheumatoid arthritis	Turbid	250–80,000	70%	Poor	30	Decreased
Group IV (infectious, inflammatory)						
Acute bacterial	Very turbid	150–250,000 (80,000)	90%	Poor	90	Positive culture for bacteria
Tuberculosis	Turbid	2,500–100,000 (20,000)	60%	Poor	70	Positive culture for *M. tuberculosis*

From Wyngaarden JB, Smith LH (eds): Cecil Textbook of Medicine, 18th ed. Philadelphia, W.B. Saunders, 1988, p 1994, with permission.

BIBLIOGRAPHY

1. Freed JF, et al: Acute monoarticular arthritis: A diagnostic approach. JAMA 243:2314–2316, 1980.
2. Goldenberg DL, Reed JI: Bacterial arthritis. N Engl J Med 312:764–771, 1985.
3. McCarty DJ, Koopman WJ (eds): Arthritis and Allied Conditions: A Textbook of Rheumatology, 12th ed. Malvern, PA, Lea & Febiger, 1993.
4. Preslar AJ, Heckman JD: Emergency department evaluation of the swollen joint. Emerg Med Clin North Am 2:425–441, 1984.
5. Smith JW: Infectious arthritis. Infect Dis Clin North Am 4:523–538, 1990.

59. RASHES

Andrea Brault, M.D., and Kristi L. Koenig, M.D.

1. How should rashes be described in terms of characteristics and size?

Characteristic	Size (cm)		
Palpable lesion	papule (<0.5)	nodule (0.5–2)	tumor (>2)
Palpable fluid-filled lesion		vesicle (<0.5)	bullae (≥0.5)
Nonpalpable lesion with color change		macule (<1)	patch (≥1)

2. Differentiate between a plaque, a wheal, and a pustule.

A **plaque** is a flat, palpable lesion that is larger than 0.5 cm. A **wheal** is an area of localized skin edema. A **pustule** is a vesicle or bullae filled with purulent material.

3. Define the secondary skin changes that occur with rashes.

Atrophy	Thinning of skin
Crusting	Dried residue
Erosions	Loss of superficial epidermis
Excoriations	Scratch marks
Fissures	Linear cracks
Keloids	Hypertrophic scars
Lichenification	Thickening or roughening of skin
Scales	Thin flakes of exfoliated epidermis
Ulcers	Deeper loss of tissue

4. Describe the rash and other clinical manifestations of disseminated intravascular coagulation (DIC).

Patients with DIC have multiple petechiae and ecchymoses (purpura), and bleeding from nasogastric and endotracheal tubes and from venipuncture sites. Remember to identify and treat the underlying cause, as DIC is always a manifestation of a serious underlying illness.

5. What type of rash is seen in asplenic patients with pneumococcal infection?

The rash consists of widespread ecchymoses and purpura. Pustules may also develop. In patients who have functional asplenia or who have had a splenectomy, a pneumococcal infection can have a fulminant course, rapidly progressing to sepsis, shock, and DIC.

6. What type of rash occurs in life-threatening *Staphylococcus aureus* infections?

Toxic shock syndrome is associated with an erythematous or sunburn-like rash that appears within hours of the onset of infection. Typically the patient is a menstruating female who presents with hypotension, fever, vomiting, diarrhea, and mild changes in mental status.

The rash of **staphylococcal septicemia** may include petechiae on the digits and extremities and a range of larger skin lesions, including necrotic, necropurulent, hemorrhagic, and even gangrenous lesions. Consider staphylococcal septicemia when you see "purulent purpura," a small area of purpura with a white purulent center. The Gram stain of aspirated material reveals staphylococcus and polymorphonuclear leukocytes.

7. Which infections can present with rash after exposure to sea water?

Vibrio vulnificus should be suspected when a patient presents with diffuse bullous lesions of the lower extremities after exposure to sea water or ingestion of raw shellfish, especially oysters. Affected persons usually have underlying liver disease or are immunocompromised. Treatment consists of tetracycline, supportive care, and aggressive wound care, including surgical debridement and occasionally amputation.

Erysipeloid is caused by *Erysipelothrix rhusiopathiae* and presents as a painful cellulitis characterized by a violaceous hue that appears about a week after exposure. Penicillin is the treatment of choice.

8. What is the appearance of the rash of meningococcemia?

Classically, it presents as 1–2-mm discrete petechial lesions on the trunk and lower extremities that may coalesce to form larger purpuric lesions. Conjunctival and buccal mucosal lesions may also be seen. It is important to fully undress the patient, as the rash often occurs in areas under pressure, such as beneath elastic bands of underwear and stockings. The number of petechiae correlates with the degree of thrombocytopenia. The rash begins on the first day of illness. Treatment includes prompt administration of IV penicillin.

9. Who said, "He who knows syphilis, knows medicine"?
Sir William Osler.

10. What is the Jarisch-Herxheimer reaction?
The Jarisch-Herxheimer reaction is a dramatic systemic response that occurs between 2 and 8 hours after the initial treatment of syphilis with penicillin and occasionally other antibiotics. It consists of the abrupt onset of fever, chills, myalgias, headache, sore throat, tachycardia, hyperventilation, vasodilation with flushing, mild hypotension, and inflammatory reaction at sites of localized spirochetal infection. It is usually self-limited and resolves within 12–24 hours. Aspirin may be used for symptomatic treatment. Be sure to warn your patients prior to treatment!

11. What diagnosis should be considered in a sexually active young person who presents with a painful joint or joints and a pustule on an erythematous base?
Be careful! The patient may have disseminated gonorrhea (GC), a serious infection. Take a thorough sexual history and obtain vaginal, urethral, throat, and rectal cultures. The lesion associated with disseminated GC begins as a papule and progresses to pustules, followed by vesicles. Characteristic lesions have an erythematous halo with grayish borders and a central white pustule. A single lesion can be diagnostic. Treatment includes penicillin or a third-generation cephalosporin for 7 days. Admission is suggested if the patient appears toxic, or there is involvement of weightbearing joints.

12. Describe a herpes zoster rash.
Herpes zoster, a painful infection caused by varicella zoster, occurs in a dermatomal distribution corresponding to a sensory ganglion. The rash has an erythematous base, with papules progressing to vesicles or bullae and then pustules over a period of 4 days. Crusts develop on the seventh to tenth day. New lesions may continue to occur for up to 1 week, and nerve involvement may occur even without the rash (zoster sine zoster). The patient often presents with pain before the rash has erupted.

13. What is the significance of a herpes zoster facial rash that extends to the tip of the nose?
When the rash extends to the tip of the nose, you must assume there is involvement of the ophthalmic branch of the facial nerve (VII 3). The eyes must be examined with fluorescein staining and a slit lamp for the dendritic lesions of corneal herpes zoster. Ophthalmologic consultation should be obtained.

14. Which rashes are associated with acquired immunodeficiency syndrome (AIDS)?
AIDS should be considered when a common rash presents with increased severity, abnormal treatment response, or abnormal location. Common examples include Kaposi's sarcoma, fulminant seborrheic dermatosis or psoriasis, chronic herpes simplex, and severe candidiasis. Kaposi's sarcoma is a purplish-red tumor that may occur anywhere on the body. Seborrheic dermatosis is described as yellow-red papules and macules that are often greasy with white, dry, scaling crusts. Psoriasis appears as papules and plaques with silver-white scaling and sharp marginations. Candidiasis is seen as a white lesion, typically on the tongue and buccal mucosa, that is easily scraped away, revealing an erythematous base.

15. What disease is associated with a herald patch?
Pityriasis rosea (PR) is a maculopapular, red, scaling eruption that usually occurs on the trunk, most commonly in patients 10–35 years old. The infectious agent is most likely a

virus. In 80% of patients, a solitary patch occurs 1–2 weeks prior to PR, hence the term "herald patch." No treatment is necessary.

16. What other test should you order to complete the differential in a patient with the rash of PR?
A VDRL or rapid plasma reagin (RPR) test should be ordered to rule out syphilis, which can have a similar appearance.

17. What rash might erupt in patients with acute rheumatic fever, glomerulonephritis, or drug reactions?
Erythema marginatum. These lesions begin as small pink or faint red macules that may be slightly raised. They expand and develop clear centers with distinct pink margins that can be serpiginous or circular. The lesions are nonpruritic and nonindurated, and blanch with pressure.

18. What is erysipelas?
A rash that generally occurs on the face and legs, erysipelas is usually caused by group A Streptococcus. It may be associated with an upper respiratory infection. The very young and the very old are the most susceptible. The rash is characterized by a rapidly expanding patch of sharply-defined erythema with a palpable edge that advances radially. When present on the face, this rash has a typical butterfly appearance. A central erythematous zone may form and subsequently rupture, leaving raw weeping areas. Treatment includes penicillin or first-generation cephalosporins.

19. What are the characteristics of the common pediatric infectious rashes?
   Erythema infectiosum—"slapped cheek" appearance and lacy reticular exanthem
   Hand-foot-mouth disease—discrete ulcerative oral lesions and maculopapular and vesicular lesions of the skin, especially on the hands and feet; caused by coxsackievirus
   Measles—maculopapular eruption starting on the upper trunk and spreading downward, later becoming confluent
   Roseola infantum—discrete macules or papules
   Staphylococcal scalded skin syndrome—tender erythematous rash that progresses to bullae, then exfoliation
   Varicella—begins as maculopapular rash that becomes vesicular, progressing to crusts in the final phase

BIBLIOGRAPHY

 1. Bates B: A Guide to Physical Examination, 3rd ed. Philadelphia, J.B. Lippincott, 1983.
 2. Emond RTD, Rowland HAK: A Colour Atlas of Infectious Diseases, 2nd ed. England, Wolfe, 1987.
 3. Fitzpatrick TB, Polano MK, Suurmond D: Color Atlas and Synopsis of Clinical Dermatology, 8th ed. New York, McGraw-Hill, 1989.
 4. Harwood-Nuss A, Linden C, Luten RC: The Clinical Practice of Emergency Medicine. Philadelphia, J.B. Lippincott, 1991.
 5. Homer C, Shulman ST: Clinical aspects of acute rheumatic fever. J Rheumatol 18:2–13, 1989.
 6. Kerle KK, Mascola JR, Miller TA: Disseminated gonococcal infection. Am Fam Physician 45:209–214, 1992.
 7. Kirchner JT: Syphilis—an STD on the Increase. Am Fam Physician 44:843–845, 1991.
 8. Koenig KL, Mueller J, Rose T: *Vibrio vulnificus*—hazard on the half shell. West J Med 155:400–403, 1991.
 9. Mandell GL, Douglas RG Jr, Bennet JE (eds): Principles and Practice of Infectious Disease. New York, Churchill Livingstone, 3rd ed., 1990.
10. Parish LC, Sehgal VN, Buntin DM: Color Atlas of Sexually Transmitted Diseases. New York, Igaku-Shoin, 1991.

XII. Environmental Emergencies

60. ELECTRICAL INJURIES AND LIGHTNING

Mark Copeland, M.D.

ELECTRICAL INJURIES

1. Who is predisposed to electrical injuries?
There is a high incidence in children under 6 years of age. Most injuries occur as a result of oral contact with electric cords, wall sockets, or extension cord outlets. Older children and adolescents are also at risk because of their risk-taking behavior, such as climbing trees or utility poles, trespassing through transformer substations, etc. The incidence then decreases throughout the teenage years and then resurges as adults enter the workforce. Serious high-voltage electrical injuries are most common in the workplace among electrical, construction, and industrial workers.

2. What factors determine the nature and severity of electrical injury?
Voltage, amperage, resistance, type of current (alternating vs. direct), surface contact, current pathway, duration of contact, and associated trauma such as falls.

3. How are voltage, amperage, and resistance related?
These three variables of electricity are related to one another according to Ohm's law:
$$I = V/R \text{ (current = voltage} \div \text{resistance).}$$

4. How are electrical injuries classified?
Electrical injuries are often classified as high voltage (>1000 volts) or low voltage (<1000 volts). High-voltage injuries are generally more serious than low-voltage injuries; however, the other factors previously mentioned can profoundly affect degree of injury.

5. What is the order of resistance of body tissues?
The following tissues are arranged in increasing order of resistance: nerves, blood vessels, mucous membranes, muscle, skin, tendon, fat, and bone. Skin resistance can be highly variable depending on its thickness, vascularity, and degree of moisture. Thick, dry skin of calloused feet and hands has the highest resistance, whereas the wet, thin skin of the lips and tongue have the lowest. Sweating and immersion in water decrease the skin's resistance.

6. How do surface contact, current pathway, and duration of contact affect the seriousness of electrical injuries?
As the cross-sectional diameter of the tissue through which a given current passes increases, less heat is generated and less damage occurs. The pathway that a current takes determines the tissues at risk. For example, current that takes a hand-to-hand pathway is more dangerous than current that takes a hand-to-foot or foot-to-foot pathway because of the potential for passage through the heart. The longer the contact with current flow, obviously the greater the injury.

7. Why is alternating current (AC) more dangerous than direct current (DC)?

AC is capable of producing ventricular fibrillation at a very low voltage (50–100 mA) because it is a repetitive fibrillatory stimulus. Furthermore, AC causes tetanic muscle contractions and may result in the victim being unable to voluntarily release the current source since the "let go" threshold is only 6–9 mA. DC tends to cause a single muscle spasm, often throwing the victim from the source, resulting in a shorter duration of exposure but increasing the likelihood of blunt injury. At the same voltage, AC tends to be three times more dangerous than DC.

8. What are the mechanisms of electrical injury?

The mechanisms are direct contact, arc, flash, thermal, and traumatic. In true electrical injuries (direct contact), the victim becomes part of the circuit. The injury reflects the passage of current through the body and is usually demarcated by entrance and exit wounds. The most destructive indirect injury occurs when a victim becomes part of an electrical arc. An electrical arc is a current spark formed between two objects of different potential that are not in contact with each other. Because the temperature of an electrical arc is extremely high (2500°C), it can cause deep thermal burns. Electrical flash burns result when current strikes the skin but does not enter the body. Secondary thermal injury may occur when a victim's clothing ignites. Traumatic injuries may occur from the violent tetanic muscle contractions associated with AC sources or being thrown from a DC source by intense single contraction of muscles.

9. Which organ systems can be damaged by electrical injury?

Electrical Injuries by Organ System

SYSTEM	INJURY
Skin	Thermal burns such as entrance and exit wounds, flexor crease burns, mouth commissure burns (risk of delayed bleeding from labial artery when the eschar separates)
Cardiac	Cardiac arrest from asystole (DC) or ventricular fibrillation (AC), other arrhythmias, nonspecific ST-T changes (common), acute MI (rare)
Vascular	Hemorrhage, arterial and venous thrombosis, ischemia
Nervous	Loss of consciousness, amnesia, confusion, disorientation, concentration and memory problems, suppression of respiratory center, seizures, paralysis, paresthesias
Musculoskeletal	Muscular pain, muscle necrosis (rhabdomyolysis), compartment syndrome, dislocations, fractures
Respiratory	Inhibition of the brainstem respiratory centers
GI	Hollow visceral and solid visceral injury (both rare), stress ulcers
Renal	Myoglobinuria, acute tubular necrosis, renal failure
Ophthalmologic	Cataracts

10. What are the most frequent causes of immediate death from electrical injuries?

Cardiac arrhythmias and respiratory arrest.

11. Which ancillary studies are helpful in the evaluation of an electrical injury?

The extent of evaluation depends on the extent of injury. All patients with evidence of conductive injury or significant surface burns should have the following tests: complete blood count, electrolytes, blood urea nitrogen, creatinine level, urinalysis, CPK and isoenzymes, and EKG. Radiographs and CT scans should be ordered when clinically appropriate.

12. What are the priorities in the prehospital treatment of electrical injuries?
The safety of the rescuers is the first priority. The source of the electricity should be turned off, if possible. The second option is to try to remove the victim from the source using well-insulated tools. Once the scene is secure, the rules of basic life support (BLS), advanced cardiac life support (ACLS), and advanced trauma life support (ATLS) should be followed, with special attention to the airway, breathing, and circulation. Cardiac monitoring is essential, as is the establishment of large-bore intravenous lines with aggressive fluid replacement. Injury to the spine should be presumed until appropriately excluded, and protective measures (cervical collar and backboard) initiated. Fractures should be splinted and burns dressed.

13. What is unique about the initial management of electrical injuries in the emergency department (ED)?
The use of traditional burn formulas is not applicable in electrical injuries, because the calculations are based solely on the affected body surface area. Surface damage in electrical injuries does not necessarily reflect the degree of deeper tissue damage. The fluid rate should be titrated to ensure a urine output of 50–100 cc/hr (1–1.5 cc/kg/hr). The objective of early aggressive fluid management is to prevent renal failure secondary to myoglobinuria. Alkalinization of the urine will further prevent the precipitation of myoglobin in the renal tubules. Intravenous mannitol and diuretics may be useful.

14. What should be the disposition of victims of electrical injury?
Purely thermal burns should be handled as such and disposition made accordingly. Asymptomatic patients with low-voltage injuries in the absence of significant burns, EKG changes, or myoglobinuria can be discharged home with appropriate follow-up. Indications for admission include all patients exposed to high-voltage conductive injury, documented loss of consciousness, cardiac arrest, EKG changes, arrhythmias, history of or significant risk factors for cardiac disease, chest pain, hypoxia, myoglobinuria, mouth commissure burns, or concomitant injury severe enough to warrant admission. For all serious injuries, consultation and transfer to a burn center should be considered.

15. What are the common pitfalls in the evaluation and management of electrical injuries?
Injuries to rescuers due to not securing the scene, neglecting the ABCs and spine immobilization, underestimating the severity (depth) of the burn, not providing adequate fluid resuscitation, and not considering potential blunt trauma injuries are the more common pitfalls.

LIGHTNING

16. What is the incidence of injury and death from lightning?
Currently it is estimated that lightning causes 150–250 deaths per year in the United States, with 4 to 5 times more injuries. Although exact numbers are unavailable, lightning is responsible for more deaths each year than any other natural phenomenon.

17. When and where are you most likely to be struck by lightning?
In the northern hemisphere, the incidence of lightning parallels the occurrence of thunderstorms during the months of May through September, with the majority occurring in the afternoon and early evening. Geographically, areas with frequent lightning strikes include the Atlantic coast, the South and Southeast, major mountain regions, and along the valleys of major river tidal basins.

18. Who is at increased risk for lightning injuries?
The most common victims of lightning are campers, sportsmen, joggers, farmers, sailors, rangers, and construction workers.

19. How often does lightning cause death or permanent morbidity?
Although only 20–30% of lightning victims die, more than 70% of the survivors will have permanent sequelae.

20. How often do lightning deaths occur in multiples?
Lightning strikes frequently involve more than one victim, with 15% of lightning deaths occurring in multiples of 2 and another 15% in multiples of 3 or more.

21. Describe the five major mechanisms of lightning injury.
   1. **Direct strike.** This occurs when the major pathway of current runs directly through the victim, resulting in the highest morbidity and mortality.
   2. **Contact.** Injury from contact occurs when lightning strikes an object or structure that is touching the victim.
   3. **Side flash or "splash."** This occurs when lightning splashes or jumps from an object through the air to the victim.
   4. **Ground current or step voltage.** This occurs as a result of lightning spreading radially through the ground and current entering the person because of potential difference in resistance between his or her feet (due to one foot being closer to the strike point than the other).
   5. **Blunt trauma or other associated trauma.** Blunt trauma may occur from the victim being thrown or by the explosive/implosive force of the lightning pathway. Other associated trauma may occur secondary to debris, or burns may occur secondary to jewelry or clothing fasteners heating up or from the ignition of clothing.

22. What makes lightning injuries different from other high-voltage injuries? Why does this matter clinically?
With lightning strikes, the average voltage may be 10–20 million volts but may be as high as 2 billion volts. However, because the duration of current flow with lightning strikes is so short (1/10,000 to 1/1,000 second), the actual amount of energy delivered is often much less than in a high-voltage injury. Lightning is considered a direct current, whereas most high-voltage injuries are caused by alternating current. The pathway is also different. As with metal conductors, the vast majority of current travels around the outside of the conductor, flashing over the outside of the victim. Although a small amount of current may leak internally and cause asystole, respiratory arrest, nervous system dysfunction, and spasm of muscles and arteries, lightning seldom causes significant burns, tissue destruction, or myoglobinuria.

23. Which organ systems can be damaged by lightning?

Lightning Injuries by Organ System

SYSTEM	INJURY
Cardiac	Asystole, arrhythmias, nonspecific ST-T changes, acute MI (rare)
Respiratory	Inhibition of the brainstem respiratory centers
Nervous	Loss of consciousness, confusion, disorientation, amnesia, autonomic dysfunction (with loss of pupillary function), coagulation of brain substance, epidural and subdural hematomas, intraventricular hemorrhage, skull fractures, seizures, transient or permanent paralysis
Skin	Feathering, linear burns, punctate burns, true thermal burns
Musculoskeletal	Muscle necrosis (rare), dislocations, fractures
Renal	Myoglobinuria (rare)
GI	Gastric atony, ileus, perforations (uncommon)
Ophthalmologic	Mydriasis, loss of light reflex, anisocoria, Horner's syndrome, cataracts
Otologic	Tinnitus, hearing loss, ruptured tympanic membranes

24. What is unique about the prehospital care of victims of lightning injury?
Unlike other mass casualty situations, efforts should be directed toward those who appear "dead" because those who show signs of life will in all probability recover. In the absence of cardiopulmonary arrest, victims are highly unlikely to die. Because the major cause of death is cardiopulmonary arrest, aggressive CPR should be attempted in all victims of lightning strike. Another unique feature is that aggressive volume resuscitation is not normally warranted, as it is for victims of electrical injuries, because muscle necrosis is rare.

25. What should be the disposition of lightning victims?
All patients with cardiac or neurologic abnormalities require admission. Those with associated trauma, burns, or rhabdomyolysis may require admission. All others may be discharged.

26. What is a common pitfall in the management of lightning injuries?
Failure to recognize that lightning injuries are not the same as high-voltage electrical injuries is one of the most common pitfalls.

27. Should an EKG be performed on all victims of electrical injury or lightning?
An EKG should be obtained for any patient who has been struck by lightning, who has sustained a full-thickness burn, or who has had direct contact with an electrical source. It is not indicated in a patient who has sustained flash, partial-thickness surface burns.

BIBLIOGRAPHY

1. Andrews CJ, et al (eds): Lightning Injuries: Electrical, Medical, and Legal Aspects. Boca Raton, CRC Press, 1992.
2. Brown BJ, Gaasch WR: Electrical injuries and lightning. Emerg Med Clin North Am 10:2, 1992.
3. Chabot DR, Gross PL: Lightning injuries. In Harwood-Nuss A, et al (eds): The Clinical Practice of Emergency Medicine. Philadelphia, J.B. Lippincott, 1991.
4. Cooper MA: Lightning injuries. In Auerbach PS, Geehr EC (eds): Management of Wilderness and Environmental Emergencies, 2nd ed. New York, McMillan, 1989.
5. Cooper MA: Lightning injuries. In Rosen P, et al (eds): Emergency Medicine: Concepts and Clinical Practice, 3rd ed. St. Louis, Mosby–Year Book, 1992.
6. Cooper MA, Johnson K: Electrical injuries. In Rosen P, et al (eds): Emergency Medicine: Concepts and Clinical Practice, 3rd ed. St. Louis, Mosby–Year Book, 1992.
7. Cwinn AA, Cantrill SA: Lightning injuries. J Emerg Med 2:379, 1985.
8. Kobernick M: Electrical injuries: Pathophysiology and emergency management. Ann Emerg Med 11:633, 1982.
9. Peters WJ: Lightning injuries. Can Med Assoc J 128:148, 1983.
10. Sosnow PL: Electrical injuries. In Harwood-Nuss A, et al (eds): The Clinical Practice of Emergency Medicine. Philadelphia, J.B. Lippincott, 1991.
11. Strasser EJ, et al: Lightning injuries. J Trauma 17:315, 1977.

61. NEAR DROWNING

Robert J. Doherty, M.D.

1. What is near drowning?
One can become easily confused by the varying terms associated with submersion accidents. **Drowning** is death by suffocation from submersion in liquid. **Near drowning** is survival for at least 24 hours following a submersion event. The **postimmersion syndrome**

is a course of progressive deterioration following initial survival from an immersion event. **Wet drowning** indicates that aspiration of water occurred during the event. **Dry drowning** indicates that asphyxia was caused by laryngospasm without aspiration.

2. How many people drown?

Each year in the United States over 8000 persons die from drowning. It is the third leading cause of accidental death in all ages. Drowning is the second leading cause of accidental death in children, exceeded only by motor vehicle fatalities. Approximately 50,000 persons annually are near-drowning victims who survive an immersion event.

3. Who drowns and why?

The incidence of drowning peaks in two groups—teenagers and toddlers. In teenagers, nearly 80% of drowning and near-drowning victims are male. Teenage males are victims because of risk-taking behavior during swimming, boating, diving, or other water-related activities. Alcohol is a contributing factor in over 60% of all teenage drownings.

Forty percent of all drowning victims are less than 4 years of age. Toddlers are at risk because of their inherently inquisitive nature and their physical inability to extricate themselves from hazards such as pools, buckets, tubs, toilets, or washers. Inadequate supervision, even for brief moments, is the primary cause of drowning in toddlers. One must always consider the possibility of abuse when evaluating a child drowning victim.

Other risk factors in all ages include seizure disorders, mental retardation, and lack of swimming skills. The increasing prevalence of swimming pools, hot tubs, pleasure craft, and outdoor sports over the last decade have all greatly increased the number of persons at risk of drowning.

4. What kills a drowning victim?

Historically, emphasis has been incorrectly placed on the significance of drowning in salt water versus fresh water due to presumed differences in the pathophysiology of the aspirated water. In fresh-water aspirations, the hypotonic fluid was thought to diffuse into the circulation, thus increasing blood volume and decreasing the concentrations of serum electrolytes. This also causes a loss of surfactant and results in alveolar collapse. Sea water was thought to pull fluid into the alveoli, decreasing the blood volume and increasing the electrolyte concentrations. This transudated fluid has the pathologic effect of pulmonary edema. In both cases there is intrapulmonary shunting, thus increasing the hypoxemia.,

Ten to twenty percent of drowning victims, however, have no aspirated water and most victims of drowning do not aspirate enough fluid to cause a significant alteration in blood volume, electrolytes, or a life-threatening pulmonary shunt due to perfusion of fluid filled alveoli. Death, therefore, is most often the result of asphyxia caused by laryngospasm and glottis closure. The aspirated water, however, is a significant pulmonary irritant and contaminant that may increase pulmonary problems in the recovery phase of a near-drowning victim.

5. What happens in a drowning?

The first event in all drownings is an unexpected or prolonged immersion. The victim begins to struggle and panic. Fatigue begins and air hunger develops. Reflex inspiration ultimately overrides breathholding. The victim swallows water and aspiration occurs causing laryngospasm that may last for several minutes. Hypoxemia worsens and unconsciousness ensues. If the victim is not promptly rescued and resuscitated, central nervous system damage begins within minutes.

6. What are the presenting symptoms?

The presenting pulmonary symptoms are varied. One may be completely asymptomatic, have a mild cough, show mild dyspnea and tachypnea, or be in fulminant pulmonary edema.

7. What is the pulmonary pathophysiology?

The central clinical feature of *all* drowning or near-drowning victims is hypoxemia caused by laryngospasm and asphyxia. The PO_2 decreases, the PCO_2 increases, and there is a combined respiratory and metabolic acidosis. If the patient is successfully resuscitated, the recovery phase is often complicated by aspirated water or vomitus. Aspiration can cause airway obstruction by particulates, bronchospasm by direct irritation, pulmonary edema from parenchymal damage, atelectasis from loss of surfactant, and pulmonary bacterial infections. Some patients may later develop pulmonary abscesses or empyema.

8. How is the cardiac system affected in drowning?

Cardiac decompensation and arrhythmias are caused by the hypoxemia and complicated by the ensuing acidosis. The heart, however, is relatively resistant to hypoxic injury and successful resumption of cardiac activity is common, but severe CNS damage often occurs. Response of the heart to therapy, particularly antiarrhythmic medications, may be limited by hypoxia, acidosis, and hypothermia. Primary therapy is aimed at reversal of those three problems.

9. What is the prehospital treatment?

The most important part of treatment of a near-drowning victim is in the prehospital phase. If a drowning victim has appropriate airway management and ventilation is rapidly established, anoxic brain injury is avoided, and prompt and full recovery is anticipated. The patient without rapid airway management and ventilation suffers irreversible anoxic brain injury and either will be unresponsive to resuscitation or have a progressively deteriorating course following initial resuscitation. Therapy must correct hypoxia, associated acidosis, and hypotension as rapidly as possible. Establish a patent airway using appropriate C-spine precautions if indicated. Apply a nonrebreather oxygen mask to patients with spontaneous respirations. Initiate bag-valve mask breathing or endotracheal intubation if indicated. Correct hypoxia and acidosis by hyperventilation with 100% oxygen. Intravenous access is needed.

10. When is endotracheal intubation indicated?

Any person with altered mentation or an inability to protect the airway needs intubation. Presence of significant aspiration or secretions usually indicate such a need. In the initially stable patient, increased PCO_2 or low PO_2 with oxygen therapy indicates that extensive pulmonary compromise may exist, and early airway management with positive pressure ventilation and positive end-expiratory pressure is appropriate.

One important point is to determine if the near-drowning event may have occurred as a result of diving into water. This patient may have suffered a cervical spine injury, and appropriate precautions should be taken to immobilize the neck prior to intubation.

11. If aspiration is suspected, what treatment is needed?

Pulmonary treatment is supportive. Close observation for signs of a developing pulmonary infection is needed. Some cases with significant aspirations may require bronchoscopy to remove particulate matter and tenacious secretions. Bronchodilator therapy with beta agonists is appropriate if bronchospasm is evident.

12. What is secondary drowning?

Secondary drowning is death due to aspiration of contaminated water with resulting pneumonitis and secondary bacterial pneumonia.

13. Is there a role for prophylactic antibiotics or glucocorticoids?

Prophylactic antibiotics and glucocorticoids are of no proven benefit. Positive sputum or blood cultures should be treated when clinically indicated.

14. Is there an indication for the use of NaHCO$_3$ during resuscitation?
No. Respiratory and metabolic acidosis should be treated by mechanical ventilation and hyperventilation.

15. What is the approach to patients with a decreased level of consciousness or coma?
Hypoxic injury leads to cerebral edema and a concomitant rise in intracranial pressure. **Cerebral resuscitation** is directed toward reducing intracranial pressure and ensuring efficient oxygen delivery. Emergency treatment of patients who appear to have suffered a severe CNS event includes controlled hyperventilation via endotracheal tube and mechanical ventilation, sedation and paralysis to reduce agitation, treatment of seizures if they occur, osmotic diuretics, and cautious fluid management. Early neurologic and neurosurgical consultation are needed. Intracranial pressure monitoring is useful. The physician must be very attentive to the possibility of cranial or spinal injuries in all boating or diving injuries. Do not forget the possibility of suicide or child abuse. If the history is in doubt, assume both a cranial and cervical injury. The possibility of toxicologic conditions should also be investigated.

16. Are glucocorticoids, barbiturate coma, or induced hypothermia indicated?
No, high-dose glucocorticoids, barbiturate coma, and induced hypothermia are unproven and remain controversial.

17. What is unique about cold-water drowning?
Cases in which victims of prolonged immersion in cold water have been successfully resuscitated without apparent neurologic sequelae are occasionally reported. The number, however, remains small. Sudden submersion in cold water theoretically induces the mammalian diving reflex in which blood is shunted from the periphery to the central core. Furthermore, the induced hypothermia causes a decrease in metabolic demand, thus reducing potential hypoxic injury in prolonged asphyxia. Cold water does have potentially deleterious effects. Most significant is the induced cardiac irritability from hypothermia. Resuscitation of hypothermic near-drowning victims should be continued until patients are adequately rewarmed (see chapter on Hypothermia).

18. What is the disposition of a near-drowning victim?
All drowning victims deserve aggressive in-hospital resuscitation until all reasonable efforts prove futile and the patient is near normothermic. All near drowning victims require close evaluation. A patient with any respiratory complaints or symptoms, chest radiograph abnormalities, or a demonstrated oxygen requirement should be closely monitored in a hospital for at least 24 hours. Similarly, any patient who received resuscitative efforts or had a reported loss of consciousness, cyanosis, apnea, or submersion greater than 1–2 minutes should be closely monitored. Patients without any symptoms and completely normal evaluation may be discharged with instructions to return immediately if respiratory distress ensues.

19. What are the most important factors in estimating a prognosis?
Grave prognostic indicators include cardiac or respiratory arrest or coma. Favorable prognostic indicators include no CPR required, no initial pulmonary complaints or coughing, and near drowning in clean (uncontaminated), cold water.

BIBLIOGRAPHY

1. Bierens JJ, et al: Submersion in the Netherlands: Prognostic indicators and results of resuscitation. Ann Emerg Med 19:1390–1395, 1990.

2. Flood TJ, et al: Childhood drownings and near drownings associated with swimming pools—Maricopa County, Arizona, 1988 and 1989. MMWR 39:441–442, 1990.
3. Haynes BE: Near drowning. In Tintinalli JE, et al (eds): Emergency Medicine: A Comprehensive Study Guide, 3rd ed. New York, McGraw-Hill, 1992, pp 688–690.
4. Knopp RK: Near-drowning. In Rosen P (ed): Emergency Medicine: Concepts and Clinical Practice, 2nd ed. St. Louis, Mosby–Year Book, 1992, pp 1013–1019.
5. Modell JH: Drowning. N Engl J Med 328:253–256, 1993.
6. Orlowski JP: The hemodynamic and cardiovascular effects of near-drowning in hypotonic, isotonic, and hypertonic solutions. Ann Emerg Med 18:1044–1049, 1989.
7. Wagner MH: Near-drowning accidents among children. Maryland Med J 39:847–850, 1990.
8. Wintemute GJ: Childhood drowning and near-drowning in the United States. Am J Dis Child 144:663–669, 1990.

62. HYPOTHERMIA AND FROSTBITE

Daniel F. Danzl, M.D.

1. What is accidental hypothermia?

Accidental hypothermia occurs when the body's "core" temperature unintentionally drops below 35°C (95°F). The preoptic anterior hypothalamus normally maintains a diurnal temperature variation within 1°C; significant pathophysiology develops below 35°C.

2. What factors are important in the epidemiology of hypothermia?

Primary accidental hypothermia results from direct exposure to the cold. Secondary hypothermia is a natural complication of many systemic disorders, including sepsis, cancer, and trauma. As a result, the mortality is much higher. Outdoor exposure is not the only threat to thermostability. Many victims are found indoors, in particular, the elderly.

3. How is body temperature normally regulated?

The normal physiology of temperature regulation is activated by cold exposure, producing reflex vasoconstriction and stimulating the hypothalamic nuclei. Heat preservation mechanisms include shivering, autonomic and endocrinologic responses, and adaptive behavioral responses.

4. What are the usual mechanisms of heat loss that predispose to hypothermia?

Radiation usually accounts for 55–65% of heat loss. Conduction and convection contribute another 15%. Moisture accelerates such heat loss; for example, conductive losses increase 25 times in cold water. The usual baseline 20–30% heat loss from respiration and evaporation is affected by the relative humidity and the ambient temperature.

5. Describe the common findings in mild, moderate, and severe hypothermia.

Mild hypothermia (32.2°–35°C) (90°–95°F) depresses the central nervous system (CNS) and increases the metabolic rate, pulse, and amount of shivering thermogenesis. Dysarthria, amnesia, ataxia, and apathy are common findings.

Moderate hypothermia (27°–32.2°C) (80°–90°F) progressively depresses the level of consciousness (LOC) and the vital signs. Shivering is extinguished as arrhythmias commonly develop. The Q-T interval prolongs, and a J wave (Osborn wave) may appear at the junction of the QRS complex and ST segment. Patients become poikilothermic and thus cannot rewarm spontaneously. A cold diuresis results from an initial central hypervolemia, which is caused by the peripheral vasoconstriction.

Severely hypothermic patients below 27°C (80°F) are comatose and areflexic, with profoundly depressed vital signs. Carbon dioxide production drops 50% for each 8°C fall in temperature, and thus there is little respiratory stimulation.

6. Which three categories do the factors predisposing to hypothermia fit into?

Factors predisposing to hypothermia either decrease heat production, increase heat loss, or impair thermoregulation.

7. What decreases heat production?

Decreased heat production is common (a) at the age extremes, (b) with inadequate stored fuel, or (c) with endocrinologic or neuromuscular inefficiency. Neonates are poorly adapted for cold, even without being subjected to emergent deliveries and resuscitations. The elderly have progressively impaired thermal perception. Anything from simple hypoglycemia to more severe malnutrition represents a threat to the core temperature. Examples of endocrinologic failure are myxedema, hypopituitarism, and hypoadrenalism.

8. What are the common causes of increased heat loss?

Increased heat loss results mainly from exposure or dermatologic problems that interfere with the skin's integrity. Poor preparation for and acclimatization to the environment can also be contributing factors.

9. How is thermoregulation impaired?

Thermoregulation can be impaired in four major ways: centrally, peripherally, metabolically, or pharmacologically. A variety of CNS processes affect hypothalamic function. Traumatic or neoplastic lesions, degenerative processes, and congenital anomalies induce hypothermia. Acute spinal cord transection extinguishes peripheral vasoconstriction, which prevents heat conservation. The abnormal plasma osmolality common with metabolic derangements, including diabetic ketoacidosis (DKA) and uremia, is an additional cause of hypothermia. Last, there are innumerable medications and toxins that can impair central thermoregulation when present in either therapeutic or toxic doses.

10. When should hypothermia be suspected?

The diagnosis is simple when a history of exposure is obvious. However, the history may not be available or helpful, and subtle presentations are far more common in urban areas. For example, ataxia and dysarthria may mimic a cerebrovascular accident or intoxication. The only safe way to avoid missing the diagnosis is to routinely measure the patient's temperature.

11. Are there decoys that confuse the physical examination?

If there is a tachycardia disproportionate for the temperature, suspect hypoglycemia, hypovolemia, or an overdose. Hyperventilation, which is inappropriate during moderate or severe hypothermia, suggests a CNS lesion or one of the systemic acidoses such as DKA or lactic acidosis. A cold-induced rectus spasm and ileus may mask or mimic an acute abdomen. Suspect an overdose or CNS insult whenever the LOC is not consistent with the temperature.

12. What options are available to measure the core temperature?

Rectal, esophageal, tympanic, and bladder temperature measurements are easily obtained. Each has it limitations. For example, the rectal temperature may lag or be falsely low if the probe is in cold feces. Esophageal temperature is falsely elevated during heated inhalation.

13. How does temperature depression affect the hematologic evaluation of patients?
Anemia will be masked because hematocrit increases 2%/1°C drop in temperature. Do not rely on leukocytosis to predict sepsis, because the leukocytes are often sequestered. Always check the electrolytes, because there are no safe predictors of the values. The increased viscosity seen with cold hemagglutination often results in either thrombosis or hemolysis, and a type of disseminated intravascular coagulation syndrome can occur.

14. Should arterial blood gases be corrected for temperature?
No. Correction implies acidosis is beneficial. An uncorrected pH = 7.4 and PCO_2 = 40 mmHg confirm acid-base balance at all temperatures.

15. What is the key decision regarding how to rewarm a patient?
The primary initial decision is whether to passively or actively rewarm the patient. Passive rewarming is noninvasive and involves simply covering the patient in a warm environment. This technique is ideal for mild previously healthy patients.

16. What conditions mandate active rewarming?
Active rewarming is necessary whenever there is cardiovascular instability or the temperature is below 32.2°C (90°F), at age extremes, or if there is neurologic or endocrinologic insufficiency.

17. What is core temperature afterdrop?
This is the commonly observed continued drop in the core temperature after initiation of rewarming. There are two explanations: (1) temperature equilibration between tissues and (2) the circulatory return of cold peripheral blood to the core.

18. Are there unique considerations and complications with active external rewarming?
The external transfer of heat to a patient is accomplished most safely when the heat is applied directly to the trunk. In chronically hypothermic patients, rapidly rewarming the vasoconstricted extremities may overwhelm a depressed cardiovascular system and result in cardiovascular collapse. Monitoring in a heated tub can be difficult, and it should be remembered that vasoconstricted skin is easily burned by electric blankets.

19. What constitutes active core rewarming?
These are techniques that deliver heat directly to the core. The options include heated inhalation, intravenous (IV) fluids, peritoneal lavage, gastrointestinal irrigation, and extracorporeal rewarming.

20. When is airway rewarming indicated?
Heated, humidified oxygen is always helpful and can be administered via mask or endotracheal tube. Heat transfer is not as significant by mask, but respiratory heat loss is eliminated while the patient is gradually rewarmed.

21. How are heated IV fluids administered?
IV fluids heated to 40°–42°C are particularly helpful during major volume resuscitations and should generally be given peripherally.

22. What are the techniques for heated irrigation?
Heat transfer from irrigation of the gastrointestinal tract is minimal. Irrigation should be considered only in combination with other techniques in severe cases. Thoracostomy tube irrigation appears to be a more promising alternative in severe cases.

23. When should heated peritoneal lavage be considered?
Double-catheter peritoneal lavage can efficiently rewarm seriously hypothermic patients. This invasive technique should generally be reserved for severely hypothermic and unstable patients when extracorporeal rewarming techniques are unavailable. Infuse 2 L of isotonic dialysate at 40°–45°C, and suction after 20 minutes.

24. When is extracorporeal rewarming indicated?
Cardiopulmonary bypass and hemodialysis can be lifesaving in cardiac arrest situations. Patients with completely frozen extremities, severe rhabdomyolysis, and major electrolyte fluxes will also be easier to manage in this manner.

25. What are the contraindications to cardiopulmonary resuscitation (CPR) in accidental hypothermia?
CPR should be initiated, unless do-not-resuscitate status is verified, lethal injuries are identified, any vital signs or signs of life are present, or the chest wall is frozen and cannot be compressed.

26. Are there unique pharmacologic considerations during hypothermia?
Protein binding increases as body temperature drops, and most drugs become ineffective. Generally avoid pharmacologic manipulation of the pulse and blood pressure.

27. What is the significance of atrial and ventricular arrhythmias?
Atrial arrhythmias normally have a slow ventricular response. They are innocent and should be left untreated. Preexistent ventricular ectopy may resurface during rewarming and can confuse the picture. Bretylium appears to be the only efficacious antiarrhythmic under hypothermic conditions.

28. What is frostbite?
Frostbite is the most common freezing injury of tissue. It occurs whenever the tissue temperature falls below 0°C. Ice crystal formation damages the cellular architecture, and stasis progresses to microvascular thrombosis.

29. Which factors predispose to frostbite?
Tissue rapidly freezes when in contact with good thermal conductors including metal, water, and volatiles. Direct exposure to cold wind (wind-chill index) quickly freezes acral areas (fingers, toes, ears, nose). A variety of conditions can impair the peripheral circulation and predispose to frostbite. Constrictive clothing and immobility reduce heat delivery to the distal tissues. Vasoconstrictive medications, including nicotine, can exacerbate cold damage, especially when coupled with underlying vascular conditions like atherosclerosis.

30. What peripheral circulatory changes precede frostbite?
Human beings possess a "life-versus-limb" mechanism that helps to prevent systemic hypothermia. Arteriovenous anastomoses in the skin shunt blood flow away from acral areas to limit radiative heat loss.

31. Before frostbite occurs, what other cutaneous events take place in the prefreeze phase?
As tissue temperatures drop below 10°C, anesthesia develops. Endothelial cells leak plasma, and microvascular vasoconstriction occurs. Crystallization is not seen as long as the deeper tissues conduct and radiate heat.

32. What happens during the freeze phase of frostbite?
The type of exposure determines the rate and location of ice crystal formation. Normally, ice initially forms extracellularly, causing water to exit the cell and inducing cellular dehydration, hyperosmolality, collapse, and death.

33. Immediately after thawing, what may occur?
In deep frostbite, progressive microvascular collapse develops. Sludging, stasis, and cessation of flow begin in the capillaries and progress to the venules and the arterioles. The tissues are deprived of oxygen and nutrients. Plasma leakage and arteriovenous shunting increase tissue pressures and result in thrombosis, ischemia, and necrosis.

34. What is progressive dermal ischemia?
This is an additional insult to potentially viable tissue that is partially mediated by thromboxane. Arachidonic acid breakdown products are released from underlying damaged tissue into the blister fluid. The prostaglandins and thromboxanes produce platelet aggregation and vasoconstriction.

35. What delayed physiologic events are observed?
Edema progresses for 2–3 days. As the edema resolves, early necrosis becomes apparent if nonviable tissue is present. Final demarcation is often delayed for more than 60–90 days.

36. What are the symptoms of frostbite?
Sensory deficiencies are always present, affecting light-touch, pain, and temperature perception. "Frostnip" produces only a transient numbness and tingling. It is not true frostbite because there is no tissue destruction. In severe cases, patients report a "chunk of wood" sensation and clumsiness.

37. What is chilblains (pernio)?
Repetitive exposure to dry cold can induce chilblains (cold sores), especially in young females. Pruritus, erythema, and mild edema may evolve into plaques, blue nodules, and ulcerations. The face and dorsum of the hands and feet are commonly affected.

38. What is trench foot?
Prolonged exposure to wet cold above freezing results in trench foot (immersion foot). Initially, the feet appear edematous, cold, and cyanotic. The subsequent development of vesiculation may mimic frostbite. However, liquefaction gangrene is a more common sequela than with frostbite.

39. How should frostbite be classified?
Classification by degrees as is done with burns is unnecessary and is often prognostically incorrect. Quite simply, superficial or mild frostbite does not result in actual tissue loss; deep or severe frostbite does.

40. What do the various signs of frostbite indicate?
The initial presentation of frostbite can be deceptively benign. Frozen tissues appear yellow, waxy, mottled, or violaceous-white. Favorable signs include normal sensation, warmth, and color after thawing. Early clear bleb formation is more favorable than delayed hemorrhagic blebs. These result from damage to the subdermal vascular plexi. Lack of edema formation also suggest major tissue damage.

41. How should tissues be thawed?
Rapid complete thawing of the part by immersion in 40°–41°C circulating water is ideal. Reestablishment of perfusion is intensely painful, and parenteral narcotics are needed in

severe cases. Premature termination of thawing is a common mistake, because an incomplete thaw increases tissue loss. Never use dry heat or allow tissues to refreeze. Rubbing or friction massage may actually be harmful.

42. What steps should immediately follow thawing?
Handle tissues gently, and elevate the injured parts to minimize edema formation. If cyanosis is still present after thawing, monitor the tissue compartment pressures. Consider streptococcal and tetanus prophylaxis. Avoid compressive dressings, and use daily whirlpool hydrotherapy. Whenever possible, defer surgical decisions regarding amputation until there are clear demarcation, mummification, and sloughing.

43. How are blisters treated?
Clear blisters may be temporarily left intact or debrided. After debridement, topical aloe vera (Dermaide) applied directly to frostbitten areas is a specific thromboxane inhibitor. When coupled with systemic ibuprofen, the strategy can minimize accumulation of arachidonic acid breakdown products. In contrast, hemorrhagic blisters should be left intact to prevent tissue desiccation.

44. Are any ancillary treatment modalities really helpful?
A variety of antithrombotic and vasodilatory treatment regimens have been tried, including medical and surgical sympathectomies. These modalities, plus dextran, heparin, and a variety of anti-inflammatory agents, have not conclusively increased tissue salvage.

45. What are some of the common sequelae of frostbite?
The most common symptomatic sequelae result from neuronal injury and abnormal sympathetic tone. Thermal misperception, paresthesias, and hyperhidrosis may become long-term complaints. Delayed findings also include epiphyseal damage, nail deformities, and cutaneous carcinomas.

BIBLIOGRAPHY

1. Danzl DF, Hedges JR, Pozos RS, et al: Hypothermia outcome score: Development and implications. Crit Care Med 17:227–231, 1989.
2. Delaney KA, Howland MA, Vassallo S, et al: Assessment of acid-base disturbances in hypothermia and their physiologic consequences. Ann Emerg Med 18:72–82, 1989.
3. Edlich RF, Chang DE, Birk KA, et al: Cold injuries. Comp Ther 15:13–21, 1989.
4. Fritz RL, Perrin DH: Cold exposure injuries: Prevention and treatment. Clin Sports Med 8:111–128, 1989.
5. Gregory JS, Flancbaum L, Townsend MC, et al: Incidence and timing of hypothermia in trauma patients undergoing operations. J Trauma 31:795–800, 1991.
6. Hamlet MP: An overview of medically related problems in the cold environment. Milit Med 152:393–396, 1987.
7. Heggers JP, Phillips LG, McCauley RL, et al: Frostbite: Experimental and clinical evaluations of treatment. J Wilder Med 1:27–32, 1990.
8. Jolly BT, Ghezzi KT: Accidental hypothermia. Emerg Med Clin North Am 10:311–327, 1992.
9. Lloyd EL: Equipment for airway rewarming in the treatment of accidental hypothermia. J Wilder Med 2:330–350, 1991.
10. Purdue GF, Hunt JL: Cold injury: A collective review. JBCR 7:331–342, 1986.

63. HEAT ILLNESS

Daryl M. Turner, M.D., and David J. Vukich, M.D., FACEP

1. What area of the brain is considered the body's thermostat for heat regulation?
The anterior hypothalamus.

2. What are four methods of transferring heat from the body to the environment?
1. **Radiation.** Infrared energy is radiated directly into the environment.
2. **Conduction.** Whenever the body touches a surface that is cooler than itself, heat is transferred to that object by conduction.
3. **Convection.** Air moving over the surface of the skin, even imperceptibly, carries heat away.
4. **Evaporation.** The water in perspiration changing from its liquid state to its gaseous state is the most effective means of heat loss to the environment.

3. What are the three organ systems primarily responsible for heat loss?
1. **Skin.** Vasodilatation and perspiration make the surface of the skin the primary location for heat loss.
2. **Cardiovascular system.** The heart is responsible for providing a substantial increase in cardiac output in order to compensate for peripheral vasodilatation and increased volumes of blood being pumped to the periphery.
3. **Respiratory system.** Some degree of evaporation cooling occurs through respiration.

4. What are heat cramps? What causes them?
Heat cramps are painful contractions of the larger muscle groups of the body, usually the calves and thighs, during or shortly after strenuous exercise in the heat. These cramps are usually caused by the replacement of water without adequate salt, resulting in a hyponatremic state in the muscles and eventually to painful contraction of the larger muscle groups.

5. How are heat cramps treated?
The treatment is the replacement of fluid and electrolyte by oral or intravenous administration of normal saline. Changes in mental status or fever are not associated with heat cramps.

6. What is heat exhaustion?
Heat exhaustion is a syndrome of volume depletion in the face of heat stress which results in mild hyperpyrexia, somatic complaints (nausea, vomiting, and light-headedness) and signs of dehydration but no alteration in mental status. The prognosis is excellent because major organ systems are minimally affected. Significant dehydration may be present and should be treated with intravenous normal saline.

7. What is the basic pathophysiologic mechanism for heat stroke?
Heat stroke results when the body's thermoregulatory mechanisms cannot overcome exogenous heat stress and body temperature rises markedly with eventual multisystem organ failure.

8. What are the two types of heat stroke? How are they manifested?
Heat stroke may be categorized as classic or exertional. **Classic heat stroke** usually involves an elderly or debilitated patient who is exposed passively to significant thermal stress. These persons generally do not have the ability to remove themselves from the heat and are exposed to it over many hours or even days. Their ability to respond to the heat stress by

cardiovascular disease, drugs, or alcohol is compromised, and their normal thermoregulatory mechanisms are overwhelmed. These victims frequently have been sweating for a prolonged length of time and are extremely dehydrated.

Exertional heat stroke occurs in a younger, usually physically fit population with normal thermoregulatory systems. Because of severe exogenous heat stress and concomitant exertional heat production, the body's heat loss mechanisms are rapidly overwhelmed. Frequently, these victims are not dehydrated and in fact may be wet with perspiration when they are seen. Nonetheless, their body temperatures are markedly elevated.

Both types of heat stress are associated with significant changes in mental status and involvement of multiple organ systems.

9. What are the pathophysiologic parameters of heat stroke?
Heat stroke is hyperpyrexia with a body temperature exceeding 40°C or 106°F with associated changes in mental status.

10. Which organ systems are primarily affected in heat stroke?
All organ systems may be affected but classically three of them predominate.

1. **Central nervous system.** Altered mental status is always present, sometimes with posturing, paralysis, or seizures. As the hyperpyrexia continues coma may eventually ensue.

2. **Cardiovascular system.** High-output congestive heart failure, pulmonary edema, and eventually complete cardiovascular collapse occur.

3. **Hepatic system.** Central lobular hepatic necrosis occurs with high temperatures.

11. What abnormal laboratory values are expected with heat stroke?
Although nearly all organ systems and laboratory values may eventually be affected, elevation of hepatic enzymes is invariable (GOT, CPT, and LDH).

12. What is the primary goal in the treatment of heat stroke?
In addition to supporting the ABCs, the most important therapeutic goal is to lower the patient's body temperature to less than 101°F within 1 hour. At the extremely high temperatures of heat stroke, the tissues literally cook, and time of hyperpyrexia equals morbidity and mortality.

13. What are the most effective means of lowering the body temperature in heat stroke?
Many methods of cooling have been attempted over the years, ranging from practical to impractical and effective to highly ineffective. Perhaps the most practical and effective method for body cooling is enhancement of evaporation. Obviously, the patient must be removed from thermal heat stress and completely disrobed. With the patient in the supine position and completely exposed, water mist is applied to the exposed skin with a handheld spray bottle. While this is being done, a fan should be directed so that air flows continuously over the moistened skin surface, dramatically enhancing evaporation. Though extremely simple, this method is very effective at reducing body temperature. Cold packs may also be placed in the groin and axillary areas, but one should avoid rubbing the skin surface with ice. Ice water baths or extremely cold cooling surfaces are contraindicated because they cause vasoconstriction of the periphery, markedly inhibiting the ability of the body to lose heat.

14. What is the prognosis associated with heat stroke?
The prognosis varies greatly with the person's age and the setting of the heat stroke. The literature reveals that young military recruits who are treated aggressively have almost no mortality, whereas inner-city elderly persons with heat stroke have a high mortality rate, approaching 30–50% in some cases. Permanent organ system damage frequently occurs,

involving the heart, central nervous system, or the kidneys through rhabdomyolysis and acute tubular necrosis.

BIBLIOGRAPHY

1. Brown WD: Heat and cold in farm workers. Occup Med State Art Rev 6:371–389, 1991.
2. Costrini A: Emergency treatment of exertional heat stroke and comparison of whole body cooling techniques. Med Sci Sports Exerc 22:15–18, 1990.
3. Horowitz BA: The golden hour in heat stroke: Use of iced peritoneal lavage. Am J Emerg Med 7:616–619, 1989.
4. Hubbard RW: Heat stroke pathophysiology: The energy depletion model. Med Sci Sports Exerc 22:19–28, 1990.
5. Knochel JP: Heat Stroke and Related Heat Stress Disorders. Chicago, Year Book Medical Publishers, 1989, pp 301–378.
6. McElroy C, Auerbach PS: Heat Illness: Current Perspectives: Management of Wilderness and Environmental Emergencies. New York, Macmillan, 1983, pp 64–81.
7. Schmidt EW, Nichols CG: Illnesses in the Clinical Practice of Emergency Medicine. J.B. Lippincott, 1991, pp 626–629.
8. Squire DL: Heat illness: Fluid and electrolyte issues for pediatric and adolescent athletes. Pediatr Clin North Am 37:1085–1109, 1990.
9. Tek DA, Olshaker JS: Hyperthermia, pulmonary edema and disseminated intravascular coagulation in an 18-year-old military recruit. Ann Emerg Med 19:715–722, 1990.
10. Vance MV: Heat Emergencies in Emergency Medicine: A Comprehensive Study Guide. New York, McGraw-Hill, 1992, pp 652–654.

64. ALTITUDE ILLNESS

Benjamin Honigman, M.D., FACEP

1. What is altitude illness?
It is a complex of symptoms brought on by the hypoxic conditions associated with travel to elevations greater than 8,000 feet (barometric pressure <560 mmHg). At this altitude, arterial blood oxygen saturation falls below 90%. Extreme altitude is >19,000 feet, whereas moderate altitude is from 8,000–12,000 feet.

2. What are the characteristics of altitude illness?
Acute mountain sickness (AMS) is manifested by headache, fatigue, dizziness, nausea or vomiting, anorexia, and insomnia. Complications are high-altitude pulmonary edema (HAPE) and high-altitude cerebral edema (HACE).

3. What is the incidence of altitude illness?
AMS, 20–50%; HAPE, 1–6%; and HACE <1%.

4. What predisposing factors are associated with altitude illness?

Rate of ascent	Exertion on arrival	Younger adults
Elevation attained	Previous symptoms of	Individual physiologic
Duration of stay at altitude	altitude illness	susceptibility

5. List the characteristics of HAPE.
Dyspnea at rest, cough, cyanosis, rales on physical exam, hypoxia, and alveolar infiltrates on chest x-ray.

6. What are the characteristics of HACE?
AMS with progressive neurologic symptoms such as ataxia and confusion, progressing to stupor and coma; CT scans may show cerebral edema.

7. What is the proposed mechanism of altitude illness?
Altitude illness is probably a spectrum of problems that share a common pathophysiologic mechanism. Hypoxemia at altitude occurs within minutes of arrival and leads to the clinical syndromes. The individual's response to hypoxemia is measured by the hypoxic ventilatory response (HVR), which in some individuals is low, producing relative hypoventilation during the acclimatization process. Altered fluid hemostasis results in fluid retention and a shift of fluid into the intracellular spaces, especially in the lung (HAPE) and brain (AMS and HACE). Hypoxemia affects the vasculature in the lung, producing uneven pulmonary vasoconstriction and capillary leak, as well as in the brain, producing increased flow and vasodilatation.

8. What is the natural course of AMS?
AMS begins hours after arrival at altitude and generally resolves within 24–48 hours with acclimatization. Rarely it will progress to HACE or HAPE.

9. How can altitude illness be prevented?
(1) Slow ascent to allow for adaptation; (2) mild to moderate exercise on first day at altitude; and (3) a diet high in carbohydrates and fluids. Acetazolamide and dexamethasone have been shown to be effective agents in the prophylaxis of AMS. It is not known whether either is useful in preventing HAPE or HACE.

10. What are the dosages of acetazolamide and dexamethasone?
Acetazolamide: 125 mg b.i.d. for 2 days prior to arrival at altitude and continued 1 day after arrival. *Dexamethasone:* 4 mg q 6 hrs for 48 hours prior to travel and 2 days after arrival.

11. What are the primary modes of therapy for AMS?
Aspirin or acetaminophen for headache and antiemetics for vomiting. If moderate symptoms occur, oxygen should be used for 24–48 hours; acetazolamide can also be effective in the treatment of moderate symptoms of AMS (250 mg t.i.d. for 2 days). If these are ineffective or symptoms progress, descent is mandatory.

12. If you are at extreme altitudes, have no oxygen, and cannot descend, is there an effective treatment for altitude illness?
Yes—a Gamow Bag.

13. What is the Gamow Bag? How does it work?
It is a portable neoprene bag that can be inflated to an 8-foot length. It can hold 1 or 2 persons and functions like a portable hyperbaric chamber. It can be inflated to 2 psi and can simulate a descent of 4,000–6,000 feet, which is usually enough to improve symptoms.

14. What is the treatment for HAPE?
Descent and oxygen for severe cases; for mild cases at altitudes of 8,000–10,000 feet, oxygen can be used as initial therapy to try to prevent the need for descent.

15. Are any pharmacologic modalities effective for HAPE?
Acetazolamide has been used and is reported to be effective anecdotally but has never been studied. Nifedipine has been used for therapy in small groups of individuals. It produces vasodilatation and improves pulmonary hemodynamics and respiratory function.

BIBLIOGRAPHY

1. Bartsch T, Maggiorini M, Ritter M, et al: Prevention of high altitude pulmonary edema by nifedipine. N Engl J Med 10:1284–1289, 1991.
2. Ellsworth AJ, Larson EB, Strickland D: A randomized trial of dexamethasone and acetazolamide for acute mountain sickness prophylaxis. Am J Med 83:1024–1030,1987.
3. Grissom CK, Roach RC, Sarquist FH, Hackett PH: Acetazolamide in the treatment of acute mountain sickness: Clinical efficacy and effect on gas exchange. Ann Intern Med 116:461–465, 1992.
4. Hackett PH, Rennie D: The incidence, importance and prophylaxis of acute mountain sickness. Lancet 2(7996):1149–1155, 1976.
5. Hackett PH, Roach RC, Sutton JR: High altitude medicine. In Auerbach PS, Geehr EC (eds): Management of Wilderness and Environmental Emergencies, 2nd ed. St. Louis, Mosby–Year Book, 1989, pp 1–34.
6. Johnson TS, Rock PB: Acute mountain sickness. N Engl J Med 319:841–845, 1988.
7. Larson EB, Roach RC, Schoene RB, Hornbein TF: Acute mountain sickness and acetazolamide. JAMA 248:328–332, 1982.
8. Reeves JR, Schoene RB: When lungs on mountains leak: Studying pulmonary edema at high altitude. N Engl J Med 325:1306–1307, 1991.
9. Scoggin CH, Hyers TM, Reeves JT, Grover RF: High-altitude pulmonary edema in the children and young adults of Leadville, Colorado. N Engl J Med 297:1269–1272, 1977.
10. Singh I, Khanna PK, Srivasta ML, et al: Acute mountain sickness. N Engl J Med 280:175–184, 1969.
11. Yaron M, Honigman B: High altitude illness. In Rosen P, et al (eds): Principles and Practice of Emergency Medicine: Concepts and Clinical Practice, 3rd ed. St. Louis, Mosby–Year Book, 1992.

65. DIVING EMERGENCIES AND DYSBARISMS

John McGoldrick, M.D.

1. Who is at risk for dysbaric injuries?

There are over 4,000,000 trained SCUBA divers in the U.S. today. This group, along with caisson workers, commercial divers, and aviators are most often subject to dysbaric injuries.

2. What are the most serious dysbaric emergencies?

Decompression sickness (DCS) and arterial gas embolism (AGE) are serious emergencies that are becoming more frequently seen in the growing population of sport SCUBA divers.

3. Why are SCUBA divers at risk for diving medical problems?

In compressed gas diving (SCUBA, self-contained underwater breathing apparatus), the diver breathes air or other gas mixtures at elevated pressures under water. Divers are exposed to a pressure environment and the problems seen can be caused by the mechanical effects of increases or decreases of pressure on the diver's body, or by the elevated partial pressures of the gases respired at depth.

4. Why do I need to understand the physics involved?

An understanding of the gas laws is helpful in understanding the pathophysiology of diving-related medical problems:

The Gas Laws

Boyle's Law: At a constant temperature, the volume of a perfect gas varies inversely with the pressure, and the pressure varies inversely with the volume. That is, the higher the pressure, the smaller the volume, and vice versa.

Charles' Law: For any gas at a constant pressure, the volume of that gas varies directly with the absolute temperature. That is, change in either volume or pressure is directly related to change in temperature.

General Gas Law: A combination of the above two laws.

$$P_1V_1/T_1 = P_2V_2/T_2$$

where P_1 = initial pressure, V_1 = initial volume, T_1 = initial temperature, P_2 = final pressure, V_2 = final volume, and T_2 = final temperature.

Dalton's Law (the law of partial pressure): The total pressure exerted by a mixture of gases is equal to the sum of the pressure of each of the different gases making up the mixture, each gas acting as if it alone were present and occupying the total volume. That is, the whole is equal to the sum of its parts.

$$P_{total} = P_x + P_y + P_z \ldots$$

Henry's Law: The amount of any given gas that will dissolve in a liquid at a given temperature is a function of the partial pressure of that gas in contact with the liquid. That is, as one dives deeper, more gas will dissolve in the body tissues.

5. Define pressure. What is the atmospheric pressure at sea level?
Pressure can be defined as force exerted on a given unit of area: pressure = force/area. Under standard conditions, atmospheric pressure at sea level equals 14.7 psi.

6. What is atmospheric absolute (ATA)?
It is another unit of pressure used where 14.7 psi equals 1 ATA. Average sea water density is such that each 33 feet of depth equals an additional atmosphere of pressure.

    1 ATA = 29.9 inches of mercury (in. Hg)
           = 760 millimeters of mercury (mmHg)
           = 33 feet of sea water (fsw)
           = 34 feet of fresh water
           = 14.7 pounds per square inch (psi)
           = 1033 grams per square centimeter (g/cm²)
           = 10.08 meters of sea water (msw)
           = 1013.3 milibars (mbar)

7. What is nitrogen narcosis?
Nitrogen narcosis (also known as "rapture of the deep") is the anesthesic-like effect that nitrogen exerts on a diver as its partial pressure increases with depth. Each 50 feet of sea water (fsw) has been equated to having the effect of one martini—hence the "martini rule." With considerable individual variation, at 100 fsw, a diver may feel light-headed and euphoric, lose dexterity and reasoning ability, and have increased reaction times. At depths greater than 300 fsw, unconsciousness can occur.

8. Can carbon monoxide present a problem for SCUBA divers?
Carbon monoxide can be a problem to divers only if the air supply is contaminated from improper placement of the compression engine exhaust, whereby carbon monoxide can be blown into the air intake of the pump when tanks are being filled.

9. What is the most common form of injury that affects divers? What causes it?

Barotrauma is probably the most common form of injury that affects divers. It is due to expansion or contraction of gas in or around the body secondary to changes in atmospheric pressure produced by ascending or descending in the water column (Boyle's law). These changes in volume in turn distort or damage the tissue surrounding the gas spaces. Barotrauma can therefore occur during descent or ascent.

10. What is middle ear squeeze?

Middle ear squeeze occurs when there is a pressure differential across the tympanic membrane. A pressure differential develops as a diver descends (or ascends) unless air is able to enter (or exit) the middle ear via the eustachian tube. As the differential pressure increases, the middle ear mucosa becomes edematous and hemorrhagic. Tympanic membrane rupture can occur. When tympanic membrane rupture occurs in the water, vertigo may result from caloric vestibular stimulation.

11. Can middle ear squeeze be prevented?

Experienced divers will use a Valsalva or Frenzel maneuver to equalize pressure in the middle ear as they descend.

12. What is the treatment for middle ear squeeze?

Depending on the severity, ear squeezes can usually be treated symptomatically with decongestants. Tympanic membrane perforations are an absolute contraindication to diving because of the risk of calorically induced vertigo.

13. What is external ear squeeze?

If air cannot freely enter or exit the external canal (because of cerumen impaction, ear plugs, or a tight-fitting wetsuit hood), the resultant negative pressure in the canal will cause the tympanic membrane to bulge outward. The lining of the canal becomes edematous and hemorrhagic, producing ear pain that does not resolve by middle ear equalization.

14. What is the treatment for external ear squeeze?

Treatment is ascent and corticosporin otic suspension for any significant external ear canal trauma.

15. What is inner ear barotrauma?

Inner ear barotrauma can occur when a pressure differential between the inner and middle ear is created, causing either an implosive or explosive round or oval window rupture. The problem usually occurs close to the surface during a difficult descent, as the middle ear differential is accentuated by a forceful Valsalva-induced increase in inner ear pressure.

16. What are the symptoms of round or oval window rupture?

The symptoms include sudden onset of severe vertigo not relieved by ascent, roaring tinnitus, nystagmus, a feeling of fullness in the affected ear, and sensorineural hearing loss. Inner ear barotrauma should be differentiated from alternobaric vertigo (which usually occurs during deep dives and is transitory), and inner ear decompression sickness (which is usually associated with deep dives using a helium and oxygen breathing mixture).

17. What is the treatment for round or oval window rupture?

Treatment consists of using antivertiginous drugs, such as droperidol, diazepam, or meclizine. Patients should be referred to an ENT surgeon for follow-up.

18. What causes alternobaric vertigo?

This condition is thought to be caused by a unilateral pressure differential between the middle and inner ears. The symptoms are transient sudden vertigo and an overwhelming feeling of disorientation. Symptoms usually last less than a minute and occur more frequently during ascent than descent. The vertigo may persist on the surface and be accompanied by nausea, vomiting, and nystagmus without tinnitus.

19. What is the treatment for alternobaric vertigo?

Alternobaric vertigo is usually transitory and usually does not require treatment. Decongestants can hasten clearing. For persisent symptoms, antiemetic and antivertiginous drugs can be used. Occasionally, a myringotomy may be necessary to relieve symptoms.

20. What other types of barotrauma are seen in diving accidents?

Pulmonary overinflation may occur when a diver is ascending in the water column and ascends too fast or fails to exhale. Constant exhalation is required to vent air from the lungs of an ascending diver to prevent pulmonary overinflation (Boyle's law). Failure to do so results in alveolar rupture with escape of air into one or more of three directions: into the mediastinum causing pneumomediastinum and interstitial emphysema; into the pleural space causing pneumothorax; and/or into the pulmonary venous system causing arterial gas embolism.

21. What are the symptoms of interstitial emphysema?

Air escaping from alveolar rupture can dissect into the mediastinal space and, from there, into the pericardium, cephalad into the neck as subcutaneous air, or caudally as retroperitoneal air. Signs and symptoms include subcutaneous air (crepitus), change in voice, Hammond's crunch, pericardial air, and dyspnea.

22. What is the treatment for interstitial emphysema?

Interstitial emphysema is usually not life threatening and can be treated symptomatically. Breathing 100% oxygen can hasten resolution. However, the presence of interstitial emphysema indicates escape of alveolar air and mandates monitoring for other more serious consequences of pulmonary overinflation.

23. What is arterial gas embolism (AGE)?

AGE is the most serious and the most fatal of all diving accidents, and is second only to drowning as the leading cause of death in sport divers. Air bubbles that enter the pulmonary venous system coalesce and travel to the left side of the heart. From the left ventricle, they may enter the coronary arteries or the cerebral circulation, causing myocardial infarction and cerebral embolism, respectively.

24. How does AGE present?

AGE occurs on ascent, and the time from alveolar rupture to initiation of symptoms is usually less than 10 minutes. Neurologic symptoms can range from subtle changes in mood or affect, visual disturbances, unilateral or bilateral muscular and sensory disturbances, to immediate unconsciousness. Other manifestations include apnea, cardiac dysrhythmia, and cardiac arrest. Sudden loss of consciousness upon surfacing must be assumed to be AGE until proved otherwise.

25. What is the treatment for AGE?

Definitive treatment of any gas embolism requires a recompression chamber. During transport, an adequate airway and proper ventilation and circulation should be assured; 100% oxygen is administered. Patients should be transported in a supine position. Ground transport is preferred, but if air transport is used, cabin altitude should be kept as close to sea level as possible.

26. What is decompression sickness (DCS)?

DCS is the result of a series of pathophysiologic responses to the evolution of dissolved tissue gases, precipitated by a change in ambient pressure. Bubbles released from solution by a too-rapid reduction in ambient pressure either obstruct blood flow, cause changes in blood chemistry, or stretch and damage tissue.

27. How do these bubbles form?

When a mixture of gases is inspired, the amount of each gas that becomes dissolved is proportional to the partial pressure of each gas (Henry's law). The eventual tissue concentration of gases also depends on the rate at which gases are either removed or metabolized. When breathing air, the dissolved tissue gas of concern is nitrogen. The oxygen component is rapidly removed by metabolism, but nitrogen is inert. Tissues with an elevated nitrogen content must release nitrogen to the blood, which transports it to the lungs for elimination. If the ambient pressure is reduced too rapidly, nitrogen cannot diffuse from tissues fast enough, the tissues become supersaturated, and some of the nitrogen comes out of solution as bubbles.

28. What happens to these nitrogen bubbles?

These bubbles can be interstitial, intralymphatic, or intravascular. They can cause symptoms mechanically (blockage of vascular flow or distortion of tissues), indirectly (endothelial damage, protein denaturation, altered blood coagulation), or a combination of the two.

29. When does DCS present?

Symptoms usually are present within 12 hours after diving: 80% of patients in one study had symptoms within 1 hour of surfacing, 95% within 4 hours. Symptoms seldom occur after 12 hours.

30. What is the clinical presentation of DCS?

DCS has classically been divided into two groups, type 1 (musculoskeletal), which presents as limb pain or with skin or lymphatic involvement. Type 2 DCS (neurologic) includes all other symptoms. DCS is an evolving condition—the patient who presents with type 1 symptoms can go on to develop more serious type 2 symptoms.

31. What is the bends?

Type 1 DCS, known as pain-only bends, presents as pain that is confined to the arms or legs and may be aggravated by movement and relieved by direct pressure on the area (as with a sphygmomanometer cuff). The pain is usually periarticular, involves the upper extremities three times as often as the lower extremities in divers, and ranges from mild discomfort (niggles) to severe pain. There should be no association with systemic symptoms and the pain should not be referred or confused with paresthesias or hypesthesias.

32. How else can type 1 DCS present?

When there are skin and lymphatic manifestations, type 1 DCS can present as pruritus alone, skin marbling, or various rashes and lymphatic symptoms. Pruritus is usually encountered only after deep chamber dives where the diver is surrounded by compressed air. Gas entering the sweat and sebaceous glands is thought to form pruritic bubbles as the diver surfaces. Pruritus is not considered a true form of DCS and resolves rapidly. It must, however, be differentiated from the tingling of paresthesias and hypesthesias of type 2 DCS.

33. How is type 1 DCS treated?
Symptoms of type 1 DCS indicate that tissue supersaturation has occurred, and may progress to type 2 DCS. Therefore, all type 1 DCS symptoms should be treated with recompression.

34. How does type 2 DCS present?
Type 2 DCS includes all other manifestations such as pain in areas other than the extremities, CNS signs or symptoms, or pulmonary manifestations ("chokes"). Pain other than in the extremities may represent referred pain from visceral sites or spinal cord involvement.

35. What is the most common type of DCS?
Spinal cord DCS is the most common type in sport SCUBA divers, whereas cerebral DCS is the most common in aviators.

36. How does spinal cord DCS present?
Paresthesia is a common presenting symptom of a spinal cord "hit" and may progress to ascending numbness, dermatomal distribution of pain, or paraplegia. Cord lesions are common in the lumbosacral area and may be associated with bladder paralysis, urinary retention, fecal incontinence, and occasionally, priapism.

37. How does cerebral DCS present?
Cerebral DCS can present as seizures, hemiplegia, scotoma, diplopia, tunnel vision, or blurry vision. Headaches are common. Soft signs include unusual fatigue, a sense of detachment, and inappropriate or uncharacteristic behavior. Any neurologic symptom can be associated with the intravascular and/or extravascular evolution of bubbles anywhere in the nervous system.

38. Are there other types of DCS?
Yes. Divers may have labyrinthine or inner ear DCS (also known as the "staggers") or pulmonary DCS (also known as the "chokes").

39. How does inner ear DCS present?
The usual symptoms include vertigo, nausea, vomiting, hearing loss, tinnitus, and nystagmus.

40. How does pulmonary DCS present?
Pulmonary DCS usually occurs within minutes of surfacing. Accumulation of bubbles within the pulmonary arterial tree can cause substernal pain, cough, and dyspnea, which can progress to respiratory failure and shock.

41. How are the various types of type 2 DCS treated?
IV fluid therapy with crystalloid is necessary in all cases of type 2 DCS because fluid loss, hemoconcentration, and increased blood viscosity promotes vascular occlusion. Diazepam or droperidol is useful in controlling the vertigo, nausea, and vomiting associated with labyrinthine DCS. Definitive treatment is recompression as soon as possible.

42. How does recompression or hyperbaric therapy work?
The three objectives in recompression therapy are (1) to reduce the size of the bubble; (2) to promote bubble reabsorption; and (3) to prevent further bubble evolution. Reduction in size is accomplished by the increase in ambient pressure. Breathing 100% oxygen washes out tissue nitrogen, enhancing diffusion by widening the nitrogen partial pressure difference.

43. What is the disposition of a patient after recompression therapy is complete?
After recompression is complete, the patient should be evaluated for admission to the hospital for further observation. Any recurrent or new symptom is automatically classified as type 2 and treated with further recompression.

44. When can people return to diving after recompression therapy?
The patient should not dive for 4–6 weeks after a type 1 DCS and at least 3–6 months following type 2 DCS. A second incident of type 2 DCS should warrant critical evaluation of the patient's fitness for further diving.

CONTROVERSIES

45. How does one distinguish between DCS and AGE?
DCS and AGE are rare but demand immediate recognition. A detailed neurologic evaluation is required in all cases. Symptoms of DCS and AGE are often difficult to distinguish. There is currently a trend away from differentiation between DCS and AGE, approaching both as decompression illnesses that require recompression. Initial treatment includes 100% oxygen, rehydration with IV crystalloid, and expeditious transport to a recompression chamber.

46. How should patients be positioned for transport to a recompression chamber after they have suffered an AGE?
The proper positioning of an air embolism patient is controversial. The head-up position can distribute air to the cerebral circulation. The head-down position can distribute more air to the coronary circulation and can increase cerebral blood flow and further increase intracranial pressure. The best compromise may be to place the patient supine with the head in a neutral position to allow unrestricted arterial and venous blood flow from the head.

BIBLIOGRAPHY

1. Arthur DC: A short course in diving medicine. Ann Emerg Med 16:689–701, 1987.
2. Francis TJ, Griffin JL, Homer LD, et al: Bubble-induced dysfunction in acute spinal cord decompression sickness. J Appl Physiol 68:1368–1375, 1990.
3. Kizer KW: Dysbaric cerebral air embolism in Hawaii. Ann Emerg Med 16:535–541, 1987.
4. Kizer KW: Management of dysbaric diving casualties. Emerg Med Clin North Am 1:659–670, 1983.
5. Kizer KW: Delayed treatment of dysbarism. JAMA 247:2555–2558, 1982.
6. Murrison AW, Francis TJ: An introduction to decompression illness. Br J Hosp Med 46:107–110, 1991.
7. Myers RA, Bray P: Delayed treatment of serious decompression sickness. Ann Emerg Med 14:254–257, 1985.
8. Neuman TS, Bove AA: Combined arterial gas embolism and decompression sickness following no-stop dives. Undersea Biomed Res 17:429–436, 1990.
9. Newman TS: Diving medicine. Clin Sports Med 6:647–661, 1987.
10. Vane KD: Mechanisms and risks of decompression. In Bove AA, Davis JC (eds): Diving Medicine. Philadelphia, W.B. Saunders, 1987.

XIII. Neonatal and Childhood Disorders

66. FEVER IN THE CHILD LESS THAN TWO YEARS OF AGE

Pamela M. Downey, M.D., FRCPC

1. What is the definition of fever?
The most frequently agreed upon parameters are an axillary temperature above 37.3°C (99°F), an oral temperature above 37.8°C (100°F), or a rectal temperature above 38.3°C (101°F). It is important to remember that the very young infant with an infectious process may be afebrile.

2. What is the best method of measuring body temperature?
The most accurate method is measurement of the distal esophageal temperature with a temperature probe. Because this is impractical, a rectal temperature is the next most accurate technique. Oral temperatures are impractical in young children.

3. How accurate is a mother's assessment of fever in her child?
Tactile skin assessment of temperature by mothers is correct in identifying the absence of fever in 94% of children. Mothers who believed their children were febrile were correct in 52% of cases.

4. Are axillary temperatures reliable?
Axillary temperatures are unreliable probably because the axillary temperature is affected by the ambient temperature. In addition, blood may be shunted from the skin surface to the core during fever onset or escalation.

5. Is tympanic membrane temperature accurate?
In spite of the ease of this method of screening for fever, it is not completely reliable.

6. Does the height of fever correlate with the presence of serious bacterial illness?
The degree of elevation of the temperature alone is a poor predictor of the presence of serious bacterial illness. Some evidence suggests that the higher the fever, the higher the incidence of serious bacterial infection. However, a temperature of <38.3°C (101°F) does not rule out the presence of a serious bacterial infection, especially in very young or immunocompromised children.

7. Which antipyretic agents should be used in the febrile child?
Aspirin has been associated with the development of Reye syndrome in children with some febrile illnesses and should not be used in the pediatric age group for the treatment of fever. Acetaminophen is effective and safe in recommended doses of 10–15 mg/kg as an antipyretic. Liquid ibuprofen (10 mg/kg) is also an effective antipyretic in children.

8. Does a clinical response to antipyretic therapy have any significance?
A recent study suggested that children who do not respond to acetaminophen by at least 0.8°C are more likely to have occult bacteremia. A child with occult bacteremia may also have a decrease in temperature and a favorable clinical response to acetaminophen. Another study revealed a positive correlation between the lack of clinical improvement with acetaminophen and the presence of meningitis.

9. Discuss the difference between bacteremia and sepsis.
Bacterial pathogens that invade the bloodstream cause both bacteremia and sepsis. Sepsis is manifested by toxicity and serious systemic signs of illness such as lethargy and hypotension. Sepsis is a manifestation of escalating invasion of the host by a virulent organism. Bacteremia is relatively asymptomatic.

10. What is the difference between primary and secondary bacteremia?
Bacteremia that occurs in association with focal disease such as pneumonia, urinary tract infections, and osteomyelitis is considered secondary bacteremia. Primary bacteremia is the isolated presence of bacteria in the bloodstream without obvious associated focal bacterial infection.

11. What is the approach to the infant under 3 months of age with fever?
Children less than 3 months of age are more likely than older children to have a serious bacterial illness when they present with a fever. Minimum assessment after a thorough history and physical exam includes lumbar puncture, complete blood count (CBC) and blood culture, urinalysis, and urine culture. Strong consideration should be given to obtaining a chest roentgenogram. Children less than 3 months of age with a fever are susceptible to different bacterial pathogens (*E. coli*, Group B streptococcus, *Listeria monocytogenes*) compared with children older than 3 months of age. Recently studies of outpatients over 4 weeks of age have identified *Hemophilus influenzae* type b, *Streptococcus pneumoniae, Neisseria meningitidis*, and Salmonella species as pathogens in addition to the three already mentioned.

12. How should a child under 3 months of age with a fever be managed?
General guidelines include admission to the hospital and initiation of antibiotic therapy until culture results are available. There has been some debate about the need for hospitalization. This controversy persists because serious bacterial infection occurs in 3–15% of such patients in spite of unremarkable physical assessment and initial laboratory evaluation. Infants less than 2 weeks of age have a higher incidence of meningitis, bacteremia, and serious bacterial illness than do infants in the second and third months of life. Recent studies have questioned the need for hospitalization of infants ≥28 days of age if they appear clinically well. It is possible that as more data become available, outpatient management with intramuscular ceftriaxone will be an accurate treatment option in this age group.

13. What are the most common causes of a fever in the child between 3 months and 2 years of age?
The clinical syndromes most often identified are viral syndromes, otitis media, or nonspecific febrile illness. Pneumonia, bacteremia, meningitis, osteomyelitis, and urinary tract infections may be difficult to detect, and clues to the presence of serious bacterial illness may be subtle. Other common causes of fever that should be sought are streptococcal pharyngitis, cervical adenitis, and superficial skin infections. In spite of a careful history and physical examination, between 3% and 10% of febrile children between the ages of 2 months and 2 years who look well and appear to have fever alone or minimal symptoms of upper respiratory infection (URI) will have bacteremia.

14. What organisms are responsible for bacteremia in a previously healthy child with a fever between the age of 2 months and 2 years?

Between 3% and 10% of children in this age group with a high fever have bacteremic infections. The organisms most commonly cultured in this age group are *Streptococcus pneumoniae* (65%), *Hemophilus influenzae* (25%), *Neisseria meningitidis* (5%), and Salmonella species (5%).

15. What is the natural history of occult bacteremia?

Bacteremia is not a benign illness. Approximately one-third of infants with occult bacteremia secondary to pneumococcus, *H. influenzae* type b, and *N. meningitidis* improve clinically and have negative blood cultures within 72 hours without treatment. Bacteremia secondary to *H. influenzae* and *N. meningitidis* is much more likely to progress to serious illness than is bacteremia secondary to *S. pneumoniae*. Severe or focal disease such as meningitis or sepsis may develop in infants. Other focal illnesses that may develop include otitis media, pneumonia, soft tissue infections, and osteomyelitis.

16. When are clinical signs of meningitis reliable?

One study found that children less then 16 months of age with bacterial meningitis may not manifest nuchal rigidity, Kernig's or Brudzinski's sign, altered sensorium, or bulging fontanelle. Meningismus may be absent in any child who is very ill regardless of the age.

17. Which children with fever require further laboratory evaluation?

The following are useful guidelines:

• In the otherwise healthy child who is over 3 months of age with a temperature ≥39.4°C (103°F), with no focus of infection identified on clinical evaluation (may have an URI or otitis media), and who looks well, CBC should be determined. A blood culture should be drawn at the same time as the CBC. If the white blood cell count (WBC) is between 4,000 and 15,000 10^9/L, the child probably has a viral illness and may be monitored at home. If the WBC is >15,000 10^9/L, a blood culture should be obtained. If the child has reliable caretakers, the patient may be discharged home with follow-up in 12–24 hours arranged.

• Any child who appears ill after appropriate antipyretic therapy should have a thorough history and physical examination. CBC, blood culture, urinalysis, and urine culture should be performed. Consideration should be given to obtaining a chest roentgenogram and a lumbar puncture after consideration of the clinical picture. Hospitalization and age-appropriate antibiotic coverage should be arranged.

• Urinalysis and culture should be performed in all children with no clinically identifiable focus of fever.

• Children who are suffering from underlying disease (malignancy, sickle cell anemia, immune deficiency, etc.), have a fever, and have no obvious focus of infection should be investigated. Recommendations include CBC, blood culture, urinalysis and urine culture, and consideration for a lumbar puncture and chest roentgenogram. The majority of these children will require hospitalization for antibiotic therapy, pending results of lab tests.

18. Which child with fever needs to be hospitalized?

• Any child who appears ill on clinical assessment and does not show marked improvement with antipyretics and rehydration should be hospitalized. Appropriate antibiotic coverage should be initiated based on the results of the evaluation.

• Children who have an unreliable caretaker or whose caretaker is not available by telephone should be considered for hospitalization.

• Children who are immunocompromised and have a fever should generally be hospitalized.

• It has been recommended that all infants less then 3 months of age who have a fever must be hospitalized. It is possible that as more data become available, treatment with intramuscular antibiotics on an outpatient basis in infants who are older than 28 days of age, look well, and have no identifiable focus will be an acceptable treatment option.

19. How do I evaluate and treat a child under 2 years of age with a fever?

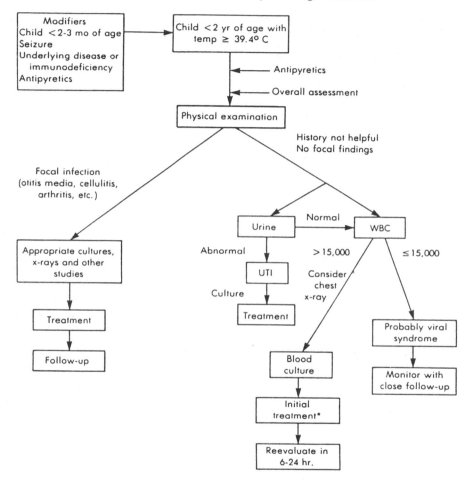

Evaluation of the febrile child under 2 yr. *Ceftriaxone 50 mg/kg/dose IM/IV; ampicillin 50–75 mg/ kg/dose IM/IV; or amoxicillin 70–75 mg/kg/24 hr q 8 hr PO. (From Rosen P, et al (eds): Emergency Medicine: Concepts and Clinical Practice, 2nd ed. St. Louis, Mosby-Year Book, 1988, with permission.)

20. What are the controversies surrounding prophylactic antibiotics in a child who has a fever but no obvious source?

There is some evidence that prophylactic oral antibiotic therapy in this group of children who clinically appear well enough to monitor at home may reduce the duration and severity of the illness. Unfortunately these studies are flawed and the data may not be reliable. Prophylactic oral antibiotics do not prevent or adequately treat serious bacterial illness. Caretakers may develop a false sense of security and ignore progression to serious illness if the child is already on antibiotics. Remember, 1 in 10 infants with a high fever is bacteremic and the risk of meningitis is increased 40 times in the bacteremic child.

The administration of parenteral antibiotics to the child who is older than 3 months of age, looks well, and has no obvious focus on clinical evaluation but who is at risk for bacteremia also requires further study. The morbidity, duration of illness, cost, adverse reactions, and the ability to prevent the development of serious bacterial illness all need to be evaluated.

Oral prophylactic antibiotics have no place in the management of the febrile infant less than 3 months of age based on present available data. A select group of infants ≥28 days of age may be safely managed on an outpatient basis with intramuscular ceftriaxone (see question 12).

21. What about the HIV-positive febrile child?

1. HIV-infected children have the usual childhood illnesses, and will have viral illnesses and otitis media as often as other children. The available data are sparse. While it is useful to know the child's immune status, a recent report notes that these children may develop *Pneumocystis carinii* pneumonia (PCP) with CD4 lymphocyte counts >450 cells/mm^3. HIV-infected children are at increased risk for bacteremia. The organisms most commonly implicated in bacteremia in HIV-infected children are *Streptococcus pneumoniae, Hemophilus influenzae* type B, and Salmonella species. Soft-tissue infections are most often caused by *Staphylococcus aureus* and *S. epidermidis.* Urinary tract infections are usually caused by *E. coli.* Patients who have been on prolonged oral antibiotics and debilitated patients are at risk for gram-negative sepsis.

2. The HIV-infected child who has a localized infection and appears well can usually be managed as an outpatient. Some localized infections and some aspects of other localized infections are peculiar to the HIV-infected child. Enlargement of the parotid gland may occur secondary to lymphocyte infiltration. The glands are enlarged, firm, and nontender. Fever, tenderness, and purulent discharge from Stenson's duct signal the onset of bacterial superinfection, usually secondary to *S. aureus.*

3. The vast majority of HIV-infected children with pneumonia are hospitalized. If PCP is a consideration, the child should be hospitalized and therapy for PCP started pending investigation. PCP is more common in children less than 18 months of age. The mortality rate for children with their first episode of PCP is 40%.

4. The HIV-infected child who presents with fever and wheezing is a diagnostic dilemma. Wheezing and rales may signal the development of routine reactive airways disease secondary to a viral illness or bacterial pneumonia, PCP, or congestive heart failure secondary to AIDS cardiomyopathy. When there is doubt, the child should be investigated for PCP.

5. Fever and diarrhea may be secondary to common pathogens as well as the organisms that plague the immunocompromised host. The child who looks well, is well hydrated, and has no blood or polymorphonuclear leukocytes in the stool may be managed as an outpatient after stool cultures have been obtained.

6. The HIV-positive child who develops fever and a rash may develop severe measles or disseminated varicella. Children with known exposures to these viral infections should receive gamma globulin or varicella zoster immune globulin.

7. The HIV-positive child who has a fever with no obvious source and appears well may be managed like the healthy child with a fever with a few exceptions. Children of any age with HIV infection may be bacteremic and should have a blood culture obtained. Prophylactic antibiotics are controversial and insufficient data exist to recommend their use.

8. The HIV-positive child who appears ill should be treated like any other ill-appearing febrile child. If PCP is suspected, appropriate therapy should be provided. Disseminated fungal infections are unusual in the HIV-infected child but should be considered if there is no response to antibiotics.

BIBLIOGRAPHY

1. Baker RC, et al: Severity of disease correlated with fever reduction in febrile infants. Pediatrics 83:1016–1019, 1989.
2. Baskin MN, O'Rourke EJ, Fleischer GR: Outpatient treatment of febrile infants 28 to 89 days of age with intramuscular administration of ceftriaxone. J Pediatr 120:22–27, 1992.
3. Dorfman DH, Crain EF, Bernstein LJ: Care of febrile children with HIV infection in the emergency department. Pediatr Emerg Care 6:305–310, 1990.
4. Jaffe DM, et al: Antibiotic administration to treat occult bacteremia in febrile children. N Engl J Med 317:1175–1180, 1987.
5. Libovitz E, Rigaud M, Pollack, et al: *Pneumocystis carinii* pneumonia in infants with the human immunodeficiency with more than 450 CD4 lymphocytes per cubic millimeter. N Engl J Med 323:531–533, 1990.
6. Mazur LJ, Mc Jones T, Kozinetz CA: Temperature response to acetaminophen and risk of occult bacteremia: A case-control study. J Pediatr 115:888–891, 1989.
7. Radetsky M: The clinical evaluation of the febrile infant. Primary Care 11:395, 1984.
8. Wasserman GM, White CB: Evaluation of the necessity for hospitalization of the febrile infant less than three months of age. Pediatr Infect Dis 9:163–169, 1990.
9. Woods ER, et al: Bacteremia in an ambulatory setting: Improved outcome in children treated with antibiotics. Am J Dis Child 1195–1199, 1990.

67. SEIZURES IN INFANCY AND CHILDHOOD

Stacie L. Ranniger, M.D.

1. What components of the history are important in the evaluation of the first-time seizure in the pediatric patient?

The history is the most important tool available to the physician in the evaluation of a seizure. Events surrounding seizure activity must be confirmed. For example, breathholding spells, seen with crying and a prolonged expiratory phase with resultant hypoxia, hyperventilation with resultant hypocalcemia, and vasovagal syncope, may precipitate brief tonic-clonic seizure activity. The age of the patient is important because the relative frequency of causes is age dependent. Pertinent past medical history, including apneic episodes, cardiac history, history of gastroesophageal reflux, and headache, will aid in the differential diagnosis. Condition prior to the seizure, including feeding problems, vomiting, diarrhea, and fever, is important. A history of head trauma should always be considered, as should the possibility of a toxic ingestion. A family history of seizure activity should be elucidated. If the seizure is believed to be febrile, the degree of temperature elevation, characterization of the febrile illness, and a complete description of the seizure must be sought. And finally, was there truly a seizure—did the child have bowel or bladder incontinence, tongue biting, and tonic-clonic movements—and what was the patient's responsiveness during and after the seizure activity?

2. What about the physical exam?

A careful neurologic examination is of paramount importance to establish any focal neurologic deficits and to determine new versus old findings. Always look for evidence of trauma to the head and rest of the body, which may clue you in to the possibility of abuse. Remember to do a funduscopic exam, looking for retinal hemorrhages, again a sign of abuse. In febrile seizures, attempt to determine the source of the fever by both history and physical exam.

3. What is a febrile seizure?

According to the National Institute of Health Consensus on Febrile Seizures, a febrile seizure is a seizure, usually occurring in children between 3 and 5 years of age, associated with fever but without evidence of intracranial infection or other defined cause. Specifically excluded in this definition, however, are children with a previous nonfebrile seizure who experience seizure with fever.

4. What features are common to febrile seizures?

The seizures are usually generalized tonic-clonic seizures that rarely last more than 15 minutes. They occur within the first 24 hours of onset of fever, during the rise of the fever curve. Neurologic sequelae are unlikely.

5. Is there a genetic predisposition to the development of febrile seizures?

In 33 to 50% of cases, there is a family history of febrile seizures.

6. What is the likelihood of further febrile seizures?

If a child experiences a febrile seizure, there is a 30% chance that he will experience a second; thereafter, the incidence remains at 30% for each succeeding febrile seizure.

7. What is the best prognosticator of future febrile seizures?

The younger the age at onset of the first febrile seizure, the more likely the risk of recurrence. According to one study, onset prior to age one was followed by recurrence in 50% of cases.

8. What is the role of antipyretic therapy in febrile seizures?

Treatment with antipyretic agents will help to prevent a second seizure during the same illness and will work toward minimizing the risk of seizures during subsequent febrile illnesses. It will also facilitate the work-up (see ch. 66, p. 247).

9. What is the relationship between a febrile seizure and future development of epilepsy?

Only a small percentage of children who have suffered a febrile seizure will go on to develop epilepsy. Those at highest risk were found to have at least two of the following risk factors. Only 2–3% with none or one risk factor developed nonfebrile seizures.
- A family history of epilepsy
- Neurologic or developmental abnormalities prior to febrile seizure
- An atypical febrile seizure, such as a prolonged or focal seizure

10. Which children should be considered for anticonvulsant prophylaxis?

Because approximately 50% of children with a single febrile seizure will not have a recurrence, even if the seizure is untreated, it is more reasonable to consider prophylaxis after a second or third febrile seizure. Prophylaxis should also be considered in the presence of abnormal neurologic development, a prolonged febrile seizure lasting longer than 15 minutes, focality to the seizure, transient or persistent neurologic deficits following seizure activity, or a history of nonfebrile seizures in a parent. Phenobarbital, at blood levels between 15 and 20 μg/ml, has been shown to decrease the number of subsequent seizures but does not eliminate them.

11. What is the ED work-up for a child with a first seizure?

In a child who has had a single febrile seizure and is neurologically normal, evaluation and treatment of the fever are usually all that is necessary. For children who are afebrile or have recurrent or focal seizures, the work-up should be dictated by the results of the history and physical exam. The work-up may include toxicologic and metabolic studies as well as head

CT scans with or without contrast material and an electroencephalogram. A lumbar puncture should be performed if a CNS infection is suspected clinically but need not be performed routinely.

12. What is status epilepticus?
Status epilepticus refers to continuous seizure activity or recurrent seizures lasting at least 30 minutes without the recovery of consciousness between attacks.

13. Why is status epilepticus considered a neurologic emergency?
Permanent brain damage or death can ensue if tonic-clonic activity lasts longer than 60 minutes. After this length of convulsive status, cell damage has been shown to occur in the hippocampus, amygdala, cerebellum, thalamus, and middle cerebral cortex. The damage is believed to be due to increased metabolic demands by continuously-firing neurons. Further damage is caused by hypoxia and the ensuing hypoglycemia, lactic acidosis, electrolyte imbalances, dehydration, and hyperthermia. Cerebral edema will progress if the convulsions are not stopped.

14. How should status epilepticus be treated in the pediatric patient?
Secure the airway, administer oxygen, and intubate as necessary. Establish IV access and obtain blood for complete blood count, electrolytes, glucose, and drug levels/toxicology screen. Monitor respirations, blood pressure, and EKG. Obtain arterial blood for determination of pH and pO_2. Administer 25% dextrose at 1 ml/kg if hypoglycemia is present, or give a 3% sodium if hyponatremic. IV or rectal diazepam should be given as soon as possible to control seizures, dosing at 0.02–0.5 mg/kg at a rate no faster than 2 mg/min to a total of 10 mg. This may be repeated two times as needed. Concurrently administer IV phenytoin at a rate of 50 mg/min to a total of 18–20 mg/kg. Seizures may occur 10–20 minutes after cessation of IV diazepam due to drug redistribution, and it may take 10–20 minutes after the start of infusion of phenytoin for anticonvulsant effects to appear; therefore the two drugs should be given concurrently.

15. What if the seizures continue?
At this point, intubate the patient if you have not already done so. Phenobarbital is the next drug option at a loading dose of 15–25 mg/kg, infusing no faster than 30 mg/min. Paraldehyde should next be considered (dilute to a 4% solution in 0.9% normal saline and infuse at a rate no faster than 1 ml/min). Finally, if seizures have not terminated within 20 minutes after the start of infusion of paraldehyde, general anesthesia and neuromuscular blockade should be considered.

BIBLIOGRAPHY

1. Behrman RE, et al (eds): Nelson Textbook of Pediatrics. Philadephia, W.B. Saunders, 1992.
2. Delgado-Escueta AV, et al: Management of status epilepticus. N Engl J Med 306:1337–1340, 1992.
3. Fleisher GR, Ludwig S: Textbook of Pediatric Emergency Medicine, 3rd ed. Baltimore, Williams & Wilkins, 1991.
4. Nelson KB, Ellenberg JH (eds): Febrile Seizures. New York, Raven Press, 1981.
5. Nelson KB, Ellenberg JH: Predictors of epilepsy in children who have experienced febrile seizures. N Engl J Med 295:1029–1033, 1976.
6. Nelson KB, Ellenberg JH: Prognosis in children with febrile seizures. Pediatrics 61:720–726, 1978.
7. Nypaver MM, et al: Emergency department laboratory evaluation of children with seizures: Dogma or dilemma? Pediatr Emerg Care 8:13–16, 1992.
8. Vining EPG, Freeman JM: Classification and evaluation of seizures. Pediatr Ann 14:730–732, 1985.
9. Vining EPG, Freeman JM: Management of nonfebrile seizures. Pediatr Rev 8:185–190, 1986.
10. Vining EPG, Freeman JM: Seizures which are not epilepsy. Pediatr Ann 14:711–727, 1985.

68. ACUTE UPPER AIRWAY OBSTRUCTION IN PEDIATRICS

Joan Bothner, M.D.

1. What are the most common causes of airway emergencies in pediatric patients?
Upper airway obstruction is a common cause of pediatric emergency department visits, accounting for approximately 15% of all critically ill patients. Infectious etiologies account for 90% of these, with viral croup accounting for 80%. Epiglottis accounts for 5% of severe cases. Other significant causes include other infectious etiologies (bacterial tracheitis, retropharyngeal space infections, tonsillar pathology, peritonsillar abscesses, mononucleosis, and diphtheria, which is rare in this current day and age and country). Traumatic etiologies must also be considered, including foreign bodies, external trauma to the neck, burns, and iatrogenia (i.e., postintubation). Congenital etiologies must be considered in young infants, and less common causes are tumors, and edema secondary to severe allergic reactions.

2. Why do pediatric patients get into trouble more easily than adults with upper airway problems?
There are several differences between the adult and the pediatric airway which are important to remember. Briefly, the tongue is large, easily displaced, and the most common cause of airway obstruction in the obtunded child. The narrowest portion of the pediatric airway is at the cricoid ring, making obstruction with subglottic pathology more likely than in adults. The most significant contribution to increased resistance with obstruction is the small radius of the pediatric larynx (remember that resistance is inversely related to the 4th power of the radius; or, in English, 1 mm of swelling in an infant airway causes big problems). A healthy child easily tolerates moderate to severe airway obstruction and will maintain his or her tidal volume almost to the point of exhaustion, at which time hypoxemia, hypercapnia, and acidosis progress rapidly, leading to cardiorespiratory arrest.

3. How can you tell where the problem is?
Stridor, which is derived from Greek, meaning "creaking," is caused by rapid turbulent flow through a narrowed airway. The sound generated depends on the degree of constriction and the localization of the obstruction. Observation of the child often offers the best clue to localization, before a cold stethoscope ever touches the chest. Supraglottic lesions, such as epiglottitis, present with inspiratory stridor, a prolonged inspiratory phase, and a muffled cry or voice. Glottic lesions also lead to high-pitched inspiratory stridor and a weak or hoarse voice. Subglottic lesions cause expiratory stridor with a normal voice and a brassy cough. A child who assumes the "sniffing position" has significant upper airway obstruction, as does a child who is dysphagic or drools. Remember that expiration should be passive and that active expiration with a prolonged expiratory time, recruitment of the accessory muscles, wheezing, and a "tripod" position is significant for severe lower airway obstruction. All that breathes noisily does not have asthma, and a few seconds of observation should make differentiation between upper and lower airway problems easy.

4. What are the signs and symptoms of a child with respiratory distress? When should I worry?
Tachycardia and tachypnea are common. Tachypnea can be roughly defined as a respiratory rate above 40 in an infant and above 30 in a child. Suprasternal retractions indicate more severe obstruction than intercostal and subcostal retractions. Warning signs of impending respiratory failure include marked retractions, decreased or absent breath

sounds, increasing tachycardia, decreasing respiratory effort or rate, decreasing stridor, and a worried or unsettled appearance. Ominous signs are decreasing level of consciousness, hypotonia, extreme pallor, head-bobbing with each breath, and decreasing heart rate. Cyanosis is an extremely late sign in upper airway obstruction. Arterial blood gases are ancillary and of limited value, and demonstrate only mild hypoxemia (as will pulse oximetry) until exhaustion causes hypoventilation. Hypercapnia and respiratory acidosis necessitate immediate intervention. Basically, the clinical state of the child should dictate intervention, with the most important parameter being mental status. A child who does not cry is not being good. The child is in big trouble.

5. Okay, the child is in trouble. What do I do?
Ensuring an adequate airway is the only priority. An attempt should be made to differentiate epiglottitis from other problems. Supplemental oxygen should be provided and the child needs to be allowed to assume a position of comfort. Remember that almost all children with an upper airway obstruction can be bag-mask-valve ventilated, and this should always be tried first in a child with respiratory failure. Oral intubation is the method of choice in a child requiring assisted ventilation. Endotracheal tube size can be estimated by looking at the child's nares, little finger, or by adding 16 to the child's age in years and dividing by 4. A smaller tube needs to be readily available because of the possibility of significant airway edema. All children have just eaten, so careful attention to prevention of aspiration is essential, including a large, working suction catheter, and cricoid pressure. A needle cricothyroidotomy can be done if an airway is otherwise unobtainable. Endotracheal tubes are uncuffed in children less than 8 years of age. Nasogastric tubes are essential because children are diaphragmatic breathers and cannot ventilate with a stomach full of air.

6. What are the signs and symptoms of croup? Who gets it, what causes it, and what do I do for it?
Croup, or laryngotracheobronchitis, is the most common cause of infectious acute upper airway obstruction. Approximately 10% of children seen with croup require admission, 1–5% require intubation, and 10 cases of croup are seen for each case of epiglottitis. Viral etiologies include parainfluenza virus type 1 (60%), other parainfluenza viruses, influenza virus type A, respiratory syncytial virus (RSV), rhinoviruses, and measles (!). The mean age of affected patients is 18 months, with a slight male predominance, and there is a seasonal increase in cases in autumn and early winter. The classic presentation is a history of a mild upper respiratory infection (URI) followed by increasing stridor with worsening at night. Temperature elevation may be significant but toxicity is minimal. Drooling is uncommon, and hoarseness and a barking cough are frequent. Croup is a clinical diagnosis; laboratory data are useless. The WBC count may be minimally elevated, and radiographic evidence, present in 40–50%, includes a distended hypopharynx with a narrowed subglottic region or a steeple sign. Treatment includes humidified air or oxygen (hypoxemia correlates with respiratory rate). Steroids are controversial, although trends toward improvement are definitely seen at 12 and 24 hours in hospitalized patients. No good studies have been done on outpatients, but evidence from the many croup studies attempted seems to suggest that dexamethasone given as a one-time dose of 0.6 mg/kg orally or parenterally is warranted. Antibiotics have no role in the management of uncomplicated croup. A child with a classic history, a barking cough, and no stridor at rest can be managed with humidified air and steroids and discharged home after a brief period of observation. Racemic epinephrine, given via nebulizer (0.5 cc in 3 cc of sterile water), is indicated for children with stridor at rest or marked increase in work of breathing, and has been shown to decrease airway obstruction. Maximum effect is seen within 30 minutes, with a rebound to baseline at 2 hours in some patients. Criteria for admission include stridor at rest, cyanosis, or other signs of significant respiratory compromise, dehydration, questionable follow-up, and,

possibly, extremes of age. Intubation is rarely needed but is the therapy of choice in respiratory failure.

7. How does croup differ from epiglottitis?

Epiglottitis classically occurs in children from 3–7 years of age, has a rapid onset with a high fever, marked toxicity, leukocytosis, drooling, dysphagia, stridor, preference for the sitting position with the head extended, and no cough. *Hemophilus influenzae* is the most common etiology, and positive blood cultures occur in 60–95% of patients. Other implicated agents include *S. pneumoniae, S. aureus,* some viruses, allergic reactions, and physical and thermal injuries. Radiographic evidence of epiglottitis includes a swollen epiglottis (the thumb sign), thickened aryepiglottic folds, and obliteration of the vallecula.

Epiglottitis is unusual in very young patients (only 4% of patients present under 1 year of age), but may present with different signs and symptoms. All studies are retrospective, but in younger patients cough is seen, there may be a URI prodrome, fever may be lacking, and there may be no drooling or preference for an upright posture. A high index of suspicion is the key. Agitation, drooling, and absence of cough are highly predictive of epiglottitis, whereas presence of a cough strongly suggests croup.

8. What is the appropriate management of a patient with suspected epiglottitis?

Do not agitate the child in any way. Blood work, IVs, and antibiotics can wait. Do not send the child to x-ray. Establishment of an airway is paramount and is ideally done in a controlled manner by an anesthesiologist with a surgeon in attendance. Elective intubation in the ED is **never** indicated, because the proper location for elective intubation is the operating room. Administer high flow humidified oxygen in order to obtain maximal alveoli oxygen saturation. Antibiotics need to be effective against *H. influenzae*; cefuroxime, ceftriaxone, and cefotaxime are all recommended after the airway is controlled. If there is obstruction, a bag-valve-mask ventilation should be initiated prior to any attempts at intubation.

9. Why do children with epiglottitis have airway obstruction?

Hypotheses include fatigue, laryngospasm, progressive swelling of the supraglottic structures, and pooled secretions.

10. What about bacterial tracheitis (membranous laryngotracheobronchitis) and retropharyngeal space infections?

Bacterial tracheitis is an uncommon but significant cause of acute upper airway obstruction. Clinically, affected children resemble children with croup but are somewhat older (mean age 4 years in some studies), have a longer prodrome, appear more toxic, and have significant cough and stridor. Etiology is unclear but is believed to be a secondary invasion of the airway after a viral insult, specifically parainfluenza, influenza, and RSV. The most common bacterial pathogen is *S. aureus*, with *H. influenzae* second. Leukocytosis is common, and radiography may demonstrate subglottic narrowing with irregular intratracheal densities and clouding of the tracheal air column. Airway management and broad-spectrum antibiotics are the mainstays of therapy. In 80% of affected patients, establishment of an artificial airway is required because of tenacious secretions, necessitating meticulous suctioning. Plugged endotracheal tubes are the most common reason for deterioration. Racemic epinephrine is of no proven benefit, and some authors feel that a lack of response differentiates bacterial tracheitis from croup.

Retropharyngeal space infections are a rare cause of pediatric upper airway obstruction but deserve mention because of the need to differentiate them from croup and epiglottitis. About 90% of all cases occur in patients less than 6 years of age. Symptoms include dysphagia, drooling, fever, nuchal rigidity with neck extension, stridor, irritability, and varying degrees of respiratory distress. Neck swelling may occur, specifically posterior adenopathy. A prodrome of a URI with a complaint of sore throat is common. This infection is thought to arise from an extension of an acute infection of the ear, nose, or throat with spread to the retropharyngeal space. Trauma to the nasopharynx (e.g., from pencils) is also a predisposing factor. Cellulitis, or inflammation of the lymph nodes in the prevertebral space, occurs first with progression to abscess formation and suppuration. Etiologic agents include *S. aureus*, various streptococcal species, gram-negative rods, and anaerobes. Diagnosis may be difficult in the young child who cannot localize pain to retropharyngeal space, and a retropharyngeal "bulge" on physical exam is often not seen. Lateral neck films are diagnostic but may be difficult to interpret depending on phase of respiration and neck position. Findings include increase in the width of the prevertebral space to greater than the AP width of the adjacent cervical vertebral body, anterior displacement of the airway, and loss of the normal stepoff at the level of the larynx. Air-fluid levels are seen after abscess formation. CT scans and barium swallow examination can also be helpful.

Treatment includes parenteral antibiotic therapy, with incision and drainage after abscess formation. Most children do not need acute airway intervention. The most common presentation is a young child who appears mildly toxic, has a URI and a fever, is alert, but who is holding his head stiffly and slightly extended. Extension of the neck seems to be most painful, versus flexion in meningitis. The child may be drooling but not in much respiratory distress. Things just don't add up, and, again, a high index of suspicion often pays off.

11. When should a foreign body be suspected?

Most patients who present with foreign-body aspiration are under 3 years of age, are rarely under 5 months of age, and are male. History of an aspiration event is absent in 30–50% of patients. The most common aspirated object is food, and most ends up in the esophagus or in the lower airways. Signs and symptoms depend on site of obstruction, and patients with foreign bodies in the upper airway present with tachypnea, stridor, retractions, voice changes, cough, and wheezing. Absence of a positive history often delays diagnosis, so foreign bodies should be suspected in children who do not respond to appropriate intervention. Plain radiographic films in upper airway obstruction can be suggestive, showing narrowing of the subglottic airway with a minimal opacity in the narrowed lumen. Fluoroscopy reveals prominent overinflation of the hypopharynx, decreased trachea diameter on inspiration, and distention of the trachea and collapse of the hypopharynx with expiration. Endoscopy is diagnostic. Immediate management obviously depends on the degree of respiratory distress, and should be minimal until respiratory failure is imminent. Basic life support measures should be tried first (remember back blows, chest thrusts, and abdominal thrusts?), followed, if unconsciousness occurs, by direct laryngoscopy with attempted removal of the foreign body by Magill forceps if it can be visualized. If this fails, bag-valve-mask ventilation and intubation should be attempted to push the offending object into a bronchus. If the child cannot be intubated, needle cricothyrotomy should be performed.

12. What about the child who has stridor and wheezing?

Think about congenital lesions in patients less than 4 months of age, especially with recurrent problems. Causes in older infants and children include foreign bodies, both in the airway and esophagus, and combinations of infectious etiologies ("status crasmaticus").

13. What are the major areas of controversy in the management of epiglottitis?

• **To look or not to look.** Most authors do not advocate visualization of the epiglottis in the ED in a child with acute stridor in whom the diagnosis of epiglottitis is considered for fear of inducing a vasovagal episode, respiratory obstruction, and cardiovascular collapse. A recent study, which directly addresses the question, found no complications in patients with epiglottitis and no missed cases, although the numbers were small. Visualization was done in the presence of an anesthesiologist in children in whom epiglottitis was strongly suspected. Visualization was first attempted by just asking the child to open his mouth, and second, with a tongue depressor in a sitting child, with careful attention not to touch the epiglottis. These maneuvers were successful in over 50% of patients. Use of a laryngoscope with the child sitting was successful in an additional 30%, and having the child lay supine was necessary in only 15%. The conclusion was that visualization is a safe and effective aid in the evaluation of the child with acute stridor. The authors do not advocate visualization for children in whom epiglottitis is strongly suspected, but more as an aid in diagnosis in questionable cases in lieu of x-rays.

• **The role of x-rays.** Children with epiglottitis may have a normal-appearing epiglottis, with distention of the hypopharynx being the only finding. X-rays are read as falsely abnormal 30% of the time by ED physicians and radiologists. Children obstruct and arrest in radiology departments. X-rays should be ordered only when someone is available who can read them correctly, when the child can be accompanied at all times, and only if the diagnosis is in doubt. Visualization saves time and money, is more sensitive and specific, and may be safer.

• **Transport.** Is establishment of an airway prior to transport necessary? This remains a controversial topic. Some centers advocate elective intubation of all transported patients. Children with epiglottitis have been safely transported without intubation, but others have had significant problems. The answer depends on many factors, including degree of respiratory distress (obviously), length of time of transport, and, most importantly, the skill in pediatric airway evaluation and management by the transporting personnel.

14. Do all patients who receive racemic epinephrine for viral laryngotracheobronchitis (croup) need to be hospitalized?

No one knows for sure but there are lots of anecdotal opinions. Most children rebound by 2 hours after a treatment. Several centers discharge patients to home after a variable observation period with no demonstrable increase in morbidity or return visits. This is currently under investigation. There seems to be a consensus that if a child requires more than one treatment, or has a minimal response, then admission is warranted.

BIBLIOGRAPHY

1. American College of Emergency Physicians and American Academy of Pediatrics: Advanced Pediatric Life Support Provider Manual, 1989.
2. Dickison AE: The normal and abnormal pediatric upper airway: Recognition and management of obstruction. Clin Chest Med 8:583–596, 1987.
3. Donelly BW, McMillan JA: Bacterial tracheitis: Report of eight new cases and review. Rev Infect Dis 12:729–735, 1990.
4. Fleischer G, Ludwig S: Textbook of Pediatric Emergency Medicine. Baltimore, Williams & Wilkins, 1988.
5. Gallagher AG, Myer CM III: An approach to the diagnosis and treatment of membranous laryngotracheobronchitis in infants and children. Pediatr Emerg Care 7:337–342, 1991.
6. Kairys SW, Olmstead EM, O'Connor GT: Steroid treatment of laryngotracheitis: A meta-analysis of the evidence from randomized trials. Pediatrics 83:5, 1989.
7. Kelley PB, Simon JE: Racemic epinephrine use in croup and disposition. Am J Emerg Med 10:182–183, 1992.
8. Lichenstein R: Retropharyngeal cellulitis: An unusual cause of respiratory distress in infancy. Pediatr Emerg Care 6:138–140, 1990.
9. Losek JD, Dewitz-Zink BA, Melzer-Lange M, Havens PL: Epiglottitis: Comparison of signs and symptoms in children less than 2 years old and older. Ann Emerg Med 19:55–58, 1990.
10. Mauro RD, Poole SR, Lockhart CH: Differentiation of epiglottitis from laryngotracheitis in the child with stridor. Am J Dis Child 142:679–682, 1988.
11. Skolnik NS: Treatment of croup: A critical review. Am J Dis Child 143:1045–1049, 1989.

69. PEDIATRIC BRONCHIOLITIS AND ASTHMA

Phyllis H. Stenklyft, M.D.

BRONCHIOLITIS

1. In what age group does bronchiolitis usually present?
Children less than 2 years old. Bronchiolitis is usually diagnosed in infants 2–6 months of age.

2. What are the clinical signs and symptoms?
Tachypnea, wheezing, nasal flaring, and retractions. These symptoms are usually preceded by 1–2 days of rhinorrhea, cough, or low-grade fever. Auscultation may reveal diffuse wheezing, prolonged expiration, and rales. Young infants may present with apnea only. Expiration may be prolonged, as with other obstructive lower respiratory illnesses.

3. What is the most common cause of bronchiolitis?
Bronchiolitis is caused by respiratory syncytial virus (RSV) in 50–75% of cases. Other less common causes are adenovirus, parainfluenza virus, enterovirus, and influenza.

4. What are the radiographic findings of bronchiolitis?
Hyperinflation and flattened diaphragms due to air trapping are the most common findings. Parahilar peribronchial infiltrates and atelectasis may also be present and indistinguishable from bacterial pneumonia.

5. List the clinical findings associated with more severe disease and the need for close follow-up or hospital admission.
1. Toxic general appearance
2. Pulse oximetry oxygen saturation of <92–95% in room air
3. History of prematurity or congenital heart disease
4. Respiratory rate >70/min
5. Atelectasis on chest radiograph
6. Age <3 months

6. What are the roles of bronchodilators, antibiotics, and steroids in the treatment of bronchiolitis?
The use of bronchodilators is controversial. Published studies are mostly inconclusive or unsupportive. Despite this lack of proven benefit, nebulized and oral sympathomimetic agents appear to be beneficial in selected cases and are commonly used in the emergency and outpatient treatment setting. Steroids have no proven therapeutic benefit. Antibiotics should be given only if bacterial pneumonia cannot be excluded on radiographic and clinical grounds.

7. When should ribavirin be used?
Ribavirin is an aerosolized antiviral agent used in selected cases of RSV-associated bronchiolitis. It decreases the severity of illness and viral shedding. Ribavirin therapy is reserved for hospitalized children with severe symptoms or chronic medical conditions. It is recommended in children with congenital heart disease, bronchopulmonary dysplasia, prematurity, and immunodeficiency.

8. Is there an association between asthma and previous RSV infection?
Yes. Approximately 30–50% of children with RSV bronchiolitis in infancy develop recurrent wheezing later in life.

9. List the differential diagnosis for an infant with new-onset wheezing.
Bronchiolitis, asthma, foreign body aspiration, pneumonia, cystic fibrosis, vascular ring or other congenital malformations, congenital heart disease with congestive heart failure, and gastroesophageal reflux. This broad differential is the logic for recommending a chest radiograph in patients with first-time wheezing.

ASTHMA

10. You have diagnosed a 3-year-old girl as having asthma. Her father, an attorney, asks the question, "What is asthma?" What is your response?
Asthma is a lung disease with the following characteristics: airway obstruction, inflammation, and hyperresponsiveness. Airway obstruction (blocking) or narrowing is responsible for the wheezing noises and cough, and is usually reversible spontaneously or with treatment. The obstruction or narrowing can be caused by swelling, excessive mucus, or muscle contraction. Inflammation is caused by special cells (mast cells, macrophages) that release substances that damage the lining of the airway. Hyperresponsiveness is constriction of the airway triggered by environmental irritants, viral respiratory infections, cold air, or exercise.

11. What is the Wood-Downes score for asthma?
It is a clinical scoring system for asthma that gives a numerical value to oxygenation, inspiratory breath sounds, use of accessory muscles, wheezing, and CNS function. It is useful to document patient progress and response to treatment.

Clinical Asthma Evaluation Score

	0	1	2
PO_2 or	70–100 in air	≤70 in air	≤70 in 40% O_2
Cyanosis	None	In air	In 40% O_2
Inspiratory breath sounds	Normal	Unequal	Decreased to absent
Accessory muscles used	None	Moderate	Maximal
Expiratory wheezing	None	Moderate	Marked
Cerebral function	Normal	Depressed or agitated	Coma

This score is designed for use in children with status asthmaticus. A score of ≥5 is thought to be indicative of impending respiratory failure. A score of ≥7 with an arterial carbon dioxide tension (PCO_2) ≥65 mmHg indicates existing respiratory failure.

From Wood DW, Downes JJ, Lecks HL: A clinical scoring system for the diagnosis of respiratory failure. Am J Dis Child 123:227, 1972, with permission.

12. Define status asthmaticus (or when do you need to admit?).
It is an acute episode of asthma that is unresponsive to usual effective treatment. Usual effective treatment has become synonymous with three nebulized beta$_2$-agonist treatments. However, with the increased use of home nebulizers, this definition is changing. All children with a poor or incomplete response to therapy should be admitted. Hospital admission should also be considered in the presence of pneumonia, lobar atelectasis, persistent vomiting, unreliable caretakers, or other adverse social situations.

13. Name the characteristics that identify children at risk for life-threatening deterioration during an exacerbation of asthma.
Prior history of life-threatening exacerbations (ICU admissions, intubation)
Children <1 year old
Less than 10% improvement in peak expiratory flow rate (PEFR) or forced expiratory volume at 1 second (FEV_1) in the ED (post-treatment)

PEFR or FEV$_1$ <25% predicted value
PCO$_2$ ≥40 mmHg
Altered mental status
Pulsus paradoxus >20 mmHg
Oxygen saturation <90% or PO$_2$ <60 mmHg
Diminished or inaudible breath sounds

14. What are the usual and ominous arterial blood gas (ABG) findings during an exacerbation of asthma?
Initially hyperventilation causes a low PCO$_2$. As airway obstruction worsens, the PCO$_2$ rises to normal or above. A PCO$_2$ of 40–45 mmHg in the presence of respiratory distress is an indication of impending respiratory failure. Hypoxemia is common but usually reverses after the patient has received oxygen. Persistent hypoxemia (O$_2$ saturation <90% or PO$_2$ <60 mmHg) is another indicator of respiratory failure. Pulse oximetry has largely reduced the need for ABGs in mild or moderate exacerbations. Blood gases are usually obtained in children with severe respiratory distress or impending respiratory failure and to measure response to treatment.

15. During an exacerbation of asthma, when should a chest radiograph be obtained? What are the findings?
A chest radiograph is indicated if pneumonia is clinically suspected, breath sounds are unequal, the patient is unresponsive to therapy, severe respiratory distress is present, or admission to an ICU is indicated. Chest radiographs commonly show hyperinflation, atelectasis, and peribronchial thickening, indicating lower airway obstruction. Approximately 25% of radiographs taken during an acute asthma attack show an abnormality other than hyperinflation. Pneumothorax is rare. Pneumomediastinum is more common in older children (age >10 years), whereas infiltrates are more common in younger children.

16. What initial ventilator settings would you recommend for a child with asthma and respiratory failure who requires mechanical ventilation?
A large tidal volume and a slow rate are usually needed to provide adequate time for exhalation, thereby preventing breath stacking and the potential for pneumothorax. A tidal volume of 15 ml/kg with a rate of 20–25 breaths/min in infants or 8–12 breaths/min in adolescents is a general starting point. Positive end-expiratory pressure (PEEP) should be avoided to prevent further risk of barotrauma. Sedation and neuromuscular blockade are usually indicated.

17. What should be included in the ED management of a child with an acute exacerbation of asthma?
    Step 1
    • Initial assessment to include vital signs, auscultation, use of accessory muscles, color, retractions, alertness, oxygen saturation, and PEFR
    Step 2
    • Oxygen to keep O$_2$ saturation >95%
    • Nebulized albuterol every 20 minutes up to 1 hour or 3 times (reassess after each treatment)
    • Begin oral steroids (prednisone, 1–2 mg/kg/dose) if no response after first nebulizer treatment or for steroid dependence
    Step 3
    • Repeat assessment
    • Good response
       PEFR >70% baseline

No wheezing, retractions, or use of accessory muscles
O_2 saturation $>95\%$
↓
Observe 1 hour or more
↓
Discharge home with reliable caretaker, patient education, medications, and follow-up instructions
Medications: albuterol, nebulized or inhaled if possible, otherwise given orally; oral prednisone, 1–2 mg/kg/day for 3–5 days
• Poor or incomplete response after 1 hour or 3 treatments
↓
Consider hospitalization or continuance of nebulizer treatments in an observation unit
Consider starting aminophylline

18. What is cough variant asthma? How is it diagnosed?
Most children present with a cough that is nocturnal, exercise induced, or cold air induced. Recurrences are often seasonal or associated with upper respiratory infections. Pulmonary function tests may be normal or abnormal (↓FEV_1, ↓PFER, ↑airway resistance). In most children, nocturnal or pre-exercise administration of a bronchodilator is therapeutic and diagnostic. A methacholine challenge test may help to diagnose older children with normal pulmonary function tests.

BIBLIOGRAPHY

1. Brunette MG, Lands L, Thibodeau LP: Childhood asthma: Prevention of attacks with short-term corticosteroid treatment of upper respiratory tract infection. Pediatrics 81:624, 1988.
2. Canny GJ, Reisman J, Healy R, et al: Acute asthma: Observations regarding the management of a pediatric emergency room. Pediatrics 83:507, 1989.
3. Chantarojahasiri T, Nicholas DG, Rogers MC: Lower airway disease: Bronchiolitis and asthma. In Rogers MC (ed): Textbook of Pediatric Intensive Care. Baltimore, Williams & Wilkins, 1987, p 204.
4. Eggleston PA, Ward BH, Pierson WE, Bierman CW: Radiographic abnormalities in acute asthma in children. Pediatrics 54:442, 1974.
5. Geelhoed GC, Landau LI, LeSouef PN: Oximetry and peak expiratory flow in assessment of acute childhood asthma. J Pediatr 117:907, 1990.
6. Goldenhersh MJ, Rachelefsky GS: Childhood asthma: Overview. Pediatr Rev 10:227, 1989.
7. Goldenhersh MJ, Rachelefsky GS: Childhood asthma: Management. Pediatr Rev 10:259, 1989.
8. Jaimovich D, Kecskes S: Management of reactive airway disease. Crit Care Clin 8:147, 1992.
9. McIntosh K: Respiratory syncytial virus infections in infants and children: Diagnosis and treatment. Pediatr Rev 9:191, 1987.
10. Shaw KN, Bell LM, Sherman NH: Outpatient assessment of infants with bronchiolitis. Am J Dis Child 145:151, 1991.
11. Yamamoto LG, Wiebe RA, Matthews WJ: A one-year series of pediatric emergency department wheezing visits: The Hawaii EMS-C project. Pediatr Emerg Care 8:17, 1992.
12. U.S. Department of Health and Human Services: Guidelines for the management of asthma. Pub. No. 91-3042, Bethesda, MD, National Institutes of Health, June 1991.

70. PEDIATRIC GASTROINTESTINAL DISORDERS AND DEHYDRATION

Benjamin A. Gitterman, M.D.

1. Are pediatric gastrointestinal (GI) problems different from adult GI problems?
Yes. Children are not little adults. The causes and management of their GI problems are often different from those in adults. Children may not be able to communicate a history as easily as adults, and you may need to use different skills in evaluating them.

2. How can a child be rapidly evaluated for dehydration?

Degree of Dehydration

	MILD (<5%)	MODERATE (5–10%)	SEVERE (10–15%)
State of consciousness	Normal	Lethargic	Lethargic to comatose
Skin turgor	Normal	Decreased	Very decreasing/tenting
Skin color	Normal	Pale/gray	Mottled
Mucous membranes	Slightly dry	Dry or "tacky"	Parched
Blood pressure	Normal	Normal or slight	Orthostatic
Pulse	Normal	Slight	Tachycardic
Capillary refill	Normal	Slow	Very slow
Fontanelle	Flat	Depressed	Sunken
Urine output	Decreased	Minimal	Anuric

3. Describe initial fluid resuscitation for a severely dehydrated child.
Children should receive 20 ml/kg of normal saline or lactated Ringer's solution over 20 minutes. A second flush of 20 ml/kg can be given just as quickly if there is no significant improvement. (The second flush usually should contain glucose, e.g., D5 normal saline).

4. What about fluid overload in a small child?
Perfusion of vital organs is of much greater concern. Fluid overload is unlikely to occur in a previously healthy child and can be managed if necessary.

5. How can I determine the weight of an infant in an emergency situation, in order to estimate fluid needs?
The "average" newborn weighs 3 kg. Birth weight generally doubles by age 5 months and triples by age 1 year.

6. How much fluid should be used after the initial fluid resuscitation?
Fluid requirements = estimated deficit + maintenance needs + ongoing losses.
In cases of isotonic dehydration:
    The deficit should be replaced ½ in the first 8 hours, ½ in the next 16 hours.
    Maintenance should be replaced evenly over 24 hours.
    Ongoing losses should be replaced as necessary.

7. How are maintenance fluids calculated?
    100 cc/kg/24 hr for the first 10 kg of body weight
    50 cc/kg/24 hr for the next 10 kg of body weight
    20 cc/kg/24 hr for the remainder of body weight

8. What if the dehydration is not isotonic?
Hypernatremic dehydration must be corrected slowly, with the deficit being replaced over 48 hours after the initial fluid resuscitation in order to avoid neurologic complications.

9. Which fluids are used for ongoing maintenance therapy after initial fluid resuscitation?
In most cases of isotonic dehydration, D5W ½ normal saline with 30 mEq of potassium (K)/liter will be effective (K^+ should be added only after the child voids). Exact calculation rather than use of standard numbers is especially important in nonisotonic cases.

10. Should hyponatremia be corrected immediately?
A symptomatic patient, such as the hyponatremic child with seizures, should be given 3% saline (0.5 mEq Na^+/ml), 4 ml/kg intravenously until symptoms stop. Immediate correction above a serum sodium of 125 is unnecessary.

11. If a dehydrated patient is acidotic, should that be corrected?
Metabolic acidosis in a dehydrated child is caused by poor tissue perfusion. Acidosis usually improves with an increase in circulating volume and subsequent improved perfusion. Although "exact" laboratory numbers are unclear, most clinicians support specific treatment of acidosis when laboratory results indicate HCO_3^- <10 mEq/L or arterial pH <7.1. At that time, $^1/_3$ to $^1/_2$ of the sodium given during the first 8 hours of resuscitation can be given as $NaHCO_3$ instead of NaCl.

12. When can children be treated with oral rehydration solutions (ORS)?
Mildly ill children can always be treated orally. Severely dehydrated children need rapid parenteral rehydration. Moderately dehydrated children should be treated primarily based on their state of consciousness and ability to retain oral fluids. Most children who present with a history of "vomiting everything" will keep down small frequent quantities offered (i.e., 1–2 teaspoons every 5 minutes, initially). Oral rehydration solutions such as Pedialyte are superior to high-sugar fluids (Gatorade or Jell-O) because of the high osmolality of the latter. Moderately dehydrated children who are treated orally, however, usually need clinical and laboratory monitoring (electrolytes, BUN, urine output).

13. How can a site of GI bleeding be identified by history?

Identification of Sites of GI Bleeding

SYMPTOM OR SIGN	LOCATION OF BLEEDING LESION
Effortless welling forth of bright red blood from the mouth	Nasopharyngeal or oral lesions; esophageal varices; lacerations of esophageal or gastric mucosa (Mallory-Weiss syndrome)
Vomiting of bright red blood or of "coffee grounds"	Lesion proximal to ligament of Treitz
Melena	Lesion proximal to ligament of Treitz. Blood loss in excess of 50–100 ml/24 hr
Bright red or dark red blood in stools	Lesion in the ileum or colon. (Massive upper GI bleeding may also be associated with bright red blood in stool.)
Streak of blood on outside of a stool	Lesion in the rectal ampulla or anal canal

Modified from Sondheimer JM, Silverman A: Gastrointestinal tract. In Hathaway WE, et al (eds): Current Pediatric Diagnosis and Treatment, 10th ed. Norwalk, CT, Appleton & Lange, 1991.

14. What are the causes of significant hematemesis in children?

Newborns—stress or gastric ulcers, hemorrhagic disease of the newborn, swallowed maternal blood

Up to age 1—esophagitis, gastric erosions, gastric and duodenal ulcers, esophageal foreign bodies

Toddlers and preschoolers—esophagitis, gastric ulcers, duodenitis

Older children and teens—all of the above, esophageal varices, Mallory-Weiss tears

15. Describe the initial management of a child with ongoing hematemesis.

A brief history and physical exam should be performed, and vital signs monitored carefully. Intravenous therapy with normal saline or crystalloid should be initiated, anticipating transfusion with packed red cells or whole blood. A nasogastric tube should be placed. Complete blood count with platelets, prothrombin, partial thromboplastin, and type and crossmatch should be obtained.

16. How should upper GI bleeding be immediately controlled?

Nasogastric lavage is still often suggested, although it is unclear if it works. The presumption is that gastric hypothermia reduces bleeding. Severe cases of persistent bleeding may be treated using intravenous vasopressin.

17. What common substances, when ingested, are mistaken for upper GI bleeding?

Jell-O, Kool-Aid, red food coloring, and various antibiotics.

18. What causes painless rectal bleeding in young children?

Meckel's diverticulum, a collection of gastric parietal cells that irritate the adjacent intestinal mucosa, may cause painless, bright red, or maroon-colored bleeding in children. It needs immediate evaluation and attention.

19. When should a foreign body be removed from the GI tract?

Foreign body ingestion in young children is common. Most small foreign bodies (coins, buttons, etc.) will pass spontaneously. Objects that lodge in the esophagus for more than 3–4 hours probably will not pass. Removal by endoscopy or, more easily, with a Foley catheter, should be considered within 12–24 hours. Round foreign bodies, straight pins, nails, etc. can safely remain in the stomach for several weeks. Button batteries, which are potentially corrosive, need early removal (24–48 hours). If a child is symptomatic, the object always needs to be removed. Surgery may be necessary to remove foreign bodies in the lower GI tract.

20. What historical clues suggest serious, life-threatening causes of vomiting in infancy?

Green bilious vomiting strongly suggests an obstruction; this history should never be taken lightly. Intermittent fits of intense pain with screaming and "bringing the knees to the chest" may suggest intussusception. Projectile vomiting in an infant 2–6 weeks old is often associated with pyloric stenosis.

21. What is unusual about the laboratory evaluation of a child with pyloric stenosis?

These infants present with hypochloremic alkalosis that results from the loss of stomach acid. Early in the presentation, the laboratory values may not yet have changed.

22. What are the presenting signs and symptoms of acute appendicitis in children?

Classic symptoms include periumbilical abdominal pain that shifts to McBurney's point in the right lower quadrant over 4–12 hours. Guarding and rebound to palpation in the right lower quadrant occur. A rectal exam may be especially tender on the right side. Preceding fever and loss of appetite are often associated. In young children, however, the signs and symptoms are often nonspecific and are further confused by the child's inability to communicate specifics. The incidence of perforation of the appendix is 30–40% in children and may be as high as 90% in children below 2 years of age.

23. Do umbilical hernias need surgical consultations?
Rarely. Most regress without treatment, although some may persist until school age. Incarceration of umbilical hernias is unusual. Covering the hernia and reducing it (with tape, coins, straps, etc.) does not change the natural course. Surgical consultation may be warranted if there is no resolution by school age.

BIBLIOGRAPHY

1. Barkin RM, Rosen PR: Emergency Pediatrics. St. Louis, Mosby–Year Book, 1990.
2. Behrman RE: Textbook of Pediatrics, 14th ed. Philadelphia, W.B. Saunders, 1992.
3. Berman S: Pediatric Decision Making, 2nd ed. Philadelphia, B.C. Decker, 1991.
4. Fleisher G, Ludwig S: Textbook of Pediatric Emergency Medicine, 2nd ed. Baltimore, Williams & Wilkins, 1988.
5. Hathaway WE, Groothuis JR, Hay WW, Paisley JW: Current Pediatric Diagnosis and Treatment, 10th ed. Norwalk, CT, Appleton & Lange, 1991.
6. Rosen P, et al (eds): Emergency Medicine, 3rd ed. St. Louis, Mosby–Year Book, 1992.
7. Silverman A, Roy CC: Pediatric Clinical Gastroenterology, 3rd ed. St. Louis, Mosby–Year Book, 1983.
8. Sleisenger MH, Fordtran JS: Gastrointestinal Disease, 4th ed. Philadelphia, W.B. Saunders, 1989.

71. COMMON PEDIATRIC INFECTIOUS DISEASES

Elaine Norman Scholes, M.D.

1. Why are we still discussing measles (rubeola)? Isn't it a disease of the past?
In the last few years there have been several outbreaks of measles in middle and high schools and on college campuses secondary to waning immunity in older children. Over 25,000 cases of measles occurred in the United States in 1991.

2. What is the mode of transmission of the measles virus?
Measles is transmitted either by direct contact with infectious droplets or by air-borne dissemination.

3. What is the incubation period for measles?
From exposure to the onset of symptoms, the incubation period is 8–12 days. It is 14 days from exposure to the onset of the rash.

4. When are patients with measles contagious?
Unfortunately, patients are contagious 1–2 days before they even become symptomatic, or 3–5 days before the rash appears until 4 days after the rash appears.

5. What are the main signs and symptoms in patients with measles?
High fever, conjunctivitis, photophobia, coryza, cough, rash, and Koplik spots.

6. What are Koplik spots? When do they appear?
They are 1–3-mm bluish-white spots on a bright red surface that appear first on the buccal mucosa opposite the lower molars and are a pathognomonic enanthem of measles. They appear on approximately the tenth day after exposure (within 48 hours following the onset of symptoms). The spots spread to involve the buccal and labial mucosa, disappearing on the second day after the onset of the rash.

7. Describe the typical rubeola rash.
A discrete red maculopapular rash first appears on the forehead, becoming coalescent as it spreads down the trunk to the feet by the third day of the illness. The rash fades in the same head-to-feet pattern as it appeared.

8. What are two frequent complications of measles?
Middle ear infections and bronchopneumonia.

9. What is subacute sclerosing panencephalitis (SSPE)?
SSPE is a rare degenerative CNS disease caused by a latent measles infection, occurring an average of 10 years after a primary measles illness. Patients have progressive intellectual and behavioral deterioration and convulsions. The disease is not contagious.

10. Describe the exanthem seen in rubella.
Numerous discrete rose-pink maculopapules first appear on the face, and, as in rubeola, spread downward to involve the trunk and extremities. On the second day the rash on the face fades, while the rash on the trunk becomes coalescent. By the third day the rash disappears, which is why rubella is also called "three-day measles."

11. What are Forchheimer spots?
Seen early in rubella, they are pinpoint red macules on the soft palate; unlike Koplik spots, they are *not* pathognomonic.

12. What is the incubation period for mumps?
16–18 days.

13. What is the period when mumps are considered contagious?
1–2 days (up to 7 days) prior to the onset of parotid swelling. Patients are no longer infectious 7–9 days after the onset of parotid swelling.

14. What are the major complications of mumps?
- Meningoencephalitis in 0.5% of cases
- Orchitis after puberty
- Sterility is rare.
- Arthritis, renal involvement, thyroiditis, mastitis, and hearing impairment are rare.

15. What is the etiologic agent in erythema infectiosum (fifth disease)?
Human parvovirus B19.

16. Describe the characteristic rash in erythema infectiosum.
Erythematous ears and a maculopapular rash on the cheeks that coalesce to form the characteristic "slapped-cheek" appearance are the initial signs of illness. One to two days later the rash spreads to the extremities with a reticular, lacelike pattern caused by central clearing of the confluent rash.

17. What is the classic presentation of roseola (erythema subitum)?
Typically a child between 6 months and 2 years (up to 4 years) of age presents with a history of high fever of 3 days' duration and mild symptoms, if any. The fever abates abruptly, followed by the appearance of a macular rash on the trunk and thighs.

18. What is the etiologic agent in roseola?
Human herpesvirus-6 (HHV-6).

19. What is the incubation period for varicella (chickenpox)?
10–20 days.

20. When is varicella contagious?
It is contagious from 1–2 days prior to the appearance of the rash until no new lesions are forming (usually 7–10 days after the appearance of the rash). The lesions do not have to be completely resolved, but all should be crusted and dry.

21. What is the mode of transmission and cause of infectious mononucleosis (IM)?
IM is transmitted through direct and prolonged contact with oropharangeal secretions. It is caused by the Epstein-Barr virus (EBV).

22. What are the clinical manifestations of IM?
- Fever lasting 1–2 weeks
- Lymphadenopathy (usually nontender, no overlying erythema, most often bilateral cervical location)
- Tonsillopharyngitis (usually an exudate is present—need to obtain a throat culture)
- Spleen or liver enlargement

23. What clinical signs are also seen in young children with IM?
Rashes, abdominal pain, upper respiratory infections with cough, failure to thrive, and early-onset otitis media.

24. In older children and adults with IM, administration of which antibiotic is correlated with a rash?
Ampicillin, by an unknown mechanism of action, can cause a rash in patients with IM. When treating streptococcal tonsillitis in patients with IM, use erythromycin instead.

25. What are the hematologic findings in IM?
A relative lymphocytosis of greater than 50% of all leukocytes and a relative atypical lymphocytosis of 10% of leukocytes are the typical findings, although the relative percentage of atypical lymphocytes in children may be lower than in adults.

26. What are heterophil antibodies?
They are serum IgM antibodies with the capability to agglutinate horse (better than sheep or bovine) erythrocytes. The ability to adsorb to beef red blood cells but not guinea pig kidney distinguishes heterophil antibodies in IM from both Forssman antibodies (found in normal serum) and the antibodies in serum sickness. A heterophil titer >40 with a good clinical history for IM strongly supports the diagnosis. It is positive in 90% of cases of IM, with few false-positive results, except in young children, in whom EBV serology is needed to establish the diagnosis.

27. What is the Monospot test?
This qualitative rapid slide test is used to detect serum heterophil antibodies in IM. It is positive in 70% of patients during the first week of illness and in 85–90% during the third

week. In children under 4 years of age, this test may be negative due to lower levels of detectable heterophil antibodies. Therefore, EBV serology, which is more sensitive, should be used in this age group.

28. What are the complications of IM?

Complications of IM

Respiratory	Airway obstruction
Hematologic	Thrombocytopenia
	Hemolytic anemia
	Granulocytopenia
Neurologic	Encephalitis, lymphocytic meningitis
	Cerebellar ataxia
	Guillain-Barré syndrome
	Transverse myelitis
	Bell's palsy
	Optic neuritis
Cardiac	Pericarditis, myocarditis
Other	Splenic rupture
	Uveitis, keratitis
	Fatal disease (familial, sporadic, other)
	Chronic disease
Infection	Tonsillar, peritonsillar abscess
	Sinusitis
	Pneumonia

From Nelson JD (ed): Current Therapy in Pediatric Infectious Disease. St. Louis, C.V. Mosby, 1986, p 158, with permission.

29. What is the treatment of uncomplicated IM?

Supportive therapy and rest are the mainstays of treatment, with emphasis on analgesia for sore throat, headaches and myalgias, oral fluids to prevent dehydration secondary to the discomfort with swallowing, and a decrease in normal activity. Patients should be given specific instructions about restriction of activity, which will vary depending on the severity of the illness and the patient's tolerance. If there is splenic enlargement, contact sports should be avoided until it has resolved.

30. What is the role of corticosteroids in the treatment of IM?

The use of steroids in upper airway obstruction may decrease the need for more invasive procedures by reducing edema and hyperplasia of the lymphoid tissue in the naso-oropharynx. There is usually improvement in 6–24 hours after administration of IV steroids. Steroids may also be useful for neurologic, hematologic, and cardiac complications. Corticosteroids have not been shown to reduce splenomegaly or the risk of rupture of the spleen.

Dexamethasone can be given parenterally if the patient is unable to take oral medication. The initial loading is 1 mg/kg/day (maximum 10 mg), followed by a dose of 0.5 mg/kg every 6 hours. The patient can be switched to oral medication when it is tolerated: prednisone, 2 mg/kg/day (maximum dose 60–80 mg/day), divided every 6–12 hours for a total of 5–7 days.

31. Which analgesic should be recommended in patients with IM?

Because aspirin inhibits platelet function, acetaminophen is the analgesic of choice.

32. How long does the patient need to worry about the risk of splenic rupture?
Rupture of the spleen usually occurs during the second or third week of the illness, if at all. Patients must avoid contact sports while the spleen is enlarged.

BIBLIOGRAPHY

1. Asano Y, Nakashima T, Yoshikawa T, et al: Severity of human herpesvirus-6 viremia and clinical findings in infants with exanthem subitum. J Pediatr 118:891–895, 1991.
2. Chetham MM, Roberts KB: Infectious mononucleosis in adolescents. Pediatr Ann 20:208–213, 1991.
3. Feigin RD, Cherry JD (eds): Textbook of Pediatric Infectious Diseases, 3rd ed. Philadelphia, W.B. Saunders, 1992.
4. Grose C: The many faces of infectious mononucleosis: The spectrum of Epstein-Barr virus infection in children. Pediatr Rev 7:35–44, 1985.
5. Hartley AH, Rasmussen JE: Infectious exanthems. Pediatr Rev 9:321–329, 1988.
6. Hathaway WE, Groothuis JR, Hay WW, Paisley JW (eds): Current Pediatric Diagnosis and Treatment, 11th ed. East Norwalk, CT, Appleton & Lange, 1993.
7. Mandell GL, Douglas RG, Bennett JE (eds): Principles and Practice of Infectious Diseases, 3rd ed. New York, John Wiley & Sons, 1990.
8. Nelson JD: Current Therapy in Pediatric Infectious Disease. St. Louis, C.V. Mosby, 1986.
9. Oski FA (ed): Principles and Practices of Pediatrics. Philadelphia, J.B. Lippincott Co., 1990.
10. Peter G (ed): Report of the Committee on Infectious Diseases, 22nd ed. Elk Grove Village, IL, American Academy of Pediatrics, 1991.
11. Sumaya CV: Epstein-Barr virus serologic testing: Diagnostic indications and interpretations. Pediatr Infect Dis 86:337–342, 1986.
12. Sumaya CV: New perspectives on infectious mononucleosis. Contemp Pediatr November 1989, pp 58–76.
13. Yamanski K, Shiraki K, Kondo T, et al: Identification of human herpesvirus-6 as a causal agent for exanthem subitum. Lancet 1:1065–1067, 1988.

72. INFREQUENT INFECTIONS IN CHILDREN

Roger M. Barkin, M.D.

1. Is it true that infrequent means unimportant?
Infectious diseases account for a significant percentage of the visits for acute illness to an emergency department (ED) by children. Although the vast majority of conditions are self-limiting and infrequent, some infections are of particular significance from the perspective of being life-threatening and requiring consideration in the differential diagnosis of many presenting complaints. It should be emphasized that a number of conditions are discussed in other sections of this book. Infections that are not multisystem are generally covered in the organ-specific chapter.

2. What are the most common findings associated with botulism in children?
Botulism results from ingestion of preformed toxins (canned vegetables, etc.), ingestion of spores in infant botulism (honey), or spore contamination of open wounds. *Clostridium botulinum* produces a neurotoxin that blocks the presynaptic release of acetylcholine following an incubation period of 12–48 hours. Clinically, patients develop symmetric descending paralysis with weakness and equal deep tendon reflexes associated with a normal sensorium. Pupils are fixed and dilated with oculomotor paralysis, blurred vision, diplopia, ptosis, and photophobia. Associated findings may include slurred speech, nausea,

vomiting, constipation, vertigo, dry mouth, dysphagia, and urinary retention. Dyspnea and rales, progressing to respiratory failure, may be noted.

3. Are there specific measures that should be initiated in the patient with botulism?
Initial management must focus upon support, airway maintenance, and monitoring. Trivalent ABE antitoxin should be administered and is available from the Centers for Disease Control (404-639-3356/2888) or local state health departments.

4. What are the distinct clinical presentations of diphtheria?
Corynebacterium diphtheriae produces an exotoxin that results in four patterns of clinical findings. The pharyngeal-tonsillar complex consists of a sore throat, fever, vomiting, dysphagia, and malaise associated with a gray, closely adherent pseudomembrane. Respiratory obstruction may develop. Less common findings include laryngeal presentation with hoarseness and loss of voice. Serosanguinous nasal discharge may persist for weeks. A sharply demarcated ulcer may develop on the skin with a membranous base. The diagnosis is confirmed by Loeffler medium and tellurite agar cultures and Gram stain.

5. How is the child with diphtheria treated?
After assuring stability of the airway and absence of associated cardiovascular dysfunction secondary to myocarditis, antitoxin should be initiated after intradermal/conjunctival tests for horse serum sensitivity. Concurrently, antibiotics should be initiated with penicillin, or with erythromycin in the penicillin-allergic patient.

6. What clinical findings must be present to make the diagnosis of Kawasaki's syndrome?
A multisystem disease, Kawasaki's syndrome is also known as mucocutaneous lymph node syndrome (MCLS). The etiology is thought to be related to lymphotropic retrovirus, although the epidemiology is undefined. The syndrome is triphasic in clinical presentation. An acute febrile episode lasts for 7–10 days with the appearance of six major diagnostic criteria, at least five of which must be present for confirmation.
  1. Fever >38.5°C (usually 38.5–40°C) for at least 5 days. The fever begins abruptly and may last as long as 23 days.
  2. Discrete bilateral, nonexudative, conjunctival infection, usually occurring within 2 days of the onset of fever and sometimes lasting 1–2 weeks.
  3. Mouth changes appearing 1–3 days after onset and possibly lasting for 1–2 weeks. Erythema, fissuring and crusting of the lips, a diffuse, oropharyngeal erythema, and strawberry tongue may be present.
  4. Peripheral changes beginning after 3–5 days and lasting 1–2 weeks. The hands and feet may be indurated. Erythema of the palms and soles is present; desquamation of the tips of fingers and toes occurs 2–3 weeks after the onset of illness.
  5. Erythematous, polymorphous rash occurs concurrently with the fever and spreads from the extremities to the trunk. It usually disappears within a week.
  6. Enlarged lymph nodes, usually cervical and over 1.5 cm.

7. What is the most significant complication of Kawasaki's disease?
The most significant complication is coronary artery disese caused by arteritis, aneurysm, or thrombosis. Other findings may include diarrhea, vomiting, hydrops of the gallbladder, leukocytosis, cough, proteinuria, arthritis, meningismus, and CSF pleocytosis.

8. What infectious conditions should be considered in the child presenting with diffuse erythroderma?
Several acute infectious entities may present with diffuse erythroderma: a scarlatiniform rash caused by group A streptococcus, *S. aureus,* or a viral illness; scalded skin syndrome

(S. aureus), toxic epidermal necrolysis or erythema multiforme caused by a variety of infections and drugs; Kawasaki's syndrome; toxic shock syndrome *(S. aureus)*; and leptospirosis.

9. How do young children present when they have infectious mononucleosis?
Caused by Epstein-Barr virus, infectious mononucleosis most frequently occurs in adolescents and young adults. Young children may have fever, diarrhea, pharyngitis, otitis media, pneumonia, lymphadenopathy, hepatomegaly, and splenomegaly. In contrast, adults more commonly have a 3–5 day prodrome of malaise, anorexia, nausea, and vomiting, which is followed by high fevers, pharyngitis, lymphadenopathy (especially cervical), and splenomegaly. The Monospot and heterophil antibody tests are usually negative in children under 5 years of age, requiring specific Epstein-Barr virus titers to make a definitive diagnosis. Serologic diagnosis can be done by measuring antibody to viral capsid antigen, which rises above 1:160 during acute infection.

10. What are the clinical characteristics of the patient with toxic shock syndrome?
Toxic shock syndrome is usually associated with *S. aureus* secondary to a toxin elaborated by the coagulase-positive organism. Findings may include:
  1. Fever over 38.9° C
  2. Rash that is diffuse, blanching, macular, erythematous, nonpruritic
  3. Desquamation 1–2 weeks after the onset of illness, particularly of the palms and soles
  4. Hypotension
  5. Involvement of three or more of the following organ systems: gastrointestinal (vomiting or diarrhea), muscular (myalgia), mucous membranes (vaginal, oropharyngeal, conjunctival hyperemia), renal (elevated BUN/creatinine, pyuria), hepatic (elevated liver function tests), hematologic (thrombocytopenia), or central nervous (disorientation, altered consciousness)

11. What are the three stages of clinical progression of the child with pertussis?
Pertussis (or whooping cough) is caused by *Bordetella pertussis*, occurring in all age groups. It peaks in late summer and early fall with an incubation period of 7–10 days. Initially patients have respiratory complaints of fever, rhinorrhea, and conjunctivitis lasting up to 2 weeks (catarrhal). The paroxysmal phase follows; a severe cough, hypoxia, unremitting paroxysms, and vomiting may occur for up to 2–4 weeks. Apnea, pneumonia, pneumothorax, seizures, and hypoxia may occur concurrently. In the convalescent phase there is an associated residual cough.

12. What are the typical stages of Reye syndrome?
Reye syndrome is an acute, noninflammatory encephalopathy with altered level of consciousness, cerebral edema without perivascular or meningeal inflammation, and fatty metamorphosis of the liver, probably secondary to mitochondrial dysfunction. It is a multisystem disease that probably has many associated etiologies, the findings often being referred to as "Reye-life syndrome." Salicylate ingestion has been incriminated. Clinically patients present with a respiratory or GI prodrome followed in several days with an encephalopathic picture that is marked by behavorial changes and a deteriorating level of consciousness. Progression of brainstem dysfunction occurs in a cephalocaudal pattern:
  0 Alert, wakeful
  I Lethargy. Follows verbal comments, normal posture, purposeful response to pain, brisk pupillary light reflex, and normal oculocephalic reflex
  II Combative or stuporous, inappropriate verbalizing, normal posture, purposeful or nonpurposeful response to pain, sluggish pupillary reaction, and conjugate deviation on doll's eye maneuver

   III   Comatose, decorticate posture and decerebrate response to pain, sluggish pupillary reaction, conjugate deviation on doll's eye maneuver

   IV   Comatose, decerebrate posture and decerebrate response to pain, sluggish pupillary reflexes, and inconsistent or absent oculocephalic reflex

    V   Comatose, flaccid, no response to pain, no pupillary response, no oculocephalic reflex

BIBLIOGRAPHY

1. American Academy of Pediatrics: Report of the Committee on Infectious Diseases. Elk Groove, IL, 1991.
2. American Heart Association Committee on Rheumatic Fever, Endocarditis, and Kawasaki Disease: Diagnostic guidelines for Kawasaki disease. Am J Dis Child 144:1210, 1990.
3. Newburger JW, Takahashi M, Beiser AS: A single intravenous infusion of gamma globulin as compared with four infusions in the treatment of acute Kawasaki syndrome. N Engl J Med 324:1633, 1991.
4. Rogers MF, Schonberger LB, Hurwitz ES, et al: National Reye's syndrome surveillance. Pediatrics 75:260, 1985.
5. Weston WL: Practical Pediatric Dermatology, 2nd ed. Boston, Little, Brown, 1985.

73. CHILD ABUSE

Merle Miller, M.D.

1. What constitutes child abuse?

Child abuse refers to a broad range of behavior on the part of caretakers that is injurious to a child. It may consist of **physical abuse**, with direct trauma to the child (sometimes referred to as nonaccidental trauma, NAT); **neglect** of basic needs of food, clothing, shelter, or parental love; or **emotional abuse**, which may retard social and psychological development. **Sexual abuse** is defined as "the involvement of dependent, developmentally immature children and adolescents in sexual activities they do not fully comprehend, are unable to give informed consent to, and that violate the social taboos of family roles."

2. How common is child abuse?

No one really knows. Estimates are complicated by varying definitions of child abuse and by reporting biases. A national study in 1987 indicated that each year 1.5% of children in the U.S. are neglected and 1% of children are physically abused. Studies show a prevalence rate of 9–10% for child abuse in children treated in the ED.

3. What are the contributing factors or warning signs of child abuse?

Child abuse occurs in all cultural, ethnic, socioeconomic, and racial groups. An abusive episode occurs in the context of the "right parent, right child, and right day." Factors contributing to the setting for abuse include socioeconomic stressors such as joblessness, homelessness, and poor social support systems. Parents involved are often those with unrealistic expectations, poor impulse control, or substance abuse. The abused child may have been unwanted, difficult to rear, or poorly bonded (premature or stepchild).

4. What are some of the important historical indicators of child abuse?

In addition to the family characteristics listed above, historical indicators of child abuse include:

- Multiple previous hospital visits
- A history of untreated injuries
- Delay in seeking medical attention
- Cause of trauma unknown according to parents
- Cause of trauma inappropriate for developmental age of child
- History incompatible with physical findings

5. Who is most commonly the perpetrator of child abuse?
In 95% of cases, the abuser is a parent.

6. What are the most common organ systems involved in ED presentation of an abused child?
Cutaneous, skeletal, and neurologic findings are most common. Up to 50% of children hospitalized for abuse present with burns, bruises, or other dermatologic findings.

7. What physical findings are clues to child abuse?
Although somewhat subjective in nature, the emotional affect and interactions between parent and child may raise the suspicion of abuse. However, the following signs are visible clues to child abuse:
- Multiple lesions in various stages of healing (bruises, fractures)
- Geometric or bilateral injuries
- Bruises in unusual locations (accidental bruises usually overlie bony prominences)
- Immersion burns (sharp demarcation, no splash marks)
- Characteristic patterns in bruises or burns (hand, iron, cord, teeth)
- Retinal hemorrhages (dilate pupil for optimal exam)
- Sudden change in neurologic status
- Failure to thrive in absence of chronic disease (weight more than two standard deviations below mean expected for age)

8. How does the presence of bruising help make the diagnosis of child abuse?
The appearance of multiple bruises at different stages of healing is highly suggestive of physical abuse and must be documented. The transition of unoxygenated blood to bilirubin and then to hemosiderin accounts for the color change.

0–2 days	swollen, tender, red-blue	7–10 days	yellow
3–5 days	blue-purple	10–14 days	brown
5–7 days	green	14–28 days	resolved

9. What fractures are suggestive of child abuse?
Fifty-six percent of fractures in children less than 1 year of age are nonaccidental. Multiple fractures of different ages and spiral fractures in preambulatory children are characteristic of child abuse. Epiphyseal separation and metaphyseal chip fractures are associated with traction, rotation, and shaking injuries and are virtually diagnostic of nonaccidental trauma. Rib and spine fractures are considered strong evidence of abuse. Increased periosteal reaction results from traction and torsional forces as a limb is grasped and pulled. However, only 20–36% of abused children will have detectable fractures.

10. What is a "skeletal survey"? Who should receive one?
A skeletal survey includes radiographs of the skull, AP views of the chest, long bones and hands, and spine films. A skeletal survey should be performed in any preverbal child in whom abuse is suspected. The radiologist should be informed of the reason for the exam. There is a high false-negative rate of skeletal surveys and repeat films or bone scans may be necessary.

11. What neurologic syndromes can result from child abuse?

The **shaken baby syndrome** refers to intracranial hemorrhage resulting from violent shaking of an infant. These children present most often with a chief complaint of respiratory distress. The diagnosis is suggested by retinal hemorrhages and xanthrochromic or bloody spinal fluid. CT or MRI scans confirm the diagnosis. Fifty percent of children who present in coma after shaking will die and half of the survivors will have significant neurologic sequelae.

12. When child abuse is suspected in the ED, what else should be considered in the differential diagnosis?

Coagulation disorders
Mongolian spots
Henoch-Schönlein purpura
Scurvy or rickets
Osteogenesis imperfecta
Folk remedies such as Vietnamese coin rubbing (C'ao Gio)
Sudden infant death syndrome (SIDS)

13. When should sexual abuse of a child be suspected?

First and foremost, sexual abuse must be investigated if the child reports it. Changes in behavior such as sleep disturbances, enuresis, poor school performance, and abdominal pain have been observed in newly identified sexually abused children. Other signs of sexual abuse include sexually transmitted disease (STD) in a prepubescent girl or genital trauma. The size of the vaginal opening, used traditionally to assess vaginal assault, is variable and positional and may not be reliable.

14. What data should be obtained in the ED when evaluating a sexually abused child?

For acute assault, the sexual assault forensic evidence kit should be utilized, including chlamydia test, gonococcus (GC) cultures of cervix, pharynx and rectum, vaginal swabs, saliva samples, pubic hair controls, blood for ABO typing, pregnancy test (if postmenarchal), and VDRL.

15. Should sexually abused children be given antibiotic prophylaxis for STDs?

Prophylactic antibiotics are probably not indicated after single assault but may be used if there is possibility of poor follow-up or high parent or patient anxiety. Victims of chronic sexual assault should be cultured initially.

16. Should all abused children be admitted to the hospital?

If medically indicated, such as for head trauma, abused children must be admitted. Otherwise, a safe disposition must be arranged, using social service or police protection for the child as necessary.

17. What is the extent of legal responsibility of an ED caregiver in caring for a child who has been abused?

The chief responsibility of ED physicians is to recognize and report child abuse. Physicians are mandated by law to notify local child protection authorities of suspected child abuse cases. Failure to do so is usually a misdemeanor of the fourth degree and is considered a malpractice of omission. The parents should be calmly informed of the report. The physician is also obligated to arrange a safe disposition for the child.

BIBLIOGRAPHY

1. American Academy of Pediatrics Committee on Child Abuse and Neglect: Guidelines for the evaluation of sexual abuse of children. Pediatrics 87:254, 1991.

2. Johnson CF: Inflicted injury versus accidental injury. Pediatr Clin North Am 37:791, 1990.
3. Ludwig S, Warman M: Shaken baby syndrome: A review of 20 cases. Ann Emerg Med 13:104, 1984.
4. Merten DF, Carpenter BLM: Radiologic imaging of inflicted injury in the child abuse syndrome. Pediatr Clin North Am 37:816, 1990.
5. Paradise JE: The medical evaluation of the sexually abused child. Pediatr Clin North Am 36:839, 1990.
6. Schmitt BD, Krugman RD: Abuse and neglect of children. In Berman RE, Kliegman RM, Nelson WE, et al (eds): Nelson's Textbook of Pediatrics, 14th ed. Philadelphia, W.B. Saunders, 1992, p 79.
7. Tercier A: Child abuse. In Rosen P, et al (eds): Emergency Medicine: Concepts and Clinical Practice, 3rd ed. St. Louis, Mosby–Year Book, 1992, pp 2717–2735.
8. Wilson EF: Estimation of the age of cutaneous contusions in child abuse. Pediatrics 60:750, 1977.

74. CONSCIOUS SEDATION OF THE PEDIATRIC PATIENT

F. Keith Battan, M.D.

1. What is the difference between sedation and conscious sedation?

Sedation refers to blunting of the level of consciousness (LOC). Conscious or light sedation refers to a minimal depression in LOC wherein the child is awake but may have droopy eyes and slightly slurred speech. The child should be able to respond to verbal command or physical stimulation and maintain protective airway reflexes. Deep sedation implies a depressed LOC from which the child is not easily aroused and protective airway reflexes are partially or totally lost. General anesthesia represents the end of this continuum. Conscious or light sedation is the optimal state for sedation of children in the emergency department (ED). Care must be taken because any sedative can result in general anesthesia if given in sufficient doses, which is not desirable in the ED due to the risk of cardiorespiratory depression and aspiration.

2. What is the difference between a sedative and an analgesic?

An analgesic treats pain, whereas a sedative or anxiolytic only relieves fear and anxiety. Some analgesics, particularly narcotics, have both sedative and analgesic properties, which make them useful for certain procedures. If a procedure is both painful and frightening (e.g., chest tube insertion), the child will benefit from both sedation and analgesia produced either by multiple or single agents.

3. Why would you want to sedate a child?

If you're reading this answer, you've obviously never tried to perform a procedure such as complicated laceration repair on a screaming, thrashing, uncooperative toddler! Children who may benefit from sedation are those undergoing painful or frightening procedures, including laceration repair, incision and drainage of abscesses, burn care, reduction of fractures or dislocations, examinations following sexual assault, and diagnostic procedures such as CT or MRI. The age group that generally benefits maximally from sedation is toddlers or preschool-age children, although older children sometimes require sedation for successful completion of a procedure. Effective ED sedation may enable the clinician to repair a wound that otherwise would require general anesthesia in the operating room. In addition to relieving pain, conscious sedation relieves excessive fear and anxiety in young patients.

4. What's wrong with "brutacaine"?

Brutacaine—simply holding the child down and performing the procedure—can result in a crying, thrashing patient whose injury is difficult to examine, explore, and repair. Continuous crying leaves the child, family, and staff exhausted and appears to onlookers as simple torture. The child is left with unpleasant memories and may fear return visits for care. This factor is particularly important for children requiring repeat procedures such as lumbar punctures or burn care. On the other hand, there is no morbidity (other than possibly psychologic) associated with brutacaine, and this method is appropriate for short, simple, uncomplicated procedures.

5. What are the characteristics of an ideal sedative?

Produce effective anxiolysis, even during painful procedures

Be safe: produce a predictable degree of sedation for a given dose and have minimal effects on airway reflexes and cardiorespiratory status

Minimize movement

Provide amnesia for the procedure

Produce no adverse interactions with other agents that may be used concurrently

Be potentially reversible

Be administered painlessly

Most importantly, have rapid onset, short duration, and rapid recovery. These factors allow the sedative to be given incrementally over a short time span (i.e., titrated) until the desired level of sedation for the particular patient and procedure is reached.

6. What is a poor sedative?

It has the converse of the characteristics outlined in question 5. One example is the combination DPT (Demerol, Phenergan, and Thorazine), or, more appropriately, mpc (meperidine, promethazine, and chlorpromazine). This combination, still used at some centers, has potential side effects of: oversedation (some children are sedated for 8 hours and are not normal for up to 36 hours); extrapyramidal reactions; life-threatening side effects such as respiratory arrest and hypotension, even at less-than-recommended doses; painful IM administration required; highly variable onset and sedative effects; and inability to titrate the dosage. The clinician must accept the sedation level achieved, which may be either inadequate or excessive. These factors make DPT an undesirable and unpredictable choice in a progressive ED.

7. What are the risks and costs associated with sedation?

• With oversedation, there is risk for: (1) loss of airway reflexes with concomitant risk of vomiting and aspiration; (2) hypoventilation with resultant hypoxia, hypercarbia, and cardiopulmonary arrest; (3) hypotension; and (4) laryngospasm.

• Use of sedative agents may entail additional costs for drugs, monitoring, and intravenous lines. Additional ED personnel and time are sometimes necessary during procedures involving sedation. However, if an OR trip is avoided by performing a procedure under conscious sedation in the ED, there can be an overall savings.

• Because of the risks involved, at least verbal informed consent should be obtained and documented on the chart.

8. What monitoring is appropriate during conscious sedation?

The best "monitor" is a skilled, dedicated observer who is not involved in the procedure and who can observe the child's LOC, response to verbal and physical stimulation, airway patency, respiratory function, and perfusion. Sedated children should not be left unobserved.

The monitoring required is dependent on the patient and the medications used. The more potent the agent, the more complete the monitoring that is required. Some agents, such as chloral hydrate, do not require monitoring other than by clinical means. Full monitoring consists of continuous cardiopulmonary monitoring, including pulse oximetry, and frequent blood pressure determinations. If single agents or combinations are used that have the possibility of serious side effects, or if deep sedation is inadvertently reached, IV access should be established and full monitoring and constant observation continued during the procedure.

Personnel and equipment to perform airway management and resuscitation must be readily available. Ideally, patients should be kept NPO for several hours before the procedure if sedatives are to be used, but this is rarely possible in an ED setting. Keep in mind the general (and usually accurate) rule that children's stomachs are always full.

9. Are there any children who should not receive conscious sedation in the ED?
Relative contraindications to conscious sedation in the ED pertain to the risk of complications, including aspiration and potential difficulty in managing the airway if that should become necessary. Children who may be better candidates for OR procedures under more controlled conditions include: unstable patients, including patients with abnormal mental status or hemodynamic instability; infants less than 6 months of age; children with abnormal airways, such as Pierre-Robin anomaly; children with cerebral palsy and abnormal swallowing mechanisms; the rare child with apnea or abnormal breathing regulation; children with seizure disorders; and children with gastroesophageal reflux.

10. What should I do if a child experiences respiratory depression or becomes poorly perfused while sedated?
Specific treatment: For narcotics and benzodiazepines, specific reversing agents are available. Naloxone (0.1 mg/kg IV, IM, ET, up to 4 mg per dose) reverses narcotic effects, and flumazenil reverses benzodiazepine overdose.

General measures: Discontinue sedative or narcotic administration. Maintain the airway and provide assisted ventilation, initially with bag-valve-mask ventilation, then with endotracheal intubation if necessary. If poor perfusion or shock is present (capillary refill time >2 seconds, cool extremities, weak pulses, poor tone, etc.), obtain vascular access and initiate treatment with a bolus infusion of 20 cc/kg of crystalloid solution.

11. Discuss the options available for conscious sedation.
1. **Midazolam** (Versed), the first water-soluble benzodiazepine, has particular usefulness in pediatrics. Its rapid onset and short duration of action make it ideal for titration of sedation level. It can be given by oral, rectal, intranasal, intramuscular, or intravenous routes. The former three routes have the advantage of painless administration. Although some clinicians believe in the maxim of "spare the needle, spoil the child," children fear injections and IVs more than any illness or injury. The pharmacokinetics of midazolam are nearly the same clinically when the drug is given intranasally, as when given intravenously and of course no injection is required. Oral and rectal administration result in relatively delayed onset, titration is difficult, and higher doses are required due to extensive first-pass hepatic metabolism. Intramuscular injections of midazolam can be combined with opioid analgesics in the same syringe if systemic analgesia is desired or they can be given sequentially by IV infusion. Intravenous administration allows optimal ability to titrate the dose to the desired sedation level and provides a "lifeline" if resuscitation becomes necessary. Children expected to undergo complicated or prolonged procedures are best sedated by this route.

2. **Barbiturates.** These agents minimize movement during the procedure, which makes them advantageous for diagnostic studies such as CT or MRI. Rectal administration of thiopental is safe and effective. Onset of action with IV administration is rapid. Potential side effects, although uncommon, include respiratory and cardiac depression and laryngospasm.

3. **Narcotics.** These analgesics, such as morphine, meperidine, and fentanyl, also have sedative effects. They can be combined with anxiolytics such as the benzodiazepines. Both desired and adverse effects, such as respiratory depression, are potentiated when given together; therefore, initial sedative doses should be reduced when combined. Fentanyl has particular usefulness in an ED setting because of its rapid onset, accurate dosing, and rapid recovery. IV administration is required. Like all narcotics, fentanyl has side effects of respiratory and cardiac depression, apnea, nausea, and vomiting. When fentanyl is given rapidly or in high doses, the "wooden-chest syndrome" (thoracic and abdominal wall rigidity) can occur. This muscular rigidity can be reversed by naloxone or neuromuscular blockade, allowing the clinician to assist respiration. Because of these potent side effects, full monitoring by continuous clinical observation, cardiorespiratory monitor, and pulse oximetry is necessary. Blood pressure should be determined every 10 minutes.

4. **Ketamine.** Ketamine is chemically related to the drug of abuse, phencyclidine (PCP), but has advantages for pediatric ED sedation. It produces sedation, a dissociative amnesia, and weak analgesia, and has the advantage of not causing cardiorespiratory depression. Time to onset of acceptable sedation is within 5 minutes in most children, and recovery time is reasonably rapid. Ketamine can be given IV but traditionally has been given IM. When ketamine is given in very large doses, side effects include random purposeless movements, nausea and vomiting, laryngospasm, and respiratory depression. Contrary to conventional reports, the rate of laryngospasm is quite low—0.017% in a recent review of 11,589 cases. Because of its sialagogue (salivation-enhancing) effects, ketamine is frequently given with atropine in the same syringe. In addition to the general contraindications listed above, ketamine should not be used in the presence of pulmonary disease, hypertension, glaucoma, psychosis, thyroid disease, or porphyria. Unpleasant emergence reactions and nightmares seem to be unusual in children. Clinical observation as well as pulse oximetry and cardiac monitoring should be continuously performed when administering ketamine.

5. **Nitrous oxide.** Pediatric dentistry uses N_2O safely and effectively. It is an excellent sedative and also has weak analgesic properties. It has no significant side effects when used as a 50/50 N_2O/O_2 mixture, but should not be used in the presence of pneumothoraces or bowel obstructions. Emesis is a risk, as in all sedated patients. Clinicians should be trained in the delivery of nitrous oxide. Clinical monitoring only is required.

Selected Agents for Conscious Sedation

	DOSE	ROUTE	MONITORING	NOTE
Nitrous oxide	30–50% NO_2	Inhalation	Clinical Oximetry	Older children able to hold mask
Midazolam	0.1 mg/kg 0.3 mg/kg 0.5 mg/kg	IV, IM IN PR, PO	Cardiac monitor Oximetry BP	Titrate to effect
Pentobarbital	4–6 mg/kg 2–6 mg/kg slowly	IM IV	Cardiac monitor	Less spontaneous movements
Ketamine	1 mg/kg 3–4 mg/kg	IV IM	Cardiac monitor Oximetry BP	Dissociative amnesia Many spontaneous movements
Fentanyl	2–4 μg/kg slowly	IV	Cardiac monitor Oximetry BP	Avoid rapid or high-dose infusions. Use with caution.

PO = oral, PR = rectal, IN = intranasal, IM = intramuscular, IV = intravenous, oximetry = continuous pulse oximetry, and BP = blood pressure taken every 10 minutes.

12. How can I successfully sedate a child?
Preparation of the child is important. Provide a calm and quiet atmosphere. Careful explanation of the procedure and the avoidance of untruths help to allay the fears of the child. Clinicians increasingly appreciate the fact that the presence of the parents in the room during the procedure decreases the child's anxiety and facilitates the procedure. After the sedative is administered, the child should be allowed to remain in a quiet, calm atmosphere, with the parents present, until the full sedative effect is achieved. If the child becomes agitated, it will subsequently be much more difficult to achieve a desirable sedation level. A trained observer should monitor the child as he or she becomes sedated. After sufficient time for the expected sedative effects to appear, gently stimulate the child to ascertain his reaction. If the child reacts with agitation and crying, and still has a normal mental status, then administer additional sedative and continue to monitor. For example, with IV or IN midazolam, if the LOC is normal and the child is still too agitated to start the procedure after 3–4 minutes, give half the initial dose and reassess the child in another 3–4 minutes. Although the initial dose of IV midazolam is 0.1 mg/kg, up to 0.7–0.8 mg/kg in repeated doses may be necessary to achieve adequate sedation. The risk of cardiorespiratory depression is generally proportional to the degree of mental status depression. Fentanyl is a notable exception. Only the amount necessary to achieve conscious sedation as described above should be used, and the child should be monitored fully for side effects. When the sedation level is judged adequate, then proceed, keeping in mind that short-acting sedatives may require re-dosing during prolonged procedures.

13. When can children who have received sedatives be discharged from the ED?
The child should have normal vital signs, be reasonably alert, be able to sit without assistance, take liquids by mouth, and respond to commands given in a normal voice. Keep in mind that some children (e.g., the author's), never respond to commands given in a normal voice!

BIBLIOGRAPHY

1. Guidelines for the elective use of conscious sedation, deep sedation, and general anesthesia in pediatric patients. American Academy of Pediatrics, Committee on Drugs, Section on Anesthesiology. Pediatrics 76:317–321, 1985.
2. Billmire DA, Neale HW, Gregory RO: Use of IV fentanyl in the outpatient treatment of pediatric facial trauma. J Trauma 25:1079–1080, 1985.
3. Diament MJ, Stanley P: The use of midazolam for sedation of infants and children. Am J Roentgenol 150:377–378, 1988.
4. Gamis AS, Knapp JF, Glenski JA: Nitrous oxide analgesia in a pediatric emergency department. Ann Emerg Med 18:177–181, 1989.
5. Green SM, Nakamura R, Johnson NE: Ketamine sedation for pediatric procedures: Part 1, A prospective series. Ann Emerg Med 19:1024–1032, 1990.
6. Hennes HM, Wagner V, Bonadio WA, et al: The effect of oral midazolam on anxiety of preschool children during laceration repair. Ann Emerg Med 19:1006–1009, 1990.
7. O'Brien JF, Falk JL, Carey BE, et al: Rectal thiopental compared with intramuscular meperidine, promethazine, and chlorpromazine for pediatric sedation. Ann Emerg Med 20:644–647, 1991.
8. Sievers TD, Yee JD, Foley ME, et al: Midazolam for conscious sedation during pediatric oncology procedures: Safety and recovery parameters. Pediatrics 88:1172–1179, 1991.
9. Terndrup TE, Dire DJ, Madden CM, et al: A prospective analysis of intramuscular meperidine, promethazine, and chlorpromazine in pediatric emergency department patients. Ann Emerg Med 20:31–35, 1991.
10. Votey SR, Bosse GM, Bayer MJ, et al: Flumazenil: A new benzodiazepine antagonist. Ann Emerg Med 20:181–188, 1991.

XIV. Toxicologic Emergencies

75. GENERAL APPROACH TO POISONINGS

Ken Kulig, M.D.

1. What are the 12 most common causes of death from acute poisoning reported to poison centers?

The 1991 annual report of the American Association of Poison Control Centers lists the following:

Category	No.	% of All Exposures in Category
Analgesics	190	0.104
Antidepressants	188	0.525
Sedative/hypnotics	97	0.166
Stimulants and street drugs	90	0.434
Cardiovascular drugs	87	0.348
Alcohols	72	0.143
Gases and fumes	49	0.188
Asthma therapies	39	0.229
Chemicals	37	0.069
Hydrocarbons	36	0.057
Cleaning substances	26	0.014
Pesticides (including rodenticides)	18	0.026

2. What is the current role of syrup of ipecac in treating acute poisoning?

Although syrup of ipecac induces vomiting within 20–30 minutes in most persons who are administered a therapeutic dose, very little poison is removed; there are more effective means of decontaminating the gastrointestinal (GI) tract. Ipecac may have a role in treating children at home, who frequently can be administered a dose soon after ingestion. By the time most patients present to a hospital, however, too much time has elapsed for syrup of ipecac to be of benefit. Its use also delays the administration of activated charcoal, which needs to be administered as quickly as possible for maximal benefit.

3. What is the current role of gastric lavage in treating acute poisonings?

Gastric lavage has the advantage over ipecac in that it works faster in emptying stomach contents, and activated charcoal can be administered down the lavage tube before it is pulled. Gastric lavage can be accomplished without prior tracheal intubation in most patients, but it is advised that airway equipment, including suction, be immediately available at the bedside. Placing the patient on his or her left side in mild Trendelenburg position will help to prevent aspiration if vomiting occurs. Nasogastric tubes are too small to remove pills or large pill fragments; whenever gastric lavage is performed, a large-bore (36- to 40-French tube in adults) should be placed through the mouth. A bite block with an oral airway will prevent the patient from biting the tube.

Gastric lavage may be contraindicated if acids or alkalis have been ingested, on the theory that the risk of esophageal perforation is excessive. Ingestion of petroleum distillates is also commonly listed as a contraindication to lavage because of the danger of causing a hydrocarbon aspiration. However, the risk of systemic toxicity if toxic material in the stomach is allowed to be absorbed must be considered. Agents such as hydrofluoric acid and chloroform, which have both local and significant systemic toxicity, cause difficult management dilemmas when ingested. It is recommended that consultation with a toxicologist be obtained in such cases.

4. What is the current role of activated charcoal?

Activated charcoal has been shown in numerous studies to be superior to gastric emptying procedures for the treatment of acute overdose. Gastric emptying procedures involve time and some risk to the patient. The time involved in lavaging the patient or in inducing emesis with ipecac is time during which drugs are being actively absorbed. By giving a dose of activated charcoal immediately upon patient presentation, the most effective means of GI decontamination has already been performed should the patient deteriorate. Not all drugs are adsorbed to charcoal, however. Those that are not include lithium, acids and alkalis, potassium, iron, and perhaps others not yet studied.

5. What if the patient is lying about the overdose? Shouldn't gastric emptying be done just to be sure?

It should always be assumed that suicidal overdose patients could be lying about what they took and when they took it. However, because activated charcoal alone is effective at preventing drug absorption and acts sooner when given without prior use of ipecac or lavage, even if the patient is not telling the truth about the overdose, the proper procedure has been done.

6. What about the asymptomatic overdose patient?

It has been advocated by some that simple observation of asymptomatic overdose patients, with treatment only if symptoms develop, is a management option. While this is probably safe for many patients who have ingested trivial overdoses, if a patient in reality ingested something quite dangerous, an opportunity to prevent absorption may have been lost if nothing is done until symptoms develop. Administering a dose of activated charcoal to all patients with a history of drug overdose is easily performed (although often messy) and helps to ensure safe and timely patient disposition.

7. Is there a role for cathartics in treating acute poisoning?

The theory behind cathartics is that they will speed up GI transit time, allowing activated charcoal to catch up with pills in the bowel, and also prevent desorption of drug from activated charcoal. A single dose of a cathartic is commonly used, although this practice is of unproven benefit. Multiple-dose cathartics should never be used because life-threatening complications from electrolyte imbalance may result. A single dose of a saline cathartic such as magnesium sulfate or magnesium citrate, or a single dose of sorbitol (approximately 1 gm/kg), is unlikely to be harmful and may be of slight benefit.

8. What is the current role of whole-bowel irrigation in the treatment of acute poisoning?

Whole-bowel irrigation uses a polyethylene glycol electrolyte solution such as GoLYTELY or Colyte, which is not adsorbed and will flush drugs or chemicals rapidly through the GI tract. This procedure appears to be most useful when radiopaque tablets or chemicals have been ingested, as their progress through the GI tract can be monitored by radiography. This procedure is also commonly used when packets of street drugs such as heroin or cocaine have been ingested and need to be passed through the GI tract as quickly as possible. The limitations of the procedure are that unless the patient is awake, cooperative, and able to sit on a commode, there is a risk of vomiting and aspiration in addition to the logistical problem of having an unconscious patient in bed with massive diarrhea.

9. What is the role of multiple-dose charcoal in the treatment of acute poisoning?

Multiple-dose charcoal has been shown to enhance the elimination of many drugs that have already been absorbed from the GI tract or that are given intravenously. This process has been called "gastrointestinal dialysis," and has been shown to be quite effective for theophylline and perhaps phenobarbital poisoning. Numerous other drugs have been shown to have their pharmacokinetics altered by multiple-dose charcoal, but it is not clear if this makes a clinical difference. Some of these drugs are listed below; new studies are being currently performed on others. For the majority of acute poisonings in which use of multiple-dose charcoal is being contemplated, it should be borne in mind that the primary reason for giving multiple-dose charcoal is to prevent absorption of drugs from the GI tract, not to enhance their elimination from the blood. In the common case of tricyclic antidepressant overdose, for example, multiple-dose charcoal should be used when large amounts of the antidepressant have been ingested to prevent its absorption but not necessarily to enhance its elimination. Many of these drugs have large volumes of distribution, and increasing elimination of the small amount present in the blood is unlikely to be of benefit.

Drugs with Altered Pharmacokinetics in Response to Multiple-dose Charcoal

Amitriptyline	Dextropropoxyphene	Meprobamate	Piroxicam
Atrazine	Diazepam	Methotrexate	Porphyrins
Carbamazepine	Digitoxin	Nadolol	Proscillaridin
Chlorpropamide	Digoxin	Nortriptyline	Quinine
Cyclosporine	Doxepin	Phenobarbital	Salicylates
Dapsone	Glutethimide	Phenylbutazone	Sotalol
Desmethyldiazepam	Imipramine	Phenytoin	Theophylline

10. Is forced diuresis of benefit in the treatment of acute poisoning?

Very few drugs are excreted unchanged in the urine, so that even increasing urine flow significantly above baseline is unlikely to be of benefit. However, by manipulating the pH of the urine by infusions of bicarbonate solution along with enhanced urine flow, in certain cases drug elimination can be increased. This is most commonly used for salicylates and phenobarbital. By placing 3 ampules of sodium bicarbonate in a liter of D5W along with potassium chloride, and infusing this solution at rates sufficient to produce at least a normal urine flow and a urine pH of 7.5 or greater, the elimination of salicylate and phenobarbital can be increased. Intake and output and urine pH should be monitored hourly with a Foley catheter in place. In the presence of pulmonary or cerebral edema, alkaline diuresis is dangerous and should not be undertaken.

There is some suggestion that alkaline diuresis will also work in a similar manner for chlorophenoxy herbicides, but acute poisonings by these agents are rare. The use of high-volume normal saline to treat lithium intoxication is common, and it is certainly important to maintain adequate urine output and serum sodium in this scenario. It is not clear, however, that forced-saline diuresis for lithium intoxication is of extra benefit over simply ensuring normal renal flow.

11. When are extracorporeal techniques such as hemodialysis or hemoperfusion indicated?

Drugs can be successfully removed by extracorporeal maneuvers only if they have relatively small volumes of distribution and hence are found in significant quantities in the circulation, as opposed to having rapid and thorough tissue distribution. This is the case for only a few drugs. In practice, the drugs most commonly dialyzed after overdose include aspirin, lithium, and perhaps theophylline. Dialysis has the advantage over hemoperfusion in that it is frequently easier and faster to get started and can correct fluid and electrolyte abnormalities as it removes drugs. Charcoal hemoperfusion may be more effective at removing drugs that are highly bound to plasma proteins, as the affinity for charcoal may be higher than the affinity for the protein carrier. The disadvantage of hemoperfusion is that unless frequently performed in skilled hands, the procedure can result in frequent canister clotting. In addition, hypocalcemia and a precipitous drop in platelet count are quite common. Drugs for which charcoal hemoperfusion is frequently employed include theophylline, phenobarbital, and a handful of other less common agents such as paraquat and amatoxin.

12. How can the diagnosis of a drug overdose be made when the patient is unconscious and history is unavailable?
The diagnosis of acute overdose is sometimes difficult to make and requires some detective work on the part of the physician. All unconscious patients should receive dextrose and naloxone (Narcan), and a positive respose to either of these is diagnostic. Whenever possible, examination of the pill bottles available to the patient is important, and it is useful to call the pharmacies where the prescriptions were filled to determine if other prescriptions were filled there for different drugs. Discovering which chemical agents were available to the patient, including street drugs, is always important. If track marks are seen, consider street drugs commonly given intravenously such as opiates, cocaine, and amphetamine. The physical examination is extremely useful in narrowing the diagnosis to a class of drug or chemicals. This concept is commonly called toxic syndromes, the most common of which are listed below.

The Most Common Toxic Syndromes

Anticholinergic

Common signs: dementia with mumbling speech, tachycardia, dry flushed skin, dilated pupils, myoclonus, temperature slightly elevated, urinary retention, decreased bowel sounds. Seizures and dysrhythmias may occur in severe cases.

Common causes: antihistamines, antiparkinsonism medication, atropine, scopolamine, amantadine, antipsychotics, antidepressants, antispasmodics, mydriatics, skeletal muscle relaxants, many plants (most notably jimson weed).

Sympathomimetic

Common signs: delusions, paranoia, tachycardia, hypertension, hyperpyrexia, diaphoresis, piloerection, mydriasis, hyperreflexia. Seizures and dysrhythmias may occur in severe cases.

Common causes: cocaine, amphetamine, methaphetamine (and derivatives MDA, MDMA, MDEA, DOB), over-the-counter decongestants (phenylpropanolamine, ephedrine, pseudoephedrine). Caffeine and theophylline overdoses cause similar findings secondary to catecholamine release, except for the organic psychiatric signs.

Opiate/Sedative

Common signs: coma, respiratory depression; miosis, hypotension, bradycardia, hypothermia, pulmonary edema, decreased bowel sounds, hyporeflexia, needle marks.

Common causes: narcotics, barbiturates, benzodiazepines, ethchlorvynol, glutethimide, methyprylon, methaqualone, meprobamate.

Cholinergic

Common signs: confusion/CNS depression; weakness, salivation, lacrimation, urinary and fecal incontinence, GI cramping, emesis, diaphoresis, muscle fasciculations, pulmonary edema, miosis, bradycardia (or tachycardia), seizures.

Common causes: organophosphate and carbamate insecticides, physostigmine, edrophonium, some mushrooms (*Amanita muscaria, Amanita pantherina*, Inocybe sp., Clitocybe sp.).

13. How can a toxicology screen and other ancillary lab tests make the diagnosis of acute poisoning?

Nontoxicologic laboratory tests that are frequently useful include the electrocardiogram, which can help diagnose overdose of trycyclic antidepressants or cardiac medications; chest radiograph, which if demonstrative of noncardiogenic pulmonary edema would make one think of salicylates or opiates; a KUB, looking for radiopaque material, which would make one suspicious of ingestion of a heavy metal, including iron, phenothiazines, chloral hydrate, or chlorinated hydrocarbon solvents. Liver function tests may help to diagnose ingestion of hepatotoxins such as acetaminophen or carbon tetrachloride. A urinalysis may demonstrate the presence of calcium oxalate crystals, suggesting the diagnosis of ethylene glycol poisoning. The acid-base status of the patient is extremely important. Persistent unexplained metabolic acidosis should always prompt the search for other diagnostic clues to aspirin, methanol, or ethylene glycol poisoning. Many other drugs can cause a persistent unexplained metabolic acidosis, including the ingestion of acids themselves, cyanide, carbon monoxide, theophylline, and others. In the work-up of persistent acidosis, a serum osmolality done by freezing point depression can be very useful if it is elevated. A difference between the measured osmolality and the calculated osmolality of greater than 10 is always significant, although a normal osmolol gap does not rule out toxic ingestion.

The toxicology screen, both blood and urine, should be done on any patient who has significant toxicity and when the diagnosis is uncertain. Alternatives to a full toxicology screen include testing discrete serum levels of the toxins in question, doing a urine qualitative test for drugs of abuse, or drawing specimens but holding them until it is determined that a toxicology screen is definitely indicated. More drugs and chemicals are *not* found on typical toxicology screens than *are* found on the screens, although the majority of drugs that are commonly ingested are found on comprehensive toxicology screens. It is important to communicate with the laboratory about which drugs are suspected, which drugs the patient takes therapeutically, and the clinical condition of the patient. Whenever there is a discrepancy between clinical suspicion and findings from toxicology screen, it is useful to communicate with the toxicology laboratory and assist them in determining if other tests are likely to be of benefit. Toxicology screens are expensive, frequently inexact, and frequently do not give all the information that is expected by the clinician. Therefore it is important to interpret the toxicology screens carefully and to know which drugs and chemicals were not screened for.

14. What are some other useful antidotes for common poisonings?

Naloxone and **dextrose** are the most common antidotes and should be given routinely to unconscious overdose patients. Intravenous administration of 2 mg of naloxone that results in awakening of the patient is diagnostic of acute opiate overdose. Lesser doses may be ineffective and should not be used unless it is known that the patient is an opiate addict and that the 2 mg dose of naloxone will precipitate withdrawal. Many drugs and chemicals can cause hypoglycemia, including ethanol, and for this reason dextrose should likewise be given.

Other common antidotes include **physostigmine** for the anticholinergic syndrome. Physostigmine should be used only when the diagnosis of the anticholinergic syndrome is certain, and should seldom if ever be used to treat tricyclic antidepressant poisoning. Seizures and bradydysrhythmias have been reported when used in this setting. A dose of 1–2 mg given slowly intravenously to an adult is usually sufficient.

Digoxin Immune Fab (Digibind) is a safe and effective antidote for digitalis glycoside poisoning and can rapidly reverse coma, dysrhythmias, and hyperkalemia, which can be life threatening. Unlike naloxone, however, Digibind does not work immediately and a full response to therapy may not be seen until approximately 20 minutes after administration. For a life-threatening digitalis overdose when the dose and the serum level are currently unknown, 10 vials of Digibind should be given.

Atropine and **pralidoxime (Protopam)** are antidotes used for cholinesterase inhibitor toxicity. This group of pesticides includes the organophosphates and carbamates, which are commonly found in even household insecticides. Atropine is used to dry up secretions, primarily pulmonary, and pralidoxime is used primarily to reverse the skeletal muscle toxicity of these agents, including weakness and fasciculations.

Flumazenil is a benzodiazepine antagonist that has been shown to be useful in cases of acute benzodiazepine overdose resulting in significant toxicity. It shouldn't be used if there has been a concomitant tricyclic overdose or if the patient is using benzodiazepines for seizure control.

BIBLIOGRAPHY

1. Hofer P, Scollo-Lavizzari G: Benzodiazepine antagonist Ro 15-1788 in self-poisoning: Diagnostic and therapeutic use. Arch Intern Med 145:663–664, 1985.
2. Hoffman RS, Smilkstein M, Goldfrank CR: Whole bowel irrigation and the cocaine body packer: A new approach to a common problem. Am J Emerg Med 8:523–527, 1990.
3. Kellerman AL, Fihn SD, Logerfro JP, et al: Impact of drug screening in suspected overdose. Ann Emerg Med 16:1206–1216, 1987.
4. Kulig KW, Bar-Or D, Cantrill SV, et al: Management of acutely poisoned patients without gastric emptying. Ann Emerg Med 14:562–567, 1985.
5. Litovitz TL, Holm KC, Bailey KM, Schmitz: 1991 Annual Report of the American Association of Poison Control Centers National Data Collection System. Am J Emerg Med 10:452–505, 1992.
6. Merigian KS, Woodard M, Hedges JR, et al: Prospective evaluation of gastric emptying in the self-poisoned patient. Am J Emerg Med 8:479–483, 1990.
7. Olson KR, Pentel PR, Kelley MT: Physical assessment and differential diagnosis of the poisoned patient. Med Toxicol 2:52–81, 1987.
8. Osterloh JD: Utility and reliability of emergency toxicologic testing. Emerg Med Clin North Am 8:693–723, 1990.
9. Smith TW, Butler VP Jr, Haber E, et al: Treatment of life-threatening digitalis intoxication with digoxin-specific Fab antibody fragments: Experience in 26 cases. N Engl J Med 307:1357–1362, 1982.
10. Tenenbein M, Cohen S, Sitar DS: Whole bowel irrigation as a decontamination procedure after acute drug overdose. Arch Intern Med 147:905–907, 1987.

76. THE ALCOHOLS: ETHYLENE GLYCOL, METHANOL, AND ISOPROPYL ALCOHOL

Louis J. Ling, M.D.

1. Why is it important to understand the metabolism of methanol?

The metabolites are the toxins and depend on alcohol dehydrogenase (AD) for their conversion from the parent methanol. Ethanol saturates AD and greatly decreases the amount of the toxin. Folate is a cofactor in the breakdown of formic acid, and, in theory, folate supplementation will maximize its metabolism. Thus, knowledge of the metabolism directs the treatment.

$$\text{Methanol} \xrightarrow{\text{AD}} \underset{\text{(toxic)}}{\text{Formaldehyde}} \rightarrow \underset{\text{(toxic)}}{\text{Formic Acid}} \xrightarrow{\text{folate}} CO_2 + H_2O$$

2. Why is it important to understand the metabolism of ethylene glycol?

As with methanol, ethanol saturates AD, inhibiting conversion of ethylene glycol into its harmful metabolites. Pyridoxine (vitamin B6) and thiamine are cofactors in the final steps to form nonharmful end-products, and should be given to ensure maximum metabolism. Oxalate crystals may not appear until late in the course of the poisoning.

Ethylene glycol

↓   alcohol dehydrogenase

Glycoaldehyde

↓

Glycolic acid   (50% excreted, causes acidosis)

↓

Glyoxylic acid   →   Alpha hydroxy beta-ketoadipate (nontoxic)

         thiamine

↓   \

        Glycine

pyridoxine

     \

        Gamma hydroxy alpha-ketoglutarate

Oxalate

    \

       Oxalomalate

(3% excreted)

crystallizes with calcium in urine, vessels

3. Why are symptoms of ethylene glycol and methanol overdose often delayed?

Because the toxicity of methanol and ethylene glycol is the result of toxic metabolites, it may take 6–12 hours for sufficient quantities of these toxic metabolites to appear and cause symptoms. The delay in onset of symptoms is even greater with concurrent ethanol intoxication.

4. How are methanol and ethylene glycol poisonings similar?

Both methanol and ethylene glycol are initially metabolized by AD. Methanol is metabolized further to formic acid and ethylene glycol is metabolized to glycolic acid, glyoxylic acid, oxalate, and several nontoxic metabolites. Because of these end-products, both poisons result in metabolic acidosis with an anion gap. Because of their low molecular weight, both increase the osmolar gap.

5. What is an anion gap?

Normal anion gap represents the difference between unmeasured anions (such as various proteins, organic acids, phosphates) and unmeasured cations (such as potassium, calcium, and magnesium). The anion gap can be calculated from the formula:

$$\text{Anion gap} = (Na^+) - (HCO_3^- + Cl^-)$$

When metabolic acidosis results from an ingestion or increase of nonvolatile acids, there are increased hydrogen ions with positive charges. Because there is an increase in unmeasured negatively-charged anions and no increases in chloride, the difference between the measured cations and anions is increased, causing an increased anion gap. The normal anion gap is about 12–14 mEq/L. The etiology of increased anion gap can be remembered by the mnemonic A MUD PILES.

A	=	Alcohol		P	=	Paraldehyde
				I	=	Iron, INH
M	=	Methanol		L	=	Lactate
U	=	Uremia		E	=	Ethylene glycol
D	=	Diabetic ketoacidosis		S	=	Salicylate

6. What is an osmolal gap?

Small atoms and molecules in solution are osmotically active and this activity can be measured by a depression in freezing point or elevation in boiling point of the solution. If there is an increase in low-molecular-weight molecules, such as methanol, ethanol, mannitol, isopropyl alcohol, or ethylene glycol, the osmolality increases more than what is calculated from the usual serum molecules. The difference between the actual measured osmolality and the calculated osmolality is the osmolal gap, and a gap greater than 10 mOsm is considered abnormal. Calculated osmolality = $2 \times Na^+$ (mEq/L) + glucose (mg/dl) / 18 + BUN (mg/dl) / 2.8 + ethanol (mg/dl) / 4.3. The inclusion of the ethanol level will exclude those patients who have an elevated osmolal gap from ethanol ingestion alone. Using SI units, the calculated osmolality is = $2 \times Na$ (mEq/L) + glucose (mmole/L) + BUN (mmole/L) + ethanol (mmole/L). The calculated osmolality is 285 ± 5 mOsm/L. A toxic ethylene glycol level of 25 mg/dl can be predicted to increase the osmolal gap 5 mOsm/L. Because of the small effects on the osmolality and the imprecision of the measurement, this test is not precise enough to be definitive. A normal osmolal gap does not exclude toxic levels of methanol or ethylene glycol. The laboratory must use the method of freezing-point depression so that volatile alcohols contributing to an osmolal gap are not boiled away during a boiling point elevation procedure.

7. How toxic are methanol and ethylene glycol?

Death has been reported after 15–30 ml (1–2 tablespoons) of methanol. However, others have survived larger ingestions. A minimum lethal dose for ethylene glycol is approximately 1–2 ml/kg, demonstrating the high toxicity of both of these poisons.

8. What are the signs and symptoms of methanol poisoning?

Methanol is a GI irritant, causing nausea, vomiting, and abdominal pain, as well as CNS intoxication with headache, decreased level of consciousness, and confusion. Ocular toxicity requires close examination for retinal edema and hyperemia of the disc, and for accurate documentation of visual acuity. The metabolic acidosis has been mentioned.

9. What is the toxicity of ethylene glycol?

There is CNS intoxication, GI irritation, and acidosis. Renal failure occurs frequently and is typically delayed in presentation. Ethylene glycol is a frequent cause of death in animals who happen upon some antifreeze and find its appearance and taste appealing. Cause of death for these animals may not be apparent because toxicity is delayed.

10. How should patients with methanol and ethylene glycol poisoning be treated?

Airway protection is paramount in patients with decreased level of consciousness or respiratory depression. Although gastric lavage might be helpful in large ingestions, small volumes and rapid absorption limit its effectiveness. Acidosis should be aggressively treated with sodium bicarbonate. Because ethanol competitively blocks the conversion of both ethanol and ethylene glycol to their toxic metabolites, it allows for elimination of the unchanged poison without injury.

11. What are the indications for ethanol therapy?
Ethanol should be used if ethylene glycol or methanol levels exceed 20 mg/dl; in the presence of acidosis, regardless of drug level; and if there is history of a toxic ingestion while awaiting confirmatory blood methanol or ethylene glycol levels.

12. How do you start and maintain ethanol treatment?
1. Maintain an ethanol level of 100–120 mg/dl:

Load	0.6–0.8 gm/kg
Maintenance	0.11 gm/kg/hr
Dialysis	0.24 gm/kg/hr

2. Oral methods:

Load	Use 20–50% solutions for load per NG tube; 2 cc/kg of 50% gives 0.8 gm/kg. Use stock pharmacy solution and dilute 1:1.
Maintain	0.11–0.13 gm/kg/hr Use 0.16 cc/kg/hr of 95% solutions but dilute with water 1:1 to avoid gastritis and give 0.33 cc/kg/hr. Increase proportionately with dialysis.

3. IV Methods

Load	Use 10% concentration (used as standard treatment for stopping labor) in D5W through a central line at 10 cc/kg.
Maintain	Use 1.6 cc/kg/hr of 10% solution. Increase proportionately with dialysis.

13. What are the indications for hemodialysis?
Dialysis is the primary treatment for these poisons and should be performed in all patients with blood levels over 50 mg/dl of methanol or ethylene glycol, when the metabolic acidosis is not correctable, with pending renal failure, or with visual symptoms in a methanol overdose. Most clinicians recommend dialysis when blood levels exceed 25 mg/dl, if dialysis is readily available.

14. How is isopropyl alcohol poisoning different from methanol and ethylene glycol poisoning?
Isopropyl alcohol is metabolized in the liver to acetone, which results in measurable ketonemia in the serum. Acetone is excreted by the kidney, resulting in ketonuria, and also is exhaled through the lungs, giving patients an acetone aroma on their breath. Because these metabolites are not acidic, isopropyl alcohol poisoning does not result in a metabolic acidosis and is far less toxic than either methanol or ethylene glycol poisoning.

15. What are the symptoms of isopropyl alcohol ingestion?
Isopropyl alcohol, commonly seen as rubbing alcohol, has a four-carbon chain compared with ethanol's two-carbon chain. Because of this, it crosses the blood-brain barrier much faster and is about twice as intoxicating as ethanol. Because it is commonly found in very concentrated solutions and is more potent, the CNS depression can occur rapidly and continue from residual poison in the stomach. Isopropyl alcohol is much more irritating to the gastric mucosa and often causes abdominal pain, vomiting, and hematemesis.

16. What treatment is advisable for isopropyl alcohol poisoning?
Generally patients need observation similar to patients intoxicated with ethanol to watch for respiratory depression. An isopropyl alcohol level is roughly equivalent to an ethanol level twice as high. However, an isopropyl level usually does not add greatly to clinical

observation. In the rare severe instance of coma or hypertension corresponding to isopropyl levels greater than 500 mg/dl, hemodialysis may be helpful because it can greatly enhance removal of isopropyl alcohol from the body.

BIBLIOGRAPHY

1. Becker CE: Methanol poisoning. J Emerg Med 1:51–58, 1983.
2. Brown LG: Ethylene glycol poisoning. Ann Emerg Med 12:501–506, 1983.
3. Dethlefs R, Naraqi S: Ocular manifestations and complications of acute methyl alcohol intoxication. Med J Aust 2:483–485, 1978.
4. Ellenhorn MJ, Barceloux DG: Medical Toxicology: Diagnosis and Treatment of Human Poisoning. New York, Elsevier, 1988.
5. Gabor PA: Ethylene glycol intoxication. Am J Kidney Dis 11:277–279, 1988.
6. Jacobsen D, Sebastian CS, et al: Effects of 4-methylpyrazole, methanol/ethylene glycol antidote, in healthy humans. J Emerg Med 8:455–461, 1990.
7. Keyvan-Larijarni H, Tannenberg AM: Methanol intoxication: Comparison of peritoneal and hemodialysis. Arch Intern Med 134:293–296, 1974.
8. Kulig K, Duff JP, et al: Toxic effects of methanol, ethylene glycol and isopropyl alcohol. Emerg Med 14–29, 1984.
9. Litovitz T: The alcohols: Ethanol, methanol, isopropanol, ethylene glycol. Pediatr Clin North Am 33:311–323, 1986.
10. McCoy HG, Cipolle RJ, et al: Severe methanol poisoning: Application of a pharmacokinetic model for ethanol therapy and hemodialysis. Am J Med 67:804–807, 1979.
11. Momont SL, Dahlberg PJ: Ethylene glycol poisoning. Wisconsin Med J September 1989, pp 16–20.
12. Spillane L, Roberts JR, et al: Multiple cranial nerve deficits after ethylene glycol poisoning. Ann Emerg Med 20:208–210, 1991.

77. ALCOHOL-RELATED DISORDERS

John A. Marx, M.D., FACEP

1. Is a patient who smells of alcohol simply intoxicated?
Perhaps, and in the majority of cases, yes. However, there is a clinically relevant differential of altered mentation in such a patient.

1. Traumatic
   Intracranial hemorrhage
   Hypotension secondary
      to hemorrhage
2. Metabolic
   Hypoglycemia
   Hepatic encephalopathy
   Hypoxia
3. Toxicologic
   Other alcohols
   Other toxins
   Disulfiram
   Disulfiram-ethanol reaction

4. Infectious
   Meningitis, meningoencephalitis
   Brain abscess
   Sepsis
5. Neurologic
   Postictal state
   Alcohol withdrawal
   Wernicke-Korsakoff syndrome

It is critical that every patient assumed to be drunk (only) receive careful initial and serial evaluations. This is neither time-consuming nor expensive.

2. Which pharmacologic agents are best for management of alcohol withdrawal?
Myriad therapies have been tested. The most widely used and time-honored mainstay is the benzodiazepine class. These should be given orally, intravenously, or in combination and titered by clinical response. No single benzodiazepine has been proclaimed the best agent. Pharmacokinetics, the presence of intermediate metabolites, and mostly physician preference are deciding factors.

Haloperidol is an appropriate adjunct for hallucinosis. Theoretical concerns over lowering seizure threshold and exacerbating hemodynamic abnormalities in this class of patients have not been substantiated.

3. What is an appropriate diagnostic work-up for alcohol withdrawal seizures?
Two issues are germane. (1) Is the story consistent with an alcohol withdrawal seizure (AWDS)? (2) Is this the initial presentation and work-up for suspected AWDS?

Typically, AWDS occur approximately 6–96 hours after the last drink and in clusters of 1 to 4. The seizures, usually grand mal, are self-limited. Notably, coincident features of withdrawal may be lacking and lateralizing findings are often present due to underlying structural pathology.

In a first-time evaluation, other causes of or contributors to seizures should be sought. Routine laboratory studies (electrolytes, glucose, magnesium, calcium, toxicologic screen) are rarely useful unless history or physical examination is suggestive. However, a noncontrast CT will help guide management. Nearly 10% of patients demonstrate traumatic, infectious, vascular, or miscellaneous abnormalities. Generally, electroencephalography is not integral to the work-up; it need not be obtained during the first visit. Lumbar puncture is indicated when meningitis, meningoencephalitis, or subarachnoid hemorrhage is suspected.

Subsequent visits demand scrupulous history and physical examination to ensure that other pathologic causes have not developed in the interim. If the presentation matches prior episodes and the findings on current neurologic exam are baseline, no other work-up, including CT, is necessary. Lingering postictal confusion warrants a check of glucose and electrolytes. If the story or examination has significantly changed or is worrisome, the clinician should start from scratch.

4. How should AWDS be managed?
Acute. Active AWDS is handled in routine fashion, i.e., assure patient safety and patent airway and administer D50, naloxone, and intravenous benzodiazepines as needed. If diagnostic evaluation is unremarkable, an observation period of 6–12 hours is optimal because additional seizures are common and will occur within this period. Use of benzodiazepines in the immediate post-seizure observation period and for 2 days thereafter likely decreases the incidence of additional seizures during this vulnerable time.

Chronic. Patients whose seizures have an elliptogenic focus (e.g., chronic subdural) should receive anticonvulsant therapy. However, compliance is typically poor. In the patient with "pure" AWDS (CT is unremarkable), chronic anticonvulsant therapy is absolutely not indicated.

5. Can AWDS be prevented?
Data support prophylactic use of benzodiazepines in the acute withdrawal period, particularly in patients with a history of alcohol withdrawal seizures during abstinence.

6. Who is at risk for alcohol-induced hypoglycemia (AIH)? What is the clinical presentation?
AIH results from two pathophysiologic processes: insufficient glycogen stores and alcohol-induced impairment of gluconeogenesis. The three groups vulnerable to AIH are chronic alcoholics, binge drinkers, and young children. AIH may occur during intoxication or up to 20 hours following the last drink.

Manifestations of neuroglycopenia (headache, depressed mental status, seizure, coma) predominate. Evidence of catecholamine excess, typical of insulin-induced hypoglycemia (tremulousness, diaphoresis, anxiety), is very unusual.

Two clinical caveats are important. Seizures are a frequent presentation in children. Localized CNS signs, including a strokelike picture, often occur in adults.

7. Must thiamine be administered prior to glucose in the alcoholic patient?

It has been widely held that delivery of glucose to a patient with marginal thiamine reserves will catapult that individual into Wernicke-Korsakoff syndrome. (1) In an alcoholic patient, AIH or hypoglycemia of any etiology is a far more likely cause of depressed level of consciousness than is Wernicke-Korsakoff syndrome. (2) The use of a rapid glucose analyzer can avoid unneeded glucose administration to patients considered at risk for inadequate thiamine stores. (3) Wernicke-Korsakoff syndrome develops over a period of hours to days. The precipitous initiation of Wernicke-Korsakoff syndrome by dextrose has not been substantiated. However, the consequences of neuroglycopenia begin within 30 minutes, can be tremendously morbid, and are easily prevented.

In alcoholic patients with known or strongly suspected hypoglycemia, administer glucose and deliver thiamine empirically as soon afterward as possible.

8. Is it dangerous to administer thiamine intravenously?

Orally administered thiamine may be poorly absorbed in the alcoholic. The intramuscular route is painful and can result in hematomas or abscesses, particularly if the patient's coagulation status is impaired. The experience with intravenous thiamine is enormous and the safety profile exceptional. It may be given as part of fluid hydration or multivitamin preparations. It can also be given in bolus infusion.

9. What causes alcoholic ketoacidosis (AKA)? How should it be managed?

This common metabolic disturbance occurs early after heavy binge drinking and is heralded by starvation and vomiting and occasionally shortness of breath (Kussmaul respirations) and abdominal pain. Ketoacidosis results from accumulation of acetoacetate and beta-hydroxybutyrate. At presentation, serum pH and bicarbonate average 7.1 and 10, respectively, with wide variation. Depressed body stores of potassium and phosphate are typical. In AKA, serum glucose is usually normal or may be low, a distinguishing feature from diabetic ketoacidosis.

Treatment consists of rehydration with dextrose-containing crystalloid, antiemetics if needed, and benzodiazepines as dictated by symptoms of withdrawal. Vitamin, potassium, and phosphate supplementation are indicated. Bicarbonate administration is rarely required and insulin therapy is proscribed. Normalization of metabolic abnormalities usually follows 12–16 hours of therapy.

10. What is the relationship between alcohol and metabolic acidosis?

Ethanol: Acute ethanol ingestion results in a mild increase in the lactate/pyruvate ratio. Clinically significant metabolic acidosis does not ensue.

Alcoholic ketoacidosis: This ethanol abstinence syndrome produces marked elevations in acetoacetate and beta-hydroxybutyrate with resultant and occasionally profound increased anion gap metabolic acidosis.

Ethylene glycol and methanol: Certain by-products of these highly toxic compounds produce increased anion gap metabolic acidosis.

Isopropyl alcohol: A significant portion of isopropyl alcohol is metabolized to acetone. This is a ketone but not a ketoacid. Thus, exposure to this alcohol can cause ketosis and ketonuria but not acidosis.

11. Which coagulopathies should be anticipated in a chronic alcoholic?

Thrombocytopenia can result from direct bone marrow depressant effects of ethanol, folate deficiency, and hypersplenism secondary to portal hypertension. Counts less than 30,000/uL due to alcohol usage alone are unlikely. Qualitative platelet defects may also occur.

Hepatocyte loss caused by chronic alcohol abuse depletes all coagulation factors save VIII, particularly II, VII, IX, and X. In addition, alcoholics often have inadequate vitamin K stores due to hepatobiliary dysfunction and poor diet. Vitamin K is a requisite cofactor for the production of factors II, VII, IX, and X. When faced with gastrointestinal hemorrhage in a chronic alcoholic, an intravenous vitamin K supplementation trial is warranted. However, the more likely culprit is hepatocellular destruction, for which vitamin K will be unhelpful. Moreover, vitamin K does not begin to restore factor levels for 2–6 hours following administration. Fresh frozen plasma provides immediate factor supplementation.

12. How should the combative alcoholic patient be managed?

When patient or staff is in jeopardy, the first step is mechanical containment of the patient. A sufficient number of competent personnel and restraint devices are necessary. A simple matter such as closed head injury, hypoxia, or a stretched bladder may be the source of distress and should be excluded.

For chemical sedation, haloperidol, a butyrophenone, is a preferred agent. It can be administered quickly (initial dose 5–10 mg IV push) and causes rapid onset of sedation (5 minutes). Repeat doses may be required. Haloperidol is not detrimental to airway patency, ventilation, or hemodynamics. The down side is a 5–10% incidence of extrapyramidal reactions that usually occur 12–24 hours following administration. This compares very favorably with the obvious dangers of benzodiazepines, narcotics, and paralytic agents.

13. When can an acutely intoxicated patient be safely discharged from the emergency department (ED)?

From a management perspective, there are two fundamental concerns. First, acute intoxication obfuscates the verification of certain diagnoses and the exclusion of others. Second, a physician who discharges an acutely intoxicated patient (read: incompetent) may be held accountable for the actions of that patient subsequent and proximate to discharge from the ED.

The conundrum lies in the definition of intoxication. Numerous tests provide tables that match serum alcohol levels with clinical findings. In truth, the degree of clinical intoxication at a specific serum alcohol is tremendously variable in accordance with the patient's chronicity and severity of drinking. A veteran with a level in excess of 500 mg/dl can look less drunk than an inexperienced teenager at 100 mg/dl.

The patient should undergo repeated examinations until the physician is comfortable that other medical concerns do not exist. Documentation of the discharge neurologic examination, including mental status and gait, is imperative. The patient may then be discharged to an appropriate environment. Serum or breath alcohol determinations can be helpful at the outset of care but are often unneeded and can be problematic when obtained at discharge.

BIBLIOGRAPHY

1. Chance JF: Emergency department treatment of alcohol withdrawal seizures with phenytoin. Ann Emerg Med 20:520–522, 1991.
2. Earnest MD, Feldman H, Marx JA, et al: Intracranial lesions shown by CT in 259 cases of first alcohol-related seizures. Neurology 38:1561–1565, 1988.
3. Eichner ER, Hillman RS: The evolution of anemia in alcoholic patients. Am J Med 50:218–232, 1971.
4. Fitzgerald FT: Hypoglycemia and accidental hypothermia in an alcoholic population. West J Med 133:105–107, 1980.

5. Frommer DA, Marx JA: Wernicke's encephalopathy. N Engl J Med 313:637–638, 1985.
6. Marx JA, Berner J, Bar-Or D, Gorayeb MJ: Prophylaxis of alcohol withdrawal seizures: A prospective study (abstract). Ann Emerg Med 15:637, 1986.
7. Miller PD, Heinig RE, Waterhouse C: Treatment of alcoholic acidosis: The role of dextrose and phosphate. Arch Intern Med 138:67, 1978.
8. Rosenbloom AJ: Optimizing drug treatment of alcohol withdrawal. Am J Med 81:901, 1986.
9. Sellers EM, Kalant H: Alcohol intoxication and withdrawal. N Engl J Med 294:757, 1976.
10. Silverstein S, Frommer DA, Marx JA, Rosen P: Parenteral haloperidol in combative patients: A prospective study. Ann Emerg Med, 1986.
11. Victor M, Adams RD, Collins GH: The Wernicke-Korsakoff Syndrome. Philadelphia, F.A. Davis, 1971.

78. ANTIPYRETIC POISONING

James C. Mitchiner, M.D.

SALICYLATE POISONING

1. What are the causes of salicylate overdose?

A salicylate overdose may be intentional or accidental. Parental administration of aspirin to a child using adult doses may cause toxicity. Pepto-Bismol, which contains 130 mg/tbsp of salicylate, is often the culprit. In adults, simultaneous ingestion of proprietary aspirin and prescription medication may lead to unintentional overdose and to the formation of gastric concretions. Dermal application of salicylic acid ointment and ingestion of concentrated methyl salicylate (oil of wintergreen; 1 tsp = 7 gm salicylate) are rare causes of acute salicylism. The minimum acute toxic ingestion is 150 mg/kg.

2. What are the characteristics of the patient who presents with an acute salicylate overdose?

Patients may present with nausea, vomiting, tinnitus, fever, diaphoresis and confusion. Hyperventilation may be mistakenly ascribed to anxiety. Patients may also present with headache or chronic pain, which prompted the ingestion of salicylate.

3. What are some signs of salicylate intoxication?

Signs include acid-base and electrolyte disturbances, dehydration, hyperthermia, GI hemorrhage, azotemia, oliguria, CNS alterations (ranging from mild confusion to seizures and coma), noncardiogenic pulmonary edema, coagulopathy, and platelet dysfunction. Hypoglycemia has been reported in children. Rarely, acute salicylate intoxication can cause rhabdomyolysis.

4. Describe the acid-base disturbances.

Salicylates are capable of producing all types of acid-base disturbances. Adults typically present with acute **respiratory alkalosis** without hypoxia, due to salicylate stimulation of the respiratory center. If the patient does have hypoxia, salicylate-induced noncardiogenic pulmonary edema or another diagnosis, e.g., pulmonary embolus, should be suspected. Within 12–24 hours after ingestion, the acid-base status in an untreated patient shifts toward an anion gap **metabolic acidosis.** Mixed respiratory alkalosis and metabolic acidosis is sometimes seen. In patients presenting with **respiratory acidosis,** concomitant ingestion of a CNS depressant should be suspected. **Metabolic acidosis** is the predominant acid-base disturbance in children, in patients who take massive amounts of salicylates, and in patients (both adults and children) who have chronic salicylate toxicity (see below). In contrast, **metabolic alkalosis** may ensue if vomiting is a prominent feature of intoxication.

5. What are some of the other metabolic disturbances seen in acute salicylate poisoning?
The patient may be dehydrated secondary to vomiting or to the diuretic effects of increased renal sodium excretion. Insensible losses are increased in patients with hyperventilation, and water and electrolyte losses may occur through diaphoresis in response to the hyperpyrexic state. Hypokalemia is due to renal excretion and alkalemia, both respiratory and metabolic (secondary to bicarbonate therapy).

6. I thought aspirin is an antipyretic. How does it cause a fever?
At a cellular level, salicylate poisoning leads to the uncoupling of oxidative phosphorylation. When this occurs, the energy obtained from O_2 reduction and NADH oxidation that is normally captured to form ATP is released as heat instead.

7. Name some features of CNS dysfunction.
Signs and symptoms of CNS dysfunction are varied and may be subtle: irritability, confusion, delirium, tinnitus, vertigo, visual hallucinations, and disorientation may progress to seizures and coma secondary to cerebral edema.

8. What are some of the hematologic abnormalities?
These are rare in an acute overdose. Features include decreased production of prothrombin (factor II) and factor VII, an increase in capillary endothelial fragility, and a decrease in the quantity and function of platelets (i.e., decreased adhesiveness).

9. How is the severity of salicylate overdose assessed?
The Done nomogram provides a guideline for assessing the severity of salicylate poisoning. This nomogram, however, is only a guideline and applicable only to salicylate levels obtained 6 hours or more after acute ingestion. It should not be used for chronic overdoses, for ingestions of enteric-coated salicylates or methyl salicylate, and in situations in which the time of ingestion is unknown. Furthermore, salicylate levels should be repeated several hours apart, **while the patient is still in the ED,** so that you can assess the trend in the severity of poisoning. This nomogram is not a substitute for serial clinical assessments.

10. Which laboratory tests are indicated?
Required laboratory tests include arterial blood gases, CBC, electrolytes, BUN, creatinine, glucose, prothrombin time, urinalysis, and a quantitative serum salicylate level. If the patient presents less than 6 hours after ingestion, a salicylate level should be repeated at 6 hours. In addition, a quantitative acetaminophen level is recommended, because many patients confuse these two antipyretics or mix both kinds in the same bottle. A limited toxicology screen, focusing on other treatable co-ingestions (opiates, barbiturates, ethanol, and cyclic antidepressants), should be performed if clinically indicated.

11. How is an acute salicylate overdose treated?
If poisoning is through dermal contact, the skin should be copiously washed with tap water. For acute ingestions, gastric lavage should be performed. A slurry of activated charcoal and cathartic (sorbitol or magnesium sulfate) should be administered either orally or by gastric lavage tube at a dose of 1 gm of charcoal per kg of body weight. Lavage may be useful even if the patient presents several hours after ingestion, because large amounts of aspirin may form gastric concretions and delay absorption for up to 24 hours. Bicarbonate containing intravenous fluids (D5 + 3 ampules $NaHCO_3$) should be administered at a rate of 10–15 ml/kg/hr. After the patient has responded with diuresis, potassium loss should be replaced with potassium chloride at a dose of 20–40 mEq/L. Patients with hyperthermia should be

cooled with a cooling blanket. Those with documented hypoglycemia should be given one ampule D50 intravenously. Patients with pulmonary edema should be treated in standard fashion, including oxygen, diuretics, intravenous nitroglycerin, and intubation, with respiratory support and positive end-expiratory pressure (PEEP) as needed.

12. Is there a role for repetitive dosing of activated charcoal?
Because of aspirin release from the aspirin-charcoal complex in the GI tract and subsequent absorption, salicylate levels may not decline significantly after a single dose of activated charcoal. Therefore, repeated doses of charcoal may be indicated to enhance elimination.

13. What is the rationale for alkaline diuresis?
Because aspirin is an organic acid, administration of bicarbonate intravenously will raise the pH of the blood and thereby "trap" salicylate ion, thus limiting the amount of salicylate that crosses the blood-brain barrier. Similarly, an alkalotic urine acts to retain salicylate ion, preventing its reabsorption by the renal tubules. The use of **forced diuresis,** however, is controversial and has been reported to cause pulmonary edema. Many authorities feel that fluid replacement should be limited to fluids that have been lost through sweat, hyperventilation, and emesis.

14. Explain the paradox of a decreasing serum salicylate concentration and increasing clinical toxicity.
The serum salicylate level by itself does not reflect tissue distribution of the drug. If the patient's blood is acidemic, salicylate acid will remain un-ionized and more will penetrate the blood-brain barrier, resulting in CNS toxicity. Therefore, salicylate levels should be interpreted in light of a concurrent blood pH; an acidotic pH is associated with toxicity regardless of the drug level.

15. What are the indications for hemodialysis?
Standard indications include persistent, refractory metabolic acidosis (pH <7.10), renal failure with oliguria, cardiac dysfunction (congestive heart failure, arrhythmias, cardiac arrest), CNS deterioration (seizures, coma, cerebral edema), or an acute salicylate level greater than 130 mg/dl 6 hours after ingestion. In addition, because ingestion of >300 mg/kg predicts severe toxicity, a nephrologist should be contacted early in anticipation of the possible need for dialysis.

16. What are the most common findings in chronic salicylate poisoning?
The main feature in chronic salicylism is change in mental status manifested by lethargy, confusion, drowsiness, slurred speech, hallucinations, agitation, or seizures. Unfortunately, because these are signs common to many other disorders, the diagnosis is frequently missed, resulting in a mortality rate as high as 25%. Many of these patients are older with a history of peptic ulcer disease, arthritis, or gastric surgery. Some have gastric outlet obstruction, resulting in delayed gastric emptying and, in some cases, formation of gastric bezoars. The latter is responsible for a slow leaching of salicylate compounds into the stomach. Serum electrolytes reveal an anion gap metabolic acidosis. The serum salicylate level may not be elevated and the Done diagram is of no use in chronic salicylate ingestions; if used, it often results in a false sense of security.

ACETAMINOPHEN POISONING

17. What are the characteristics of acetaminophen overdose?
Acetaminophen is the drug most commonly involved in acute analgesic ingestions, either as a single agent or in combination with various over-the-counter cough and cold remedies.

Early diagnosis of acute (phase I) acetaminophen toxicity is important because early symptoms may be subtle; the onset of hepatotoxicity, the major manifestation, is delayed by several days following ingestion. Failure to recognize and treat toxicity within 16 hours of ingestion results in significant morbidity and mortality. *The main issue in treatment is the prevention of hepatotoxicity.*

18. Outline four phases of acetaminophen overdose.
Phase I begins within hours of ingestion and is marked by anorexia, nausea, vomiting, and diaphoresis (some patients may be completely asymptomatic). These physical findings are obviously associated with a multitude of other disorders, which accounts for the diagnostic difficulty in the recognition of acetaminophen poisoning. Phase II begins 24–72 hours after ingestion and includes abnormalities in liver function tests and right upper quadrant abdominal pain. Phase III starts 3–5 days after ingestion and includes features of advanced hepatotoxicity, including jaundice, hypoglycemia, coagulopathy, and encephalopathy. The SGOT level is often greater than 1000 IU/L. Myocardiopathy and renal failure due to acute tubular necrosis may also be present. Phase IV begins 1 week after ingestion and for most patients is marked by a gradual return of laboratory values to normal levels, provided phase III damage is not permanent or lethal.

19. What are the CNS manifestations of acute acetaminophen poisoning?
There are none. Abnormalities in mental status or level of consciousness should be attributed to other drugs (e.g., salicylates, opiates, propoxyphene) or to other disease states.

20. Describe the pathophysiology of acetaminophen toxicity.
Acetaminophen is metabolized primarily by the liver. About 90% of it is conjugated with glucuronic or sulfuric acid to form nontoxic compounds that are excreted in the urine. About 2% of the drug is excreted unchanged, also in the urine. The remainder is metabolized by the cytochrome P-450 mixed function oxidase system. This involves formation of a toxic intermediary compound, which is rapidly conjugated with hepatic glutathione. The resulting conjugate is further metabolized and its byproducts are excreted in the urine. Because the liver normally has a fixed amount of glutathione, this compound is rapidly depleted in an acute overdose situation. The toxic intermediary then accumulates, unmetabolized, and binds to the sulfhydryl groups of hepatic enzymes. The result is an irreversible centrilobular hepatic necrosis.

21. How is hepatotoxicity predicted?
In an adult, acute ingestion of 7.5 gm or 140 mg/kg is generally predictive of hepatotoxicity. Certain drugs such as cimetidine and ethanol (in *acute* ingestion; see below) compete with acetaminophen for metabolism by the P-450 pathway, thereby offering some protection from hepatotoxicity. On the other hand, certain drugs such as phenytoin and phenobarbital may induce the P-450 enzymes, allowing a greater percentage of acetaminophen to be metabolized to the toxic intermediary and increasing the risk of toxicity. The most accurate predictor of hepatotoxicity is the serum acetaminophen level obtained between 4 and 25 hours after ingestion. The Rumack-Matthew nomogram, which plots serum concentration against hours post-ingestion, is the standard reference for predicting hepatotoxicity in an *acute* overdose.

22. Why is hepatotoxicity in children rare?
No one really knows. Toxicity in children is rare, even when toxic levels of acetaminophen are found. One theory holds that acetaminophen metabolism in children shows a preference for alternative pathways other than the P-450 system. The conversion from "juvenile" to "adult" metabolism occurs between 6 and 9 years of age.

23. Is the serum half-life helpful? Are serial serum acetaminophen levels helpful?
In general, the serum half-life is not as reliable in predicting toxicity as is the acetaminophen level 4 hours after ingestion. If an accurate estimate of the time of ingestion cannot be obtained, however, the half-life may be useful. The half-life can be calculated by knowing the acetaminophen level at initial presentation to the ED and 4 hours later; if the second level is greater than half of the first level, liver toxicity is likely.

24. What is the role of alcohol in acetaminophen hepatotoxicity?
It depends on whether the alcohol ingestion is acute or chronic. **Acute ethanol ingestion** is thought to decrease the risk of hepatotoxicity through competition with acetaminophen for metabolism by the P-450 pathway. This results in decreased production of the toxic intermediary and therefore decreases the risk of hepatic necrosis. **Chronic alcoholism,** on the other hand, induces the P-450 enzymes such that increased amounts of the toxic intermediary are formed with increased susceptibility to centrilobular necrosis. Clinically, hepatotoxicity may occur when chronic alcoholics ingest amounts only slightly above the therapeutic range, i.e., 4–6 gm/day. Findings include marked elevations of aminotransferase levels and elevated prothrombin times. In chronic acetaminophen poisoning, the nomogram is not helpful in predicting toxicity.

25. Which laboratory tests are helpful?
If the serum acetaminophen level is in the toxic range on the nomogram, additional blood should be obtained for a CBC, electrolytes, BUN, glucose, prothrombin time, and liver function tests. A *limited* toxicology screen should also be ordered, with attention to treatable concomitant ingestions such as salicylates, opiates, barbiturates, ethanol, and cyclic antidepressants. If the acetaminophen level is within the toxic range, liver function tests and prothrombin time should be repeated daily while the patient is receiving treatment.

26. How is acetaminophen poisoning treated?
If the patient presents within 2 hours of ingestion, gastric lavage should be performed. Activated charcoal (1 gm/kg) mixed with sorbitol or magnesium sulfate should be administered by gastric lavage tube. If the patient presents more than 2 hours after ingestion, he or she should be given the charcoal/cathartic orally without lavage, unless there is reason to suspect a concomitant ingestion of an anticholinergic compound that would delay gastric emptying. The specific antidote is *N*-acetylcysteine (NAC; Mucomyst). This agent is a glutathione substitute with a high therapeutic/toxic safety ratio. It works best if given within 16 hours of ingestion. It should not be given indiscriminately and should be administered only if the nomogram predicts toxicity on the basis of a timed serum acetaminophen level. It is given orally after dilution 1:5 with water or a beverage such as soda pop or juice. This produces a 20% solution, which is given as a loading dose of 140 mg/kg, followed by a maintenance dose of 70 mg/kg every 4 hours for 17 additional doses. If the patient vomits a dose within 1 hour, the dose should be repeated.

27. What is the controversy surrounding the use of intravenous NAC?
Because palatability of NAC is poor and vomiting is common, intravenous NAC has been used in an attempt to obviate GI side effects and increase compliance. NAC is approved for IV administration in Canada and Europe, and the IV route is actually the preferred route in Great Britain. It is available in the United States only on an investigational basis. However, because enteral administration of NAC leads to direct delivery of the drug to the liver by the portal vein and thus concentration in the target organ, some investigators feel that the oral route has a theoretical advantage over the IV route. Adverse reactions, which occur in as many as 14% of patients, include angioedema, flushing, bronchospasm, hypotension, tachycardia, and urticaria.

28. Is there a critical window in time to administer NAC?
Patients who present up to 24 hours after ingestion with toxic levels predicted by the nomogram should receive NAC. Beyond 24 hours, however, most authorities believe that NAC is not helpful in prevention of hepatotoxicity. The patients should have supportive care and should be considered for hepatic transplantation.

29. How does activated charcoal affect NAC absorption?
Although activated charcoal is capable of adsorbing NAC, the overall clinical effect is unclear. Some authorities have recommended increasing the loading dose of NAC by 40% to offset this effect. On the other hand, there is usually an interval of several hours between administration of charcoal and receipt of a 4-hour acetaminophen level before the decision to use NAC is made. Experimental coadministration of activated charcoal and NAC has not been shown to affect NAC pharmacokinetics.

30. What is the treatment for chronic acetaminophen toxicity?
Any alcoholic presenting with abnormal liver function tests who is taking acetaminophen chronically in therapeutic or higher doses should be suspected of having acetaminophen hepatotoxicity. NAC should be started immediately and continued as long as hepatic enzymes are elevated. Theoretically, the risk of toxicity should be less than in the acute overdose because the liver has had a chance to regenerate depleted glutathione stores.

IBUPROFEN POISONING

31. What are the characteristics of ibuprofen overdose?
Ibuprofen is readily available as an over-the-counter medication used in the treatment of mild to moderate pain and fever. It is also available in prescription form as Motrin, Rufin, and Medipren. Symptoms are usually seen within 4 hours of ingestion and more likely to be serious in children. Toxicity is limited in patients who ingest less than 100 mg/kg, whereas patients, primarily children, who ingest more than 400 mg/kg may be at risk for more severe symptoms.

32. What are the primary symptoms of ibuprofen toxicity?
GI symptoms include nausea, vomiting, abdominal pain, and hematemesis. Nephrotoxicity is manifested as acute renal failure secondary to interstitial nephritis. CNS toxicity (seen mostly in children) appears as somnolence, apnea, seizures, and coma. Severe metabolic acidosis and thrombocytopenia have also been reported.

33. When should a serum ibuprofen level be obtained?
Because the serum ibuprofen level does not correlate with clinical symptoms, there is no role for this test in decision making.

34. Describe the treatment for ibuprofen toxicity.
Treatment is directed at alleviating symptoms and supportive care. The patient should be given activated charcoal, 1 gm/kg, mixed with sorbitol or magnesium sulfate. Ipecac should be reserved for pediatric ingestions. If hematemesis is present or there is blood in the stool, a nasogastric tube should be placed; if blood is present, the stomach should be irrigated with saline. A limited toxicology screen to search for other readily treatable toxins (salicylates, acetaminophen, opiates, barbiturates, cyclic antidepressants, and ethanol) is recommended. Convulsions should be treated with intravenous diazepam. Renal and hepatic function tests should be ordered. Children with ingestions of greater than 400 mg/kg should be observed in the hospital. Forced diuresis, alkalinization, and hemodialysis are not indicated.

BIBLIOGRAPHY

Salicylate Poisoning

1. Bogacz K, Caldron P: Enteric-coated aspirin bezoar: Elevation of serum salicylate level by barium study. Am J Med 83:783–786, 1987.
2. Goldfrank LR, Bresnitz EA, Hartnett L: Salicylates. In Goldfrank LR, et al (eds): Goldfrank's Toxicologic Emergencies. Norwalk, CT, Appleton and Lange, 4th ed. 1990, ch 23.
3. Hillman RJ, Prescott LF: Treatment of salicylate poisoning with repeated oral charcoal. Br Med J 291:1472, 1986.

Acetaminophen Poisoning

4. Ekins BR, Ford DC, Thompson MIB, et al: The effect of activated charcoal on *N*-acetylcysteine absorption in normal subjects. Am J Emerg Med 5:483–487, 1987.
5. Rumack BH: Acetaminophen overdose in young children. Am J Dis Child 138:428–433, 1984.
6. Smilkstein MJ, Bronstein AL, Linden C, et al: Acetaminophen overdose: A 48-hour intravenous *N*-acetylcysteine treatment protocol. Ann Emerg Med 20:1058–1063, 1991.
7. Smilkstein MJ, Knapp GL, Kulig KW, et al: Efficacy of oral *N*-acetylcysteine in the treatment of acetaminophen overdose: Analysis of the national multicenter study (1976–1985). N Engl J Med 319:1557–1562, 1988.

Ibuprofen Poisoning

8. Hall AH, Smolinske SC, Conrad FL, et al: Ibuprofen overdose: 126 cases. Ann Emerg Med 15:1308–1313, 1986.
9. Howland MA, Weisman RS, Goldfrank LR: Nonsteroidal anti-inflammatory agents. In Goldfrank LR, et al (eds): Goldfrank's Toxicologic Emergencies. Norwalk, CT, Appleton and Lange, 1990, ch 24.

79. SEDATIVES AND HYPNOTICS

Jeffrey Brent, M.D., Ph.D.

1. "Sedative" vs. "hypnotic"—what's the difference?

For our purposes, there really is not a difference. Technically, sedatives are tranquilizing agents that should induce a state of calm. Hypnotics, on the other hand, should induce sleep. In reality, all of these agents tend to act by similar mechanisms and the distinction between them is artificial. They are tranquilizing drugs and, in sufficient quantity, can cause depression of the central nervous system.

2. Which medications fall into this category?

A variety of unrelated tranquilizers are generally referred to as sedatives/hypnotics: benzodiazepines, barbiturates, chloral hydrate, glutethimide, ethchlorvinyl, meprobamate, and buspirone. Of these, the ones used most frequently are benzodiazepines and barbiturates. The distinction is somewhat artificial because other agents, such as ethanol, have similar effects. In addition, a large group of drugs and toxins in toxic amounts can produce decreased mental status.

3. How do sedative/hypnotic overdoses present clinically?

Although there is some variation from agent to agent, the common thread is a depressed mentation. Frequently this depression is associated with hypotension, both from vasodilatation and direct depression of cardiac activity, decreased gut motility, hypothermia, and respiratory depression.

4. Should I be thinking of anything else in patients who present in this way?

You sure should! Do not be fooled by first impressions. Any patient who presents with depressed mental status should be thoroughly evaluated for *any* of its potential causes. (See ch. 5, p. 19, "Altered Mental Status and Coma.")

5. How is sedative/hypnotic overdose treated?

The mainstay of management is supportive care. Be sure to serially monitor respirations, airway, and blood pressure. Assessment includes securing airway, breathing and circulation (ABCs), including intravenous lines and cardiac monitors for patients who are showing any clinical effects, GI decontamination, empirical administration of naloxone and dextrose, and a thorough history and physical examination to rule out other causes. A few tricks can be used with certain specific agents, but you have to read further to find out what they are.

6. What is the best way to decontaminate the GI tract following sedative/hypnotic overdose?

The key to preventing further drug absorption is activated charcoal administered in an initial total dose of approximately 1 gm/kg. A dose of cathartic such as sorbitol, magnesium sulfate, or magnesium citrate may be given along with it. There is probably a role for giving several doses of charcoal in major poisonings. These can be administered every 4 hours. Never give more than 1 dose of cathartic. All doses beyond the first should always be given in a simple aqueous suspension. Sedative/hypnotics often have an inhibitory effect on GI motility and therefore multiple doses of activated charcoal should not be given in the absence of bowel sounds, in the presence of radiologic evidence of an ileus, or if there is abdominal distention clinically.

Orogastric lavage is an effective adjunct to GI decontamination for most poisonings, particularly if done early. Beyond an hour after the overdose, it becomes unlikely that there will be significant amount of drug in the stomach and thus one can expect little benefit of lavage beyond this time frame.

7. Is there a role for measuring specific drug levels or doing toxicology screens in these patients?

Sometimes. If patient is awake and alert, with a normal examination, stating that he or she overdosed on a sedative/hypnotic, there is nothing to be gained from a screen. Even verification that the patient has some drug in his or her system is irrelevant because clinically no significant amount is present. Specific drug levels can be both difficult to obtain and interpret. They are generally not useful for sedative/hypnotic overdose except in the case of phenobarbital poisoning. In distinction to the patient who is alert, any patient with a depressed mental status should probably have a drug screen unless the cause is definitively known. Do not forget, however, that in *any* patient with a history of *any* drug overdose, no matter how trivial, an acetaminophen level must be obtained.

8. How are these drugs cleared from the body?

In general, most drugs are eliminated by hepatic metabolism or urinary excretion. The overwhelming majority of sedative/hypnotic drugs are cleared by the former route. Because they have low rates of renal clearance, there is little benefit to trying to increase elimination by this route—even doubling or tripling low values still gives a low value. The one prominent exception to this rule is phenobarbital, for which urinary excretion is predominant, which has important implications in the treatment of phenobarbital poisoning.

9. Is there a way to enhance the clearance of sedatives/hypnotics?

In general, there is not, but there are exceptions. Remember, absorption of virtually all of these agents can be decreased by the use of oral activated charcoal. Techniques that enhance clearance of certain drugs are urinary alkalinization, multiple-dose activated charcoal, and extracorporeal drug removal techniques.

Urinary alkalinization is effective in the case of phenobarbital poisoning. Raising the pH to greater than 7.3 can have as much as a tenfold effect on renal drug elimination.

Multiple-dose activated charcoal has been shown not only to prevent absorption but also actually to reduce the amount of certain circulating drugs, a phenomenon referred to as "gastrointestinal dialysis." This technique can be used with phenobarbital and appears to work with meprobamate poisoning as well.

Extracorporeal drug removal techniques are useful for molecules with small volumes of distribution. Hemodialysis can be used to remove significant amounts of phenobarbital, chloral hydrate, and meprobamate. Hemoperfusion may also be used with chloral hydrate and meprobamate poisoning.

10. A patient has depressed mental status and a "vinyl-like" odor on the breath. What does that mean?
A vinyl-like odor in association with a sedative/hypnotic overdose suggests poisoning by the drug ethchlorvynol. This drug is a sedative/hypnotic that is used much less commonly now than in the past. The clinical course of intoxication by this drug involves depressed mental status and coma, often lasting for a prolonged period of time. Treatment is supportive.

11. Following a drug overdose, a patient is unconscious with widely dilated pupils. What drug should you think of?
Glutethimide. This drug is a sedative/hypnotic that was popular in the late 1950s but is now uncommon. Unusual features of glutethimide poisoning include prolonged and fluctuating coma and anticholinergic features such as widely dilated pupils.

12. Are there special considerations in chloral hydrate poisoning?
Chloral hydrate poisoning presents with signs and symptoms that are typical of sedative/hypnotic overdose. Most of its effects are mediated through its metabolite trichloroethanol. Atrial and ventricular arrhythmias, particularly tachyarrhythmias, may occur with chloral hydrate poisoning and thus these patients need intensive cardiovascular monitoring.

13. Are there any specific antidotes for sedative/hypnotic poisoning?
Only flumazenil for benzodiazepine overdose.

14. How does flumazenil work?
Flumazenil is a specific competitive inhibitor of benzodiazepines at the benzodiazepine receptor.

15. What is the correct dose of flumazenil?
For symptomatic benzodiazepine overdose, 0.5–10 mg of flumazenil administered IV over 1 minute will reverse the effects of benzodiazepines. However, flumazenil has a half-life of approximately 1 hour and therefore the benzodiazepine effect may recur once the flumazenil has worn off.

CONTROVERSY

16. Should flumazenil be administered empirically to all patients with depressed mental status?
For: Flumazenil is a relatively safe drug that may provide a diagnostic clue to benzodiazepine poisoning if a comatose patient has a response. This may save an extensive and

expensive work-up and potentially avoid the need for intubation prior to establishment of the diagnosis.

Against: Flumazenil is expensive, and administering it to all patients with depressed mental status would be costly. Benzodiazepine overdoses have little long-term morbidity and deaths are rare. A positive response to flumazenil does not guarantee a diagnosis of benzodiazepine poisoning. Awakening may occur in patients who have depressed mental status from either ethanol intoxication or hepatic coma. However, the response to flumazenil in the latter conditions is much less predictable than in benzodiazepine poisoning.

There are conditions in which it would be undesirable to administer flumazenil. Patients who have toxic amounts of tricyclic antidepressants in their systems may be more vulnerable to seizures if flumazenil is administered, particularly if it is a mixed antidepressant and benzodiazepine overdose. If flumazenil is inadvertently administered to a patient who is benzodiazepine dependent, acute withdrawal may occur.

BIBLIOGRAPHY

1. Amrein R, Leishman B, Bentzinger C, Roncari G: Flumazenil in benzodiazepine—Antagonism actions and clinical use in intoxications and anaesthesiology. Med Toxicol 2:411–429, 1987.
2. Osborn H, Goldfrank LR, Howland MA, et al: Barbiturates and other sedative hypnotics. In Goldfrank LR, et al (eds): Goldfrank's Toxicologic Emergencies, 4th ed. Norwalk, CT, Appleton and Lange, 1990, pp 449–463.
3. O'Sullivan GF, Wade DN: Flumazenil in the management of acute drug overdosage with benzodiazepines and other agents. Clin Pharmacol Ther 42:254–259, 1987.
4. Prischl F, Donner A, Grimm G, et al: Value of flumazenil in benzodiazepine self-poisoning. Med Toxicol 3:334–339, 1988.
5. Winchester JF: Barbiturates, methaqualone, and primidone. In Haddad LM, et al (eds): Clinical Management of Poisonings and Drug Overdose, 2nd ed. Philadelphia, W.B. Saunders, 1990, pp 718–730.

80. MUSHROOMS, HALLUCINOGENS, AND STIMULANTS

Atkinson W. Longmire, M.D., FACEP, and Donna L. Seger, M.D., FACEP

1. Why are stimulants, hallucinogens, and mushrooms grouped together?

The three groups have these things in common: (1) they may be used recreationally, (2) they may cause CNS stimulation, and (3) they may cause hallucinations.

MUSHROOMS

2. What are the most dangerous mushrooms?

Amatoxin-containing mushrooms. Amatoxins are highly toxic peptides that are found in the Amanita and some Galerina species. One *Amanita phalloides* mushroom may contain enough amatoxin to be lethal.

3. How do the symptoms differ?

Most nonlethal mushrooms produce vomiting and diarrhea soon after ingestion. These patients are treated with IV fluids and have a good outcome. However, the more deadly amatoxin-containing mushrooms cause abdominal pain, vomiting, and diarrhea 10–12 hours after ingestion. Liver function tests should be obtained in patients with delayed symptoms. If the patient is clinically stable after 12 hours, further liver function tests may be done on an outpatient basis. The patient may subsequently be asymptomatic prior to onset of liver failure 3 or 4 days after ingestion.

4. What treatment is available for amatoxin-containing mushrooms?
Ipecac-induced emesis is useful if used within the first 2 or 3 hours after ingestion. Supportive care with special attention to fluids, electrolytes, and glucose is the mainstay of therapy.

5. Are these the only mushroom syndromes?
No. Many different syndromes may result following mushroom ingestion. Some of these, with some possible treatments, are listed below.

Syndromes After Mushroom Ingestion

ONSET	SYMPTOMS	TOXIN	TREATMENTS
Over 6 hours	GI	Amatoxin	Fluids/glucose
	GI, CNS, methemo-globinemia	Monomethyl-hydrazine	Fluids, pyridoxine, methylene blue
Under 2 hours	GI	Multiple	Fluids
	Hallucinations	Psilocybin	Supportive
	Cholinergic	Muscarine	Supportive
	Anticholinergic	Ibotenic acid Muscimol	Supportive
	Antabuse reaction	Coprine	Avoid alcohol

HALLUCINOGENS

6. What are hallucinogens?
Hallucinogens are drugs that cause hallucinations. Many drugs, including stimulants, antidepressants, antihistamines, atropine, theophylline, heavy metals, bromides, and solvents, can cause hallucinations, but the specific hallucinogens described in this chapter are the illegal drugs LSD, marijuana, and phencyclidine.

7. What are typical presentations of patients with ingestions of hallucinogens? What is life threatening?
Besides hallucinations, these patients may have increased heart rate, temperature, and blood pressure. Unlike patients with an anticholinergic overdose who are hallucinating, patients who have ingested LSD, marijuana, or phencyclidine are diaphoretic with moist mucous membranes. Life-threatening conditions are hyperthermia, rhabdomyolysis, seizures, and arrhythmias.

8. What is "supportive care" for hallucinogen ingestion?
Reassurance and "talking down" are often used in patients intoxicated with LSD or marijuana. *Note:* Do not attempt to "talk down" a phencyclidine-intoxicated patient; he is potentially dangerous to himself and to others. Phencyclidine is a dissociative anesthetic that decreases pain perception. It also induces rage, aggressive behavior, and suicide. Intravenous diazepam may be required for sedation. Intramuscular haloperidol lowers the

seizure threshold, but may be used when extreme agitation or psychosis indicates the need for an antipsychotic drug. Elevated serum creatinine kinase and rhabdomyolysis occur secondary to intense muscle activity and myoglobinuria. Fluid replacement, alkalinization and maintenance of urinary output is imperative to prevent renal damage.

STIMULANTS

9. How are overdoses from stimulants different?

Cocaine and amphetamines are more likely to cause cardiotoxicity such as dysrhythmias and ischemic cardiac damage. Intracranial hemorrhage may occur—it is more frequent with amphetamines and is secondary to increased blood pressure. Tachycardia is a prominent presenting sign of cocaine and amphetamine use. Cocaine toxicity can progress rapidly, with seizures and arrhythmias occurring within minutes of cocaine use.

10. What is free-base cocaine?

Cocaine usually arrives in this country as cocaine hydrochloride. It is often converted back to its alkaloid form, or free-base, with an alkaline solution and a solvent. Crack cocaine is a form of free-base that is made with baking soda and water. Free-base cocaine is resistant to pyrolysis and can be smoked.

11. What is the significance of chest pain after use of cocaine?

Pneumothorax or pneumomediastinum may occur following a Valsalva maneuver when smoking cocaine. Myocardial infarction has followed intranasal, intravenous, and smoked cocaine, even in young patients with normal coronary arteries.

12. Should my diagnosis be based on a toxicology screen?

Au contraire! These screens vary from hospital to hospital. Often LSD, amphetamines, and, of course, mushrooms, are not included on a toxicology screen. Toxicology screens are best used for confirmation of clinical impressions and should not be used alone to make treatment decisions. When requesting such screens, be specific about your clinical suspicions in order for the laboratory to perform the proper screens.

BIBLIOGRAPHY

1. Barish P, Tintinalli J, Shields RO: Designer drugs and amphetamines. In Haddad LM, et al (eds): Clinical Management of Poisoning and Drug Overdose. Philadelphia, W B. Saunders, 1990, pp 770–780.
2. Brent J, Kulig K, Rumack BH: Mushrooms. In Haddad LM, et al (eds): Clinical Management of Poisoning and Drug Overdose. Philadelphia, W.B. Saunders, 1990, pp 581–590.
3. Derlet RW, Rice P, Horowitz Z, et al: Amphetamine toxicity: Experience with 127 cases. J Emerg Med 7:157–161, 1989.
4. Ellenhorn MJ, et al (eds): Medical Toxicology: Diagnosis and Treatment of Human Poisoning. New York, Elsevier, 1988, pp 625–641, 643–661, 663–672, 673–685, 763–777, 1209–1291.
5. Goldfrank LR, Hoffman RS: The cardiovascular effects of cocaine. Ann Emerg Med 20:165–175, 1991.
6. Goldfrank LR, Kirstein RH: Amphetamines. In Goldfrank LR, et al (eds): Goldfrank's Toxicologic Emergencies. Norwalk, CT, Appleton and Lange, 1990, pp 509–515.
7. Hurlbut KM: Drug-induced psychoses. Emerg Med Clin North Am 9:31–52, 1991.
8. Leikin JB, Krantz AJ, Zell-Kanter M, et al: Clinical features and management of intoxication due to hallucinogenic drugs. Med Toxicol Advers Drug Exp 4:324–350, 1989.
9. Milhorn HT: Diagnosis and management of phencyclidine intoxication. Am Fam Physician 43:1293–1302, 1991.
10. Parish RC, Doering PL: Treatment of Amanita mushroom poisoning: A review. Vet Hum Toxicol 28:318–322, 1986.

11. Szara S: Marijuana. In Haddad LM, et al (eds): Clinical Management of Poisoning and Drug Overdose. Philadelphia, W.B. Saunders, 1990, pp 737–748.
12. Shepherd SM, Jagoda AS: Phencyclidine and the hallucinogens. In Haddad LM, et al (eds): Clinical Management of Poisoning and Drug Overdose. Philadelphia, W.B. Saunders, 1990, pp 749–769.

81. OPIOIDS

Roy Purssell, M.D., FRCPC

1. I know that opioids cause coma, respiratory arrest, and miosis, and that the antidote is naloxone. Is there anything else I should know?
Yes! Patients who have taken an overdose of opioids can present with mydriasis, ventricular arrhythmias, and seizures. Some opioids can precipitate the life-threatening serotonin syndrome. To learn about these and other interesting characteristics of opioids, read on.

2. What do the terms opium, opiate, opioid, and narcotic mean?
Opium is a mixture of alkaloids, including morphine and codeine, extracted from the opium poppy. An **opiate** is a natural drug derived from opium (heroin, codeine, morphine). An **opioid** is any drug that has opium-like activity. This includes the opiates and all synthetic and semisynthetic drugs that interact with opioid receptors in the body. The term narcotic is nonspecific. It originally meant any drug that could induce sleep.

3. What is the typical presentation of opioid poisoning?
The classic triad of opioid poisoning is central nervous system depression, respiratory depression, and miosis. Patients who have overdosed on opioids are hyporeflexic and have decreased bowel sounds. They may be hypotensive, hypothermic, and bradycardic.

4. How should a patient with respiratory compromise caused by opioid overdose be treated?
Resuscitation must take precedence over the administration of naloxone. The patient's respiration must be supported with a bag-valve-mask until the opioid antagonist is administered. If there is an inadequate response to naloxone, the patient should be intubated.

5. What is the appropriate dose of naloxone?
The recommended initial dose of naloxone for adults and children with CNS and respiratory depression is 2.0 mg IV. If the patient has CNS depression only, it is reasonable to start with a smaller dose (0.4 mg to 0.8 mg IV). If there is no response to a smaller dose, 2.0 mg can be given. Patients who are regular opioid users may develop symptoms of opioid withdrawal after receiving naloxone. Opioid withdrawal is unpleasant to the patient but is not life threatening. It is sensible to titrate the dose of naloxone to reverse respiratory and CNS depression without precipitating withdrawal.

6. Does naloxone have to be given intravenously?
No. If it is difficult to start an intravenous line, naloxone can be given intramuscularly if the patient does not have hypotension. It can also be given down the endotracheal tube or injected sublingually into the venous plexus under the tongue. Naloxone is not effective orally.

7. Do all patients respond to 2.0 mg of naloxone?
No. Larger doses of naloxone may be required to reverse the effects of codeine, diphenoxylate (Lomotil), propoxyphene (Darvon), pentazocine (Talwin), and the fentanyl derivatives. If an opioid overdose is suspected and the patient does not respond to the initial 2.0 mg of naloxone, repeat 2.0-mg doses of naloxone can be administered every 3 minutes until a response is noted or 10 mg has been given. If there is no response to 10 mg of naloxone, it is unlikely that the diagnosis is an isolated opioid overdose.

8. Do patients often become resedated after the effects of naloxone wear off?
The duration of action of intravenous naloxone is 20–60 minutes. Many opioids produce clinical effects that last 3–6 hours. Although the duration of action of most opioids is much longer than that of naloxone, resedation is relatively uncommon.

9. How should recurrent sedation and respiratory depression due to a long-acting opioid be treated?
A naloxone infusion should be started. Giving repeated doses of naloxone to an opioid-dependent patient may cause the patient to fluctuate between symptoms of withdrawal and CNS depression.

10. How is a naloxone infusion set up?
The dose of naloxone necessary to reverse the respiratory depressant effects of the opioid overdose should be determined clinically. A continuous intravenous infusion of two-thirds of the initial bolus dose should be given each hour. If the patient develops symptoms of opioid withdrawal or resedation, the infusion rate should be adjusted accordingly. A simple way to mix up the infusion is to add 10 mg of naloxone to a 250-cc bag of normal saline. A rate of infusion of 25 cc/hr will then deliver 1.0 mg of naloxone per hour.

11. Should naloxone be administered empirically to every patient with altered mental status?
Yes. Naloxone is a safe medication. Although most cases of opioid overdose can be diagnosed clinically, some cases may be atypical. Treatment with naloxone may be useful both diagnostically and therapeutically.

12. Do all cases of opioid intoxication present with miosis?
No. Mydriasis or normal pupils can occur in conjunction with opioid overdose in the following situations:
- Overdose of meperidine, morphine, propoxyphene, or pentazocine
- Diphenoxylate-atropine (Lomotil) poisoning
- Coingestion of other drugs
- After the use of naloxone
- Hypoxia
- Prior institution of mydriatic drops

13. Why may a patient under treatment with oral meperidine for chronic pain present with seizures?
The seizures may be caused by normepiridine, a metabolite of meperidine. Normeperidine has excitatory effects on the CNS and can cause agitation, tremors, myoclonus, and seizures. Normeperidine levels will be elevated in the following situations:
(1) repetitive administration of meperidine by the oral route, as meperidine has significant first-pass metabolism;
(2) renal failure; and
(3) use of drugs that induce hepatic enzymes.

14. Which opioids can cause seizures?
Seizures have been reported in the following situations:
1. Intravenous use of fentanyl or sufentanil
2. Overdose of propoxyphene or pentazocine
3. Use of meperidine
4. Opioid withdrawal in infants
5. High doses of intravenous morphine administered to infants

15. Is it appropriate to give dextromethorphan or meperidine to patients on monoamine oxidase inhibitors (MAOIs)?
No. These combinations of drugs may precipitate the life-threatening serotonin syndrome. This syndrome is characterized by agitation, restlessness, irritability, headache, muscle rigidity, hyperpyrexia, hypotension, seizures, coma, and death. The syndrome may be indistinguishable from malignant hyperthermia or the neuroleptic malignant syndrome. The syndrome occurs unpredictably. Increased serotonin levels occur because MAOIs decrease serotonin metabolism, and meperidine and dextromethorphan block neuronal reuptake of serotonin, resulting in serotonin excess at the neuronal synapse. The treatment includes rapid cooling and cardiovascular support. Neuromuscular paralysis may be necessary.

16. Are any opioids safe to use for a patient on MAOIs?
If a patient on MAOIs must be treated with opioids, morphine is the recommended drug, as less is known about the potential interaction of other opioids with MAOIs. However, coma, respiratory compromise, and hypotension can occur after the administration of standard doses of opioids to patients on MAOIs. MAOIs inhibit the hepatic microsomal enzymes responsible for opioid metabolism. If used at all, opioids should be administered in small increments with careful monitoring.

17. Which opioid can produce ventricular arrhythmias, a wide QRS complex, mydriasis, and seizures?
Propoxyphene has a membrane depressant (quinidinelike) effect, similar to that of the cyclic antidepressants. Large doses of intravenous naloxone, up to 10 mg, may be required to reverse the CNS effects of propoxyphene. Naloxone will not reverse the cardiotoxic effects of propoxyphene, although it may play a role in the treatment of seizures. Cardiac conduction defects and ventricular arrhythmias should be treated with antiarrhythmic positive inotropic agent, defibrillation, and temporary cardiac pacing as required.

18. Which antidiarrheal agent can cause significant toxicity if ingested by children?
Diphenoxylate-atropine (Lomotil). (The Canadian product contains diphenoxylate only.) This drug can cause signs of atropine overdose (CNS excitement, hypertension, flushed dry skin) or opioid overdose (CNS and respiratory depression). Contrary to popular belief, mydriasis is rare. Coma and respiratory depression can present up to 12 hours after ingestion and may recur up to 24 hours after ingestion. Children are sensitive to the toxic effects of diphenoxylate-atropine. **Any child that has taken even one Lomotil tablet should be carefully observed for 24 hours.**

19. What is a "designer drug"?
Designer drugs, synthesized in illicit laboratories, are slightly different from the parent compound. The initial impetus to synthesize these drugs was a legal loophole that existed prior to passage of explicit legislation. Before this legislation was enacted in 1986, no laws

could be applied to a drug until it was isolated, studied, and scheduled. However, designer drugs continue to be synthesized.

20. Which designer drug has been associated with a syndrome similar to Parkinson's disease?
MPTP (1-methyl-4-phenyl-1,2,5,6 tetrahydropyridine). This compound was produced accidentally during the synthesis of MPPP, a meperidine analogue, when the chemist decided to take short cuts in the manufacturing process. MPTP is cytotoxic for dopaminergic neurons in the substantia nigra. The syndrome is almost identical to Parkinson's disease, is permanent, and occurs after a single ingestion of MPTP.

21. Which designer drug is 6,000 times as potent as morphine?
3-Methyl fentanyl. The fentanyl analogues are short-acting opioids that are pharmacologically similar to morphine. They are sold as synthetic heroin and are referred to by such names as "China White" and "Persian White." These drugs are very potent and over 100 deaths have been attributed to their use in California alone.

BIBLIOGRAPHY

1. Ford M, Hoffman RS, Goldfrank LR: Opioids and designer drugs. Emerg Med Clin North Am 8:495–511, 1990.
2. Goldfrank LR, Weisman RS, Errich JW, Lo MW: A dosing nomogram for continuous intravenous naloxone. Ann Emerg Med 15:566–570, 1986.
3. Handel KA, Schamben JL, Salamone FR: Naloxone. Ann Emerg Med 12:438–445, 1983.
4. Hoffman JR, Schriger DL, Luo JS: The empiric use of naloxone in patients with altered mental status: A reappraisal. Ann Emerg Med 20:246–252, 1991.
5. Jerrard DA: Designer drugs: A current perspective. J Emerg Med 8:733–741, 1990.
6. McCarron MM, Challoner KR, Thompson GA: Diphenoxylate-atropine (Lomotil) overdose in children: An update (report of eight cases and review of the literature). Pediatrics 87:694–700, 1991.

82. ANTIDEPRESSANTS: CYCLICS AND NEWER AGENTS

Russell U. Braun, M.D., Eric Isaacs, M.D., and Marc J. Bayer, M.D.

1. How are cyclic antidepressants classified? What are the newer antidepressants?
The cyclic antidepressants (CA) are classified as tricyclics, tetracyclics, and structural analogs (dibenzoxazepines). The newer agents include fluoxetine, trazodone, and bupropion. These newer agents were developed to reduce adverse side effects and possible toxicity from the standard cyclic antidepressants. Imipramine and amitriptyline are the prototype tricyclics because there are three rings (a central ring bonded to two benzene rings). All tricyclics contain a side chain with a varied number of methyl groups. The demethylation of imipramine, amitriptyline, or doxepin converts these tertiary amines to active secondary amines (desimipramine, nortriptyline, and protriptyline). The most toxic of these agents are the tertiary tricyclic amines. Antidepressants can be subdivided according to their major mechanism of action:

Mechanism of Action of Antidepressants

GROUP	MECHANISM OF ACTION	GENERIC EXAMPLES
I Tricyclic Tetracyclics Dibenzoxazepines	Block reuptake of norepinephrine (NE)	Imipramine (Tofranil) Maprotiline (Ludiomil) Amoxapine (Ascendin) Doxepin (Sinequan)
II Bicyclic	Block reuptake of serotonin	Fluoxetine (Prozac)
Triazolopyridine	Serotonin receptor antagonist	Trazodone (Desyrel)
III Unicyclic	Block dopamine (DA) reuptake	Bupropion (Wellbutrin)
IV Monoamine oxidase inhibitors	Elevate CNS NE & DA	Phenelzine (Nardil) Isocarboxazid (Marplan) Tranylcypramine (Parnate)
V Lithium	Not well understood	

2. What are the epidemiologic characteristics associated with antidepressant overdoses?
Pharmaceutical overdoses in the U.S. numbered over 812,000 cases for 1991, of which antidepressant overdoses numbered over 35,000. Amitriptyline was the most frequent CA ingested (18%), followed in order by imipramine, doxepin, and nortriptyline. Women aged 20–40 are most commonly involved in antidepressant overdoses. Mortality has been reduced substantially over the last 15 years from 15% to a current rate of 1–3%. However, antidepressants were still the #1 cause of ingestion-related deaths in 1990. The newer antidepressants accounted for significantly less morbidity and mortality compared with tricyclics.

3. How do antidepressants work to treat depression?
One theory holds that depression is related to a deficiency of particular neurotransmitters, such as norepinephrine, serotonin, and dopamine. CAs act to increase the amounts of catecholamines by decreasing neuronal uptake of norepinephrine, while the newer agents block the reuptake of serotonin or dopamine.

4. What are the three major mechanisms of CA toxicity?
   1. **Anticholinergic:** Anticholinergic effects of CA ingestions include supraventricular tachycardia, hallucinations, seizures, and coma. Signs and symptoms are listed below:

Clinical Presentations of Cyclic Antidepressant Overdose

	CVS	CNS	ANTICHOLINERGIC
SYMPTOMS	Dizziness	Confusion	Blurred vision Dry mouth
SIGNS	Cond. blocks QRS widening Hypotension Arrhythmias Cardiac arrest	Delirium Agitation Extrapyramidal Myoclonus Seizures Coma	Tachycardia Mydriasis Decreased bowel sounds Urinary retention Hyperthermia/hypothermia

2. **Quinidine-like:** The quinidine-like effects of CA toxicity, manifested by decreased cardiac contractility, hypotension, and ventricular dysrhythmias, are characteristic of all type 1A antiarrhythmics (quinidine, procainamide, and disopyramide).

3. **Alpha-adrenergic Blockade:** Peripheral alpha-receptor blockade may lead to hypotension.

5. What is the anticholinergic syndrome?

The anticholinergic syndrome includes hyperthermia, blurred vision, dry mouth, skin flushing, hallucinations, and tachycardia. These effects may be summarized by the phrase: "Hot as a hare, blind as a bat, dry as a bone, red as a beet, and mad as a hatter." Other substances that cause anticholinergic symptoms are antihistamines, phenothiazines, scopolamine, belladonna, jimson weed, nightshade, and *Amanita muscaria* mushrooms.

6. What is the clinical presentation of CA ingestions?

CA ingestions may present with initial signs and symptoms such as sinus tachycardia, slurred speech, dry mouth, and drowsiness, which may rapidly progress to lethargy, hallucinations, and the life-threatening complications of coma, seizures, hypotension, and arrhythmias.

7. What is the clinical course of CA toxicity?

The major clinical signs and symptoms of toxicity (coma, seizures, arrhythmias, and hypotension) occur within several hours of ingestion. The symptomatology may range from mild to severe, but in one review of CA fatalities, all patients developed major signs of toxicity within 2 hours. A review of over 2,500 cases identified the incidence of various clinical findings as follows: tachycardia (51%), coma (35%), increased QRS duration (21%), hypotension (14%), seizures (8%), and arrhythmias (6%).

8. Are there any reliable indicators that predict the severity of CA toxicity?

There is anecdotal evidence to suggest a relationship between a widened QRS duration (>120 ms) and the subsequent development of ventricular arrhythmias. Hypotension is an ominous sign and needs to be treated aggressively. Seizures have been associated with an increased mortality.

9. What is the general approach to management of antidepressant overdoses?

Patient stabilization after an acute ingestion is paramount, including management of the ABCs and supportive care. The patient should be given oxygen and the altered mental status protocol of thiamine, glucose, and naloxone (if indicated). After stabilization, GI decontamination followed by administration of charcoal with a cathartic is recommended. Persons with CA overdose are at risk of developing an ileus from anticholinergic effects. Use of serial dosed charcoal administration is controversial and may put the patient at risk for bowel obstruction. One must be cautious during stabilization and GI decontamination because patients can rapidly lose consciousness, placing them at risk for aspiration. For this reason, ipecac is contraindicated and endotracheal intubation should be considered prior to gastric lavage in patients with a decreased level of consciousness. These patients require constant cardiac monitoring with intravenous access. A Foley catheter may be necessary because of the risk of urinary retention.

10. Should antidepressant drug levels be ordered when CA overdose is suspected?

Antidepressant drug levels are not helpful and have not been shown to be a reliable predictor of toxicity.

11. What diagnostic test ordering is helpful with an antidepressant overdose?

An EKG is essential in the evaluation of a patient with CA overdose. Any prolongation of the intervals should be considered a sign of tricyclic cardiotoxicity. Because of the potential for polydrug ingestions with any overdose, one may need to consider other toxins. Obtaining acetaminophen and aspirin levels is recommended. Generally, a full urine and serum toxicology screen is not indicated because of the low yield and cost ineffectiveness. Results of toxicology screens are often delayed and rarely change patient management.

12. What other drug ingestions can mimic those of CAs?
Flexeril (cyclobenzaprine), structurally similar to amitriptyline, was developed in 1961 as an antidepressant and is now prescribed as a muscle relaxant. Tegretol (carbamazepine) is structurally similar to imipramine but causes less toxicity in cases of overdose.

13. What are the treatment recommendations for cardiovascular system (CVS) toxicity?
Arrhythmias: Sodium bicarbonate is the drug of choice for treatment of ventricular dysrhythmias. The mechanism of action of sodium bicarbonate is unclear, but may be related to reduced sodium channel blockade and increased plasma protein binding of CAs (decreasing the amount of circulating free drug). Hyperventilation is also useful as an adjunctive measure to increase plasma pH. The dose of bicarbonate is 1–2 mEq/kg and may be repeated to maintain an arterial pH of 7.5. Alkalinization may be maintained via constant IV infusion of sodium bicarbonate added to maintenance fluids. Lidocaine is effective for ventricular tachycardia but may decrease cardiac contractility. Phenytoin has been used in first-degree atrioventricular block and intraventricular conduction defects. Phenytoin may be used to treat ventricular dysrhythmias that do not respond to alkalinization or lidocaine. Group 1A antiarrhythmics (quinidine, procainamide, and disopyramide) are contraindicated because of their synergistic effects on cell membranes, enhancing antidepressant toxicity. Physostigmine is contraindicated for the treatment of ventricular arrhythmias. Sinus tachycardia and supraventricular arrhythmias usually do not require specific treatment more than supportive care.

Hypotension: Hypotension should be initially treated with fluids and Trendelenburg positioning. Bicarbonate may be useful if hypotension does not respond to the above. Vasopressors should be used with caution, as they may increase ventricular irritability. Norepinephrine and phenylephrine are the vasopressors of choice because of their primary alpha-adrenergic effect.

Widened QRS: Bicarbonate is useful in narrowing a widened QRS (>120 ms), which may confer a cardioprotective effect.

14. What are the treatment recommendations for central nervous system (CNS) toxicity?
Hallucinations: Physostigmine has been shown to reverse hallucinations; however, as it may precipitate seizures and asystole, it is not generally recommended. Neuroleptics should be avoided because they may lower the seizure threshold.

Coma: Imipramine, amitriptyline, doxepin, and trazodone are the most sedating of the antidepressants. Supportive care with aggressive airway management is fundamental. Coma lasting greater than 24 hours is rare and suggests further complications of a coingestant or inadequate GI decontamination.

Seizures: Seizure activity related to CA toxicity is usually brief. Benzodiazepines and phenobarbital are recommended for management of seizures. Phenytoin may be used as a third-line drug.

15. Which patients should be admitted after antidepressant overdose?
All patients with antidepressant overdoses should be monitored and observed for at least 6 hours. In one series of fatal CA ingestions, all patients developed signs of major toxicity within 2 hours and died within 24 hours of arrival. There are reports of patients with delayed complications after initial improvement. However, these patients either presented with major signs of toxicity or they did not have adequate GI decontamination or

assessment of bowel motility. Patients with persistent signs of toxicity, such as tachycardia, QRS widening, mental status changes, and ileus, should be admitted to a monitored unit.

16. How do the newer antidepressants differ from tricyclic antidepressants?
Fluoxetine and trazodone appear to have less CNS and CVS toxicity than the traditional CAs. Although bupropion has less CVS toxicity, there is concern about the risk of seizures with this drug. To date, there is limited experience on the toxicology of the newer antidepressants in the overdose setting. However, the cardiovascular toxicity appears to be less with these newer agents.

CONTROVERSIES

17. What are the most current controversies related to antidepressant ingestion?
Physostigmine: Physostigmine is a reversible cholinesterase inhibitor and thus counteracts many of the peripheral and central anticholinergic effects of antidepressant toxicity. Physostigmine has been shown to reverse altered mental status, coma, and supraventricular and sinus tachycardias, but may cause seizures, cholinergic crisis, or cardiac arrest. At this time, we do not recommend the use of physostigmine, particularly in the presence of an antecedent conduction delay.

Bicarbonate: Sodium bicarbonate administration narrows a widened QRS (>120 ms), reverses hypotension, and treats ventricular arrhythmias. The cardioprotective effect of bicarbonate has been postulated based on the above cardiac effects. Some researchers have suggested that widened QRS (>120 ms) is associated with an increased risk for the development of ventricular arrhythmias. In vitro studies have supported the use of sodium bicarbonate for prevention of ventricular arrhythmias, but to date there are no controlled human studies on its efficacy with this particular use.

BIBLIOGRAPHY

1. Bessen HA, Niemann JT, Haskell RJ, et al: Effect of respiratory alkalosis in tricyclic antidepressant overdose. West J Med 139:373–376, 1983.
2. Callaham M, Kasrel D: Epidemiology of fatal tricyclic antidepressants: Implications for management. Ann Emerg Med 14:1–9, 1985.
3. Ellenhorn M, Barceloux D: Medical Toxicology. New York, Elsevier, 1988.
4. Foulk GE, Albertson TE, Walby WF: Tricyclic antidepressant overdose: Emergency department findings as predictors of clinical course. Am J Emerg Med 4:496–500, 1986.
5. Fromer DA, Kulick KW, Marx JA, et al: Tricyclic antidepressant overdose. JAMA 20:75–80, 1987.
6. Hoffman JR, McElroy CR: Bicarbonate therapy for dysrhythmia and hypotension in tricyclic antidepressant overdose. West J Med 134:60–64, 1981.
7. Krishel S, Jackimczyk K: Cyclic antidepressants, lithium and neuroleptic agents. Emerg Med Clin North Am 9:53–86, 1991.
8. Litovitz TL, Bailey KM, et al: 1991 Annual Report of AAPCC National Data Collection System. Am J Emerg Med 10:452–505, 1992.
9. Moore JL, et al: Toxicity of fluoxetine in overdose. Am J Psychiatry 147:1089, 1990.
10. Niemann JJ, Bessen HA, Rothstein RJ, et al: Electrocardiographic criteria for tricyclic antidepressant cardiotoxicity. Am J Cardiol 57:1154–1159, 1986.
11. Smilkstein JM: As the pendulum swings: The saga of physostigmine. J Emerg Med 9:275–277, 1991.
12. Stephen JM, Ghezzi L, et al: Post-triathalon delirium. J Emerg Med 9:265–269, 1991.
13. Weber JJ: Seizure activity associated with fluoxetine therapy. Clin Pharmacol 8:296–298, 1989.

83. HYDROCARBON POISONING (PETROLEUM DISTILLATES)

Ernest Stremski, M.D., and Louis Ling, M.D.

1. What are hydrocarbons?

Hydrocarbons are distillation products of crude oil. Although all petroleum distillates are hydrocarbons, all hydrocarbons are not derived from petroleum. They may be produced synthetically or distilled from other sources such as wood tars (i.e., pine oils). They are classified as **aliphatic:** straight or branched-chain carbon links that are fully or incompletely saturated to hydrogen atoms; **aromatic:** contain cyclic benzene ring(s); or **halogenated:** hydrogen atoms have been substituted with halide anions (Br, Cl, F, or I).

2. What types of symptoms do these agents cause?

Aspiration of these agents may lead to "chemical pneumonitis." Gastrointestinal (GI) absorption of hydrocarbons plays a minimal role in the development of pulmonary toxicity. Pulmonary toxicity is the result of direct tracheal instillation of the hydrocarbon. Attempts at swallowing a hydrocarbon may produce gagging and impair protective airway reflexes, resulting in influx of the agent into the trachea. Further migration down the airways produces acute inflammation, hemorrhage, edema, and loss of surfactant activity. Progression of the inflammatory response may lead to excessive intraluminal secretions, peribronchial edema and cellular infiltration, nonuniform atelectasis, obstructive emphysema, bronchospasm, interstitial edema, and alveolar consolidation. These anatomic abnormalities contribute to ventilation/perfusion (V/Q) mismatch and resultant hypoxemia.

Certain hydrocarbons cause unique toxicity if systemically absorbed. Toxic effects include transfer across the blood/brain barrier, producing CNS depression or excitation, bone marrow suppression, hepatic or renal toxicity, and cardiac arrhythmias. When coupled with heavy metals (e.g., lead), hydrocarbons may produce heavy metal intoxication.

3. Which characteristic of a hydrocarbon most increases the risk of aspiration?

Hydrocarbons are classified according to viscosity and volatility. Viscosity is the property that most increases the risk of aspiration. The viscosity of a hydrocarbon is determined by the time it takes to flow a specified distance through a calibrated diameter, measured in SSU units (Sabolt seconds universal). Low-viscosity agents (SSU <60) have less resistance to flow and are capable of spreading over the epiglottis and into the larynx. The agents that are more likely to be aspirated are mineral seal oils, mineral spirits, kerosene, turpentines, naphthas, gasoline, and aromatics. Less likely to be aspirated are agents with a high viscosity (>100 SSU), such as waxes, paraffins, jellies, greases, and lubricating oils.

4. What is important about volatility?

Volatility refers to the tendency of a liquid to become a gas. Vapors released from highly volatile hydrocarbons (primarily with low molecular weight and aromatics) may displace oxygen, resulting in a diminished inspired oxygen. Individuals working in enclosed areas with volatile hydrocarbons may experience symptoms from hypoxia.

5. What is the incidence of hydrocarbon toxicity? Who is at highest risk?

The American Association of Poison Control Centers collected data on 1,837,939 human poisonings in 1991. Exposures to hydrocarbons (fuels and oils) accounted for 3.5% of all human exposures, or 63,536 cases. Children less than 6 years of age accounted for 30,645 cases, of which 99.7% were considered accidental. Ingestion by toddlers remains the number one cause of reported human exposure to hydrocarbons. Of the recorded 63,536 cases in 1991, approximately 95% had no or "minimal" symptoms directly attributable to the exposure. There were a total of 36 deaths, and 104 patients developed undefined "major" toxicity.

6. What are the signs and symptoms of hydrocarbon poisoning?

The severity of symptoms is highly dependent on the degree of pulmonary aspiration. Following attempts at oral ingestion, patients may immediately experience paroxysmal coughing in an effort to clear the airway. Nausea, emesis, and variable degrees of respiratory distress may ensue. Physical signs initially may be absent yet progress to cyanosis, mottling or dusky appearance of the skin, tachycardia, tachypnea, stridor, salivation, grunting, nasal flaring, retractions, hemoptysis, fever, rales, or wheezing. The presence or absence of a hydrocarbon odor on the breath is unreliable in determining whether aspiration has occurred. Symptoms may rapidly resolve or progress to significant respiratory distress. Hypoxia may lead to CNS excitation (hallucinations, agitation, confusion) and CNS depression (lethargy, coma). Direct pulmonary toxicity (V/Q mismatch) is the primary cause of hypoxia; however, volatilization of hydrocarbons may produce hypoxia from displacement of oxygen. Extreme hypoxia may lead to arrhythmias, hypotension, seizures, and cardiopulmonary arrest.

7. How likely are patients to require hospitalization?

The majority of patients who ingest hydrocarbons do not develop clinical or x-ray evidence of pneumonia. Even in patients with initial chest x-ray findings, the vast majority do not develop significant pulmonary complications. In one series of 950 cases of hydrocarbon ingestion in children, there were only two deaths and only seven patients exhibited progressive worsening of pulmonary disease. The development of symptoms or an abnormal chest x-ray occurred within 6–8 hours of the ingestion in all these patients.

8. What types of x-ray changes are most likely?

Initial chest x-rays may be normal in 60% of patients who develop symptomatic pulmonary disease. Radiographic abnormalities may be present within 30 minutes of aspiration and include perihilar densities, linear/basilar atelectasis, extension of interstitial infiltrate, early alveolar infiltrate, lobar consolidation, and lobar atelectasis. Early (6–8 hours) abnormalities may lead to further progression. Pleural effusions, pneumothorax, pneumomediastinum, pneumopericardium, and pneumatoceles may develop.

9. Which patients should be admitted?

Patients who are asymptomatic and have a normal physical examination following hydrocarbon exposure may be discharged home. However, they should be given instructions to return immediately if they develop respiratory, GI, or CNS symptoms. Symptoms usually occur within 6–8 hours. Patients who are symptomatic or who have positive findings on physical examination should have a chest x-ray, and oxygen saturation should be measured. Such patients should be admitted for observation and treatment. Other considerations for admission include ingestion of hydrocarbons with unique systemic toxicity, such as pesticides or carbon tetrachloride.

10. Are toxicology screens helpful?

No. Standard toxicology screens do not identify hydrocarbons and are not indicated in the diagnosis of hydrocarbon pneumonitis.

11. What about other laboratory studies?

Pulse oximetry is useful for monitoring these patients. Patients who develop desaturation during the observation period require supplemental oxygen and admission. Serial arterial blood gases (ABGs) may be used to follow severely symptomatic patients. Secondary bacterial infections may occur along with the primary chemical pneumonitis. Although an initial cell count with differential may be elevated solely on the basis of the chemical pneumonitis, serial cell counts along with respiratory tract cultures (endotracheal tube aspirate, sputum) and blood cultures may help to diagnose a secondary bacterial infection.

12. What is the appropriate management of hydrocarbon pneumonitis?

Initial treatment is aimed at assessment of pulmonary symptoms and measurement of oxygen saturation. Chest films may be taken after assessing and securing the airway. Supraglottitis with upper respiratory tract obstruction may occur, particularly if the hydrocarbon was heated. Otherwise, treatment is primarily supportive. Oxygen should be administered to patients with desaturation or respiratory difficulty. Increased oropharyngeal secretions or gastric emesis may develop from chemical irritation and require suctioning and clearing from the airway. Petroleum distillates are not caustic, so upper airway and esophageal burns are unlikely. Bronchospasm may be treated with aerosolized and parenteral bronchodilating agents.

13. What are the indications for intubation?

Indications for controlled endotracheal intubation are severe respiratory distress, persistent alveolar-arterial oxygen gradient despite high-flow oxygen administration, or CNS depression leading to respiratory acidosis or inability to maintain airway protective reflexes. Both obstructive and restrictive lung disease may occur with chemical pneumonitis. Therefore ventilatory management may require frequent reassessment and change. The development of edema, consolidation, and atelectasis may worsen V/Q mismatch. Positive end-expiratory pressure (PEEP) may be useful for ventilating these patients. The restoration of functional residual capacity by PEEP may allow for lower inspired FiO_2 concentrations. However, excessive PEEP may lead to pneumothorax and pneumomediastinum in individuals with obstructive lung disease.

14. What else is of concern?

Hydrocarbons should be assessed for the presence of other dangerous additives that may induce other toxicity (e.g., isopropyl alcohol in pine oil cleaners may lead to CNS depression and ketosis). Specific hydrocarbon agents may also cause toxicity that requires administration of an antidote (e.g., nitrobenzene leading to methemoglobinemia).

CONTROVERSIES

15. Does gastrointestinal decontamination help to prevent pulmonary toxicity?

Multiple animal studies have shown that gastric absorption of hydrocarbon does not lead to chemical pneumonitis. Only when extremely large quantities (>18 cc/kg) of hydrocarbon are placed in an animal's stomach does enough gastric absorption occur to produce pneumonitis. Direct instillation of hydrocarbon into the portal vein as well was found not to produce pneumonitis. Induced emesis and gastric lavage both carry the risk of aspiration of gastric contents. Activated charcoal does not bind petroleum distillates well. The risks of induced emesis and gastric lavage probably outweigh the benefits when ingestion of a simple petroleum distillate is less than 2 cc/kg, a typical accidental swallow for a toddler. Emesis is certainly contraindicated when the patient exhibits altered mental status, is unable to protect the airway, the ingested agent is caustic, or the ingested agent produces rapid mental status changes (e.g., camphorated oils). However, hydrocarbons may possess potential for serious systemic toxicity or contain toxic additives. If the quantity of the substance ingested equates to a toxic dose, then gastric lavage with a controlled airway should be considered. Gastric lavage may be considered if ingestion of a simple petroleum distillate was greater than 2 cc/kg (adult suicidal ingestion).

16. What are the most dangerous hydrocarbons?
Ingestion of multiple substances along with a hydrocarbon may warrant the use of gastric lavage and/or administration of enteral activated charcoal. These substances can be remembered with the mnemonic CHAMP:

C = Camphor
H = Halogenated (as little as 10 cc of CCl_4 may lead to acute hepatic failure)
A = Aromatics
M = Metals
P = Pesticides

17. Are prophylactic antibiotics and steroids indicated for hydrocarbon pneumonitis?
Prophylactic administration of steroids and antibiotics is not currently recommended. Animal studies have shown that antibiotic treatment did not change the rate or type of bacterial organisms recovered from lung tissue. Groups that also received dexamethasone had a significant increase in bacterial lung contamination.

A human study of 71 children with a history of hydrocarbon ingestion and admission to the hospital with radiographic evidence of pulmonary abnormalities were randomized to placebo or methylprednisolone/penicillin for 3 days. No difference in respiratory rate, pulse rate, and days of hospitalization, or radiographic changes were found. There were, however, only 3 cases of severe pneumonitis. There were no deaths. Although large, prospective, controlled human trials are lacking, available data suggest that the prophylactic use of steroids and antibiotics is not warranted following hydrocarbon aspiration. Serial use of cell counts and bacterial cultures may be used to determine if antibiotics are needed for secondary bacterial infection.

BIBLIOGRAPHY

1. Anas N, Namasonthi V, Ginsburg CM: Criteria for hospitalizing children who have ingested products containing hydrocarbons. JAMA 246:840, 1981.
2. Arena JM: Hydrocarbon poisoning: Current management. Pediatr Ann 16:879, 1987.
3. Dice WH, Ward G, Kelley J, et al: Pulmonary toxicity following gastrointestinal ingestion of kerosene. Ann Emerg Med 11:138, 1982.
4. Litovitz TL, Bailey KM, Schmitz KM, et al: 1991 Annual Report of the American Association of Poison Control Centers National Data Collection System. Am J Emerg Med 10:452, 1992.
5. Marks MI, Chicione L, Legere G, et al: Adrenocorticosteroid treatment of hydrocarbon pneumonia in children—a cooperative study. J Pediatr 81:366, 1972.
6. Mullin LS, Ader AW, Daugherty WC, et al: Toxicology update. Isoparrafinic hydrocarbons: A summary of physical properties, toxicity studies and human exposure. J Appl Toxicol 10:135, 1990.
7. Reyes de la Rocha S, Cunningham JC, Fox E: Lipoid pneumonia secondary to baby oil aspiration: A case report and review of the literature. Pediatr Emerg Care 1:74, 1985.
8. Scalzo AJ, Weber TR, Jaeger RW, et al: Extracorporeal membrane oxygenation for hydrocarbon aspiration. Am J Dis Child 144:867, 1990.
9. Seger DL: The hydrocarbon controversy. Emergency Medicine Survey. Baltimore, Williams & Wilkins, 1984.
10. Truemper E, Reyes de la Rocha S, Atkinson SD: Clinical characteristics, pathophysiology, and management of hydrocarbon ingestion: Care report and review of the literature. Pediatr Emerg Care 3:187, 1987.

84. PESTICIDES AND OTHER CHOLINERGICS

Loi E. Graham, M.D.

1. What are the two classes of cholinergic pesticides?

The cholinergic pesticides are the organophosphates and carbamates. These two classes differ in their chemical structures and in the fact that the organophosphates are irreversible cholinesterase inhibitors, whereas the carbamates are reversible cholinesterase inhibitors. The signs and symptoms of poisoning with organophosphates and carbamates are almost identical except that carbamates have a shorter and less severe toxicity and do not produce CNS toxicity because they penetrate the CNS only poorly.

2. Where and how do these pesticides effect their toxicity?

There are two main types of cholinesterases in the body—red blood cell or true cholinesterase (acetylcholinesterase), found in erythrocytes, nervous tissue, and skeletal muscle, and plasma cholinesterase (pseudocholinesterase), a hepatic protein found in the plasma, heart, pancreas, liver, and brain. Under normal conditions there is rapid hydrolysis of acetylcholine by cholinesterase after neurochemical transmission at autonomic and neuromuscular synapses. In organophosphate poisoning, phosphate radicals covalently bind to an active serine site on the enzyme, rendering it inactive. This inhibition of cholinesterase action allows an accumulation of acetylcholine at synapses, resulting in overstimulation, and later, disruption of transmission in the CNS, parasympathetic nerve endings, some sympathetic nerve endings, somatic nerves, and autonomic ganglia.

3. What is the difference with carbamates?

With carbamates, carbamylation of cholinesterase occurs, and this bond spontaneously breaks within 48 hours with regeneration of cholinesterase to the active form.

4. What is the mechanism that keeps the process going?

Binding of the organophosphates and the acetylcholinesterase forms a short-lived intermediate compound that undergoes partial hydrolysis and the loss of a substituent group. The result is a stable inhibited enzyme. Without intervention, signs and symptoms of intoxication persist until enough new acetylcholinesterase is synthesized in 22–30 days to destroy the excess acetylcholine. The mechanism of producing the inactive enzyme is known as "aging," which is believed to fix an extra charge to the protein, causing an alteration of the active site and thereby preventing regeneration. Hydrolysis of the inactive enzyme is slow and clinically unimportant. Many of the more recently produced organophosphates are less tenacious inhibitors of acetylcholinesterase, and the active enzyme is more spontaneously dissociated.

5. How are organophosphates and carbamates metabolized?

Most of these compounds are well absorbed from the conjunctiva, skin, lungs, and GI tract. Once absorbed, they undergo extensive biotransformation with both the route and the rate of metabolism being highly species specific and dependent on the different types of attached groups. The enzymes involved use a nicotinamide adenine dinucleotide phosphate (NADPH) and cytochrome P_{450}-mediated mono-oxygenases to provide the necessary oxygen and electrons to produce polar (water-soluble) metabolites, which can be detected 0.5–2 days after exposure.

6. What are the clinical effects?

When large amounts of acetylcholine accumulate at the cholinergic synapses, initial stimulation and then exhaustion of the synapses occur. Compensatory inhibition by dopaminergic and GABA (gamma-aminobutyric acid)-mediated pathways counteracts the excessive cholinergic activity. These pathways are thought to be antagonized by organophosphates, and so CNS dysfunction and seizures are produced independently of the effect on brain acetylcholinesterase. The clinical effects can be divided into two categories: acute and delayed.

Acute effects
    1. **CNS effects**—will lead to initial stimulation and then depression of all activity, and coma.
    2. **Muscarinic effects**—due to enhancement of parasympathetic activity on smooth muscle.
    3. **Nicotinic effects**—accumulation of acetylcholine at the motor endplates and autonomic ganglia causes persistent depolarization of skeletal muscles.

Delayed effects
    Delayed neurotoxicity
    1. **Delayed psychopathologic-neurologic lesions** involving neurobehavioral, cognitive, and neuromuscular functions may develop and persist for several months following exposure to high concentrations of organophosphates. In addition, there may be depressive disorders of vital functions (syncopal attacks) lasting 5–10 years.
    2. An **intermediate syndrome** may occur 24–96 hours after the cholinergic crisis, with the major effect being weakness of muscles supplied by the cranial nerves (e.g., respiratory muscles) and cranial nerve palsies. There is increased risk of death from respiratory depression, which responds to ventilatory support and atropine.
    3. In **organophosphate-induced neurotoxicity (OPIN),** development of flaccidity and muscle weakness in the limbs proceeds to spasticity, hyperreflexia, and hypertonicity indicative of damage to the pyramidal tracts. The accompanying biochemical lesion is the inhibition of a neuronal carboxylase–neuropathic target esterase (NTE) that appears to have a role in lipid metabolism in neurones. The histologic lesion is a wallerian degeneration or "dying back" of axons. The onset is about 10–21 days after exposure.

7. When are symptoms expected after exposure to organophosphates?
Onset of symptoms is determined by the nature and quantity of the product and the route of exposure. Symptoms can occur as early as 5 minutes with massive exposure or be delayed 40–48 hours if a very lipid-soluble product such as fenthion is involved. By 12 hours, most organophosphates will cause symptoms, and after 24 hours another diagnosis should be entertained.

8. What are the signs and symptoms?
Signs and symptoms are the result of excess acetylcholine and manifest as CNS, muscarinic, and nicotinic symptoms.
    1. **CNS symptoms** include agitation, drowsiness, seizures, depression of the cardiorespiratory center, and death.
    2. **Muscarinic symptoms** are the hollow organ parasympathetic effects and involve the eyes (lacrimal glands, pupils, and ciliary body), the heart, bronchial tree, and sweat glands.
    3. **Nicotinic symptoms** reflect the ganglionic and somatic motor effects and include muscle fasciculations, muscle weakness with areflexia, and even paralysis. Weakness of respiratory muscles can result in respiratory failure. The pulse and blood may be increased and the pupils dilated. In any case, the symptoms displayed depend on the relative dominance of muscarinic and nicotinic effects.

9. Is there a mnemonic to describe the symptoms of cholinergic excess?
The mnemonic DUMBELS can be used.

D   =   Diarrhea
U   =   Urination
M   =   Meiosis
B   =   Bronchospasm
E   =   Emesis
L   =   Lacrimation
S   =   Salivation

10. How is the diagnosis made?
A history is helpful but not always available. A garlic odor may be detected. The presence of a combination of the characteristic CNS, muscarinic, and nicotinic effects are the main aids. Meiosis characteristically occurs, but in 10% of cases mydriasis is present. Pancreatitis can present in organophosphate poisoning because the pancreatic acinar glands have cholinergic innervation, so their rate of secretion is enhanced.

11. Which laboratory tests should be obtained?
The confirmatory laboratory tests are the measurement of the decrease in the activity of red blood cell acetylcholinesterase (RBCAChE) and plasma cholinesterase (PChE). Though the RBCAChE level is a more accurate reflection of the activity of the toxicant, the PCheE is technically easier to obtain, is depressed before AChE, and recovers earlier as well.

12. What factors affect these levels?
Low levels of PChE may occur in liver disease, infection, use of some drugs (e.g., morphine), and as a genetic deficiency. Factors affecting the life of circulating erythrocytes can affect the AChE activity.

13. Are there other laboratory studies needed?
Other studies include CBC, liver function tests, creatinine, BUN, electrolytes, glucose amylase, EKG, ABG, and chest x-ray.

14. What abnormalities may be seen on laboratory tests?
Abnormalities include hyperglycemia and glycosuria, acetonuria, and albuminuria. The blood may show a leukocytosis with a left shift and reduction of monocytes, lymphocytes, and eosinophil counts. The EKG may show ST-T wave changes, QT prolongation, and PVCs. The EEG may show changes similar to those of temporal lobe seizures.

15. What is a typical presentation?
The person poisoned with organophosphates is likely to have a depressed level of consciousness associated with pinpoint pupils, respiratory distress, diaphoresis, and a smell of pesticides on the clothes or breath.

16. What is the emergency management?
Emergency management consists of effective supportive care and the use of specific antidotes. The ways to address these include:
   1. Establish an airway as necessary and oxygenate.
   2. Respiratory distress, if present, may be due to excessive secretions, bronchospasm, pulmonary edema, chemical pneumonitis, aspiration, ARDS, muscle weakness, or paralysis. ABGs and chest x-ray are part of the initial assessment. **Note:** The use of theophylline is contraindicated in this setting.
   3. Establish intravenous access. Most circulatory problems due to the poisoning will be addressed with the use of specific antidotes—atropine and oximes.

4. Institute specific therapy.

    a. Atropine: adults, 3–4 mg IV; children, 0.05 mg/kg IV. Repeat dosage until signs of mild atropinization appear (dilated pupils, warm red skin, tachycardia). Large amounts of atropine (10–20 gm) may be needed over 24 hours.

    b. Pralidoxime (2-PAM): adults, 1–2 gm IV; children, 23–30 mg/kg IV given over 3–5 minutes.

5. Decontamination: all the clothes should be removed and the skin washed thoroughly with water and a mild soap, care being taken to include the hair and under the nails. If the patient is seen after 6 hours postingestion, gastric decontamination is not useful.

17. What other cholinergics are particularly dangerous?
The chemical warfare agents were first used during WWI. These are extremely potent, longlasting anticholinesterases, and include the G agents: tabun (GA), sarin (GB), soman (GD), and agent VX. The estimated median dose of sarin is 1 mg, and that of VX is 0.4 mg. The G agents are volatile and do not penetrate intact skin, but absorption is greatly increased through broken skin. The nonvolatile agent VX has dermal toxicity equaling that of the vesicant sulfur mustard.

18. What is the effect of exposure to the chemical warfare agents?
Respiratory exposure to the volatile nerve agents leads to a rapid onset of clinical symptoms within 2–3 minutes, with a peak effect at 20–30 minutes. Intense cholinergic symptoms are present. Death usually results from respiratory failure due to a combination of excessive secretions, bronchospasm, muscle paralysis, and respiratory center dysfunction.

19. What treatment is effective?
The treatment is similar to that for pesticide toxicity and consists of cholinergics with central (benactyzine and scopolamine) and peripheral (atropine) activity. Pralidoxime is not effective against soman (GD); obidoxime is used. The onset and progression of symptoms are so rapid that immediate use of a preloaded syringe intramuscularly by the person exposed is necessary. The treatment sequence set out by the U.S. Army is antidotes first, airway and circulation management, decontamination, and then treatment of any other life threats.

20. What are the classes of cholinesterase inhibitors?
There are three broad classes of cholinesterase inhibitors:

    1. **Organophosphates**—e.g., isoflurophate, echothiophate, pesticides such as malathion and parathion, and toxins such as sarin.

    2. **Carbamates**—e.g., pyridostigmine, physostigmine, neostigmine, and pesticides like carbaryl.

    3. **Quaternary amines**—e.g., edrophonium, ambenonium, and demecarium.

    Physostigmine, a tertiary amine, is nonionized and lipophilic and can easily traverse the blood-brain barrier. This ability led to the widespread use of the drug as an awakening agent in many cases of anticholinergic excess. It can reverse the central and peripheral effects of cyclic antidepressant overdose. Because the development of seizures, heart block and asystole have complicated some cases, use in the treatment of cyclic antidepressant overdose is to be avoided. Some toxicologists believe that physostigmine has been given bad press because of misuse.

    Pyridostigmine, a quaternary carbamate, is used to (1) treat myasthenia gravis, (2) terminate the action of neuromuscular blocking agents in anesthesia, and (3) pretreat by the Armed Forces in the threat of nerve agent exposure to improve the postexposure survival achieved by the antidotal therapy.

    The other cholinesterase inhibitors are used in the treatment of myasthenia gravis and eye disorders, including glaucoma.

BIBLIOGRAPHY

1. Berkenstadt H, et al: Combined chemical and conventional injuries: Physiological, diagnostic and
   therapeutic aspects. Isr Med Sci 27:623–626, 1991.
2. deKort WL: The use of atropine and oximes in acute organophosphate poisoning. Clin Toxicol
   26:199–208, 1988.
3. Ellen MJ, Barceloux DG: Medical Toxicology. New York, Elsevier, 1988.
4. Goldfrank LR (ed): Goldfrank's Toxicological Emergencies. Norwalk, CT, Appleton & Lange,
   1990.
5. Koelle GB: Organophosphate poisoning: An overview. Fundam Appl Toxicol 1:129–134, 1981.
6. Minton NA, Murray VSG: A review of organophosphate poisoning. Med Toxicol 3:355–378, 1988.
7. Olson KR (ed): Poisoning and Drug Overdose. Norwalk, CT, Appleton & Lange, 1990.
8. Tafuri J, Roberts J: Organophosphate poisoning. Ann Emerg Med 16:193–202, 1987.

85. CORROSIVES

Marsha D. Ford, M.D., FACEP

1. Which agents are classified as corrosives and can cause injury?

Ingestion of alkaline or acidic materials produces the majority of caustic injuries to the gastrointestinal (GI) tract in the U.S. Alkaline substances are bases that release hydroxide ions upon dissociation in water, whereas acids liberate hydronium ions with water contact. The alkaline and acidic materials may be in either liquid or solid form.

2. What tissue injuries are caused by alkaline and acidic corrosive preparations?

Alkalis produce liquefaction necrosis, with destruction of protein and collagen, tissue dehydration, saponification of fat, and blood vessel thrombosis. This process can penetrate some or all layers of the esophagus and stomach. The injuries are classified by endoscopists according to the degree of penetration:

First-degree burn: superficial erythema, edema

Second-degree burn: erythema, blistering, superficial ulceration, fibrinous exudate

Third-degree burn: deep ulceration, friability, eschar formation, perforation

Acids produce coagulation necrosis, with damage to the columnar epithelium, submucosa, and muscularis mucosa. The injury is covered by a coagulum consisting of damaged tissue and thrombosed blood vessels. In mild to moderate cases, this coagulum may inhibit further penetration of acid and protect the deeper muscular layers. In severe cases, full-thickness injuries with perforation can occur. Acid burns are classified using a five-grade system:

Grade 0:   normal

Grade 1:   edema, mucosal hyperemia

Grade 2a: superficial ulcerations, mucosal friability, blisters

Grade 2b: grade 2a findings plus circumferential ulceration

Grade 3:   multiple, deep ulcerations and extensive necrosis

3. Are injuries produced by alkaline caustic agents limited to the esophagus?

No. Many studies suggesting a relative sparing of the stomach in ingestions of alkalis were performed in children, in whom the ingestions were accidental and involved small amounts of material. Both hemorrhage and perforation of the stomach and small intestine have been reported with ingestion of large amounts of alkaline caustic substances. Thus, when the ingestion is known or suspected to be large, the stomach and small intestine must also be evaluated.

4. What injuries have been reported with the ingestion of household ammonia or bleach?
These common household cleaners generally cause problems only if aspirated or ingested in large amounts. Ingestion of household bleach (sodium hypochlorite) usually produces no injury or mild esophageal burns. Two cases of esophageal injury requiring surgical repair have been reported in patients who were re-exposed to the sodium hypochlorite when they vomited. Complications reported with large ingestions of household ammonia include severe esophageal burns and perforation, acute respiratory distress syndrome (ARDS), gastric necrosis, airway obstruction due to supraglottic edema, and death.

5. What clinical signs and symptoms indicate the presence of a significant (> first degree or grade 1) GI tract injury?
The presence or absence of oropharyngeal burns cannot be used to determine the presence or absence of a significant upper GI tract lesion.
Alkalis: In small children suspected or known to have ingested a caustic alkaline substance, the presence of drooling, vomiting, or stridor may indicate a significant esophageal lesion. In a retrospective study of 79 pediatric patients by Crain et al., the presence of two or more of these signs predicted all the patients who were found to have significant esophageal lesions on endoscopy. All patients who presented with stridor had a significant esophageal lesion. These findings may be used as general guidelines to determine the need for endoscopy in the pediatric population, although the decision ultimately depends upon the clinician's suspicion of a significant upper GI tract burn.
Endoscopy is recommended for all adult patients, regardless of the presence or absence of symptoms, because these ingestions are often deliberate and may involve large amounts of caustic substance, and these patients may have significant injuries with few or no symptoms immediately apparent.
Acids: Dysphagia and odynophagia have been closely associated with acid-induced esophagitis. Signs and symptoms referable to significant gastric injuries are less reliable, with epigastric pain, tenderness, or both being reported in fewer than half the patients. GI tract hemorrhage and perforation may occur rapidly. Systemic effects such as metabolic acidosis, disseminated intravascular coagulation (DIC), hyponatremia, and hypotension may develop. Aspiration of acid can produce stridor, upper airway obstruction, and ARDS.

6. How should patients with suspected caustic injury be managed initially?
Airway management is the first priority because pharyngeal or laryngeal burns can compromise airway patency. Immediate endotracheal intubation should be performed for life-threatening respiratory compromise. Less acute cases with stridor need ENT examination to evaluate the hypopharynx, cords, and larynx, basing the decision to intubate on the presence and severity of burns. Patients should be kept NPO and given intravenous (IV) crystalloids and opioid analgesics for pain control. Corticosteroids may decrease laryngeal edema.
Alkalis: Gastric evacuation and/or neutralization therapies are contraindicated. The efficacy of H2-blocker drugs remains unknown, and antibiotics should be used only for known infection or concomitantly with corticosteroid therapy (see Controversy below). Patients with second-degree and third-degree burns should be admitted.
Acids: Gastric emptying is recommended via a nasogastric (NG) tube to decrease gastric mucosal exposure and systemic absorption of acids. Again, neutralization is contraindicated. Corticosteroids should not be given because their efficacy is unproved and their use may mask signs of peritonitis. Laboratory tests include coagulation studies and blood type and cross-match.

7. What are the indications for emergency endoscopy?

Alkalis: All pediatric patients with presenting signs and symptoms indicative of upper GI tract burns more serious than first degree should undergo endoscopy within 12–24 hours after ingestion. All adults with known or suspected alkali ingestion should have endoscopy during the same time frame.

Acids: Endoscopy should be performed immediately in all cases of known or suspected acid ingestion because the findings will help to determine the necessity of acute surgical intervention.

8. What are the contraindications and potential complications of endoscopy?

For injuries caused by acids and alkalis, evidence of GI tract perforation rules out the use of diagnostic endoscopy. In the presence of severe hypopharyngeal burns, a flexible scope may be inserted through a rigid endoscope to minimize the risk of hypopharyngeal perforation. Alternatively, limited evaluation may be accomplished with a water-soluble contrast radiographic study.

Alkalis: Traditionally, diagnostic endoscopy is terminated at the first deep, penetrating, or circumferential burn of the esophagus. However, development of the flexible endoscope and realization that alkaline caustic substances can produce life-threatening gastric and small intestinal injuries have led to more aggressive endoscopic examination. Panendoscopy of the upper GI tract, to include stomach and duodenum, should be performed in all cases of alkali ingestion that meet the criteria for endoscopy. The skill of the endoscopist determines whether endoscopy proceeds past the level of a deep esophageal burn.

Acids: Panendoscopy of the upper GI tract is the standard, given the predilection of acids to produce life-threatening gastric burns.

9. When is immediate surgical intervention indicated?

Alkalis: Surgery may be required for life-threatening GI hemorrhage or GI tract perforation, although some esophageal perforations have been managed successfully with drainage and antibiotics. Exploratory laparotomy for direct visualization of the stomach may be necessary when severe gastric injury is suspected, and severe esophageal burns preclude gastric endoscopic examination.

Acids: Immediate surgery is indicated for GI tract perforation and when endoscopy reveals grade 3 burns with full-thickness necrosis of the esophagus or stomach. In the latter case, surgical drainage of the acid remaining in the stomach, with resection of nonviable tissue, may prevent further tissue damage and the systemic complications that may occur with perforation.

10. What complications and clinical sequelae may occur?

Ingestions of alkalis and acids may be complicated by GI tract perforation or hemorrhage, chemical pneumonitis, ARDS, and strictures of the upper respiratory or GI tract.

Alkalis: Esophageal squamous cell carcinoma may develop at the site of the stricture, with a latency period ranging from 9–71 years. Patients who develop strictures must be monitored lifelong for the development of carcinoma.

Acids: Metabolic acidosis, hypotension, or DIC can complicate these ingestions. As with alkali ingestions, malignancies can arise in stricture sites, mandating lifelong monitoring. Additionally, severe gastric burns with subsequent scarring can result in (1) achlorhydria and diminished/absent intrinsic factor, and/or (2) dumping syndrome secondary to a small, immobile stomach.

CONTROVERSY

11. Should corticosteroids be used in the treatment of alkali-induced esophageal burns?

For: When used in conjunction with esophageal dilation therapy for established strictures, corticosteroids begun immediately after injury may decrease the incidence of surgical repair of the esophagus. In studies by Haller and Tewfik, using a combination of corticosteroid and esophageal dilation therapies, no surgical repair was required in 14 patients who developed esophageal strictures. In Anderson's study, which used dilation therapy for all esophageal strictures, a trend toward less surgical repair of the esophagus was noted in the corticosteroid-treated group.

Against: Traditionally, early corticosteroid therapy was thought to decrease esophageal stricture formation. Analysis of comparable studies in the literature reveals the severity of the burn, rather than the use of corticosteroids, to be the major determinant of stricture formation. Anderson et al. prospectively randomized 60 children with alkali-induced esophageal burns to treatment with or without corticosteroids. In this study, the development of strictures correlated better with burn severity than with the therapeutic regimen, and they concluded corticosteroids were of no benefit in preventing stricture formation.

BIBLIOGRAPHY

1. Anderson KD, Rouse TM, Randolph JG: A controlled trial of corticosteroids in children with corrosive injury of the esophagus. N Engl J Med 323:637, 1990.
2. Crain EF, Gershel JC, Mezey AP: Caustic ingestions: Symptoms as predictors of esophageal injury. Am J Dis Child 138:863, 1984.
3. Dilawari JB, Singh S, Rao PN, et al: Corrosive acid ingestion in man: A clinical and endoscopic study. Gut 25:183, 1984.
4. Estrera A, Taylor W, Mills LJ, et al: Corrosive burns of the esophagus and stomach: A recommendation for an aggressive surgical approach. Ann Thorac Surg 41:276, 1986.
5. Ford M: Alkali and acid injuries of the upper gastrointestinal tract. In Hoffman RS, Goldfrank LR (eds): Critical Care Toxicology. New York, Contemporary Management in Critical Care, 1991, pp 225–244.
6. Haller JA, Bachman K: The comparative effect of current therapy on experimental caustic burns of the esophagus. Pediatrics 34:236, 1964.
7. Hawkins DB, Demeter MJ, Barnett TE: Caustic ingestion: Controversies in management: A review of 214 cases. Laryngoscope 90:98, 1980.
8. Middelkamp JN, Ferguson TB, Roper CL, et al: The management and problems of caustic burns in children. J Thorac Cardiovasc Surg 57:341, 1969.
9. Middelkamp JN, Cone AJ, Ogura JH, et al: Endoscopic diagnosis and steroid and antibiotic therapy of acute lye burns of the esophagus. Laryngoscope 71:1354, 1961.
10. Tewfik TL, Schloss MD: Ingestion of lye and other corrosive agents: A study of 86 infant and child cases. J Otolaryngol 9:72, 1980.
11. Webb WR, Koutras P, Ecker RR, et al: An evaluation of steroids and antibiotics in caustic burns of the esophagus. Ann Thorac Surg 9:95, 1970.
12. Zargar SA, Kochhar R, Nagi B, et al: Ingestion of corrosive acids: Spectrum of injury to upper gastrointestinal tract and natural history. Gastroenterology 97:702, 1989.

86. BITES AND STINGS

Lee W. Shockley, M.D., FACEP

1. What is a snakebite?
Equal parts of Yukon Jack and Rose's Lime Juice, but that is not important now.

2. What is a dry snakebite?
It is not a snakebite made with vermouth; it is a bite in which no venom was introduced.

3. What are the chances of a bite from a snake causing a dry bite? How can you tell?
About 25% of all bites from venomous snakes in the United States do not result in envenomation. Quick observations helpful in determining whether envenomation has taken place include the presence of fang marks that ooze nonclotting blood with surrounding ecchymosis and severe burning pain. These signs combined with microhematuria are characteristic of severe envenomation and a poor prognosis.

4. What are the clinical signs of Crotalidae (pit viper) envenomation?
The rapid onset of edema with slow spreading (80%), pain out of proportion to the puncture (72%), weakness (65%), lightheadedness (52%), nausea (48%), erythema at the bite site (53%), bleeding diathesis (52%), lymphangitis, hypotension, shock, diaphoresis, chills (58%), paresthesias, taste changes, and fasciculations (33%).

5. What is the grading system for envenomation from pit viper bites?
Trivial (Grade 0): local signs only; no systemic symptoms
Minimal (Grade 1): local signs and perioral paresthesias only without other systemic signs
Moderate (Grade 2): manifestations beyond the local reaction; significant systemic symptoms and laboratory abnormalities (hemoconcentration, decreased fibrinogen, decreased platelets)
Severe (Grade 3): manifestations involving the entire extremity or part with serious systemic symptoms and significant laboratory abnormalities
Very Severe (Grade 4): manifestations of systemic symptoms and rapid progression, CNS symptoms, shock, or seizures

6. How does the grade of envenomation help in making therapeutic decisions?
Trivial envenomation needs local wound care and tetanus prophylaxis only. Minimal envenomation may require antihistamines as well. Moderate envenomation should be treated with antivenin for bites from rattlesnakes and coppermouths, but treatment is controversial and should be decided case by case. If antivenin is to be used for a moderate envenomation, 2–4 vials should be used. A severe or very severe envenomation requires the use of antivenin and may require 5–15 (or more) vials.

7. What is the "pit" that distinguishes the pit viper?
It is a thermoreceptor organ located halfway between the snake's eye and nostril. It appears as a small indentation.

8. What is pit viper antivenin?
The only commercially available Crotalidae polyvalent antivenin is from Wyeth-Ayerst Laboratories. It is horse antisera to four snake venoms: *Crotalus atrox, Crotalus adamanteus, Crotalus terrificus* and *Bothrops atrox*. All pit viper venom (rattlesnakes, copperheads, and moccasins) share antigenicity with the venom of these species.

9. What is the incidence of serum sickness after the administration of horse antivenin? When does it happen and how is it treated?
Up to 75% of patients who receive some antivenin and nearly 100% of patients receiving 70 ml or more develop serum sickness. It occurs within 24 days of the administration of antivenin. The treatment of choice is parenteral corticosteroids.

10. How is antivenin dosing altered for children? Why?
The amount of venom children receive is the same as for adults; therefore they receive a greater toxic load per body weight, have less body water to dilute the toxin, and have less

inherent resistance to the effects of the venom. Thus the dose of antivenin per kilogram needs to be higher for children than adults.

11. What is the importance of the coloring of coral snakes? What are the active components of its venom? How is coral snake envenomation treated?
This small, thin, brightly colored snake is venomous; however, the king snake, which is nonvenomous, has similar but not identical coloration:
"Red on yellow, kill a fellow" (coral snake)
"Red on black, venom lack" (harmless snake)
Coral snake venom blocks acetylcholine receptors and can cause slurred speech, ptosis, dilated pupils, dysphagia, and myalgias. Death is from progressive paralysis and respiratory failure. Envenomation is treated with neostigmine (2.5 mg every 30–60 minutes) and equine antivenin.

12. Where can one obtain information about antivenin for the treatment of bites from exotic snakes?
Try a local zoo or aquarium. Many keep antivenin on hand for bites from snakes in their collections. In addition, many antivenins are polyvalent and can be used for similar species. The Oklahoma Poison Control Center keeps the National Antivenin Index, which lists all of the antivenins available in the United States. Their phone number is (405) 271-5454. In addition, possession of many of these species is restricted by law and, therefore, these cases should be reported to the authorities.

13. What types of reactions occur from Hymenoptera stings (bees, wasps, and ants)?
There are two types of reactions—toxic and anaphylactic. The toxic reaction is a nonantigenic response to the venom characterized by vomiting, diarrhea, light-headedness, and syncope. There may also be headache, fever, drowsiness, involuntary muscle spasms, edema without urticaria, and occasionally convulsions. Information about anaphylactic reactions can be found elsewhere in this book.

14. What is a stinger?
Cognac and white creme de menthe, but that is also not important now. Try to keep your mind on the subject.

15. How should a honeybee stinger be removed?
Honeybees almost invariably leave their stinger and venom sac in the victim. It should not be squeezed with fingers or tweezers during removal, but rather scraped out. This should be done as soon as possible as the venom sac continues to pulse venom after it has been detached from the bee.

16. What are the clinical signs of Lactrodectus envenomation (black widow spider bite)?
The initial bite is usually not particularly painful. The systemic signs and symptoms begin after a latent period of 10–60 minutes. Muscle cramps and spasms accompanied by pain and fever are typical manifestations. Diffuse abdominal muscle spasms may mimic the boardlike rigidity of an acute, surgical abdomen. Facial muscle spasm, lacrimation, photophobia, and swollen eyelids can cause the characteristic facies lactrodectisima. There may be headache, lightheadedness, nausea, vomiting, diaphoresis, and dysphagia in severe envenomations. Hypertensive crisis may be precipitated.

17. What is the treatment for the muscle spasms caused by Lactrodectus envenomation?
The slow intravenous injection of 10 ml of 10% calcium gluconate usually relieves the muscle cramps, headache, and paresthesias. This may need to be repeated at 2–4-hour

intervals. Narcotics, benzodiazepines, and muscle relaxants, sometimes in large doses, may give additional symptomatic relief.

18. What are the characteristic signs of a Loxosceles bite (brown recluse or fiddleback spider)?

After the bite, which often may not be painful, there is a latent period of 1–4 hours, followed by the development of a painful reddish blister surrounded by a blue-white halo (the "bull's eye" lesion). There may be chills, malaise, and a scarlatiniform rash. During the next 3–6 days, the lesion becomes hemorrhagic and spreads with a central area of necrosis. Healing is slow and may require debridement and skin grafting to treat large areas of skin necrosis. There have been cases of intravascular hemolysis following such bites.

19. Are mygalomorph spider bites (tarantulas) particularly dangerous?

On the whole, these bites tend to be of low toxicity with a mild, briefly-active venom causing local symptoms only. However, the most dangerous mygalomorphs are the funnel-web spiders of southeastern Australia. These spiders can cause a significant envenomation with intense local pain, nausea, vomiting, diaphoresis, salivation, muscle twitching, confusion, and severe dyspnea. Coma, cardiopulmonary failure, and death have been known to occur after such bites.

20. What are the chances of envenomation from a scorpion bite? What are the active components of its venom? What are the signs of envenomation?

There is no chance of envenomation from the bite (trick question); they do not envenomate by their bite but rather their sting. The paired venom glands are located in the last of the five abdominal segments (the "tail"). The principal toxins are polypeptides and low-molecular-weight proteins, histamine, and indole compounds (including serotonin). The sting is acutely painful. Later, systemic manifestations may develop, including salivation, diaphoresis, perioral paresthesias, dysphagia, gastric distention, hyperactivity, diplopia, nystagmus, visual loss, incontinence, penile erection, hyperreflexia, opisthotonos, seizures, hypertension, pulmonary edema, and respiratory arrest. The majority of scorpions that inhabit the United States are of low toxicity with stings comparable to bee stings.

21. How do I treat jelly fish or other coelenterate stings?

Acetic acid (vinegar) applied continuously for at least 30 minutes. Alcohol, in the form of 40% isopropyl alcohol, perfume, aftershave lotion, or high-proof liquor (see questions 1 and 14), is a good second choice. Alcohol may stimulate the nematocysts to release their venom, but this has not been shown to be clinically significant. Immersion of the affected extremity in hot water may be of some benefit (following alcohol or acetic acid decontamination). The nematocysts that remain in the skin can then be removed by applying shaving cream, talc, baking soda, or flour, and by shaving the area.

22. In an urban emergency practice, what is the most commonly encountered bite wound? Why is it potentially very dangerous? How should it be treated?

The most common bite wound is that caused by another human being. A human bite that occurs when the fist of one opponent strikes the teeth of a second opponent is known as a "fight bite." Usually this involves the knuckles of the dominant hand. The importance of this injury is that the laceration can involve the extensor tendon and its bursa, the superficial and deep fascia, and the joint capsule. These structures are contaminated with oral flora at the time of the injury and are notorious for becoming infected. There are at least 42 species of bacteria in human saliva. The most frequently cultured organism from fight bites is Streptococcus, followed by *Staphylococcus aureus* (usually penicillin-resistant): 31% of these wound infections are due to gram-negative organisms and 43% are due to mixed gram-negative and gram-positive organisms. Up to 29% of these infections may be due to a facultatively anaerobic gram-negative rod, *Eikenella corrodens*. This organism is typically resistant to the semisynthetic penicillins, clindamycin, and the first-generation cephalosporins. However, it is usually sensitive to penicillin and ampicillin. These wounds should be meticulously cared for, with special attention given to a thorough exploration and irrigation. The choice of antibiotic(s) should consider the polymicrobial nature of these infections.

BIBLIOGRAPHY

1. Auerbach PS, Halstead BW: Hazardous marine life. In Auerbach PS, Geehr EC (eds): Management of Wilderness and Environmental Emergencies. St. Louis, Mosby, 1989, pp 213–259.
2. Callaham ML: Domestic and feral mammalian bites. In Auerbach PS, Geehr EC (eds): Management of Wilderness and Environmental Emergencies. St. Louis, Mosby, 1989, pp 310–351.
3. Doan-Wiggins L: Animal bites and rabies. In Rosen P, et al (eds): Emergency Medicine: Concepts and Clinical Practice, 3rd ed. St. Louis, Mosby, 1992, pp 864–875.
4. Ennik F: Deaths from bites and stings of venomous animals. West J Med 133:463–468, 1980.
5. Milton SA: Arthropod envenomation. In Auerbach PS, Geehr EC (eds): Management of Wilderness and Environmental Emergencies. St. Louis, Mosby, 1989, pp 270–304.
6. Otten EJ: Venomous animal injuries. In Rosen P, et al (eds): Emergency Medicine: Concepts and Clinical Practice, 3rd ed. St. Louis, Mosby, 1992, pp 875–892.
7. Rest JG, Goldstein EJC: Management of human and animal bite wounds. Emerg Med Clin North Am 3:117–126, 1985.
8. Wasserman G: Wound care of spider and snake envenomations. Ann Emerg Med 17:1331–1335, 1988.
9. Wingert WA: Venomous snake bites. In Auerbach PS, Geehr EC (eds): Management of Wilderness and Environmental Emergencies. St. Louis, Mosby, 1989, pp 352–378.

87. SMOKE INHALATION

Richard E. Wolfe, M.D.

1. What causes death in fire victims?
Although incineration would have been a good guess, 50–80% of deaths occurring during fires result from smoke inhalation.

2. Why is smoke so lethal?
Carbon dioxide and carbon monoxide, the major components, are responsible for a drop in the concentration of ambient oxygen from 22% to 5–10%. Carbon monoxide and more rarely hydrogen cyanide block the uptake and utilization of oxygen, leading to severe tissue cellular hypoxemia. Depending on fuel, temperature, and rate of heating, smoke contains a wide variety of toxins. Soot may act as a vehicle in transporting these toxic gases to the lower respiratory tract where they dissolve to form acids and alkali. Removal of the soot is impaired by action of certain of these toxins on respiratory cilia, leading to severe, delayed pneumonia. Thermal injury is unusual because the upper respiratory tract is very efficient in heat exchange and cools the air before it reaches the vocal cords.

3. How should smoke inhalation victims be managed in the field?
All victims of smoke inhalation should be placed on 100% nonrebreather mask as soon as possible, even if they are asymptomatic. Although not as effective as hyperbaric oxygen, this method will dramatically accelerate washout of carbon monoxide. Endotracheal

intubation should be performed for respiratory distress. If the patient sustained a loss of consciousness or has altered mentation, transport to a hyperbaric facility should be strongly considered.

4. Why is hyperbaric therapy beneficial in smoke inhalation?

Providing increased oxygen to poorly functioning mitochrondrial enzymes, inhibited by carbon monoxide and cyanide, is one rationale for hyperbaric therapy. Furthermore, hyperbarics decrease the average half-life of carbon monoxide from 300 minutes (room air) to 80 minutes (100% nonrebreather mask) to 23 minutes (HBO at 3 atmospheres). Although no prospective controlled clinical human studies have been done, animal studies suggest that neurologic sequelae from carbon monoxide intoxication are decreased by prompt use of hyperbarics.

5. What should I ask about the fire?

Ask if the patient was trapped in a closed space because significant inhalation injury will not occur in an open area. Try to determine what material was burning. The fuel is of prime importance in determining the composition of smoke and the risk to the patient. For example, in the Cleveland Clinic fire in 1929, 123 deaths were linked to poisoning from oxides of nitrogen released by the burning of nitrocellulose x-ray films.

Hydrogen Cyanide—Combustion of wool, silk, nylons, and polyurethanes found commonly in furniture, and paper.

Aldehydes, Acrolein—Wood, cotton, paper, and plastic materials

Hydrogen Chloride, Phosgene—Pyrolysis of chlorinated polymers; polyvinal chloride (wire insulation materials), chlorinated acrylics, and wall, floor, and furniture coverings.

Oxides of Nitrogen—Nitrocellulose film

Sulfur Dioxide, Hydrogen Sulfide—Rubber

6. How helpful is the physical examination in determining which patients have significant injury from smoke inhalation?

Not very helpful. Singed nasal hair is present in only 13% of patients with smoke inhalation. Although facial burns occur in 66% of patients with pulmonary burns, 86% of hospitalized patients with facial burns have no pulmonary injuries. Auscultatory findings and bronchorrhea are often absent initially. Sooty sputum is present in only 50% of smoke inhalation victims. Hoarseness is present in less than 25%.

7. How should asymptomatic patients be managed?

Provide comprehensive discharge instructions on when to return. Although the physical examination cannot reliably rule out complications such as delayed noncardiogenic pulmonary edema or pneumonia, ancillary studies and observation are not cost effective. The patient should be instructed to return to the ED if shortness of breath, chest pain, or fever occur.

8. If the patient's pulse oximetry is normal, will arterial blood gas (ABG) analysis yield additional information?

It is of some use in detecting significant carbon monoxide poisoning. However, the ABGs are not good discriminators of inhalation injury. Although the alveolar-arterial gradient is highly correlative in detecting smoke inhalation, it does not predict the extent of injury. If your laboratory directly measures (not calculated) oxygen saturation on the ABG, a drop in saturation with a normal PaO_2 suggests carbon monoxide poisoning. A high carboxy-hemoglobin level obtained with the blood gas is a good indication of significant exposure to carbon monoxide. A normal level, however, does not rule out carbon monoxide poisoning if the exposure occurred several hours before.

9. Should I get a chest x-ray on all patients with a history of smoke inhalation?
No. The chest x-ray offers little benefit in the ED. Chest radiographs are normal immediately after smoke inhalation injury and abnormalities will appear only on a delayed basis. Therefore a chest x-ray is not indicated in asymptomatic patients and, at best, only as a baseline in symptomatic patients.

10. Can I use the standard burn formula for intravenous fluids if smoke inhalation is present?
Patients with both cutaneous and inhalation injuries pose a difficult problem, as their fluid requirements are usually greater, and yet, because of leaky capillaries, they are much more likely to develop membrane permeable pulmonary edema. IV fluids must therefore be guided by regular clinical reevaluation (breath sounds, oxygen saturation, urinary output, vital signs) rather than by formulas. Swan-Ganz monitoring may be required.

11. Are hyperbarics the only available therapy for cyanide poisoning?
No. All EDs are required to stock the Lilly cyanide antidote kit, and hydrocobalamin may soon be made available for use in the U.S.

12. How does the Lilly cyanide antidote kit work?
Cyanide binds to the ferric ions, blocking the mitochondrial cytochrome oxidase pathway and cellular respiration. The cyanide antidote kit acts in two ways to limit this. First, nitrites generate methemoglobin, creating heme-ferric ions to compete for cyanide with mitochondrial ferric ions. Sulfur transferase (rhodanase) binds cyanide molecules to sulfur-forming thiocyanate, which is nontoxic and eliminated in the urine. Thiosulfate accelerates this process by increasing available sulfur molecules.

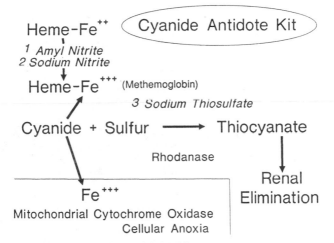

13. How do I administer the cyanide antidote kit?
Amyl nitrite pearls are used in patients without IV access. The pearl is placed close to a breathing patient's mouth (broken in gauze or placed into the lip of a face mask) for 30 seconds out of each minute, with a new pearl every 3–4 minutes. If the patient is apneic, break the pearl inside the resuscitation bag. The full amount of a 10-cc ampule in adults, or 5–10 mg/kg of sodium nitrite, is administered intravenously over 4 minutes. This is followed by 12.5 gm of intravenous thiosulfate.

14. When should I use the cyanide antidote kit?
Generally the kit is administered to patients with coma, seizures, hypotension, and acidosis with a clear history of cyanide inhalation or ingestion. Cyanide poisoning may be suspected

in smoke inhalation, but there is no immediate definitive means to differentiate cyanide toxicity from carbon monoxide poisoning. Furthermore, the amyl nitrite capsules and sodium nitrite both cause methemoglobinemia, which will exacerbate systemic hypoxemia from carbon monoxide poisoning. Therefore, if cyanide poisoning is suspected in an unstable patient, use only the sodium thiosulfate portion of the kit.

CONTROVERSY

15. Are steroids indicated in smoke inhalation?

It was initially assumed that if the tracheobronchial inflammatory response could be prevented or at least decreased by the anti-inflammatory action, edema would be decreased and surfactant would be maintained. It was also postulated that pulmonary fibrosis would be reduced after the acute injury. These beliefs were initially supported by early experimental studies. However, later animal experiments and clinical trials could not demonstrate increased survival with the use of steroids. Notably, Moylan and Alexander, in a randomized prospective trial, showed a fourfold increase in mortality in the steroid-treated group. Other retrospective studies added to the argument against steroids. These studies, however, have examined only the use of repeated doses of steroids throughout the hospital course. The use of a single bolus dose when the patient presents to the ED has not been studied and may be beneficial in reducing smoke induced bronchospasm. At present, routine administration of steroids in the ED is not indicated.

BIBLIOGRAPHY

1. Blinn DL, Slater H, Goldfarb W: Inhalation injury with burns: A lethal combination. J Emerg Med 6:471–473, 1988.
2. Cohen MA: Inhalation of products of combustion. Ann Emerg Med 12:628–631, 1983.
3. Hall AH, Rumack B: Cyanide poisoning. In Harwood-Nuss A (ed): The Clinical Practice of Emergency Medicine. Philadelphia, J.B. Lippincott, 1991.
4. Hoffman RS: Toxic inhalations. In Rosen P, et al (eds): Emergency Medicine: Concepts and Clinical Practice, 3rd ed. St. Louis, Mosby–Year Book, 1992.
5. Moylan JA, Alexander LG: Diagnosis and treatment of inhalation injury. World J Surg 2:185–191, 1978.
6. Phillips AW, Cope O: Burn therapy. II. The revelation of respiratory tract damage as a principal killer of the burn patient. Ann Surg 155:1–19, 1962.
7. Robinson NB, Hudson LD, Riem M: Steroid therapy following isolated smoke inhalation injury. J Trauma 22:876–879, 1982.
8. Surveyer JA: Smoke inhalation injuries. Heart & Lung 9:825–832, 1980.

XV. Gynecology and Obstetrics

88. PELVIC INFLAMMATORY DISEASE

Alexander T. Trott, M.D.

1. What is pelvic inflammatory disease (PID)?

PID is an acute clinical syndrome caused by the spread of microorganisms from the vagina and cervix to the organs of reproduction. The organisms are most commonly sexually transmitted. PID can involve the endometrium (endometritis), fallopian tubes (acute salpingitis), ovaries (oophoritis), and surrounding pelvic peritoneum (peritonitis). Any structure, either alone or in combination, can be involved. The inflammatory response can range from the very mild to the very severe.

2. Who is at risk for the disease?

Sexually active women between the ages of 15 and 19 are at highest risk. The risk is increased by the number of sexual partners and coital frequency. People in lower socioeconomic groups are at greater risk, but the disease strikes at all levels of society. The method of contraception can either lower or increase the risk. Oral contraceptives lower both the risk and the severity of infection, if it does occur. The intrauterine device, on the other hand, increases the risk of infection. Operative procedures such as dilatation and curettage (D&C), hysterosalpingography, and legal abortion may increase the risk of PID.

3. What are the microbiologic causes?

In recent years, *Chlamydia trachomatis* has overtaken *Neisseria gonorrhoeae* as the most common organism. In 30% of cases, both organisms are present. Other organisms that can cause PID are *Mycoplasma hominis* and *Ureaplasma urealyticum*. In recurrent and chronic PID, gram-negative bacteria such as *Escherichia coli* and anaerobes may be the causative organism.

4. Can patients have more than one sexually transmitted disease (STD)?

The presence of one STD does not preclude another. Patients with PID can have syphilis, and all patients being evaluated for an STD should have a serologic test for syphilis. Vaginitis, a mild vaginal infection caused by candida, trichomonas, or gardnerella, may be associated with PID. Women who have vaginal discharge or itching require testing for chlamydia and gonorrhea in addition to a microscopic exam of the vaginal secretions for the common causes of vaginitis.

5. What are the signs and symptoms?

The classic signs and symptoms of PID are lower abdominal pain and vaginal discharge accompanied by fever, abdominal tenderness, and tenderness of the cervix and adnexa. However, the minority of patients with laparoscopically proven PID present in this manner. More commonly, patients have lower abdominal pain of varying severity with mild to moderate pelvic organ tenderness. The presence of vaginal discharge and fever is variable. Extensive tubal inflammation and damage can occur in the face of a mild clinical presentation, most commonly when the infection is due to *C. trachomatis*. In fact, abdominal uterine bleeding or dysuria alone may be the only clinical evidence of PID.

6. What other diseases should be considered?

When examining a woman in whom PID is suspected, other diseases must be considered because they share similar symptoms and signs. The most important of these diseases are ectopic pregnancy and acute appendicitis. Ovarian tumors, pelvic endometriosis, and uterine fibroids are also included in the differential diagnosis. In a small number of patients, the etiology of pelvic pain is never diagnosed in spite of intensive testing.

7. Which diagnostic tests should be performed?

During the evaluation of the patient with suspected PID, a beta-hCG pregnancy test, urinalysis, and complete blood count are recommended. Urinalysis may reveal a urinary tract infection (UTI) as a possible cause of the patient's symptoms or a coexistent UTI. The white blood cell count can help to indicate the severity of infection. If the pregnancy test is positive, an ultrasound is recommended to diagnose or rule out ectopic pregnancy. Ultrasound is also indicated if a tubo-ovarian abscess is suspected. *C. trachomatis* and *N. gonorrhoeae* cultures should be obtained in all patients with PID. There is no reliable test to exclude PID short of laparoscopy.

8. What are the consequences of PID, particularly if it is unrecognized and untreated?

Women who have PID are 2–7 times more likely to have ectopic pregnancy in the future. There has been a significant increase in occurrence of ectopic pregnancy in recent years as a result of PID. Infertility is another serious sequela of PID and is directly proportional to the number of pelvic infections and the severity of infection. One of the most troublesome sequela of PID is chronic abdominal pain, which may eventually require a hysterectomy to resolve.

9. Who should be treated?

Because the consequences of unrecognized and untreated PID can be severe, overtreatment of sexually active women with pelvic organ symptoms is recommended. Only 30% of patients with PID have the classic textbook symptoms. Women with mild or atypical symptoms should be treated empirically with a full course of antibiotics. Response to antibiotics and close follow-up will help to resolve the diagnosis. The presence of *N. gonorrhoeae* or *C. trachomatis* on culture confirms the diagnosis but their absence does not exclude it.

10. Who should be hospitalized?

Some authorities recommend hospitalization of all patients in whom PID is suspected in order to provide intensive initial antibiotic therapy. Hospitalization is not always practical; therefore, the Centers for Disease Control's guidelines for hospital admission are: (1) the diagnosis is uncertain (appendicitis cannot be ruled out), (2) pelvic abscess is suspected, (3) the patient is pregnant, (4) severe illness is present (high fever, peritoneal signs, vomiting), (5) the patient is an adolescent, (6) the patient has failed outpatient therapy.

11. What are the recommended antibiotic regimens for PID treatment?

Outpatient

Cefoxitin 2 g IM *plus* **probenecid**, 1 g orally, concurrently *or* **ceftriaxone** 250 mg IM *or* equivalent **cephalosporin** *plus*

Doxycycline 100 mg orally 2 times a day for 10–14 days *or*

Tetracycline 500 mg orally 4 times a day for 10–14 days.

Alternative Regimen for Patients Who Do Not Tolerate Doxycycline/Tetracycline*

Substitute **erythromycin** 500 mg orally 4 times a day for 10–14 days.*

Inpatient
   One of the following:

Recommended Regimen A
   Cefoxitin 2 g intravenously (IV) every 6 hours **or cefotetan*** IV 2 g every 12 hours ***plus***
   Doxycycline 100 mg orally or IV every 12 hours.

   The above regimen is given for at least 48 hours after the patient clinically improves.
After discharge from hospital, doxycycline 100 mg orally 2 times a day should be continued
for a total of 10–14 days.

Recommended Regimen B
   Clindamycin IV 900 mg every 8 hours ***plus***
   Gentamicin loading dose IV or IM (2 mg/kg of body weight) followed by a
   maintenance dose (1.5 mg/kg) every 8 hours.

12. Does the presence of an intrauterine pregnancy effectively rule out PID?

Once the gestational sac is large enough to form an effective barrier to ascending infection
(at 6 weeks), new-onset PID is extremely unlikely. However, recurrent PID can be
exacerbated by microorganisms present in the tubes even after the sac has become an
effective barrier. Because of increased blood flow to the pelvic organs during pregnancy,
clearance of infectious agents is more efficacious. Overall, presence of an intrauterine
pregnancy should lead to the search for other causes of pelvic pain.

13. Does a history of tubal ligation preclude the diagnosis of PID?

No, but generally these patients are clinically more symptomatic and may be septic. Because
the tubal lumens are blocked, a more severe infection is necessary to cause peritoneal
involvement.

14. Is cervical motion tenderness diagnostic of PID?

Cervical motion tenderness can be elicited in any patient with an acute peritoneal inflammatory process. Thus it may be present in patients with ectopic pregnancy, intraperitoneal
bleeding, appendicitis, and adnexal torsion, among others. The **chandelier sign** is the term
commonly applied to cervical motion tenderness to describe the pain experienced when
peritoneal motion is elicited.

15. Summarize the principles of management of acute PID.

Principles of Management of Acute PID

• Rule out pregnancy	• Reassess patient in 48–72 hours after
• Use standard clinical criteria to guide—	initiating treatment
not dictate—diagnosis	• Identify, treat/refer sexual partners
• Err on side of "overdiagnosis" of PID	• Screen and treat lower genital infections in
to prevent sequelae	both men and women
• Treat early and with broad-spectrum	• Encourage the use of a barrier contraceptive
antibiotics	with spermicide

From Shafer MA, Sweet RL: Pelvic inflammatory disease in adolescent females. Adolescent Medicine:
State of the Art Reviews. Philadelphia, Hanley & Belfus, 1990, pp 545–564.

BIBLIOGRAPHY

1. Centers for Disease Control Report: Pelvic inflammatory disease: Guidelines for prevention and
   management. MMWR 40(RR-5):1–25, 1991.
2. Holmes KK, Mardh PA, Sparling PF, et al (eds): Sexually Transmitted Diseases, 2nd ed. New
   York, McGraw-Hill, 1990.

3. Judson FN: The importance of co-existing syphilitic, chlamydial, mycoplasmal and trichomonal infections in the treatment of gonorrhea. Sex Transm Dis 6:112–119, 1979.
4. Kahn JG, Walker CK, Washington AE, et al: Diagnosing pelvic inflammatory disease: A comprehensive analysis and considerations for developing a model. JAMA 266:2594–2604, 1991.
5. Mogabgab WJ: Recent developments in the treatment of sexually transmitted diseases. Am J Med 91(Suppl 6A):140–144, 1991.
6. Petersen HB, Galaid EI, Zenilman JM: Pelvic inflammatory disease: Review of treatment options. Rev Infect Dis 12(Suppl 6):656–664, 1990.
7. Rolfs RT: "Think PID." New directions in prevention and management of pelvic inflammatory disease. Sex Transm Dis 18:131–132, 1991.
8. Washington AE, Aral SO, Wolner-Hanssen P, et al: Assessing risk for pelvic inflammatory disease and its sequela. JAMA 266:2581–2585, 1991.

89. SEXUAL ASSAULT

David Magid, M.D.

1. What is the legal definition of sexual assault?

Rape is the carnal knowledge of a victim (male or female) without consent through compulsion by use of fear, force, or threat of force or fraud. Carnal knowledge can consist of complete coitus to slight penile penetration, intentional fondling or touching, or coercing the victim to fondle or touch the assailant's genitals. Lack of consent is an important aspect of the crime unless the victim is a minor, intoxicated, asleep, or mentally incompetent.

2. How common is sexual assault?

Because of underreporting, the exact incidence of sexual assaults is difficult to determine, although sexual assault is considered to be the fastest-growing violent crime in the U.S. It has been estimated that 1 in 5 women will be raped during their lifetime, but less than 10% will report the crime.

3. Why is it important for the ED physician to be knowledgeable about sexual assault?

The ED is the most common place that sexual assault victims present for acute medical care and forensic evidence gathering.

4. What information should be elicited in the patient history?

A directed history of the assault to aid in medical treatment as well as for evidence collection should be obtained. The date, time, and location of the assault as well as the type and details of sexual acts should be recorded. In addition to a general medical history, the physician should determine birth control usage, date and time of last voluntary intercourse, last menstrual period, and history of recent gynecologic symptoms or disorders prior to the assault.

5. What should be done in the physical exam?

The purpose of the physical exam is to detect injuries requiring treatment and to meticulously record data that might support the claim of assault. All patients should be examined carefully for evidence of scratches, bruises, lacerations, teeth marks, or any other signs of trauma that might support the victim's lack of consent. The gynecologic exam should include a thorough search for contusions, abrasions, lacerations, bleeding, or tenderness. In cases of rectal penetration, a careful rectal exam should be performed, looking for perianal fissures or lacerations and, if blood is present, anoscopy or sigmoidoscopy should be done to explore the possibility of any internal injuries.

6. What additional evidence should be obtained?

Specimens to detect sperm or semen may serve as evidence to prove sexual contact and possibly indicate the assailant's identity. Vaginal and saliva samples (and rectal samples when appropriate) should be obtained. Swabs of semen deposits on the skin should also be collected. If there is suspicion of semen stains on the patient, a Wood's lamp can be used because semen fluoresces. The clothing the victim wore as well as any foreign matter such as loose hair, fibers, or vegetation that may be found on the victim should be collected. Hair samples should be plucked from the victim for comparison to loose hairs or those obtained from the crime scene. A system must be in place in order to preserve the chain of evidence.

7. What is the risk of pregnancy after sexual assault?

The risk of getting pregnant from a sexual assault is about 1%.

8. What are the current options for pregnancy prophylaxis?

The physician should determine that no preexisting pregnancy exists by obtaining a serum pregnancy test before initiating pregnancy prophylaxis. A variety of high-dose estrogen preparations are available, which act to prevent pregnancy by altering the endometrial lining so as to prevent implantation. These preparations should be given within 72 hours of the assault. The most widely used is oral norgestral and ethinyl estradiol (Ovral), 2 tablets at presentation followed by 2 tablets in 12 hours. Patients should be warned about nausea as a side effect, along with possible vaginal spotting. Because these preparations are not foolproof, patients should be warned of failure rates and be advised to seek medical attention if menses is delayed.

9. What is the risk of contracting a sexually transmitted disease (STD) from sexual assault?

Prospective studies suggest that the risk of contracting a new chlamydia or gonorrhea infection from a sexual assault is about 3%. The risk of contracting HIV infection from sexual assault is unknown but is believed to be significantly lower than 1%.

10. What additional laboratory studies are indicated?

All patients should have specimens taken from those areas in which sexual contact was made. Cultures for chlamydia and gonorrhea and serology for syphilis should be obtained at the time of the assault. If the patient does not receive prophylactic antibiotics in the ED, then chlamydia and gonorrhea cultures should be repeated 2 weeks after the assault and syphilis testing should be repeated 6 weeks after the assault. Victims who are concerned about potential HIV transmission should be referred to the health department or some other organization where counseling and confidential HIV antibody testing are performed.

11. Is empirical antibiotic treatment of sexual victims indicated?

For many sexual assault victims the possibility of contracting an STD as a result of the assault is very disturbing. These patient concerns, coupled with the fact that follow-up by sexual assault victims has traditionally been very poor, led many emergency physicians to offer patients antibiotic prophylaxis effective against gonorrhea, chlamydia, and incubating syphilis. One effective combination includes IM ceftriaxone followed by doxycycline or erythromycin for 7 days. New oral antibiotics effective in a single dose against gonorrhea (cefixime) and chlamydia (azithromycin) may supplant the above regimen. Even in cases in which empirical antibiotic therapy is given, cultures for chlamydia and gonorrhea and serology for syphilis should be obtained at the time of the assault. Epidemiologic studies have shown that sexual assault victims are at high risk for preexisting infection; baseline cultures are important for control of the STD epidemic through confidential contact tracing.

12. What are special characteristics of male sexual assault?

The male sexual assault victim should be treated similarly to female victims. Special attention should be paid to the mouth, genitals, anus, and rectum.

13. What are special characteristics of pediatric sexual assault?

In pediatric sexual assault, the assailant is often known to the victim and there is often a history of repetitive assaults. In addition to documenting signs of acute trauma, the physician should look for signs of recurrent abuse such as healed hymenal tears, a large vaginal opening, a vaginal discharge, or relaxed rectal sphincter tone. Gynecologic examination should take into account the nature of the assault and the age of the child. In the evaluation of a small child in whom a speculum exam is indicated, a nasal speculum may be used in place of a vaginal speculum. Sometimes, because of the emotional state of the child, the vaginal or rectal examination must be done under general anesthesia. The child should be protected from further abuse by admission to the hospital or immediate referral to the appropriate social service agency.

Prophylactic antibiotics are not generally indicated when sexual abuse of children is suspected. The baseline infection rate in children is significantly lower than in adults. The presence of an STD in a child is strong evidence that abuse has occurred; therefore, it is important to document the presence of the infection before treatment is instituted. In the child, chlamydia and gonorrhea cultures should be obtained from the vagina instead of the cervix.

14. What are the important aspects of follow-up care?

Follow-up medical care should ensure (1) that any physical injuries have healed properly, (2) the adequacy of pregnancy prophylaxis, (3) proper treatment of STDs, and (4) referral for psychological counseling.

15. What forms of emotional trauma do sexual assault victims experience?

The development of a posttraumatic stress disorder with its attendant manifestations of sleep disturbances, guilt feelings, memory impairment, and detachment from the world and other people can occur in the days to weeks after the event. Long-term psychological sequelae in the form of the **rape trauma syndrome** can occur as well. The rape trauma syndrome has an initial short-term phase of disorganization that lasts days to weeks and is characterized by a wide range of emotional behaviors, followed by period of reorganization that lasts months to years and is characterized by depression, flashbacks, anxiety, and sexual dysfunction. Many communities have rape crisis centers with social workers and volunteers who are trained to provide counseling for sexual assault survivors. Physicians should be aware of the availability of such services so they can recommend them to their patients.

BIBLIOGRAPHY

1. Braen GR: Sexual assault. In Rosen P, et al (eds): Emergency Medicine: Concepts and Clinical Practice, 3rd ed. St. Louis, Mosby–Year Book, 1992, pp 2003–2012.
2. Hochbaum SR: The evaluation and treatment of the sexually assaulted patient. Emerg Med Clin North Am 5:601–622, 1987.
3. Hoelzer M: Sexual assault. In Tintinalli J, et al (eds): Emergency Medicine: A Comprehensive Study Guide, 3rd ed. New York, McGraw-Hill, 1992, pp 398–402.
4. Hoffman G: Sexual assault. In Harwood-Nuss A, et al (eds): The Clinical Practice of Emergency Medicine. Philadelphia, J.B. Lippincott, 1991, pp 305–308.
5. Jenny C, Hooton TM, Bowers A, et al: Sexually transmitted diseases in victims of rape. N Engl J Med 322:713–716, 1990.
6. Kombernick ME, Seifert S, Janders AB: Emergency department management of the sexual assault victim. J Emerg Med 2:205–214, 1985.
7. Soules MR, Pollard AA, Brumm J, et al: The laboratory's rule in investigating rape. Am J Obstet Gynecol 130:142–147, 1978.
8. Tintinelli JE, Hoezler M: Clinical findings and legal resolution in sexual assault. Ann Emerg Med 14:447–453, 1985.

90. SPONTANEOUS ABORTION

Ellen M. Dugan, M.D.

1. What is abortion?
Abortion is termination of pregnancy prior to achieving fetal weight or maturity compatible with survival—less than 20 weeks' gestation or less than 500 gm fetal weight.

2. What is the incidence of spontaneous abortion?
Approximately 15–20% of pregnancies between 4 and 20 weeks will undergo spontaneous abortion.

3. What is the most common morphologic finding in early spontaneous abortion?
The most common finding is an abnormality of development of the embryo, the fetus, or the placenta. Chromosomal abnormalities are seen most commonly—50–60% of early spontaneous abortions are associated with a chromosomal abnormality. An abnormality in the number of chromosomes is more common than structural abnormalities.

4. When do most spontaneous abortions occur?
1–3 weeks after the death of the conceptus.

5. Describe the pathology of spontaneous abortion.
There is hemorrhage into the decidua basalis with subsequent necrotic changes in the area of implantation. The ovum becomes partially or completely detached, then acting as a foreign body in the uterus, stimulating contractions, and resulting in expulsion of contents.

6. What is a threatened abortion?
When any vaginal bleeding or bloody discharge appears in the first half of pregnancy. There may or may not be cramping or backache. The cervical os is closed.

7. Besides a threatened abortion, what else causes vaginal bleeding in the first half of pregnancy?
Ectopic pregnancy, vaginal ulcers, trophoblastic disease, cervical erosion, cervical polyps, cancer, and decidual reactions of the cervix.

8. What is a blighted ovum?
It is an ovum with no visible fetus in the sac. The embryo is degenerated or absent with fluid surrounding it when the sac is opened.

9. What is the treatment for threatened abortion?
1. Examination
2. Restricting physical activity
3. Restricting sexual intercourse
4. Following serial quantitative beta-hCGs. If they decrease, the prognosis is poor
5. If bleeding persists, do serial Hct/Hgb
6. If bleeding is profuse, causing hypotension, evacuation is necessary.

10. What are the earliest symptoms of an abortion?
Bleeding or spotting usually starts first, followed by crampy abdominal pain.

11. What is the prognosis with bleeding accompanied by pain?
Poor. There is no treatment regimen that influences the course of a threatened abortion.

12. Describe the sonographic findings in a healthy pregnancy.
There is a distinct, well-formed gestational ring, with central echoes indicating a fetal pole. A sac with no central echoes from an embryo or fetus implies, but it does not prove, death of the conceptus. Serial sonograms are important to follow the progression of lack of fetal growth.

13. What is an inevitable abortion?
An inevitable abortion occurs when there is rupture of the membranes in the presence of cervical dilatation with bleeding and/or pain.

14. What is an incomplete abortion?
It is the incomplete passage of products of conception from the uterus, the protruding of tissue from the cervical os, or persistent bleeding and cramping after the passage of tissue.

15. What is the treatment for an incomplete abortion?
Dilatation and curettage or suction curettage with local cervical anesthesia.

16. What is a missed abortion?
In a missed abortion, the conceptus dies but is not passed, with retention of dead products of conception in utero for 4–8 weeks or more. Uterine size decreases and symptoms of pregnancy regress. Most usually abort spontaneously.

17. What is the danger of prolonged retention of products of conception?
The danger is the occurrence of disseminated intravascular coagulation. Therefore, laboratory studies for coagulation defects (i.e., PT, PTT, fibrinogen, and fibrin split products) need to be obtained.

18. What is a complete abortion?
A complete abortion is passage of the entire conceptus with cessation of pain and bleeding.

19. Do diagnostic radiographs cause spontaneous abortion?
No! Diagnostic radiographs (less than 10 rads) place a pregnant woman at little to no increased risk. Therapeutic radiation and antineoplastic agents *do* increase the incidence of spontaneous abortion.

20. Is impaired psychological well-being associated with early fetal loss?
The association has been proposed but not proved.

21. What is a septic abortion?
A septic abortion may be associated with any spontaneous abortion as an infectious process manifested by endometritis, parametritis, and/or peritonitis.

22. What are the symptoms of a septic abortion?
   1. Malodorous discharge from the cervix or vagina
   2. Pelvic and abdominal pain
   3. Fever
   4. Uterine tenderness
   5. Hypothermia may be an indication of endotoxic shock.

23. List the etiologies of spontaneous abortion.

1. Chromosomal abnormalities: most common autosomal trisomy 51.9%.
2. Risk increases with increased maternal parity and increased maternal and paternal age.
   The frequency increases from 12% in females <20 yrs to 26% in females >40 yrs.
3. Conception within 3 months after a live birth.
4. Systemic disease of the mother (e.g., diabetes mellitus, cancer, hypo- or hyper-thyroidism)
5. Autoimmune mechanisms: antiphospholipid autoantibodies
6. Laparotomy: The closer the surgery to the pelvic organs, the greater the risk of spontaneous abortion.
7. Uterine defects
   - *Acquired*
     Leiomyomas: the location is more important than the size. Submucous fibroids are more dangerous.
     Intrauterine adhesions: synechiae or Asherman's syndrome secondary to curettage.
   - *Developmental*
     Abnormal mullerian duct formation or fusion. May be secondary to diethylstilbestrol use.
     Septate, bicornate, or unicornate uterus.

24. Is the drug isotretinoin (Accutane) safe for use in pregnancy?

No! It has been associated with spontaneous abortion and fetal abnormalities. Do **not** use in pregnancy or in women planning to become pregnant.

25. Has use of oral contraceptives been associated with spontaneous abortion?

No. Oral contraceptives taken either before or during pregnancy have not been associated with spontaneous abortion.

26. Is trauma a major factor associated with spontaneous abortion?

No. Fetuses are well protected by maternal structures and amniotic fluid from minor falls or blows, but penetrating trauma such as a gunshot wound or stab wound is dangerous to the fetus.

27. Name drugs, chemicals, and/or noxious agents associated with spontaneous abortions.

1. Cigarettes
2. Alcohol (at high exposure range)
3. Contraceptive agents (conception with an IUD in place increases the risk of spontaneous abortion)
4. Environmental chemicals (anesthetic agents, arsenic, aniline, benzene, ethylene oxide, formaldehyde, and lead)

28. Is exposure to spermicide prior to or after conception deleterious to a pregnancy?

No.

29. Define cervical incompetence.

Cervical incompetence is painless dilatation of the cervix during the second trimester, followed by spontaneous rupture of membranes, with subsequent expulsion of uterine contents.

30. Name the drug used to prevent Rh immunization.

Rh immune globulin or Rhogam. A woman who is aborting and is Rh negative should receive a 300-μg dose of Rh immune globulin.

BIBLIOGRAPHY

1. Cohen-Overbreek TE, Hop WCJ, et al: Spontaneous abortion rate and advanced maternal age: Consequences for prenatal diagnosis. Lancet 336:27–29, 1990.
2. Cunningham FG, MacDonald PC, Gant NF: Williams' Obstetrics, 8th ed. Norwalk, CT, Appleton & Lange, 1989, pp 489–499.
3. Gabbe SG, Niebyl JR, Simpson JL: Obstetrics Normal and Problem Pregnancies, 2nd ed. New York, Churchill Livingstone, 1991, pp 783–807.
4. Jones HW III, Wentz AC, Burnett LS: Novak's Textbook of Gynecology, 11th ed. Baltimore, Williams & Wilkins, 1988, pp 341–350.
5. Pernoll ML(ed): Current Obstetric and Gynecological Diagnosis and Treatment, 7th ed. Norwalk, CT, Appleton & Lange, 1991, pp 300–308.
6. Rosenberg L, et al: Breast cancer in relation to the occurrence and time of induced and spontaneous abortion. Am J Epidemiol 127:981–989, 1988.
7. Scott JR, et al: Danforth's Obstetrics and Gynecology, 6th ed. Philadelphia, J.B. Lippincott, 1990 pp 209–220.
8. Wichit Srisuphan PH, Bracken MB: Caffeine consumption during pregnancy and association with late spontaneous abortion. Am J Obstet Gynecol 154:14–20, 1986.

91. ECTOPIC PREGNANCY

Jean Abbott, M.D.

1. What is an ectopic pregnancy?

An ectopic pregnancy (EP) is one in which implantation of the gestational sac occurs outside of the uterus. In most cases, the pregnancy is located in the fallopian tubes, but EPs can occur on the ovary (0.1%), intraabdominally (1.5%), within the cervix (0.1%), or in the interstitial or cornual portion of the uterus (2%). EP occurs in approximately 1 in 60 pregnancies in the United States, although the risk is higher in older women and minorities. Common risk factors for EP are prior pelvic inflammatory disease (PID), prior ectopic pregnancy, tubal ligation, IUD use, and prior pelvic surgery.

2. Why is the risk of EP increasing so much?

The risk of EP has quadrupled in the past 20 years. The major identified risk factor is prior tubal infection (PID), which can be seen histologically in 50% of patients with EP. Other structural abnormalities of the fallopian tubes and host abnormalities that discourage implantation in the endometrium are believed to cause some cases of ectopic implantation. New technology, such as artificial fertilization, ovulation stimulation, and surgical procedures that result in salvage of potentially abnormal fallopian tubes, may also contribute to the increased incidence.

3. What is the risk of heterotopic (combined intrauterine and ectopic) pregnancy?

The classic risk of combined ectopic and intrauterine pregnancy has been cited as 1 in 30,000 pregnancies. Recent estimates, however, put the risk at closer to 1 in 4,000 and the chances in infertility patients with pregnancy stimulation or embryo transfer procedures may be much higher.

4. How often is a routine pregnancy test positive in the patient with EP?

Sensitivity of serum or urine pregnancy tests in EP depends on the threshold of the test. Human chorionic gonadotropin (hCG), measured in all modern pregnancy tests, is secreted from the time of implantation, about 7–8 days after implantation of the fertilized ovum. Because hormone levels are frequently lower in EP than in normal pregnancy (owing to impaired growth in the ectopic location), a sensitive qualitative pregnancy test is required to accurately detect the pregnancy. Qualitative pregnancy tests positive at a level of 10–50 mIU/ml (International Reference Preparation, IRP) are positive in almost 99% of patients with ectopic pregnancy. If the test threshold is 300–400 mIU/ml (IRP), 10–20% of EPs may be falsely negative. Serum and urine tests both provide similar accuracy for qualitative testing if their thresholds are similar.

5. What clinical symptoms are useful to increase suspicion of an EP?

The classical picture of EP is of vaginal bleeding, pelvic or abdominal pain, prior missed menses, and an adnexal mass. Unfortunately, this is neither sensitive nor specific. Missed menses occur in only 85% of EP patients. Vaginal bleeding may occur only when the growing pregnancy begins to fail, and pain may also occur later. Adnexal masses are palpated in only 50% of patients, even under anesthesia; they may represent the corpus luteum of the pregnancy rather than the ectopic gestation itself. EP should be suspected in every woman who presents with a clinical complaint related to pregnancy in the first trimester, although the risk in different clinical settings may vary considerably. Patients at high risk for EP are those with first-trimester pregnancy and either pelvic pain or risk factors for EP.

6. Why are corpus luteum cysts frequently confused with EPs?

The corpus luteum of the ovary, originating from the graafian follicle, supports the pregnancy with secretion of hCG and progesterone during the first 6–7 weeks of gestation, and may become cystic, growing to 5 cm diameter or more. Cyst rupture can occur in the first trimester, giving rise to a patient in early pregnancy with a clinical picture of sudden pain, unilateral peritoneal findings, adnexal tenderness, and perhaps even a mass.

7. What is the risk of EP in a patient with painless vaginal bleeding?

Although the risk of EP is low in patients with painless bleeding in the first trimester, occasionally women with EP present this way initially. Although use of ultrasound to locate all pregnancies in the first trimester in the ED is not feasible or necessary, instructions should be given to all women as if they could have an EP until an intrauterine pregnancy (IUP) is proved by ultrasound, auscultation of fetal heart sounds, or tissue diagnosis of an abortion.

8. What is the role of sonography in the evaluation of EP?

Sonographic location of early pregnancy continues to make great technologic advances. With transabdominal sonography (TAS), the normal fetal sac can be seen by about 6 weeks after the last menstrual period (beta-hCG of 6,500 mIU/ml) and fetal heart motion by 8 weeks. Ectopic gestations are rarely seen, and EP is suspected when an IUP is not seen at the expected gestational age or quantitative hCG level. With the improved resolution of transvaginal sonography (TVS), intrauterine gestational sacs normally can be visualized at 5 weeks from the last menstrual period (5,000 mIU/ml 1st IRP) and fetal heart motion by 7 weeks (beta-hCG level of about 17,000 mIU/ml 1st IRP). Many sonographic results are indeterminate and must be repeated in a few days to a week to provide definitive diagnosis of either IUP or EP.

9. What is the relative usefulness of TAS vs. TVS in the patient with possible EP?

Along with providing earlier detection of normal IUPs, TVS provides a greater chance of seeing ectopic gestations. In some studies, up to half of EPs were seen directly with TVS, and a far smaller number of total patients studied to rule out EP have indeterminate results.

10. What is the role of quantitative hCG? Should it be a "stat" test in every patient with possible EP?

Beta-hCG levels double every 2–3 days during the first 7–8 weeks of normal pregnancies. Because many women do not know the date of their last menstrual period, quantitative levels may be useful to estimate gestational age and correlate with expected sonographic findings (see above). In addition, failure to double levels during the first 7 weeks indicates the pregnancy is failing—either within the uterus or at an ectopic site. Such a failed pregnancy is likely to be ectopic if D&C fails to detect villi or if no products of conception are found at the time of miscarriage. Although single quantitative beta-hCG levels are available in some EDS on a stat basis, next-day follow-up is usually necessary anyway in the stable patient, and such data can be interpreted then in light of sonographic results and the patient's clinical picture.

11. What is the role of culdocentesis?

Sonography has obviated the need for culdocentesis in most instances. Sonography, however, is most likely to be indeterminate in very early pregnancy, and culdocentesis, which is painful but relatively accurate, may be useful to detect EP in such circumstances. While up to 20% of aspirations from culdocentesis may be dry and give no information, over 90% of the remainder are positive, even in women with subacute presentations and without signs of peritonitis. Culdocentesis is indicated in patients who are unstable and simply need rapid confirmation of intraperitoneal bleeding, or in EDs in which sonography is not readily available but diagnosis needs to be made relatively urgently.

12. Does every patient with bleeding or pain in the first trimester require ultrasound before discharge from the ED?

The unstable patient should probably have a rapid culdocentesis and a trip to the operating room. Urgent sonography should be reserved for patients with acute pain, significant risk factors, or other reasons for a high index of suspicion for EP. For the majority of patients who must continue to be managed with the uncertainty that they could be harboring an EP, it is useful to schedule sonography in the subsequent few days, particularly because daytime sonographic studies are frequently more complete and accurate. If all first-trimester complaints are treated as EP until proved otherwise, then patients should receive careful instructions to return if they develop pain and can be safely scheduled for later ultrasound.

13. What are the ultrasound findings in patients with suspected EP?

Ultrasound Findings in the Patient with Suspected Ectopic Pregnancy

Indicative of IUP	Suggestive of ectopic gestation
"Double" ring sign	Cul-de-sac fluid without IUP
"Double" gestational sac	Adnexal mass* without IUP
Intrauterine fetal pole	
Intrauterine fetal heart activity	Indeterminate
	No intrauterine findings
Diagnostic of ectopic gestation	Single gestational sac
Ectopic fetal heart activity or	Multiple intrauterine echoes
Ectopic fetal pole	

* Complex mass most suggestive of EP, but cyst can also be seen with EP.
From Abbott J: Complications related to pregnancy. In Rosen P, et al (eds): Emergency Medicine: Concepts and Clinical Practice, 3rd ed. St. Louis, Mosby–Year Book, 1992, pp 1972–2002, with permission.

14. What is the management of possible EP?

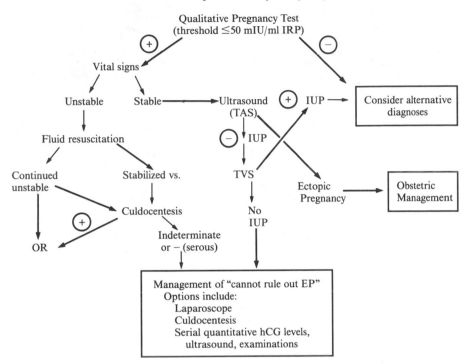

Management of possible ectopic pregnancy. TAS, transabdominal sonography; TVS, transvaginal ultrasonography. Adapted from Abbott J: Complications related to pregnancy. In Rosen P, et al (eds): Emergency Medicine: Concepts and Clinical Practice, 3rd ed. St. Louis, Mosby–Year Book, 1992, pp 1972–2002, with permission.

15. Should patients with EPs ever be discharged from the ED?

Certainly persons with significant pain or signs of significant blood loss require admission. Observation may be useful in stable patients with worrisome symptoms or risk factors or expected poor compliance to facilitate rapid sonography, quantitative hCG interpretation or specialist consultation. In specific circumstances, patients may be followed on an outpatient basis. Conservative outpatient treatment modalities, even when a woman has a known EP, are becoming more common in the 1990s. Expectant management or chemotherapy for women with few symptoms and low hormonal levels is becoming standard and should be directed by the patient's obstetrician. The role of ED caretakers is to consider the diagnosis, make every effort to exclude or make the diagnosis of EP expeditiously, let the patient be aware of the differential diagnosis and signs that should be of concern to her, and ensure access to close follow-up care for this potentially serious problem.

BIBLIOGRAPHY

1. Abbott JT, Emmans L, Lowenstein SR: Ectopic pregnancy: Ten common pitfalls in diagnosis. Am J Emerg Med 8:515, 1990.
2. Abbott JT: Ectopic pregnancy. In Rosen P, et al (eds): Emergency Medicine: Concepts and Clinical Practice, 3rd ed. St. Louis, Mosby–Year Book, 1992.

3. Cacciatore B, Stenman UH, Ylostalo P: Comparison of abdominal and vaginal sonography in suspected ectopic pregnancy. Obstet Gynecol 73:770, 1989.
4. Mishell DR: Ectopic pregnancy. In Herbst AL, et al (eds): Comprehensive Gynecology, 2nd ed. St. Louis, Mosby–Year Book, 1992.
5. Ory SJ: New options for diagnosis and treatment of ectopic pregnancy. JAMA 267:534, 1992.
6. Romero R, et al: The value of adnexal sonographic findings in the diagnosis of ectopic pregnancy. Am J Obstet Gynecol 158:52, 1988.
7. Romero R, et al: The value of serial human chorionic gonadotropin testing as a diagnostic tool in ectopic pregnancy. Am J Obstet Gynecol 155:392, 1986.
8. Timor-Tritsch IE, et al: The use of transvaginal ultrasonography in the diagnosis of ectopic pregnancy. Am J Obstet Gynecol 161:157, 1989.

92. THIRD-TRIMESTER VAGINAL BLEEDING

John M. Howell, M.D., FACEP

1. What are the sources of third-trimester vaginal bleeding?
Sources include the vagina, cervix, and uterus.

2. List the causes.
Etiologies are placenta previa, placental abruption, marginal sinus rupture, "bloody show," local trauma, and cervical polyps and lesions.

3. What are the life-threatening causes?
Placenta previa, placental abruption, and uterine rupture.

4. What is the frequency of placenta previa?
This abnormality occurs in less than 1% of pregnancies.

5. Describe placenta previa.
Placenta previa occurs when the placenta implants on or near the cervical os. Total coverage of the cervical os by placenta is called complete placenta previa, whereas subtotal coverage is termed partial placenta previa. Marginal placenta previa occurs when the margin of the placenta approaches but does not occlude the cervical os.

6. Why is it dangerous?
Vaginal penetration or manipulation of the placenta during a pelvic examination may rupture blood vessels and cause massive hemorrhage, which in turn may cause maternal or fetal demise.

7. How is placenta previa diagnosed?
Ultrasound is 93 to 98% accurate in locating the placenta. Placenta previa is frequently diagnosed early in pregnancy and followed with serial ultrasound studies until delivery. Occasionally, gravid women present with vaginal bleeding and an undiagnosed placental abnormality.

8. What is the clinical presentation?
If vaginal bleeding occurs, it is generally painless and bright red in color. Palpation of the fetus is not difficult. Fetal heart tones are clearly heard and there is no coagulopathy.

9. How is placenta previa treated?

Do not perform a pelvic examination unless you are in the operating room or delivery suite with an experienced obstetrician; life-threatening bleeding may occur if the placenta is inadvertently manipulated. Place the patient on her left side in the recumbent position. In patients who are hemodynamically stable with small amounts of bleeding, start an IV line and admit the patient for ultrasound, serial maternal vital signs, and fetal monitoring. In selected cases, delivery is delayed to optimize fetal development. If serious vaginal bleeding occurs, start two large-bore IV lines, administer oxygen, monitor fetal heart tones, and admit the patient for delivery.

10. Define placental abruption (aka abruptio placentae).

Placental abruption is the premature separation of the placenta from its insertion on the uterine wall.

11. What is the incidence of placental abruption?

It occurs in 0.2 to 0.5% of pregnancies.

12. Why is it dangerous?

A large amount of blood may collect between the placenta and the uterine wall, causing maternal shock and fetal demise.

13. What is the clinical presentation?

Abruption occurs spontaneously or after mild, moderate, or severe trauma. The uterus is very firm or hard, and the patient reports severe abdominal pain. Hypertension may or may not occur, and vaginal bleeding may not be present. If vaginal bleeding does occur, the blood is dark red in color. This presentation is in contrast to the painless, bright red bleeding of placenta previa. The presence of additional blood in the uterus makes palpating the fetus and measuring fetal heart tones difficult. Coagulopathy may occur.

14. How is it diagnosed?

Ultrasound. However, a clinical diagnosis is made when the mother or fetus are in danger and the signs and symptoms reflect placental abruption.

15. Describe the treatment.

Start two large-bore IV lines and administer oxygen. Monitor fetal heart tones and the mother's vital signs frequently. Obtain clotting studies to diagnose coagulopathy. If the patient is stable, arrange an immediate ultrasound. Take unstable patients directly to the operating room or delivery suite for delivery.

16. Define uterine rupture. What is the frequency?

It is a grave complication of late pregnancy in which the uterus ruptures, usually during contractions. Uterine rupture occurs in 0.05% of pregnancies.

17. Why is it dangerous?

Intraabdominal bleeding is life threatening. Maternal mortality is 8% and fetal mortality about 50%.

18. State the two anatomic classifications of uterine rupture.

The uterus is either scarred or not scarred. Uterine scarring is caused by prior hysterotomy, cesarean section, and curettage.

19. What are the proximate causes?
Excessive intrauterine pressures during oxytocin stimulation or a difficult labor with cephalopelvic disproportion, weakening of the uterine wall due to multiparity, and placenta percreta (extension of villi through the uterine myometrium).

20. Describe the clinical presentation.
Sudden abdominal pain and shock late in pregnancy are usually associated with uterine contractions. There is scant vaginal bleeding and the abdomen is remarkably tender.

21. What is the treatment?
Start two large-bore IV lines and administer oxygen with immediate transfer to the operating room or delivery suite for laparotomy and hysterectomy. Ultrasound may be necessary in selected cases to distinguish uterine rupture from placental abruption.

22. Describe non–life-threatening causes of third-trimester vaginal bleeding.
"Bloody show" is a pink mucous discharge caused by cervical changes that precedes labor by several hours to a week. The cervix is prone to hemorrhage during late pregnancy, and local trauma from vaginal penetration, including intercourse, may cause bleeding. Cervical erosions or preexisting polyps produce limited bleeding. Marginal sinus rupture is a premature separation of the placenta limited to the placental margin.

BIBLIOGRAPHY

1. Eden RD, Parker RT, Gall ST: Rupture of the pregnant uterus: A 53-year review. Obstet Gynecol 68:671–674, 1986.
2. Gorodeski IG, Bahari CM: The effect of placenta previa localization upon maternal and fetal-neonatal outcome. J Perinat Med 15:169–177, 1987.
3. Lavery JP: Placenta previa. Clin Obstet Gynecol 33:414–431, 1990.
4. Lowe TW, Cunningham FG: Placental abruption. Clin Obstet Gynecol 33:406–413, 1990.
5. Scott JR, Disaia PJ, Hammond CB, et al (eds): Danforth's Obstetrics and Gynecology, 6th ed. Philadelphia, Harper and Row Publishers, 1990, pp 553–566.

93. PREECLAMPSIA AND ECLAMPSIA

Robert S. Van Hare, M.D.

1. Is every pregnant patient with hypertension considered preeclamptic or eclamptic?
No. Hypertension during gestation can be divided into four categories: (1) preeclampsia/eclampsia; (2) chronic hypertension; (3) chronic hypertension with superimposed pre-eclampsia; and (4) late or transient hypertension. Preeclampsia/eclampsia and chronic hypertension with superimposed preeclampsia pose the greatest threat to fetal and maternal well-being. Chronic hypertension is simply hypertension of whatever cause that predates the pregnancy; it accounts for one-third of all cases of hypertension in pregnancy. Late or transient hypertension consists of mild or at most moderate elevation of blood pressure near term but may herald the development of essential hypertension later in life.

2. How does toxemia of pregnancy fit into this categorization?
It is a general term referring to the specific entities of preeclampsia and eclampsia and is defined as the onset of hypertension, proteinuria, or edema or a combination of them after the 20th gestational week.

3. Define preeclampsia.

Preeclampsia is acute elevation of blood pressure ($>$140/90, $>$30 torr elevation in systolic blood pressure, or $>$15 torr elevation in diastolic blood pressure above baseline levels) accompanied by proteinuria (1 gm/L in a random specimen or more than 3 gm/L in a 24-hour collection). The third traditional requirement is generalized edema, no longer recognized by many authorities.

4. What is the etiology of preeclampsia/eclampsia?

This is an easy question to answer correctly, because if you do not know the answer, you are right! One theory suggests that alteration in prostaglandin metabolism is responsible for the disorder, but the exact cause is unknown.

5. What is the incidence of preeclampsia/eclampsia?

Preeclampsia can be found in 5–10% of all pregnancies.

6. Who is predisposed to preeclampsia/eclampsia?

Preeclampsia/eclampsia occurs most commonly in young primiparous and older multiparous females. Diabetes, multiple gestation, hydatidiform mole, and fetal hydrops are also predisposing factors.

7. Is there a role for outpatient management of preeclampsia?

No. Clinical evaluation of the preeclamptic is inaccurate in predicting which patients may develop eclamptic seizures. Furthermore, the blood pressure of the preeclamptic patient can quickly escalate to dangerous levels. Obstetric consultation is essential and admission usually indicated due to the potential maternal and fetal risks.

8. What are some of the signs of severe preeclampsia?

Rising blood pressure $>$160/110, heavy proteinuria ($>$5 gm/L in 24 hours), oliguria, headache, visual disturbances, apprehension, pulmonary edema, right upper quadrant pain, hemolytic anemia, elevated liver enzymes, thrombocytopenia, and hyperreflexia may be found in a severely preeclamptic patient.

9. What is the most frequent cause of death in preeclampsia/eclampsia?

Central nervous system (CNS) disorders account for the majority of maternal deaths. CNS abnormalities include cortical and subcortical hemorrhages, microinfarctions, cerebral edema, subarachnoid hemorrhage, and large intracerebral hematomas.

10. Define eclampsia.

Simply, eclampsia is the development of seizures (generalized motor type) or coma in a patient with preeclampsia. It carries a grave prognosis.

11. Does a patient have to be pregnant to become eclamptic?

No, but this is a trick question. A preeclamptic patient may worsen after delivery (technically no longer pregnant) and develop late postpartum eclampsia, which usually occurs in the first 24–48 hours postpartum but which may not present until several weeks after delivery.

12. What is the treatment for the preeclamptic/eclamptic patient?

If preeclampsia develops after 34 weeks' gestation, and the fetus has adequate pulmonary maturity, delivery is the definitive treatment. Prior to 34 weeks, delivery may be postponed if one can adequately control blood pressure and there are no signs of impending eclampsia. Depending on ethical considerations, delivery is also indicated at any gestational age if the patient has severe preeclampsia or impending eclampsia. Prior to delivery, blood pressure must be controlled and seizure prophylaxis initiated.

13. What are the current prophylaxis and treatment of eclamptic seizures?

Prophylaxis should be considered in all preeclamptic patients during risk periods: labor, delivery, and 24 hours postpartum. Although controversy continues, magnesium sulfate still is the drug of choice of obstetricians in the U.S. A loading dose is 4–6 gm magnesium sulfate in a 10% solution infused slowly over 5–10 minutes. The maintenance dose is 1–2 gm/hr intravenously.

14. Is magnesium sulfate the standard of care worldwide?

No. In Europe, Great Britain, and Australia, phenytoin and benzodiazepines are used much more frequently than magnesium is in the treatment of eclamptic seizures. Unfortunately, good controlled studies have not been performed to "settle" this controversy. Emergency physicians need to establish a therapeutic management plan that is acceptable to both consulting obstetricians and neurologists.

15. What are the risks of magnesium therapy?

Excessive magnesium sulfate can lead to loss of reflexes (>8 mEq/L), hypotension, and eventual respiratory arrest (>12 mEq/L). One must monitor reflexes; when they disappear, the infusion must be stopped. If magnesium toxicity ensues, it should be treated with 10 cc of 10% calcium gluconate slow intravenous (IV) push.

16. How do you control the elevated blood pressure of preeclampsia/eclampsia?

Although magnesium sulfate is reported to be of some benefit in lowering blood pressure, hydralazine (10–20 mg slow IV push or 0.5–1.0 mg/hr constant infusion) is the drug of choice. Labetalol is a second-line drug. Diazoxide can be used in the rare patient with severe hypertension unresponsive to hydralazine or labetalol or both. In a life-threatening situation unresponsive to prior measures, nitroprusside may be used, but only for a short duration due to the risk of fetal cyanide toxicity. Nifedipine is advocated by some authors; diuretics are contraindicated.

17. What is the HELLP syndrome?

*H*emolysis, *E*levated *L*iver enzymes, and *L*ow *P*latelet count. Described in 1982, it is controversial whether it is a variant of preeclampsia/eclampsia or a separate complication of pregnancy. It occurs in older multiparous patients, with maternal and perinatal mortality reaching 24% and 64%, respectively. It should be managed in the same manner as severe preeclampsia.

18. What are the clinical manifestations of the HELLP syndrome?

The majority of patients usually present before term complaining of epigastric and right upper quadrant pain, nausea or vomiting, and nonspecific viral-syndrome-like symptoms. Some give a history of malaise for the past few days prior to presentation. Hypertension and proteinuria may be absent or minimal.

19. What are the primary differential diagnoses of the HELLP syndrome?

The differential diagnosis includes many entities ranging from gastroenteritis and hyperemesis gravidarum to gallbladder and peptic ulcer disease. A more specific differential includes acute fatty liver of pregnancy, hepatitis, thrombotic thrombocytopenic purpura, disseminated intravascular coagulation (caused by sepsis, hypovolemia, hemorrhage, etc.), and hemolytic uremic syndrome.

20. What is an acute life-threatening complication of the HELLP syndrome?
Any patient who presents with shoulder pain, shock, evidence of massive ascites, or a pleural effusion may have a ruptured or unruptured subcapsular liver hematoma. Even appropriate management results in over 50% mortality.

BIBLIOGRAPHY

1. Barron WM: Hypertension. In Barron WM, Lindheimer MD (eds): Medical Disorders During Pregnancy. St. Louis, Mosby–Year Book, 1991.
2. Barton JR, Sibai BM: Care of the pregnancy complicated by HELLP syndrome. Obstet Gynecol Clin North Am 18(2):165, 1991.
3. Kaplan PW, Lesser RP, Fisher RS, et al: A continuing controversy: Magnesium sulfate in the treatment of eclamptic seizures. Arch Neurol 47:1031, 1990.
4. Lindheimer MD, Katz AI: Preeclampsia: Pathophysiology, diagnosis, and management. Annu Rev Med 40:233, 1989.
5. Martin JN, Stedman CM: Imitators of preeclampsia and HELLP syndrome. Obstet Gynecol Clin North Am 18(2):181, 1991.
6. Remuzzi G, Ruggenenti P: Prevention and treatment of pregnancy-associated hypertension: What have we learned in the last 10 years? Am J Kidney Dis 18(3):285, 1991.
7. Scott VB: Complications of pregnancy. In Rosen P, et al (eds): Emergency Medicine: Concepts and Clinical Practice, 3rd ed. St. Louis, Mosby–Year Book, 1988.
8. Sibai BM: The HELLP syndrome (hemolysis, elevated liver enzymes, and low platelet): Much ado about nothing? Am J Obstet Gynecol 162:311, 1990.
9. Sibai BM: Magnesium sulfate is the ideal anticonvulsant in preeclampsia-eclampsia. Am J Obstet Gynecol 162:1141, 1990.

XVI. Trauma

94. MULTIPLE TRAUMA

Richard Kingsland, M.D., and Peter Rosen, M.D.

1. What is multiple trauma?

Multiple trauma is significant injury to more than one major body system.

2. Can severity of injury be determined at the scene?

No. A variety of different trauma scales and scoring devices have been developed to quantify the extent of injury. These devices are imperfect, however, and in order to maintain an acceptable safety margin, systems need to over-triage potential multiple-trauma victims. Transport to a trauma center should be based upon the mechanism of injury, underlying disease, physiologic parameters such as alterations in vital signs and neurologic status, and the presence of obvious multiple organ system injury.

3. What is "mechanism of injury"?

The mechanism of injury refers to the events and conditions that lead to both known and unknown traumatic injuries. Significant mechanism of injury is associated with a higher likelihood of multiple trauma. Less obvious mechanism is of greater concern with increasing age or the underlying disease. For example, a 70-year-old patient with ankylosing spondylitis is much less able to tolerate blunt trauma to the spinal column and pelvis than is a healthy person.

Examples of Significant Mechanisms of Injury

Blunt Trauma		Penetrating Trauma
Automobile accidents	Automobile-pedestrian accidents	Gunshot wounds to
Fatality at the scene	High speed	head, neck, torso
Passenger ejection	Damage to exterior of vehicle	Stab wounds to neck,
Vehicle rollover	Falls	torso
Significant interior	Greater than 1 story	
damage	(12–15 feet)	

4. What are the first steps in managing multiple trauma in the ED?

- Activate the trauma resuscitation team.
- Designate a trauma captain and call for O-negative blood if indicated by prehospital course.
- Transfer the patient from the ambulance stretcher or other conveyance to the ED resuscitation bed.
- Quickly obtain a history of the accident, including the mechanism of injury.
- Obtain vital signs while the patient is being undressed.
- Assess the ABCs and intervene as necessary.
- Draw blood for type, cross-matching, and baseline laboratory testing.

5. How should the patient be undressed?

Because immobilization is necessary until the spine can be cleared, all movement should be avoided. To obtain complete visualization rapidly while protecting the spine, simply cut the clothes away. Keep in mind that one of the purposes of clothing removal is to rid the patient of objects that can cause further damage, such as shards of broken glass, bits of metal, or weapons.

6. What are the ABCs (and D) of trauma?

Airway. Airway patency is evaluated by listening for vocalizations, asking for the patient's name, and looking in the patient's mouth for signs of obstruction (blood, emesis, or foreign debris). The trauma captain must determine if the patient needs active airway management and verify that supplemental oxygen is being continuously administered to all patients who do not require immediate intubation.

Mandatory Indications for Airway Management in Trauma
- Massive facial injuries
- Head injury with Glasgow Coma Scale less than 8
- Penetrating injury to the cranial vault
- Missile penetrating injury to the neck
- Blunt injury to the neck with expanding hematoma or alteration of the voice
- Multisystem trauma with persistent shock

Relative Indications for Airway Management in Trauma
- Upper airway obstruction from any cause
- Any patient with injuries impairing ventilation
- Flail chest with increasing respiratory rate or deteriorating oxygenation
- Any patient with one or more rib fractures who is going to need a ventilator or a general anesthetic
- Patients with bilateral pneumothorax
- Bilateral missile penetrating injuries of the thorax
- Patients with continuing hemothorax that recurs or does not respond to tube thoracostomy
- Patients with severe hypovolemic shock

Breathing. Ventilation is assessed by observing for symmetric rise and fall of the chest and by listening for bilateral breath sounds over the anterior chest and axillae. The chest should be gently palpated for subcutaneous air and bony crepitus. Oxygen saturation should be monitored continuously. The trauma captain then determines the need for chest tubes and ventilatory support.

Circulation. Circulatory function is assessed by noting the patient's mental status, skin color and character (cool and clammy vs. warm and dry), vital signs, and presence or absence of radial, femoral and carotid pulses. Continuous EKG monitoring should be started. Prehospital vascular access and type and amount of volume infused are assessed. The trauma captain then determines whether additional vascular access or volume of crystalloid is needed and if blood should be administered.

Disability. The patient's neurologic status should be assessed (level of consciousness and gross motor function). An initial ED Glasgow Coma Scale rating should be ascertained.

7. What type of intravenous access should be established in a patient with major trauma?

At least two large-bore (16 gauge or greater) IV lines should be placed. Forearm or antecubital veins are the preferred sites for initial access. Although subclavian and internal jugular lines allow central venous pressure monitoring, this rarely provides access for high volume IV infusions unless a Cordis introducer is left in place. Therefore, these routes should be used only if no other access exists and lines should be placed on the ipsilateral side of the chest trauma unless a subclavian vascular injury is suspected. Femoral lines and cutdowns are indicated in patients with a dropping blood pressure in that large volume infusions will be needed quickly.

8. Where should cutdowns be performed?
Cutdowns are most easily performed at the ankle. The distal saphenous vein can be found between the anterior tibialis tendon and the medial malleolus.

9. What parameters should be monitored in multiple trauma victims?
Vital signs, neurologic status, and, if possible, oxygen saturation and central venous pressure should be carefully monitored. Hypothermia adversely affects outcome and core temperature can drop rapidly when the patient is disrobed and receives large quantities of cold intravenous fluid. Tachypnea is a sensitive sign of both hypoxia and acidosis and should be accurately measured rather than estimated. Ability to mentate, skin color and character, and urinary output over time should be monitored as well.

10. When should blood be administered?
O-negative (universal donor) blood should be reserved for patients who are in arrest from hypovolemic shock. If 40 cc/kg of crystalloid is rapidly infused and there is no significant improvement in the patient's circulatory status, type-specific noncrossmatched blood should be administered. For more details, see ch. 4 on "Shock."

11. Are laboratory tests useful?
Not very, although all major trauma victims should have a clot sent for type and cross-match. Baseline values of hematocrit and serum amylase may be useful in detecting occult injuries and preexisting anemia. Urinalysis should be performed to detect hematuria. Many trauma centers obtain an extensive trauma panel, which may be useful if the patient requires surgery or has underlying disease. However, no laboratory test defines injury, and the trauma panel is of little use in determining initial management, disposition, or need for surgery.

Initial Laboratory Tests in Multiple Trauma

CBC	Clot for type and cross-match
Electrolytes	Urinalysis
BUN, creatinine	Blood alcohol as indicated
Glucose	Toxicology screen as indicated
Prothrombin and partial thromboplastin times	Amylase

12. What is the secondary survey?
The secondary survey is the complete physical examination performed after the ABCs have been assessed and stabilized. This survey includes assessment of the chest, abdomen, pelvis, back, and extremities. A repeat neurologic examination and rectal examination should also be performed. The purpose of the rectal examination is to determine if there is gross blood in the rectum, if there is adequate sphincter tone and sensation, and if the prostate gland is in a normal position.

13. Which radiologic studies need to be obtained immediately?
Once the patient is stabilized, portable radiographs of the lateral cervical spine, the chest, and the pelvis should be obtained. In gunshot wounds, portable films in two planes may be needed to determine the location of the bullet.

14. How do I prioritize diagnostic tests?

Prioritization is based on potential life threats. After external hemorrhage is controlled, diagnosing intraperitoneal hemorrhage takes precedence. Unless an indication for immediate laparotomy is present, the patient should undergo diagnostic peritoneal lavage or abdominal CT scan to assess the intraperitoneal cavity. Following these procedures, attention should be focused on ruling out correctable intracranial hemorrhage such as a subdural or an epidural hematoma. Finally, based on the mechanism of injury and the initial course, other specialized studies to evaluate the aorta and the retroperitoneum should be performed.

95. MAXILLOFACIAL TRAUMA

Steven Dominguez, M.D.

1. What is maxillofacial trauma?

Maxillofacial trauma is injury to the anatomic area bounded inferiorly by the mandible, superiorly by the scalp, and laterally from ear to ear. Trauma ranges from a simple abrasion, contusion, laceration, fracture, or burn (contact and/or inhalation) to any combination of the above. Structures in the face include skin, fat, muscles, nerves, arteries, veins, bones, cartilage, teeth, eyes, and mucous membranes.

2. What is the primary concern in a patient with maxillofacial trauma?

Of the essential ABCs of resuscitation (airway, breathing, circulation), the airway is the primary concern. Significant facial trauma may cause swelling or distortion of the airway. Elective intubation is more prudent than emergent surgery to secure an airway. Endotracheal intubation should be considered early in patients with significant midface or mandibular trauma, especially if they exhibit any signs of airway distress. Stridor is the classic sign of an upper airway obstruciton, from either a foreign body or edema of the tongue, oropharynx, hypopharynx, or larynx. Edema of the soft tissues progresses rapidly, compromising both the patient's airway and the physician's ability to visualize the vocal cords, and often necessitates a cricothyrotomy.

3. What is a blow-out fracture?

A blow-out fracture, which involves the orbital floor, is produced by a direct blow to the orbit. Classic signs include diplopia (secondary to entrapment of the inferior rectus muscle), hypesthesia of the infraorbital nerve, and enophthalmos (posterior displacement of the globe, noted after resolution of edema). Diplopia is noted most frequently by having the patient follow and count fingers on upward gaze. This fracture requires ophthamologic evaluation for associated orbital trauma (hyphema, retinal detachment, closed-angle glaucoma, blindness) despite an initially normal fundoscopic exam.

4. Where are Le Fort fractures?

Le Fort fractures are midface fractures diagnosed by pulling on the maxilla and noting which part of the midface moves. **Le Fort 1**, a transverse fracture just above the teeth, allows movement of the maxilla en bloc. **Le Fort 2**, a pyramid fracture with its apex just above the bridge of the nose and extending laterally and inferiorly through the infraorbital rims, allows movement of the maxilla, nose, and infraorbital rims. **Le Fort 3**, the most serious of the Le Fort fractures, represents complete cranofacial disruption and involves fractures of the zygoma, infraorbital rims, and maxilla.

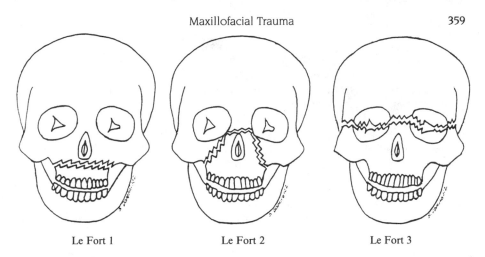

Le Fort 1   Le Fort 2   Le Fort 3

Classification of true Le Fort fractures. Typically patients with Le Fort fractures present with a combination of the above.

Cerebrospinal fluid (CSF) leaks, although occult in presentation, result in significant morbidity if unrecognized and should be assessed by checking for glucose with a Dextrostix or by observing for a halo ring on the gurney linen. Cervical spine injury should be suspected, given the force necessary to produce a midfacial fracture.

5. How do I approach the patient with nasal trauma?
Nasal trauma, although common, must be approached in a manner that allows elucidation of the mechanism of injury (windshield, fist), immediate findings (loss of consciousness, epistaxis, rhinorrhea, deformity), and risk for late sequelae (saddlenose deformity, meningitis).

6. When are nasal x-rays indicated?
Nasal fractures are typically a clinical diagnosis without the need for routine x-rays. Physical examination may reveal swelling, angulation, bony crepitus, deformity, pain on palpation, epistaxis, and periorbital ecchymosis. If the mechanism of injury and the physical examination indicate significant force, then facial films to rule out other associated fractures (orbital, frontal sinus, and cribriform plate) should include lateral and occlusal views of the nasal bones. However, even the severest nasal fracture may not be revealed on x-ray. Therefore, if the exam is compatible with a fracture and the x-ray is negative, then the fracture is presumed to be present and reevaluation is necessary after resolution of edema (typically 4–7 days) for accurate diagnosis.

7. What is the initial treatment for a nasal fracture?
Initial treatment consists of a thorough history and physical exam as well as reduction (if possible) and treatment of septal hematoma (if present). Early reduction of an angulated fracture is performed by exerting firm, quick pressure with both thumbs toward the midline. This can be done without analgesia and with a relatively small and fleeting amount of discomfort to the patient.

8. What is a septal hematoma? Why is it important?
A septal hematoma is a collection of blood between the mucoperichondrium and the cartilage of the septum; if left undrained, it may result in septal abscess, necrosis, and permanent deformity. Incision and drainage of the hematoma are indicated, followed by nasal packing, antistaphylococcal antibiotics (prophylaxis for toxic shock syndrome), and prompt referral.

9. What is the significance of continued epistaxis?

The nasal mucosa is a heavily vascular structure prone to profuse initial bleeding that is usually self-limited. Continued epistaxis suggests associated fractures of the ethmoid or frontal sinuses or a CSF leak. Anterior or posterior packs should be placed carefully to avoid further displacement of the bony fragments; surgical consultation is recommended.

10. When should a consultation be obtained for a nasal fracture?

Immediate consultation is suggested for nasal fractures with associated facial fractures, CSF rhinorrhea, and sustained epistaxis. Displaced or angulated nasal fractures require reduction by either the open or closed techniques.

11. How is a frontal sinus fracture diagnosed?

Frontal sinus fracture, the third most common facial fracture, should be suspected in patients with maxillofacial or anterior skull trauma. A careful history and physical exam should define supraorbital nerve anesthesia, anosmia, CSF rhinorrhea, subconjunctival ecchymosis, crepitus, and pain on palpation. Plain x-rays should include Waters, posteroanterior, and lateral sinus upright films. The preferred modality is CT scanning in the coronal plane to ascertain if there is unmistakable involvement.

12. How are frontal sinus fractures treated?

Patients with **nondisplaced anterior wall fractures** may be discharged on appropriate antibiotics, with instructions to avoid further forehead trauma and Valsalva maneuvers and to return within 1–2 weeks for repeat x-rays and surgical evaluation. Patients with **displaced anterior wall and sinus floor fractures** require admission and antibiotic therapy before surgical exploration. Patients with **posterior wall fractures** require antibiotics and immediate neurosurgical consultation.

13. What are the classic zygoma fractures?

The zygoma is the second most commonly fractured facial bone, with the mandible being the most common. Clinical findings in a zygoma fracture involve the structures to which the bone contributes in facial function. Zygoma fractures have been classified into three basic types:

    1. **Arch:** The bone is fractured in two places and displaced medially. Pain and trismus are caused by bony arch fragments abutting the coronoid process of the mandible. Because the masseter muscle originates on the zygoma, any movement causes further arch disruption.

    2. **Tripod:** The most common zygoma fracture involves the rim, arch, and infraorbital rim, producing deformity, pain, epistaxis, infraorbital nerve hypesthesia, inferior rectus muscle entrapment, and diplopia on upward gaze as well as other ophthalmic symptoms.

    3. **Body:** Fracture of the body of the zygoma, which involves the clinical signs and symptoms of the tripod fracture, results from severe force and leads to exaggerated malar depression.

14. Which radiologic studies assist in the diagnosis of zygoma fractures?

Plain x-ray views should include Waters, Caldwell, submentovertex, and exaggerated Waters. CT scans are the preferred preoperative modality, given the high level of resolution in imaging the infraorbital rim and floor fracture and structures. Fluid in a maxillary sinus without initial radiologic evidence of an infraorbital floor fracture is presumed to be blood secondary to occult fracture until proved otherwise.

15. When is a CT scan indicated in the evaluation of maxillofacial trauma?

High-resolution, thin-cut CT scanning is the preferred modality for the elucidation of the bony and soft-tissue destruction inherent in maxillofacial trauma. Depending on the pathology, plain x-rays may reveal the fracture, whereas CT allows better understanding of both the fracture and its consequences.

16. How do I recognize an injury to Stenson's duct?
Stenson's (parotid) duct arises from the parotid gland and courses from the level of the external auditory canal (superficial) through the buccinator muscle to open at the level of the upper second molar. Any laceration at this level may involve the parotid gland, parotid duct, or buccal branch of the facial nerve. Laceration of the parotid system is recognized by a flow of saliva from the wound or bloody drainage from the duct orifice. Careful exploration reveals whether the flow is from the parotid gland or duct. The buccal branch of the facial nerve travels in close proximity to Stenson's duct; injury leads to drooping of the upper lip, which indicates a possible parotid duct injury.

17. When should closure of a facial laceration be deferred?
Closure of facial lacerations in the ED depends on the severity of facial and systemic injuries. Complex lacerations in patients needing operative intervention should be cleansed with normal saline, covered with dampened gauze, and deferred for intraoperative closure. Closure of the highly vascular tissues of the face may be delayed routinely up to 24 hours and in some cases up to 2 weeks. Wounds involving the facial nerve, lacrimal duct, and avulsions should be referred upon presentation to a plastic surgeon for definitive care.

18. Where do I start in closing a lip laceration?
A cosmetic and anatomic closure begins with approximating the vermilion border with a nonabsorbable suture.

19. What are the clinical signs of an inhalation injury in a facial burn?
Significant inhalation thermal injury is suspected if the patient exhibits facial burns, stridor, singed nasal and facial hairs, carbonaceous deposits and sputum, oropharyngeal mucosa edema, and altered mental status. Aggressive intervention, including endotracheal intubation and transfer to a burn center, is recommended.

20. Why is silver sulfadiazine relatively contraindicated in the treatment of facial burns?
Silver sulfadiazine is a topical sulfonamide with a pH of 6.5. Sulfadiazine is released slowly, with resultant low systemic levels. It is an effective agent in inhibiting gram-negative and gram-positive bacteria, with the exception of Pseudomonas, Serratia, Proteus, and other resistant organisms. Use on facial burns is not recommended because this antibiotic has been shown to delay wound healing. The recommended agents are Polysporin, Bacitracin, or Mycitracin. The status of tetanus immunization should also be determined.

BIBLIOGRAPHY

1. American College of Surgeons: Advanced Trauma Life Support Course Manual. Lincoln, NE, Subcommittee on ATLS, American College of Surgeons, 1988, pp 201–214.
2. Boswick JA (ed): The Art and Science of Burn Care. Gaithersburg, MD, Aspen Publishers, 1987, pp 47–51.
3. Cummings CW, et al (eds): Otolaryngology: Head and Neck Surgery. St. Louis, C.V. Mosby, 1986, pp 611–637, 1015–1026.
4. Hendler BH: Maxillofacial fractures. In Tintinalli JE (ed): Emergency Medicine: A Comprehensive Study Guide, 2nd ed. New York, McGraw-Hill, 1988, pp 599–611.
5. Lee KJ: Essential Otolaryngology, 4th ed. New York, Medical Examination Publishing Co., 1987, pp 299–313.
6. Papay FA: Rigid endoscopic repair of paranasal sinus cerebrospinal fluid fistulas. Laryngoscope 99:1195–1201, 1989.
7. Smith RG: Maxillofacial injuries. In Harwood-Nuss A (ed): The Clinical Practice of Emergency Medicine. Philadelphia, J.B. Lippincott, 1991, pp 337–342.

96. SPINE AND SPINAL CORD TRAUMA

Robert M. McNamara, M.D., FACEP

1. What are the most common causes of spinal injury?
Almost half of all spinal injuries are due to motor vehicle accidents. Falls are the next most common cause, followed by firearm and recreational activities such as diving and tackling.

2. What percentage of patients with a vertebral column fracture or dislocation present with neurologic impairment?
Overall, only 14–15% of all spinal column fractures or dislocations cause neurologic deficit. However, injury to the cervical spine has a higher rate of neurologic compromise than lower spine injuries.

3. If the majority of spinal injuries do not cause neurologic injury, why is their management so important?
Unfortunately, studies have shown that a significant percentage of patients suffer permanent neurologic injury caused by improper medical care due to inadequate suspicion of injury, improper patient immobilization and handling, errant radiographic interpretation, poor quality radiographs, or being misled by completely normal radiographs despite a definite injury.

4. Why do you not want your patient to contribute to the above statistics?
Spinal cord injury with resultant permanent paralysis is one of the single most devastating catastrophes. It generally affects young healthy people; the financial, social, and psychological sequelae are enormous to the patient and the patient's family.

5. Who is at risk and how should one approach the patient with potential spinal injury?
The most important issue to establish is whether the patient's mental status is normal. If pain perception is altered by alcohol, drugs, head injury, shock, or other causes, injury is assumed to be present. A helpful reminder in potential spine injury is that "a proper history is A MUST:

A	=	Altered mental state. Check for drugs, alcohol.
M	=	Mechanism. Does the potential for injury exist?
U	=	Underlying conditions. Are high-risk factors for fractures present?
S	=	Symptoms. Is pain or paresthesia part of the picture?
T	=	Timing. When did the symptoms begin in relation to the event?

7. What are the underlying conditions of concern?
Less force is required to cause fractures in elderly than in younger patients. Rheumatoid arthritis can lead to subluxation problems at C_1 and C_2, whereas patients with Down's syndrome may lack normal development of the odontoid. Certainly a patient with osteopetrosis or metastatic bone cancer should raise concern about possible fracture.

8. What parameters should be assessed on physical exam?
The two key areas of focus are the spine itself and the neurologic exam. The spine is palpated to assess for tenderness, deformity, and muscle spasm. Because the examiner feels only the posterior elements of the vertebrae, a fracture may be present despite a lack of tenderness. The neurologic exam should include motor, sensory, and some aspect of posterior column function (position, vibration). In the unconscious patient, the only clues may be poor rectal tone, priapism, absence of deep tendon reflexes, or diaphragmatic breathing.

9. If the history or physical exam suggests a potential spine injury, how would you immobilize the patient?
When lumbar or thoracic injuries are suspected, the patient is strapped to a long wooden board. A long or short board is also used for potential cervical spine injuries; the patient's forehead is taped to the board to prevent neck flexion. Cervical collars are frequently used in combination with boards because they can help to reduce flexion and extension.

10. Do all patients with a suggestive mechanism require radiographs of the spine?
If the mechanism creates the potential for spinal injury and the patient has altered mental status, it is mandatory to exclude the diagnosis. Radiographs in the alert, nonintoxicated patient are controversial, but most feel that patients without neck pain or tenderness and with normal neurologic exams do not require radiographs. Some add the ability to perform a full active range of motion without pain as another criterion for omitting radiographs. Others feel that the presence of another significantly painful injury requires radiographs, regardless of symptoms related to the spine.

11. Which radiographs should be obtained initially in potential spinal injuries?
Cross-table lateral radiographs are generally the first films ordered because they can be taken without moving the patient. Depending on the stability of the patient, they are taken either in a portable fashion or in the radiology suite.

12. If the cross-table lateral film of the cervical spine is normal, can the patient be mobilized?
Only with great risk. Although this view detects most major injuries, it misses up to 18% of cervical spine injuries. The most important missed injuries are at the C_1–C_2 level. A view of this area (the odontoid or open-mouth view) is recommended before movement of the patient.

13. How is the lateral cervical spine film interpreted?
The first rule is to count all seven cervical vertebrae and be sure that the top of T_1 is visible on the film. Next, follow the ABC'S:

A = Alignment. Check for a smooth line at the anterior and posterior aspect of the vertebral bodies and the spinolaminal line from C_1 to T_1

B = Bones. Carefully check each vertebral body to ensure that the anterior and posterior heights are similar (>3 mm difference suggests fracture); follow the vertebrae out to the laminae and spinous process.

C = Cartilage. Check the intervertebral joint spaces and the facet joints.

S = Soft-tissue spaces. Look for prevertebral swelling, especially at C_2–C_3 (more than 5 mm), and check the predental space, which should be <3 mm in adults and <5 mm in children.

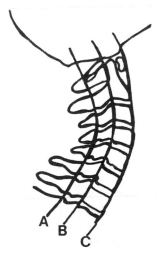

Curve of alignment. *A*, Spinolaminal line; *B*, posterior cervical bodies; *C*, anterior cervical bodies.

14. What are the indications for flexion-extension views of the cervical spine?
Flexion-extension views are generally used if ligamentous injury is suspected. Included are patients with severe neck pain and normal routine cervical radiographs or those with suspicious but not clearly abnormal radiographs. Flexion-extension views should be performed only in alert, cooperative patients and must be supervised by a physician.

15. When would more complex imaging of the cervical spine, such as tomograms or computed tomography (CT), be considered?
Such studies are useful if plain radiographs are inconclusive or difficult to interpret. If neurologic deficit is present, CT is useful to identify correctable problems such as hematomas or disc fragments within the spinal canal. Because multiple injuries are present in two-thirds of patients with a cervical spine injury, these studies should be considered in all patients with at least one identified injury.

16. Describe Jefferson's fracture, hangman's fracture, and clay-shoveler's fracture.
    (1) Jefferson's fracture is a burst fracture of the ring of C_1 that occurs from axial loading.
    (2) A hangman's fracture describes a disruption of the posterior arch of C_2.
    (3) A clay-shoveler's fracture refers to a fracture of the spinous process that is classically caused by forceful cervical extension.

17. Describe the incomplete cord syndromes or injuries.
    Anterior cord syndrome results in loss of function in the anterior two-thirds of the spinal cord. Findings include loss of voluntary motor function as well as pain and temperature sensation below the level of injury, with preservation of the posterior column functions of position and vibration. The key issue is the potential reversibility of this lesion if a compressing hematoma or disc fragment can be removed. Hence, this condition requires immediate neurosurgical consultation.
    Central cord syndrome results from injury to the central portion of the spinal cord. Because more proximal innervation is placed centrally within the cord, this lesion results in greater involvement of the upper extremities than of the lower extremities. The mechanism of injury is hyperextension of a cervical spine with a cord space narrowed by congenital variation, degenerative spurring, or hypertrophic ligaments. This syndrome can occur without actual fracture or ligamentous disruption.
    Brown-Sequard syndrome is a hemisection of the spinal cord, usually from penetrating trauma. Contralateral sensation of pain and temperature is lost, whereas motor and posterior column functions are absent on the side of the injury.

18. What is the significance of sacral sparing and spinal shock?
Sacral sparing refers to the preservation of any function of the sacral roots, such as toe movement or perianal sensation. If sacral sparing is present, the chance of functional neurologic recovery is good. **Spinal shock** is a temporary concussivelike condition in which cord-mediated reflexes, such as the anal wink, are absent. The extent of cord injury—and hence prognosis—cannot be determined until these reflexes return.

19. What are the general principles of emergency treatment in the patient with spinal injury?
Obviously, the general principles of trauma resuscitation must be followed as necessary. Specific issues related to the cervical spine include preventing a worsening of the injury by proper immobilization and cautious patient handling. The patient with a cervical spine injury may not be able to maintain an adequate tidal volume because the intercostal muscles are nonfunctional. Hence the respiratory status must be carefully monitored. Gastric and bladder decompression are indicated early in the care of these patients. Overhydration is to be avoided. The absence of pain below the level of injured spinal cord can mask other injuries.

20. What is the status of steroids in acute spinal cord injury?
The recently published results of the Second National Acute Spinal Cord Injury Study indicate improved neurologic outcomes in patients with spinal cord injuries when methyl-prednisolone is given in bolus doses of 30 mg/kg, followed by 5.4 mg/kg/hr for 23 hours. Treated patients were not cured but demonstrated greater preservation of neurologic function, which can make a world of difference in the ability to lead a more normal life.

21. What can physicians do to prevent spinal injuries?
As motor vehicle accidents are the leading cause, one can work to reduce problems such as driving under the influence of alcohol or drugs and to encourage the use of safety belts (ejected accident victims are at very high risk for cervical spine injury). Diving and tackling injuries can be reduced by proper public education. Because handgun violence is increasing, physicians need to voice their opinions on this issue.

BIBLIOGRAPHY

 1. Bracken MB, Shepard MJ, Collins WF, et al: A randomized, controlled trial of methylprednisolone or naloxone in the treatment of acute spinal-cord injury. N Engl J Med 322:1405–1411, 1990.
 2. Lewis LM, Docherty M, Ruoff BE, et al: Flexion-extension views in the evaluation of cervical spine injuries. Ann Emerg Med 20:117–121, 1991.
 3. Mahoney BD: Spinal injuries. In Tintinalli JE (ed): Emergency Medicine: A Comprehensive Study Guide. New York, McGraw-Hill, 1992, pp 922–927.
 4. McNamara RM, Heine E, Esposito B: Cervical spine injury and radiography in alert, high-risk patients. J Emerg Med 8:177–182, 1990.
 5. Podolsky S, Baraff LJ, Simon RR, et al: Efficacy of cervical spine immobilization methods. J Trauma 23:461–464, 1983.
 6. Reid DC, Henderson R, Saboe L, et al: Etiology and clinical course of missed spine fractures. J Trauma 27:980–986, 1987.
 7. Riggins RS, Kraus JF: The risk of neurologic damage with fractures of the vertebrae. J Trauma 17:126–132, 1977.
 8. Streitwieser DR, Knopp R, Wales LR, et al: Accuracy of standard radiographic views in detecting cervical spine fractures. Ann Emerg Med 12:538–542, 1983.
 9. Wales LR, Knopp RK, Morishima MS: Recommendations for evaluation of the acutely injured cervical spine: A clinical radiologic algorithm. Ann Emerg Med 9:422–428, 1980.
10. Williams CF, Bernstein TW, Jelenko C: Essentiality of the lateral cervical spine radiograph. Ann Emerg Med 10:198–204, 1981.

97. HEAD TRAUMA

Edward Newton, M.D., FACEP

1. What types of head injury commonly present to the emergency department (ED)?
There is a whole spectrum of head injury ranging from minor scalp lacerations to lethal massive brain injury. These injuries occur with a higher propensity in certain groups of patients.

Concussion	Intracerebral hemorrhage
Skull fracture	Diffuse cerebral edema
Brain contusion	Posttraumatic infarction
Subdural hematoma	Brain herniation syndrome
Epidural hematoma	Axonal shear injury
Subarachnoid hemorrhage	

2. Which groups of patients are at particular risk from head injury?

Because of their relatively large head size and compressibility of the skull, **infants** are more prone to brain injury than adults. Because the skull sutures have not yet fused, the head can expand and open fontanelles will bulge outward, accommodating proportionately larger volumes of blood before intracranial pressure (ICP) increases. However, this is offset by relatively smaller ventricles and cisterns. The net effect is an unfavorable pressure/volume curve compared with adults. In the **elderly**, cerebral atrophy stretches the bridging veins from the dura to brain parenchyma, making these veins vulnerable to tearing from deceleration forces. **Alcoholics** are at risk because of the greater frequency of head trauma, cerebral atrophy, and bleeding diathesis from lack of liver-dependent clotting factors. Finally, patients who are taking anticoagulants or who have **coagulation disorders** will obviously bleed much more actively than patients with normal coagulation.

3. What is a cerebral concussion?

A concussion is a traumatic transient loss of central neurologic function (loss of consciousness, transient amnesia, confusion, disorientation, visual changes, etc.) without any gross cerebral abnormalities.

4. What is the postconcussive syndrome?

Although the patient may appear completely neurologically intact following recovery from a concussion, there are common sequelae of this type of injury. Patients frequently report severe headaches, dizziness, inability to concentrate, and irritability. These symptoms may persist for several months following a single concussion. Treatment is supportive and the long-term prognosis is good. Boxers and others who sustain repeated concussions or knockouts may develop permanent neurologic deficits ("punch drunk").

5. How do you detect cerebrospinal fluid (CSF) leaks caused by basilar skull fractures?

CSF can be distinguished from blood by the presence of a double-ring sign when applied to filter paper or a bed sheet. CSF migrates further than blood, forming a target shape with blood in the center and blood-tinged CSF forming a ring outside the clot. CSF rhinorrhea can be detected by checking the glucose content of the fluid with Dextrostix or glucometer. CSF contains approximately 60% of serum levels of glucose; nasal mucus does not contain glucose. However, these bedside tests are not highly sensitive or specific in detecting CSF leaks.

6. How are CSF leaks treated?

CSF leaks through tears in the dura are generally managed conservatively. The use of prophylactic antibiotics is controversial. They have never been shown to reduce the incidence of meningitis in this condition to a level of statistical significance. In fact, they may select for drug-resistant organisms. Patients must be followed closely until the dural tear heals because of the risk of meningitis. Dural tears that fail to close spontaneously over 2–3 weeks usually require operative repair.

7. How does a patient with an epidural hematoma present?

Epidural hematomas are present in 5–10% of patients with severe head injury. The classic pattern is that a patient loses consciousness from the initial concussion, gradually recovers over a few minutes, and enters the "lucid interval" wherein he may be virtually completely intact neurologically. During this interval, blood is building up from the lacerated artery, usually the middle meningeal artery, and eventually enough blood accumulates so that the brain is compressed and begins to shift. This process is accompanied by a second reduction in the level of consciousness and pupillary and motor signs of herniation. However, this classic pattern occurs in only a minority of patients with epidural hematoma. Many patients remain unconscious from the moment of first impact, or, in milder cases, they may not develop elevated ICP at all. The characteristic CT scan appearance of an epidural hematoma is a hyperdense lenticular collection of blood which indents adjacent brain parenchyma.

8. How does a subdural hematoma present?

Subdural hematoma may be acute, subacute (6–20 days), or chronic (more than 20 days after trauma). Acute subdural hematomas are associated with a high incidence of underlying brain injury. The classic presentation varies with the severity of this underlying injury, but commonly patients present with a diminished level of consciousness, headache, and focal neurologic deficits corresponding to the area of brain injury. If sufficient bleeding occurs, ICP increases and herniation may occur. The characteristic appearance of an acute subdural hematoma on CT scan is a collection of hyperdense blood in a crescent-shaped pattern conforming to the convexity of the hemisphere.

At times the initial injury causes a small amount of bleeding and is undetected or unreported by the patient. The subdural hematoma then undergoes lysis over a period of several days and organizes into an encapsulated mass. Subacute or chronic subdural hematoma is a difficult clinical diagnosis because symptoms are vague and common (e.g., persistent headache, difficulty concentrating, lethargy, etc.) and the trauma may have been forgotten. Even the CT scan diagnosis is difficult because the subdural hematoma may become isodense and indistinguishable from surrounding brain. Chronic subdural hematomas appear as lucent collections of fluid in the same pattern as the acute type.

9. What is axonal shear injury?

Axonal shear injury occurs during abrupt deceleration because white matter and gray matter have different densities, resulting in different rates of deceleration. This produces a shearing force that may tear axons at the white/gray interface, resulting in coma or other severe neurologic derangements. The CT scan may appear totally normal because there is little intitial bleeding or edema. MRI of the brain is a more sensitive tool in detecting these injuries in the subacute phase but is currently impractical in the acute phase.

10. What is the herniation syndrome?

Herniation is caused by increased ICP. Because the cranium is a rigid structure, pressure varies with the volume of its contents. Approximately 10% of intracranial volume is blood, another 10% is CSF, and the remainder is brain parenchyma and intracellular fluid. An increase in any of these components by tumor, hydrocephalus, bleeding, etc., will cause a predictable response. In the case of trauma, accumulation of blood increases the vascular component and compresses the other compartments. Initially CSF is forced into the spinal canal, and the ventricles and basilar cisterns collapse. Once this has occurred, ICP rises steeply and the brain parenchyma shifts away from the accumulating blood and herniates through one of several spaces, producing a neurologic catastrophe primarily by compressing the brainstem.

11. Discuss the four common herniation syndromes.

1. **Uncal herniation.** The uncus is the most medial portion of the hemisphere and thus is often the first structure to shift below the tentorium, which separates the hemispheres from the midbrain. As the uncus is forced medially and downward, the ipsilateral III cranial nerve is compressed, producing pupillary dilatation, ptosis, and oculomotor paresis. Approximately 10% of the time, the opposite III nerve is involved. As herniation progresses, the ipsilateral cerebral peduncle and pyramidal tract are compressed, resulting in contralateral hemiplegia. Further progression leads to brainstem compression and respiratory and cardiac arrest. In the vast majority of cases, the bleed is located on the same side as the

dilated pupil and the side opposite hemiplegia. Transtentorial herniation of this type is by far the most common variety.

2. **Central herniation.** Occasionally, hematomas located at the vertex or frontal lobes cause simultaneous downward herniation of both hemispheres through the tentorium. Symptoms are similar to uncal herniation except that bilateral motor weakness will also occur.

3. **Cingulate herniation.** Rarely, the cingulate gyrus is forced medially beneath the falx by an enlarging lateral hematoma, causing compression of the ventricles and impairing cerebral blood flow.

4. **Posterior fossa herniaton.** Hematoma in the posterior fossa can produce herniation either upward through the tentorium or downward through the foramen magnum. In the latter case, coma and brainstem dysfunction may occur rapidly and with little warning.

12. What is the ED treatment for increased ICP?

The following are proved and effective mainstays of therapy:

1. **Hyperventilation.** Hyperventilation is the single most effective and rapid treatment for elevated ICP. Carbon dioxide (CO_2) is one of the main determinants of cerebrovascular tone. High levels cause cerebrovascular vasodilatation; low levels produce vasoconstriction. In an effort to limit vascular congestion and edema formation following brain injury, patients are hyperventilated until the PCO_2 reaches 25 mmHg. This has been determined to be the optimal PCO_2 for producing cerebral vasoconstriction while still maintaining adequate perfusion to the brain. Lower levels of PCO_2 vasoconstrict and limit cerebral blood flow to the point that cerebral hypoxia begins to occur, exacerbating rather than improving the injury. In order to accomplish this degree of hyperventilation, it is necessary to paralyze and intubate the patient, making certain that the neck is protected from movement by in-line stabilization during intubation. Adjustments in minute volume of ventilation should be made according to ABG results, with the optimal PCO_2 being 25 mmHg.

2. **Diuresis.** The use of an osmotic diuretic such as mannitol (0.5–1.0 gm/kg IV over 15 minutes) or loop diuretics such as furosemide (0.5–1.0 mg/kg IV) is also effective in reducing brain edema. Infusion of mannitol creates an osmotic gradient between the intravascular space and the extracellular fluid (ECF), drawing fluid from the ECF, and thereby reducing brain water content and ICP. Mannitol is then filtered by the kidneys, producing systemic dehydration. Clinical experience and animal studies seem to support the concomitant administration of osmotic diuretics and volume resuscitation in patients with hypovolemic shock.

3. **Barbiturates.** Conscious patients who are paralyzed for intubation must also be sedated. The ideal agent for this purpose is a short-acting barbiturate, which lowers ICP, prevents seizures, and decreases cerebral metabolism. However, such agents cannot be used when the patient is hypotensive because barbiturates will further lower blood pressure. In these cases, a reversible agent such as morphine sulfate (0.1 mg/kg) or lorazepam (0.01 mg/kg) is preferred since they can be reversed quickly by appropriate antagonists if adverse effects on blood pressure or cardiac output are noted.

4. **Elevation of the head of the bed.** Providing the patient is not in shock and has no unstable vertebral injury, elevation of the head of the bed to 30° can reduce ICP by up to 6 mmHg. The patient's neck should be kept straight to allow maximal cerebral venous drainage.

13. What is different about intracranial hemorrhage in infants?

Infants may bleed intracranially sufficient to produce hemorrhagic shock, whereas in adults and older children, another source of bleeding is inevitably responsible for hypotension.

14. If a patient has a normal CT scan following head trauma, is it completely safe to discharge him home?

Nothing is completely safe. There are well-documented instances of delayed epidural and subdural bleeding many hours after injury. Consequently, although it is generally safe to discharge such patients, head injury instructions should be given to responsible family members and the patient should be instructed to return immediately if symptoms worsen. If the patient is socially isolated or unreliable, a judgment has to be made regarding the seriousness of the mechanism of injury and the risk of discharge. Intoxicated patients should be kept under observation until their mental status can be properly evaluated.

15. Since CT scan is available, is there any role for plain skull films?

In many ways the usefulness of plain radiographs of the skull has been far outstripped by more informative imaging modalities such as CT and MRI. Skull films still have certain indications in evaluation of the following:

- Penetrating trauma (GSWs)
- Suspected depressed skull fracture
- Suspected basilar skull fracture
- As part of the skeletal survey for suspected child abuse
- In patients with prior craniotomies, shunts, etc.

BIBLIOGRAPHY

1. Eisenberg HM, Aldrich EF (eds): Management of head injury. Neurosurg Clin North Am 2:1–501, 1991.
2. Feldman Z, Kanter MJ, Robertson CS, et al: Effect of head elevation on intracranial pressure, and cerebral blood flow in head-injured patients. J Neurosurg 76:207–211, 1992.
3. Hockberger RS, Schwartz B: Blunt head injury: A spectrum of disease. Ann Emerg Med 15:202–207, 1986.
4. Israel RS, Marx JA, Moore EE, et al: Hemodynamic effects of mannitol in a canine model of concomitant increased intracranial pressure and hemorrhagic shock. Ann Emerg Med 17:560–566, 1988.
5. Lehman LB: Intracranial pressure monitoring: A contemporary view. Ann Emerg Med 19:295–303, 1990.
6. Little NE: Postconcussion syndrome. Emerg Med Aug. 15, 1988, pp 30–44.
7. Livingston DH, Loder PA, Koziol J, et al: The use of CT scanning to triage patients requiring admission following minor head injury. J Trauma 31:483–489, 1991.
8. Masters SJ, McClean PM, Arcarese JS, et al: Skull x-ray examinations after head trauma: Recommendations by a multidisciplinary panel and validation study. N Engl J Med 316:84–90, 1987.
9. Redan JA, Livingston DH, Tortella NJ, et al: Value of intubating and paralyzing patients with suspected head injury in the emergency department. J Trauma 31:371–375, 1991.
10. Rosner MJ, Daughton S: Cerebral perfusion pressure management in head injury. J Trauma 30:933–941, 1990.
11. Stein CS, Young GS, Talucci RC, et al: Delayed brain injury after head trauma: Significance of coagulopathy. Neurosurgery 30:160–165, 1992.

98. TRAUMATIC OPHTHALMOLOGIC EMERGENCIES

Hal Thomas, M.D.

1. What are the two most time-critical emergencies in ophthalmology?
Central retinal artery occlusion and chemical burns to the eyes.

2. What is the treatment for a chemical burn of the eye?
Immediate copious irrigation of the eyes (for at least 20 minutes). If you receive a phone call from a patient at home or from the paramedics, irrigation should be initiated before transport to the emergency department (ED).

3. How do you know when you have irrigated the eye enough?
Nitrazine paper can be used to ensure that the pH has been corrected to normal. This usually requires at least 3 L of normal saline in each eye and continuous irrigation for 20 minutes. Alkalis, which cause the most damaging burns, tend to adhere to the tissue of the eye and are remarkably difficult to remove completely with irrigation. After irrigation, emergent ophthalmologic consultation is indicated.

4. What is the significance of pain from an eye injury that is not relieved with topical anesthesia?
Complete symptomatic relief with topical anesthesia implies a superficial injury involving only the cornea. If a patient still has significant pain after application of anesthetic drops, a deeper injury (often traumatic iritis) must be suspected, even in the presence of an obvious superficial injury.

5. List 9 potential injuries that must be considered in a patient sustaining a blunt injury to the eye.

Blowout fracture of the floor of the orbit	Lens dislocation	Traumatic iritis
Corneal abrasion	Traumatic mydriasis	Ruptured globe (rare after blunt injuries)
Anterior hyphema	Vitreous hemorrhage	
	Retinal detachment	

6. What is the most common eye injury seen in the ED?
Corneal abrasion with or without a superficial foreign body.

7. How is corneal abrasion diagnosed?
The anesthetized eye can be stained with fluorescein and illuminated by an ultraviolet or Wood's lamp; corneal defects fluoresce bright yellow/orange. Visual acuity should be checked and the eye inspected, with particular emphasis on the anterior chamber to look for an anterior hyphema. A funduscopic examination for evidence of vitreous hemorrhage or retinal detachment, a visual field examination (also for evidence of retinal detachment), and testing of extraocular movement should also be performed.

8. What is the treatment for a corneal abrasion?
The mainstay of treatment for corneal abrasion is a double eye patch to limit ocular motion and continued irritation of the denuded cornea. Because this injury is extremely painful, narcotic analgesics are indicated. **Never dispense topical anesthesia from the ED.** One frequently overlooked aspect of therapy is the instillation of a cycloplegic, usually

cyclopentolate (Cyclogel), to relieve the ciliary spasm that commonly accompanies this injury. Patients also need evaluation for tetanus prophylaxis.

9. What is the most common location of an ocular foreign body?
Foreign bodies are often lodged just beneath the upper eyelid along the palpebral conjunctiva. The eyelid needs to be everted with a cotton swab to examine this area adequately. Conjunctival foreign bodies should be suspected when a number of vertical linear streaks are noted on the cornea with fluorescein examination.

10. What is the proper treatment for a corneal foreign body?
First, topical anesthesia is applied, usually proparacaine. Nonembedded foreign bodies should be removed with a sterile moist Q-tip. Embedded foreign bodies are removed with a 27-gauge needle or eye spud; the involved eye is patched with a double patch. Most metallic foreign bodies leave a residual rust ring that should be removed in approximately 24 hours, after the cornea has softened.

11. What is an anterior hyphema?
An anterior hyphema is a collection of blood in the anterior chamber of the eye; it is seen as a layering of cells that pool along the bottom of the eye when the patient is sitting upright. When the patient is lying down, a hyphema is not easily recognized; it may appear as a diffuse haziness of the anterior chamber. Very small hyphemas, termed microhyphemas, may be identified only with a slit-lamp.

12. How is an anterior hyphema treated?
A degree of controversy surrounds the treatment of hyphemas. The standard in the past was to admit all patients for bed rest; today the dominant tendency is toward outpatient management. Complications include rebleeding, glaucoma formation (particularly in black patients with sickle-cell trait), and corneal staining. The patient should be kept upright, the eye patched, and ophthalmologic consultation initiated, at least by phone.

13. What physical findings lead to the suspicion of a blowout fracture?
Classic findings with a blowout fracture (fracture of the inferior orbital wall with herniation of the eye contents into the maxillary sinus) are (1) decreased sensation over the inferior orbital rim, extending to the edge of the nose, secondary to compromise of the inferior orbital nerve; (2) enophthalmos, or a sunken appearance of the eye, which may be masked by edema; and (3) paralysis or limitation of upward gaze (manifested as diplopia), due to entrapment of the inferior rectus muscle.

14. What is traumatic mydriasis?
It is an efferent pupillary defect manifested by a dilated (in most instances irregular) pupil that does not react to direct or consensual light, usually as a result of minor trauma to the eye. Because such a patient is at risk for other more serious eye injuries, a careful eye examination is mandatory. The possibility of uncal herniation secondary to intracranial injury should be considered if level of consciousness is decreased in the presence of a perfectly round, nonreactive, unilateral, dilated pupil. If level of consciousness is unaltered, this is most likely an isolated ocular injury.

15. Why is a history of hammering metal on metal important in a patient presenting with an eye complaint?
Often a small, high-velocity fragment penetrates the globe with minimal or no physical findings. This injury, which can cause inflammation weeks later, is diagnosed with soft-tissue films or a CT scan of the globe.

16. Which eyelid lacerations should be repaired by an ophthalmologist or plastic surgeon?
- Those involving the lid margin or gray line
- Those involving the tear duct mechanism along the lower eyelid
- Those involving the tarsal plate or levator muscle

17. When should penetration of the globe be suspected?
The pupil is usually misshapen, pointing in the direction of the penetration. The globe may appear soft due to decreased intraocular pressure. Intraocular pressure should not be tested if a penetrating injury is suspected because the test promotes extrusion of aqueous humor.

18. What is the significance of a subscleral (subconjunctival) hemorrhage?
Subscleral hemorrhages are perfectly benign and often occur spontaneously with complete resolution over 2–3 weeks. When associated with trauma, other, potentially more serious eye injuries should be suspected and ruled out.

19. Which traumatic ophthalmologic injuries require immediate ophthalmologic consultation?
- Chemical burns of the eye, particularly with corneal opacification
- Perforation of the globe or cornea
- Lens dislocation
- Orbital hemorrhage with increased intraocular pressure
- Lacerations involving the lid margin, tarsal plate, or tear duct

20. Which ophthalmologic injuries require urgent ophthalmologic consultation (within 12–24 hours)
Anterior hyphema, blowout fracture, and retinal injuries.

21. What is solar keratitis?
Also known as flash burns or snow blindness, solar keratitis is a corneal injury secondary to overexposure to ultraviolet light. Diagnosis is made with fluorescein staining, which shows multiple punctate lesions of the cornea. Treatment consists of resting the eyes with adequate narcotic analgesia. Spontaneous resolution can be expected in 12–24 hours.

BIBLIOGRAPHY

1. Mathews J, Zun LS: Ophthalmologic emergencies and ocular trauma. Emerg Clin North Am 6:1, 1988.
2. Ostler HB: Risk of tetanus from corneal injuries. JAMA 260:553, 1988.
3. Sklar DP, et al: Topical anesthesia of the eye as a diagnostic test. Ann Emerg Med 18:1029–1033, 1989.
4. Talbot EM: A simple test to diagnose iritis. BMJ 295:812–813, 1987.
5. Wilson TW, et al: Outpatient management of traumatic microhyphemas. Ann Ophthalmol 22:366–368, 1990.

99. NECK TRAUMA

Jeffrey J. Schaider, M.D.

1. Is neck trauma a complicated topic?
Yes. The lack of bony protection makes the anterior neck especially vulnerable to severe, life-threatening injuires. The exposed anatomic structure of the neck, which contains many vital parts of the vascular, airway, and gastrointestinal systems, provides a fertile ground for debate and a myriad of opinions about modality of treatment.

2. What is the most urgent concern in the initial management of neck trauma?
Airway and hemorrhage control are the most urgent concerns. Always remember that airway management comes before anything else discussed in this chapter. Early endotracheal intubation is indicated for any patient with existing or potential airway compromise. Delay in airway management increases the difficulty of intubation because of swelling and compression of the anatomic structures. If severe damage to the larynx and cricoid cartilage makes endotracheal intubation impossible, tracheostomy is preferred over cricothyrotomy for airway management. Bleeding should be controlled with pressure rather than with blind clamping. The wound should be examined to determine whether it has violated the platysma. However, injudicious probing of the wound may be dangerous because a vascular structure that has ceased to bleed may then resume, when its tamponade is released, with disastrous consequences.

3. What common findings indicate significant neck injury?
Injuries involving the vascular system result in hematomas, bleeding, pulse deficit, shock, and neurologic deficit due to arterial interruption. Laryngeal trauma causes voice alteration, airway compromise, subcutaneous emphysema, crepitus, and hemoptysis. Signs and symptoms of esophageal disruption include pain and tenderness in the neck, resistance of the neck to passive motion, crepitation, dysphagia, and bleeding from the mouth or nasogastric tube. The diagnosis of esophageal disruption is difficult because of injuries to other overlying structures. Ancillary testing must be employed to assist in the diagnosis of these injuries.

4. What are the signs and symptoms of blunt carotid artery trauma?
The diagnosis of blunt carotid trauma is also difficult. Twenty-five to 50% of patients have no external signs of trauma. Delayed neurologic signs are the rule rather than the exception; only 10% of patients have symptoms of transient ischemic attacks or strokes within 1 hour of injury. Most patients develop symptoms within the first 24 hours, but 17% develop symptoms days or weeks after injury. Horner's syndrome due to stretching and compression of the sympathetic ganglia may also occur. Other patients may present with a hematoma or bruit over the lateral neck.

5. What are the main controversies regarding management of penetrating neck trauma?
The main controversy lies in the management of penetrating neck trauma that violates the platysma. Some physicians and surgeons advocate mandatory exploration for penetrating neck wounds, whereas others use the approach of selective management.

6. What is mandatory exploration for penetrating neck wounds?
All patients who have wounds that penetrate the platysma muscle in the neck are explored surgically to determine the presence or absence of injury to the deeper structures in the neck. Some ancillary diagnostic testing (angiography, esophagraphy, esophagoscopy, laryngoscopy) may be performed preoperatively, depending on the location of the wound and the stability of the patient.

7. What are the advantages of mandatory exploration for penetrating neck wounds?
During the 1940s mandatory exploration was instituted for all penetrating wounds that violate the platysma. This policy reduced mortality significantly and remained the only mode of therapy until the mid-1970s. Proponents of mandatory exploration warn of the catastrophic complications from delayed treatment and missed injuries. They also point out that neck exploration is relatively simple and that a negative exploration has low morbidity and mortality.

8. What are the disadvantages of mandatory exploration for penetrating neck wounds?
Because the negative exploration rate (no injuries found at surgery) is 50%, the cost of the operation and added length of hospital stay are unwarranted. A significant number of these operations could be avoided with the selective approach to neck exploration.

9. Describe the theory behind the selective surgical management of penetrating neck wounds.
With the improved sensitivity and specificity of ancillary diagnostic testing (angiography, CT, esophagography, esophagoscopy, laryngoscopy), a nonoperative approach to a select group of patients, based on physical exam and results of ancillary tests, is safe. The selective approach has significantly reduced the negative exploration rate.

10. What are the three anatomic zones of the neck?
Zone I is the area below the sternal notch. Zone II extends from the sternal notch to the angle of the mandible. Zone III extends from the angle of the mandible to the base of the skull. Some authors raise the border between zone I and zone II to the cricoid cartilage from the sternal notch.

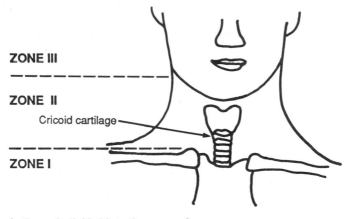

11. Why is the neck divided into three zones?
The location of the injury plays a major role in assessing the need for angiography. All zone I injuries require angiography to determine the integrity of the thoracic outlet vessels. In stable but symptomatic patients needing surgery, angiography should be performed preoperatively because positive findings necessitate a thoracotomy before neck exploration.

The familiar anatomy of zone II, coupled with relative ease of surgical exposure, minimizes the need for angiography in symptomatic patients undergoing surgery. Some authors observe asymptomatic patients with penetrating injuries without angiography. Others perform angiography on asymptomatic patients to detect occult injuries and involvement of vertebral vessels prior to observation.

The management of zone III injuries remains controversial because of the complex anatomy of the area as well as the difficulty in obtaining adequate exposure. Most authors agree that for asymptomatic patients not undergoing surgery, angiography is necessary to assess the status of the internal carotid artery and the intracerebral circulation. For symptomatic patients, preoperative angiography is helpful because high internal carotid artery injuries are difficult to visualize at operation and may require carotid artery ligation and concomitant extracranal/intracranial bypass.

12. Which diagnostic studies are important in suspected laryngeal injuries?

Soft-tissue cervical radiographs may demonstrate a fractured larynx, subcutaneous air, or prevertebral air. CT accurately identifies the location and extent of laryngeal fractures. Flexible laryngoscopy provides valuable information regarding the integrity of the cartilaginous framework and the function of the vocal cords. CT should be performed when the diagnosis of a laryngeal fracture is still suspected in spite of a negative examination of the endolarynx or when flexible laryngoscopy cannot be performed (e.g., the intubated patient).

13. Are diagnostic studies necessary in suspected esophageal injuries?

Diagnostic studies are essential in the diagnosis of esophageal injuries. Soft-tissue cervical radiographs may demonstrate subcutaneous emphysema or an increased prevertebral shadow. Chest x-ray findings include pleural effusion, pneumothorax, mediastinal air, and mediastinal widening. Esophageal contrast studies should be performed initially with Gastrografin; if negative, they should be repeated with barium to increase diagnostic yield. Radiographic imaging is difficult because of the high false-negative rate. Esophagography has a 30–50% false-negative rate and should be followed by esophagoscopy in patients with suspected esophageal injury. No one study can exclude esophageal perforation; rather, a combination of physical signs, plain and contrast radiographs, and esophagoscopy should be used to make the diagnosis.

BIBLIOGRAPHY

1. Asensio JA, Valenziano CP, Falcone RE, Grosh JD: Management of penetrating neck injuries: The controversy surrounding zone II injuries. Surg Clin North Am 1:267, 1991.
2. Fakhry SM, Jacques PF, Proctor HJ: Cervical vessel injury after blunt trauma. J Vasc Surg 8:501, 1988.
3. Fuhrman BM, Stieg FH, Buerk CA: Blunt laryngeal trauma: Classification and management protocol. J Trauma 30:87, 1990.
4. Glatterer MS, Toon RS, Ellestad C, et al: Management of blunt and penetrating external esophageal trauma. J Trauma 25:784, 1985.
5. Golueke PJ, Goldstein AS, Sclafani JA, et al: Routine versus selective exploration of penetrating neck injuries: A randomized prospective study. J Trauma 24:1010, 1984.
6. Jurkovich GJ, Zingarelli W, Wallace J, Curreri PW: Penetrating neck trauma: Diagnostic studies in the asymptomatic patient. J Trauma25:819, 1985.
7. Meyer JP, Barrett JA, Schuler JJ, Flanigan P: Mandatory vs selective exploration for penetrating neck trauma. Arch Surg 122:592, 1987.
8. Miller RH, Duplechain JK: Penetrating wounds of the neck. Otolaryngol Clin North Am 24:15, 1991.
9. Narrod JA, Moore EE: Initial management of penetrating neck wounds—a selective approach. J Emerg Med 2:17, 1984.
10. Richardson JD, Simpson C, Miller FB: Management of carotid artery trauma. Surgery 104:673, 1988.
11. Schaefer SD: Use of CT scanning in the management of the acutely injured larynx. Otolaryngol Clin North Am 24:31, 1991.
12. Schild JA, Denney EC: Evaluation and treatment of acute laryngeal fractures. Head Neck 11:491, 1989.
13. Wood J, Fabian TC, Mangiante EC: Penetrating neck injuries: Recommendations for selective management. J Trauma 29:602, 1989.

100. CHEST TRAUMA

Robert C. Jorden, M.D.

1. How should the patient with chest trauma be approached?

One must immediately identify actual or potential life threats based on the clinical evaluation. This evaluation consists of the standard inspection, auscultation, and palpation.

Inspection. Completely undress the patient and visually inspect the entire chest, which necessitates rolling over a supine patient. Look for a flail chest (paradoxical movement of the chest wall) and sucking chest wounds. Identify the exact location, number, and type (i.e., penetrating or blunt) of wounds.

Auscultation. Listen for diminished or absent breath sounds and bowel sounds in the chest. The latter may indicate a pneumothorax, a large hemothorax, a tension pneumothorax, or diaphragmatic rupture with herniation of abdominal contents into the chest.

Palpation. It is important to palpate the chest wall carefully to detect bony crepitus and subcutaneous emphysema. The former indicates a major blow to the chest with rib fractures and the potential for underlying organ damage, and the latter, depending on location, is indicative of pneumothorax or pneumomediastinum.

2. What is a flail chest?

A flail chest occurs when a segment of the chest wall becomes unattached from the rest of the chest. It occurs in one of three settings: (1) two or more ribs are broken in two or more places; (2) more than one rib is fractured in association with costal cartilage disarticulation; or (3) the costal cartilages on both sides of the sternum are disarticulated, resulting in a sternal or central flail segment. The significance of a flail chest lies in the tremendous force that caused it and the near certainty of associated intrathoracic injuries.

3. What is the treatment for a flail chest?

The condition of the underlying lung generally dictates the treatment. Underlying pulmonary contusion and resultant hypoxemia indicate the need for intervention. In general a flail chest should be treated supportively; if the patient is doing well and tolerating the flail (i.e., blood gases do not show hypoxemia or hypercarbia), only supplemental oxygen is indicated. However, if the patient is in respiratory distress either clinically or as indicated by blood gas analysis, then intubation and positive pressure ventilation should be initiated. Positive pressure ventilation results in uniform expansion of the chest from within and stabilizes the flail segment.

4. What significant history should be obtained from the victim of a motor vehicle accident?

What was the nature of the accident (rollover, head-on collision, etc.)? Was the patient wearing a seat belt? Was the steering wheel or windshield broken? Was there substantial vehicular damage? When a frontal deceleration mechanism is operative, one should consider not only chest wall injuries and pulmonary contusion but two other specific entities—myocardial contusion and aortic rupture.

5. How is myocardial contusion diagnosed and treated?

Unfortunately, there is no gold standard for the diagnosis of myocardial contusion. Many modalities have been used in the attempt, including the EKG, radionuclide scanning, cardiac enzyme analysis, and echocardiography. Because a contusion rarely causes serious arrhythmias or compromises cardiac output, there is a trend away from aggressive monitoring of patients based on mechanism only. Instead, most recommend using the EKG and the clinical assessment as a screening device. A normal EKG in the absence of hemodynamic instability precludes the need for extended monitoring and probably effectively rules out a clinically significant contusion. An abnormal EKG or unexplained hypotension may merit further diagnostic evaluation, such as echocardiogram or radionuclide scan. Treatment is symptomatic, with arrhythmia control and measures to optimize cardiac output.

6. How can anyone survive a ruptured aorta?
Approximately 85–90% of patients with aortic rupture do indeed die and they do so before medical aid reaches them. Ten to 15% survive because not all three layers of the aorta are ruptured; the adventitia remains intact and temporarily contains the hemorrhage. Left untreated, however, this injury results in complete rupture and exsanguination, usually in hours to days, but may be delayed for years in the form of a pseudoaneurysm rupture.

7. What is the mechanism of a traumatic aortic tear?
The thoracic aorta is particularly susceptible to deceleration because the arch is a movable structure that is anchored in two places—the aortic root and the ligamentum arteriosus (just distal to the takeoff of the left subclavian artery). In frontal or transverse deceleration, the aortic arch continues to move forward, resulting in shearing forces applied at the points of fixation, with a tear usually occurring just distal to the left subclavian artery. Vertical acceleration-deceleration injuries such as falls may result in a tear of the ascending aorta with coronary artery compromise or acute pericardial tamponade.

8. How is aortic rupture diagnosed and treated?
The most useful screening tests for aortic rupture are a standard upright chest radiograph and an aortogram. An abnormal-appearing or widened mediastinal silhouette is the most useful clue to the diagnosis. Other suggestive findings include deviation of the nasogastric tube to the right, an apical cap, a left pleural effusion, loss of the aortic window or the left pleural stripe, and depression of the left mainstem bronchus.

There are three important caveats to interpretation of the mediastinal width. (1) In the supine position, the mediastinum may falsely appear wide (greater than 8 cm at a 100-cm distance to the x-ray tube). One must therefore exercise caution in interpreting supine chest films. (2) The second caveat relates to a subjective interpretation of the silhouette. If it just does not quite look right, it is best to accede to clinical suspicion and further evaluate the aorta. (3) Finally, even in the absence of radiographic findings, an aortic rupture can be present. If clinical suspicion is strong enough based on mechanism and clinical findings, an angiogram should be performed. Dynamic chest CT scanning and transesophageal ultra-sonography are currently being studied and may be used in the future to aid in making this diagnosis.

9. How is penetrating chest trauma managed?
There is no simple answer to that question. Multiple diagnostic and therapeutic approaches exist depending on the location of the chest wound and the nature of the wounding implement.

10. What is the significance of the location of the wound?
Wound location dictates the clinical approach by virtue of the organs at risk. From a functional standpoint, wounds are categorized as central, peripheral, thoracoabdominal, and those in adjacent areas (abdomen and neck). Anatomically speaking, central wounds are located anteriorly (bordered by the midclavicular lines, the clavicles superiorly, and the costal margins inferiorly). All other wounds are considered peripheral; they are either lateral (bordered by the midclavicular lines, the posterior axillary lines, the axilla, and the costal margins) or posterior (bordered by the posterior axillary lines, the shoulders, and the

costal margins). Thoracoabdominal wounds are those in the inferior positions of all three anatomic areas. The inferior portions are defined by the nipple line anteriorly, the sixth rib laterally, and the tip of the scapulas posteriorly. Any wound below these landmarks is considered thoracoabdominal.

11. How are penetrating wounds of the central region managed?
Patients who are grossly unstable require an emergent thoracotomy with no ED work-up. Stable patients should be monitored closely while a diagnostic work-up (consisting of aortography, an esophagram ± esophagoscopy, and possibly bronchoscopy) is performed. If the work-up is negative, observation for 24–48 hours is appropriate; if positive, surgical intervention is needed.

12. What are the indications for ED thoracotomy?
Clear indications for ED thoracotomy include a victim of penetrating chest trauma who arrests in the ED or en route to the hospital or who has arrested at the scene and still has some sign of life (pulse, respirations, or reactive pupils) and does not require prolonged CPR.

13. What are the radiographic findings of a tension pneumothorax?
There should not be any because this diagnosis should be made on clinical grounds and treatment undertaken before a film is obtained. If a film is obtained, a hyperlucent, over-expanded hemithorax with an evident pneumothorax and a mediastinal shift to the opposite side would be observed.

14. What are the clinical signs of a tension pneumothorax?
Clinical findings include respiratory distress, an overexpanded hemithorax, hyperresonance to percussion, absent or markedly diminished breath sounds, tracheal shift away from the pneumothorax (the trachea must be palpated above the sternal notch; it is not appreciated on inspection), tachycardia, subcutaneous emphysema, and hypotension. In addition, in patients who are intubated and are being bag ventilated, increasing resistance to ventilation (requiring more manual pressure to insufflate air into the lungs) is often the earliest sign of tension pneumothorax.

15. Why does tension pneumothorax cause hypotension?
The mediastinal shift compromises vena caval blood return to the heart. The severely altered preload results in hypotension.

16. What is the treatment for a tension pneumothorax?
Immediate reduction in the intrapleural pressure on the affected side is appropriate therapy. For patients in extremis, the best way to accomplish this goal is the quickest method; that is, placement of a 14-gauge over-the-needle catheter into the fifth intercostal space between the anterior and midaxillary lines followed by aspiration with a 50-cc syringe. After vital signs improve, the procedure should be followed immediately by tube thoracostomy, which is the definitive treatment. For patients who are stable, aspiration need not precede insertion of a chest tube.

17. When should pericardial tamponade be suspected?
Acute pericardial tamponade is a clinical condition that results from the accumulation of blood and clots in the pericardial space. When pericardial pressure exceeds cardiac filling pressure, shock and ultimately death rapidly ensue. It should be suspected in any patient with a penetrating wound of the chest (particularly in the central area) who develops hypotension, tachycardia, and elevated CVP after tension pneumothorax has been treated or ruled out. The most accurate means of diagnosing pericardial blood is bedside ultrasonography.

18. How is acute pericardial tamponade treated?
The proper course of action in an unstable patient is pericardiocentesis followed by immediate transfer to the operating room for definitive therapy. If vital signs are lost in the ED, an immediate thoracotomy is indicated. In stable patients with impending tamponade, the presence of pericardial blood can be confirmed by bedside echocardiography. In unstable patients, diagnosis is confirmed by response to therapeutic interventions.

19. Should all patients with a stab wound of the chest be admitted to the hospital?
Patients with peripheral wounds not in the thoracoabdominal area who are stable and have an initial chest film that is normal usually do not require admission. They should, however, be observed in the ED and have a repeat film and hematocrit done in 4–6 hours. If repeat studies are normal, the patient may be discharged.

20. Are peripheral gunshot wounds that cross the mediastinum handled differently?
Determining missile trajectory based on entry wound and final resting position or exit wound is not always accurate. Nevertheless, if the estimated trajectory does traverse the mediastinum, these patients require a more thorough diagnostic evaluation while they are observed as inpatients. They should undergo the same work-up as patients who have sustained a penetrating injury of the central chest.

21. How are thoracoabdominal wounds managed?
By virtue of their low chest location, such wounds risk injury to the infradiaphragmatic, intraperitoneal, and retroperitoneal organs. Unfortunately there is no clear consensus on how to manage these patients. Some recommend observation alone, basing surgical intervention on positive physical findings. Others use diagnostic peritoneal lavage (DPL) with a lowered red blood cell criteria (greater than 5,000 or 10,000 red cells as opposed to the usual 50,000–100,000). Posterior thoracoabdominal wounds are particularly difficult to evaluate because retroperitoneal injuries are predominant and they are undetected by peritoneal lavage. Observation with a variable diagnostic work-up is recommended. Some merely observe, whereas others recommend adding an intravenous pyelogram (IVP), DPL, abdominal CT scan, contrast-enhanced CT enema (CECTE), or varying combinations of these alternatives. The CECTE adds rectally instilled contrast material to the usual intravenous and oral contrast agents given during abdominal scanning. The goal is early diagnosis of an occult colon injury. Although data are limited, the technique is promising and gaining popularity.

BIBLIOGRAPHY

1. Baxter BT, Moore EE, Moore JB: Emergency department thoracotomy following injury: Critical determinants for patient salvage. World J Surg 12:671–675, 1988.
2. Borlase BC, Moore EE, Moore FA: Penetrating wounds to the posterior chest: Analysis of exigent thoracotomy and laparotomy. J Emerg Med 7:445–447, 1989.
3. Durham LA, Richardson RJ, Wall MJ, et al: Emergency center thoracotomy: Impact of prehospital resuscitation. J Trauma 32:775–779, 1992.
4. Lorenz HP, Steinmetz B, Lieberman J, et al: Emergency Thoracotomy: Survival correlates with physiologic status. J Trauma 32:780–788, 1992.
5. Mayron R, Gaudio FE, Plummer D: Echocardiography performed by emergency physicians: Impact on diagnosis and therapy. Ann Emerg Med 17:150–154, 1988.
6. Merlotti GJ, Dillon BC, Lange DA: Peritoneal lavage in penetrating thoraco-abdominal trauma. J Trauma 28:17–23, 1988.
7. Moore JB, Moore EE, Thompson JS: Abdominal injuries associated with penetrating trauma in the lower chest. Am J Surg 140:724–730, 1980.
8. Phillips T, Sclafani SJ, Goldstein A: Use of the contrast-enhanced CT enema in the management of penetrating trauma to the flank and back. J Trauma 26:593–601, 1986.

9. Richardson JD, Flint LM, Snow NJ: Management of transmediastinal gunshot wounds. Surgery
    90:671–676, 1981.
10. Weigelt JA, Aurbakken CM, Meier DE, et al: Management of asymptomatic patients following
    stab wounds to the chest. J Trauma 22:292–294, 1982.

101. ABDOMINAL TRAUMA

Robert A. Read, M.D., and Ernest E. Moore, M.D.

1. What is the difference in pathophysiology between blunt and penetrating trauma?
Blunt trauma results from a combination of crushing, stretching, and shearing forces. The
magnitude of these forces is proportional to the mass of the objects, rate of change in
velocity (acceleration and deceleration), direction of impact, and elasticity of the tissues.
Injury results when the sum of these forces exceeds the cohesive strength and mobility of
the tissues and organs involved. Additionally, high-energy transfer to the abdomen induces
a pronounced rise in intraabdominal pressure that can produce hollow viscus rupture or
solid-organ burst injuries. Compression of abdominal contents against the thoracic cage or
spinal column may result in visceral crush injuries, and abrupt shearing forces may avulse
organs from their vascular pedicles. The injuries produced are a constellation of tissue
contusions, abrasions, fractures, or organ ruptures. Penetrating injuries result from the
dissipation of energy into tissue along the path of the offending projectile. Typically,
injuries result in localized tears or contusions of involved organs. The magnitude of injury
depends on the penetrating object (i.e., knife vs. bullet) as well as the trajectory.

2. What is the difference in pathophysiology between stab wounds and gunshot wounds?
Stab wounds typically produce clean lacerations of contiguous structures along the path of
penetration. Although critical structures may be involved, the physical damage is limited
and generally requires only debridement and hemostasis or primary repair. In contrast,
injuries from firearms are more extensive and are defined by the weapon and trajectory as
well as the tissues traversed. The wounding potential of a projectile is largely determined by
the kinetic energy (KE) imparted to the tissue. The KE of a missile is proportional to its
mass (M) and velocity (V):

$$KE = \frac{MV^2}{2}$$

An increase in the mass of a given missile by a factor of 2 doubles its KE, whereas the same
increment in velocity quadruples the KE. The efficiency of energy dissipation in tissue for
a given projectile is determined by its physical characteristics and pattern of flight. Soft lead
or hollow-tip projectiles are prone to mushrooming, fragmentation, and tumbling, which
make them more destructive than fully jacketed spiraling projectiles. Low-velocity weapons
produce injury predominantly by direct crush and tearing, whereas high-velocity missiles
induce variable tissue cavitation as well. The extent of cavitation is governed by the rate of
energy dissipation and physical characeristic of the tissues involved. Solid, inelastic organs
such as the liver, spleen, and brain are more susceptible than the relatively pliant lung and
skeletal muscle. The shotgun fires a group of pellets that disperse as a function of distance
and length or taper of the gun barrel. Shotguns vary in the number and size of pellets per
load; at close range (<7 meters) the predominant determinant of wounding potential is the
aggregate KE of the pellets. Because of the spherical shape of the pellets, however, velocity
dissipates rapidly at greater distances.

3. What are the common injury patterns produced by blunt abdominal trauma?

A working knowledge of injury patterns and factors that influence their presentation is helpful in the initial treatment of multisystem trauma. Blunt injuries usually represent energy transfer to underlying visceral and vascular structures in the anatomic region sustaining the directed impact. Specific examples of these patterns are listed below.

Patterns of Blunt Abdominal Injury

DIRECT IMPACT	RESULTANT INJURIES
Right lower rib fractures	Liver, gallbladder
Left lower rib fractures	Spleen, left kidney
Mid-epigastric contusion	Duodenum, pancreas, small bowel mesentery
Lumbar transverse process fracture	Kidney, ureter
Anterior pelvic fracture	Bladder, urethra

4. What are the common patterns of injury associated with penetrating abdominal wounds?

Penetrating injuries typically follow the tract or trajectory of the inflicting instrument and thus involve contiguous structures.

Patterns of Penetrating Abdominal Injury

REGION	MOST CONSPICUOUS WOUND	ASSOCIATED INJURIES
Right upper quadrant	Liver	Diaphragm, gallbladder, right colon
Left upper quadrant	Spleen	Diaphragm, stomach, pancreas (tail), left kidney
Mid-epigastric	Stomach	Pancreas (body)
	Duodenum	Diaphragm, vena cava
	Portal vein	Hepatic artery, common bile duct
	Superior mesenteric artery	Pancreas (neck), left renal vein, abdominal aorta
Pelvis	Iliac artery	Iliac vein, bladder, rectum

5. What are the key aspects of the history and physical examination in the initial evaluation of abdominal trauma?

Historical details are important in establishing the tempo, sequence, and extent of early diagnostic efforts. After blunt trauma, the size of motor vehicles, their velocity and direction of impact, the use of lap and shoulder restraints, associated steering wheel and windshield damage, and patient ejection are critical facts to glean from prehospital providers. The initial physical examination is conceptually divided into the primary and secondary survey. The primary survey is a rapid search for immediate life-threatening injuries, whereas the secondary survey is a compulsive examination that includes a systematic review for signs of potential occult injury. Abdominal and thoracic trauma should be considered as a unit because the dome of the diaphragm rises to the fourth intercostal space during full expiration, thus rendering the upper abdominal contents at risk for injury after impact to the lower chest. Gentle pressure over the lower ribs helps to establish the presence of fractures; fractures of the left and right lower ribs involve a 20% chance of splenic injury and a 10% chance of hepatic injury, respectively. The physical findings most often associated with internal injury are abdominal tenderness and guarding; rebound tenderness and rigidity are relatively infrequent. Most importantly, 20–40% of patients with serious intraabdominal injury in the context of multisystem trauma may be asymptomatic.

6. Which diagnostic tools are most useful for the initial evaluation of blunt abdominal trauma?

1. **Diagnostic peritoneal lavage (DPL)** is a safe and inexpensive method to rapidly identify life-threatening intraperitoneal hemorrhage. Despite the widespread popularity of CT scanning in the U.S. and of ultrasonography in Europe and Japan, we believe DPL remains the gold standard for evaluation of the critically injured in spite of its inherent limitations and a morbidity rate of about 1%. Significant complications, which occur most frequently with the closed technique, include perforations of the small bowel, mesentery, bladder, and retroperitoneal vascular structures. Previous abdominal surgery, morbid obesity, and portal hypertension are relative contraindications for DPL. In patients with previous midline abdominal incisions, DPL can be performed through a left lower quadrant transverse incision, although this approach is technically more challenging. Moreover, intraabdominal adhesions can loculate both the lavage fluid and free blood, increasing the chance of a false-negative study. Finally, DPL does not sample the intact retroperitoneum and may not adequately reflect isolated small-hollow visceral or diaphragmatic perforations.

2. **Computed tomography (CT)** plays an important role as a diagnostic adjunct in the early evaluation of abdominal and pelvic injuries. Limitations center on timely completion, availability of experienced radiologists, equipment variability, patient cooperation, and the necessity for oral and IV contrast-enhancement agents. Indeed, several prospective clinical studies have confirmed these concerns by comparing CT to DPL in acutely injured patients. On the other hand, CT has the unquestionable virtue of injury specificity. Clearly, select patients with isolated injuries to the liver or spleen can be managed expectantly based primarily on CT findings and physiologic information. In practice, CT should complement DPL. Four groups of patients are particularly suitable for CT scanning: (1) patients with delayed (>12 hours) presentation who are hemodynamically stable and do not have overt signs of peritonitis; (2) patients in whom DPL results are equivocal and repeated physical examination is unreliable or untenable (e.g., those who require prolonged general anesthesia for neurosurgical or orthopedic procedures; patients with altered mental status from head injury, drugs, or alcohol; or patients with spinal cord injury); (3) patients in whom DPL is difficult to perform (e.g., morbid obesity, portal hypertension, or previous laparotomies); and (4) patients at high risk for retroperitoneal injuries in whom the DPL is unremarkable (e.g., the unrestrained, intoxicated driver who strikes the steering column or a patient with postinjury hyperamylasemia). In addition, CT is valuable for defining the extent and configuration of complex pelvic fractures. However, it must be emphasized that CT scanning may not demonstrate blunt pancreatic fractures in the first 6 hours after injury and cannot be relied on for early detection of hollow visceral perforation.

3. **Ultrasonography (US)** is becoming more popular for initial evaluation of blunt abdominal trauma, in part because quality ultrasound machines are now portable. US is currently used routinely in EDs through Japan and Germany, and the recent experience in the U.S. affirms that it is about 95% sensitive to significant hemoperitoneum. The procedure is safe, particularly for the injured pregnant patient, because it does not employ ionizing radiation or contrast media. US, however, cannot reliably stage solid-organ injuries or reliably assess hollow visceral perforation. Moreover, its accuracy is compromised by the presence of lower rib fractures, extensive soft-tissue injuries, or dressings. Nonetheless, in the future, US will assume a significant role in the initial evaluation of posttraumatic hemoperitoneum and thus is likely to supplant DPL in certain instances.

4. **Laparoscopy.** Laparoscopy will have a place in the evaluation and definitive treatment of the acutely injured with the development of new technology. In the past, laparoscopy has been limited by the time required to perform the examination, the need for

specialized equipment, and the necessity for general anesthesia. Several studies confirm the accuracy of laparoscopy, under local anesthesia, in identifying diaphragmatic injuries, and a number of authors have described successful laparoscopic hemostasis for hepatic wounds. The major limitations relate to comprehensive examination of the small bowel and the posterior recesses of the abdomen and retroperitoneum.

7. What are the DPL indications for exploratory laparotomy after blunt trauma?

The peritoneal tap is considered positive if >10 ml of free blood is aspirated. Otherwise, 1 L of warmed 0.9% sodium chloride is infused (15 ml/kg in children). If the clinical condition permits, the patient is rolled from side to side to enhance intraperitoneal sampling. The saline bag is then lowered to the floor for the return of lavage fluid by siphonage. A minimal recovery of 75% of lavage effluent is required for the test to be considered valid. The fluid is sent for laboratory analysis of red blood (RBC) and white blood (WBC) cell counts, levels of lavage amylase (LAM) and lavage alkaline phosphatase (LAP), and presence of bile. The criteria for positive DPL are outlined below. In the context of blunt abdominal trauma, significant visceral damage is encountered in $>90\%$ of patients in whom the RBC count exceeds $100,000/mm^3$ but in $<2\%$ of those in whom the count is under $20,000/mm^3$. RBC counts between $20-100,000/mm^3$, however, may reflect serious injury in 15–35% of cases and merit further diagnostic evaluation. Occasionally, an elevated WBC count (>500 mm^3), LAM, or LAP signals an otherwise occult intestinal injury. The contents of a perforated viscus evoke migration of leukocytes into the peritoneal cavity, but this response may be delayed for several hours after injury. Conversely, an isolated WBC count exceeding $500/mm^3$ in a DPL performed promptly after injury is often nonspecific. If the initial WBC count is elevated, repeat the DPL in 4 hours and perform a laparotomy only if the count remains elevated. In fact, a lavage enzyme amylase is more accurate in the detection of hollow visceral injury; an LAM >20 IU/L combined with an LAP >3 IU/L has a specificity $>95\%$ for small bowel perforation.

Criteria for Positive DPL After Abdominal Trauma

INDEX	POSITIVE	EQUIVOCAL
Aspirate		
Blood	>10 ml	—
Fluid	Enteric contents	—
Lavage		
RBCs	$>100,000/mm^3$	$>20,000/mm^3$
WBCs	—	$>500/mm^3$
Enzyme	Amylase >20 IU/L and Alkaline phosphatase >3 IU	Amylase >20 or Alkaline phosphatase >3 IU
Bile	Confirmed biochemically	—

8. Which diagnostic tests are most useful for the initial evaluation for penetrating abdominal wounds?

The management of penetrating abdominal wounds is dichotomous. Gunshot wounds (GSWs) warrant mandatory laparotomy, whereas stab wounds (SWs) can be managed selectively. Only two-thirds of SWs to the anterior abdomen penetrate the peritoneal cavity and only one-half of those entering the peritoneum produce injuries requiring laparotomy. Consequently, the first diagnostic question is whether the SW traverses the peritoneum. Local wound exploration, performed under local anesthesia in the ED, answers this question reliably. In fact, patients with an unequivocally negative wound examination can be discharged. If peritoneal violation has occurred, the next question is whether significant intraabdominal injury is involved. DPL has proved to be exceedingly useful in the decision for laparotomy in this scenario.

9. What are the indications and interpretation of DPL after penetrating trauma?

The DPL indications for laparotomy are somewhat controversial, but most authorities recommend the same criteria employed for blunt trauma. However, because of a proportionally higher number of isolated intestinal perforations after an SW, DPL has a 5% false-negative rate. Thus, all patients with a negative lavage are admitted for at least 24 hours of observation and undergo prompt exploration if signs of peritoneal irritation ensue. Fortunately, most injuries missed by the initial DPL are isolated small bowel perforations, which are usually recognized within 12 hours and, if managed promptly, yield minimal additional morbidity. Lower chest SWs are associated with a 15% risk of abdominal injury because the diaphragm rises to the midchest during deep expiration. In addition, unrecognized diaphragmatic rents pose a lifelong threat because the continuous negative pleuroperitoneal pressure gradient encourages visceral herniation into the pleural cavity, which results in strangulated intestine. The physical examination of pateints with thoracoabdominal trauma is notoriously inaccurate. Consequently, DPL is recommended for all lower thoracic wounds. However, blood loss may be minimal after perforation of the diaphragm; therefore, the RBC threshold for laparotomy is lowered to 5,000/mm³. In addition, thoracoscopy may prove to have a role in the evaluation of lower thoracic SWs with associated RBC counts between 1,000–5,000 mm³.

10. In summary, how are the management priorities different for penetrating versus blunt abdominal trauma?

Initial management of penetrating abdominal trauma (see figure below) can be distilled to three elements: (1) aggressive resuscitation for any sign of hypovolemia, (2) directed physical examination, and (3) quick diagnostic studies with appropriate therapeutic interventions.

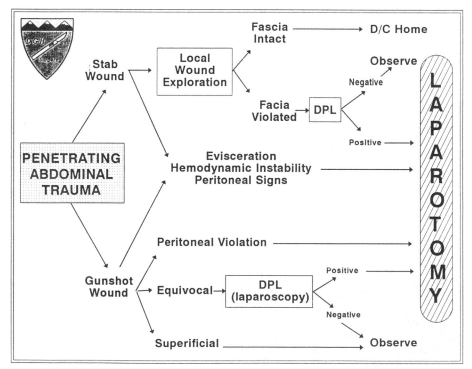

Management priorities for penetrating abdominal trauma.

In contrast, the initial management of blunt abdominal trauma (see figure below) consists of (1) gathering pertinent information from the patient, paramedics, flight nurses, and family; (2) systematic physical examination; and (3) directed laboratory as well as diagnostic studies, performed in a fashion dictated by the patient's physiologic status.

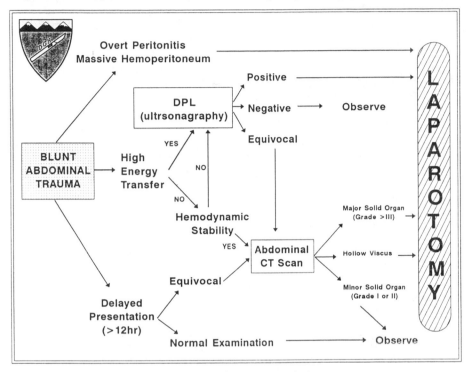

Management priorities for blunt abdominal trauma.

11. What are the concerns in a pregnant patient with abdominal trauma?

Pregnancy alters both the susceptibility to blunt injury and the physiologic response to injury. The gravid uterus occupies the pelvis and lower abdomen and hence is vulnerable to a variety of insults from direct blows or seatbelt injuries. These insults result in a spectrum of injuries from minor soft-tissue contusions to uterine wall disruption or placental abruption and potential exsanguination as well as fetal loss. The significance of relatively minor injuries mandates an aggressive posture in the early evaluation of pregnant patients. We routinely employ DPL (open technique) while simultaneously evaluating the gravid uterus with ultrasound, noninvasive fetal monitoring, and amniocentesis. Hemodynamic instability, uterine rupture, placental abruption, fetal distress, or a bloody amniocentesis indicates the need for emergent abdominal exploration and uterine evacuation with the rare possibility of hysterectomy.

12. What about the pediatric patient?

Pediatric trauma provides unique challenges because of patient size and different injury patterns. The elasticity of the child's lower rib cage and the relative large size of the abdominal cavity increase susceptibility to intraabdominal injury. Blunt injuries are commonly minor, with modest liver or splenic fractures that are self-limited. Fortunately pancreatic fractures and intestinal perforations are infrequent in children. Despite the enthusiasm for nonoperative management, an aggressive operative policy is warranted in the context of pediatric multisystem trauma because of the child's limited physiologic reserve. Although grossly positive DPLs in hemodynamically stable children can be further elucidated by CT scan to verify solid-organ injury amenable to expectant care, abdominal exploration is undertaken promptly for hemodynamic instability, need for ongoing blood transfusions, or DPLs positive by enzymes.

BIBLIOGRAPHY

1. American College of Surgeons Committee on Trauma: Advanced Trauma Life Support Course. Chicago, American College of Surgeons, 1991, pp 111–130.
2. Feliciano DV, Mattox KL: Small intestine injuries. In Moore EE, Eiseman B, Van Way CW (eds): Critical Decisions in Trauma. St. Louis, Mosby–Year Book, 1984, p 206.
3. Ivatury RR, Simon RJ, Weksler B, et al: Laparoscopy in the evaluation of the intrathoracic abdomen after penetrating injury. J Trauma 33:101–109, 1992.
4. Marx JA, Moore EE, Jorden RC, et al: Limitations of computed tomography in the evaluation of acute abdominal trauma: A prospective comparison with diagnostic peritoneal lavage. J Trauma 25:933, 1985.
5. Moore EE: Critical decision-making in management of acute hepatic injury. Am J Surg 148:712, 1984.
6. Moore EE, Mattox KL, Feliciano DV (eds): Trauma, 2nd ed. Norwalk, CT, Appleton & Lange, 1991, pp 81–96.
7. Moore EE, Moore FA: Immediate enteral nutrition following multisystem trauma—a decade experience. Am Coll Nutr 10:633, 1991.
8. Pickhardt B, Moore EE, Moore FA, et al: Operative splenic salvage in the adult—a decade perspective. J Trauma 29:1386, 1989.
9. Read RA, Moore EE: Abdominal and pelvic trauma. In Copeland EM, Howard R, Warshaw A, et al (eds): Current Practice of Surgery. New York, Churchill Livingstone, 1992.
10. Rothenberger DA, Quattlebaum FW, Zabel J, et al: Blunt maternal trauma: A review of 103 cases. J Trauma 18:173, 1978.
11. Rothenberg S, Moore EE, Marx JA, et al: Selective management of blunt abdominal trauma in children—the triage role of peritoneal lavage. J Trauma 27:1101, 1987.
12. Tso P, Rodriguez A, Cooper C, et al: Sonography in blunt abdominal trauma: A preliminary progress report. J Trauma 33:39–44, 1992.

102. HEMORRHAGE FROM PELVIC FRACTURES

Robert A. Read, M.D., and Ernest E. Moore, M.D.

1. Why do I need to know about pelvic fractures?

Major pelvic fractures, which are among the most challenging injuries encountered in the emergency department (ED), result from high-energy transfer, most commonly from motor vehicle, auto-pedestrian, and motorcycle accidents. Consequently, patients frequently present with multisystem trauma and potentially critical injuries. Life-threatening hemorrhage from pelvic fractures occurs in a minority of patients but remains the leading cause of early death. Control of pelvic hemorrhage can be frustrating because of the complex nature of the injury and the extensive interconnecting vascular channels that are difficult to access and control technically.

2. How are pelvic fractures classified?

Multiple classification systems have been developed based on a variety of perspectives, including injury mechanism, bone involvement, fracture stability, or location. One classification system incorporates direction of impact, magnitude of force, and fracture geography. Anteroposterior (AP) impact fractures are associated with symphyseal diastasis and sacroiliac (SI) disruption. Similarly, the vertical shear (VS) injury consists of displaced fractures of the anterior rami and posterior columns, including SI dislocation. These two patterns are generally associated with major blood loss, predominantly from the internal iliac system bridging the anterior surface of the SI joint and, because of the force encountered, multiple associated injuries. On the other hand, lateral compression (LC) fractures are encountered in side impacts, typically following a T-bone motor vehicle accident. Because LC injuries result in compression of posterior ligaments and local vasculature rather than disruption, they are not usually associated with massive pelvic blood loss.

3. What is the approach to the patient with a pelvic fracture?
The evaluation of patients with complex pelvic fractures begins with the primary trauma survey (ABCs) and rapid evaluation of the patient's overall status. Life-threatening associated injuries are evaluated simultaneously with systematic assessment of the pelvic fractures. The physical examination directed at the pelvis includes manual compression of the bony pelvis and inspection of the perineum, rectum, and vagina for ecchymosis, ongoing bleeding, and open wounds. Plain roentgenograms of the pelvis are a priority in the patient with suspected fracture, although anteroposterior and inlet views may not reflect the full magnitude of bony instability. Hemodynamically stable patients may be further evaluated with computed tomography. However, patients with complex fractures and significant associated injuries require vigilant monitoring, active resuscitation, and appropriate diagnostic interventions before they leave the ED. Often these patients mandate rapid ED triage, coordinated interventions by radiology and orthopedics, and early transfer to the intensive care unit (ICU) with advanced capabilities.

4. Which abdominal injuries are associated with pelvic trauma?
Nearly 90% of patients with significant pelvic fractures have associated injuries. Associated abdominal injuries occur in approximately 15–20% of patients and increase with the magnitude and direction of force on impact (i.e., fracture classification). The relative frequency of abdominal injuries associated with major pelvic fractures is listed below.

Relative Frequency of Intraabdominal Injuries
Associated with Major Pelvic Fractures (%)

	ANTERO-POSTERIOR	LATERAL COMPRESSION	VERTICAL SHEAR	COMBINED MECHANICAL
Spleen	20	0	25	12
Liver	10	0	7	5
Bowel	15	15	5	5
Kidney	1	1	4	4
Bladder	5	0	1	10
Vascular	25	25	5	5
Retroperitoneal hematoma	50	60	50	25

From Dalal S, et al: J Trauma 29:981, 1989, with permission.

5. Which physical findings are specifically associated with major pelvic trauma?
Anterior pelvic instability, perineal hematomas, or blood at the urethral meatus are associated with urethral lacerations and bladder disruptions. These physical signs mandate aggressive urologic examination, including a retrograde cystourethrogram and commensurate therapy. Similarly, vaginal or rectal blood is strong evidence for laceration of these structures. Although the treatment for vaginal lacerations is somewhat unclear, open pelvic

fractures with rectal tears portend profound septic complications and consequently require aggressive interventions centered on fecal diversion, perineal debridement, and wide presacral drainage.

6. What are the source and site of bleeding from major pelvic fractures?
Uncontrolled hemorrhage is the leading cause of early death in patients with complex pelvic fractures. Massive bleeding is most frequently associated with SI disruption from vertical shear or AP compression fractures. Of note, the most frequent source of bleeding is venous. The arterial vessels likely to produce rapid bleeding are branches of the internal iliac; particularly common is the superior gluteal. Pubic diastasis and anterior fractures may also result in significant blood loss, notably from vesicular branches of the pudendal artery. Branches of the corresponding veins in these distributions and the lumbosacral venous plexus contribute significantly to retroperitoneal and pelvic hemorrhage.

7. What is the role of pneumatic antishock garments (PASG) in the management of patients with pelvic fractures?
Controversy continues to surround the use of PASG in prehospital trauma care, specifically in urban areas within short transport times. However, there is general agreement that PASG has a useful role in the acute management of pelvic fractures. Relatively low-pressure inflation, even in hemodynamically stable patients, is advocated to provide temporary splinting and tamponade of ongoing venous hemorrhage. This approach is particularly useful in patients with complex fractures or hemodynamic instability during prehospital transport, ED triage and resuscitation, or inhospital transport to radiology, the operating room, and ICU.

8. What is the role of external fixation in the acute management of pelvic fractures?
External fixation of complex pelvic fractures in the ED is becoming standard. Compression of the fractured pelvis decreases fracture mobility and limits expansion of the pelvic ring and hence may contribute to tamponade of ongoing hemorrhage. The most favorable situation is the AP "book-open" fracture, i.e., disruption of the anterior ligaments of the SI joint with symphyseal diastasis. In this setting, the external frame can close the book, reducing the overall pelvic volume. More complex fractures, including complete SI disruption (i.e., VS injury) may also benefit from early fracture stabilization, but fixation is not as complete because of the instability of the posterior column.

9. What is the role of diagnostic peritoneal lavage (DPL) in the early evaluation of pelvic fractures?
With significant blood loss, early recognition of an extrapelvic source is imperative; the risk of active intraperitoneal visceral bleeding is 20–30%. Thus DPL is an integral part of the initial evaluation. It is performed at the infraumbilical ring to avoid the dissecting pelvic hematoma; if results are negative, the catheter can be left in place to facilitate serial lavages as other diagnostic procedures are completed.

10. When should patients with pelvic trauma undergo laparotomy?
A grossly negative DPL reliably excludes life-threatening intraperitoneal blood loss. A grossly positive aspirate in a hemodynamically unstable patient, however, mandates emergent abdominal exploration because aspiration of >20 ml of gross blood is associated with a 95% chance of active splenic, hepatic, or mesenteric hemorrhage. A grossly negative tap but cell-count positive lavage must be interpreted cautiously because as many as 20% are falsely positive from a ruptured pelvic hematoma or trivial hepatic or splenic injury. In the stable patient, CT scanning should be used in conjunction with serial lavage to clarify the source of bleeding after the immediate life-threatening problems have been addressed.

11. How is continued pelvic bleeding managed in these patients?
The patient with ongoing hemorrhage, despite the PASG, demands a critical triage decision. The unstable individual with a grossly positive DPL should undergo laparotomy because of the high probability of solid visceral or major vascular injury. In the patient with a positive lavage by red blood cell count, the pelvic bleeding should be managed first. The key decision is whether to employ skeletal fixation or selective pelvic arterial embolization; thus prompt consultation of orthopedic and interventional radiology specialists is imperative.

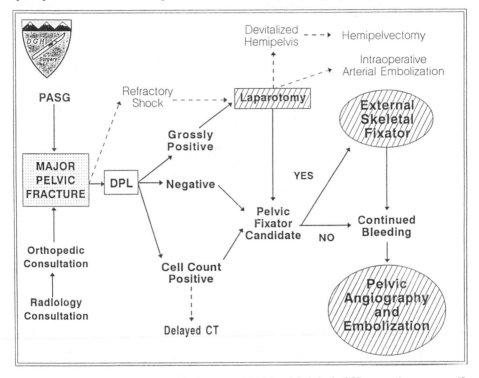

12. How frequently are rectal injuries associated with pelvic injuries? How are they managed?
Approximately 5% of pelvic fractures are associated with rectal injuries. These complex injuries result in a high mortality rate due to septic complications. The current management principles are based on accumulated war-time experience, which has proved the efficiency of fracture stabilization, hemorrhage control, and fecal diversion with rectal washout, perineal debridement, and pelvic drainage via the presacral space.

13. What is rectal washout?
With the identification of a rectal injury in association with a pelvic fracture, the patient undergoes a diverting colostomy (usually sigmoid) with exclusion of the distal colon and rectum. The anal sphincters are gently dilated and the excluded distal colon and rectum copiously irrigated until gross fecal material has been removed. This technique has been shown to significantly reduce morbidity and mortality in critically injured patients.

14. What are the common urologic injuries associated with pelvic fractures?
Pelvic fractures usually cause posterior (above the urogenital diaphragm) urethral tears, as opposed to anterior lesions, which are typically associated with perineal straddle trauma (see ch. 103). If urethral disruption is suspected, Foley catheterization should be deferred until a retrograde urethrogram can be obtained. The ED management of complete urethral

disruption is transcutaneous suprapubic cystostomy. Displaced pelvic rami fractures may also perforate the extraperitoneal bladder. Hematuria is absent in >10% of such patients, and the ability to void does not exclude the injury. Gravity flow cystography with 250 ml of contrast material and postvoiding views should be performed in patients with displaced anterior pelvic fractures.

15. What are the major causes of death following pelvic trauma?
The overall mortality from pelvic trauma ranges from 5–30%. Early mortality results from uncontrolled hemorrhage, refractory shock, or associated multisystem injuries. Delayed mortality is most frequently due to septic complications and may be as high as 50% in the subset of patients with open pelvic fractures.

BIBLIOGRAPHY

1. Burgess AR, Eastridge BJ, Young JWR, et al: Pelvic ring disruptions: Effective classification system and treatment protocols. J Trauma 30:848, 1990.
2. Cryer HM, Miller FB, Evers BM, et al: Pelvic fracture classification: Correlation with hemorrhage. J Trauma 28:973, 1988.
3. Latenser BA, Gentilello LM, Tavver AA, et al: Improved outcome with early fixation of skeletally unstable pelvic fractures. J Trauma 31:28, 1991.
4. Moreno C, Moore E, Rosenberger A, et al: Hemorrhage associated with pelvic fracture—a multispecialty challenge. J Trauma 26:987, 1986.
5. Mucha P: Pelvic fractures. In Moore EE, Mattox KL, Feliciano DV (eds): Trauma, 2nd ed. Norwalk, CT, Appleton & Lange, 1991, pp 553–569.
6. Panetta T, Sclafani SJA, Goldstein AS, et al: Percutaneous transcatheter embolization for massive bleeding from pelvic fractures. J Trauma 25:1021, 1985.
7. Poole GV, Ward EF, Muakkassu FF, et al: Pelvic fracture from major blunt trauma: Outcome is determined by associated injuries. Ann Surg 213:532, 1991.
8. Read RA, Moore EE: Abdominal and pelvic trauma. In Copeland EM, Howard R, Warshaw A, et al (eds): Current Practice of Surgery. New York, Churchill Livingstone, 1992.
9. Richardson JD, Harty J, Amin M, Flint LM: Open pelvic fractures. J Trauma 22:533, 1982.
10. Shannon FL, Moore EE, Moore FA, McCroskey BL: Value of distal colon washout in civilian rectal trauma—reducing gut bacterial translocation. J Trauma 28:989, 1988.

103. GENITOURINARY AND PELVIC TRAUMA

Joanne Edney, M.D.

1. What are the primary mechanisms of renal trauma?
Blunt traumatic injuries caused by direct impact or severe deceleration represent more than 80% of all renal injuries, whereas penetrating injuries, generally from gunshot or stab wounds, account for 20%. Renal injury should be suspected in the presence of lower posterior rib fractures, transverse process fractures of the upper lumbar spine, acute scoliosis, flank tenderness or ecchymoses, or hematuria.

2. Name the two true genitourinary emergencies.
Uncontrolled hemorrhage and renal pedicle injuries resulting in ischemia. The kidneys move to a limited degree on the vascular pedicle. Victims with a complete severance of the renal pedicle usually exsanguinate at the scene. Deceleration injuries may cause shearing of the major renal vessels, leading to thrombosis and subsequent ischemia. Early diagnosis and surgical intervention are critical for salvage of the affected kidney. However, in the

multiple-trauma patient the guidelines of the advanced trauma life support (ATLS) program should be followed, focusing initially on the airway, breathing, and circulation (ABCs) and life-threatening thoracic and abdominal injuries.

3. Describe the general classifications of renal injury.
1. **Renal contusion:** bruise or minor tears of renal tissue with intact renal capsule.
2. **Renal laceration:**
   a. **Minor:** superficial cortical parenchymal disruption with damage to capsule
   b. **Major:** deep laceration to corticomedullary junction or involving collection system or major intrarenal vessels (includes fragmentation or shattering of kidney and renal pelvis rupture)
3. **Renal pedicle injury:** intimal tear, laceration, or occlusion of main or segmental renal arteries or veins

4. What is the clinical course of these injuries?
Almost all renal contusions and minor lacerations heal spontaneously with bed rest and observation. Treatment of major laceration is controversial and should be left to the urologist. Renal pedicle injuries and shattered kidneys require early surgical intervention.

5. What are the roles of intravenous pyelography, selective angiography, and computed tomography in the evaluation of renal trauma?
Intravenous pyelography (IVP) is a good screening test to rule out significant blunt renal trauma and isolated ureteral injury. However, abnormal or indeterminate IVPs require additional studies to define the injury. Renal arteriography is indicated in the presence of a suspected pedicle injury, major kidney fractures, or segmental areas of nonrenal enhancement. Computed tomography (CT) is clearly superior to IVP in defining the severity and extent of injury and has become the modality of choice for definitive evaluation of the renal parenchyma. Increasing data suggest that CT may also be an accurate method of diagnosing renal artery injuries, thereby decreasing the need for arteriography. However, CT is insensitive for detecting an isolated ureteral injury.

6. When should ureteral trauma be suspected?
Ureteral injury should be suspected in the presence of penetrating injuries in proximity to the ureter. Hematuria may be absent. IVP identifies the injury. Blunt ureteral trauma is usually associated with other intraabdominal injuries and is often diagnosed intraoperatively.

7. Describe the most reliable method to diagnose bladder injuries.
Bladder rupture is established with a retrograde cystogram. Proper technique is important. The bladder should be filled with 300 cc of contrast material through the indwelling catheter. A flat anteroposterior abdominal roentgenogram is obtained both after instillation of contrast and after drainage. A false-negative study due to incomplete filling of the bladder is the most common error.

8. What are the indications for retrograde cystography?
Retrograde cystography is indicated if bladder rupture is suspected. The most frequent clinical findings associated with bladder injury are gross hematuria, pelvic fractures, and lower abdominal tenderness.

9. What are the associated clinical findings in bladder injury?
Approximately 10% of all pelvic fractures are associated with bladder or urethral rupture. Lower abdominal compression, as seen with lapbelt and steering wheel injuries, may rupture the distended bladder without injuring the pelvic girdle. Gross hematuria is present

in more than 95% of patients with bladder rupture after blunt trauma. Penetrating trauma with any degree of microscopic hematuria should be evaluated for genitourinary injury. If the wound is in the vicinity of the bladder, a cystogram should be performed. Asymptomatic blunt trauma with microscopic hematuria is controversial.

10. What are the contraindications to urethral catheterization in the traumatized patient?
Catheterization should not be performed in a patient with suspected urethral injury because a partial tear may be converted into a complete tear, and the risks of infection and further damage are increased. Of patients with urethral injury, 80–90% have blood at the urethral meatus. Scrotal and perineal hematomas or a high-riding prostate on rectal exam are other signs of urethral rupture. Therefore, patients with these findings should not be catheterized until a retrograde urethrogram is performed to rule out urethral injury.

11. How is a retrograde urethrogram performed?
The urethrogram is obtained using a #12-Fr urinary catheter secured in the meatal fossa by inflating the balloon to approximately 3 cc. Alternatively, a catheter-tipped syringe may be used. Standard water-soluble contrast material (25–30 ml) is injected under gentle pressure as the anteroposterior and oblique views are taken.

12. What is a penile fracture?
Penile fracture refers to a sudden tear in the tunica albuginea with subsequent rupture of the corpora cavernosum. It occurs only in the erect penis and is usually associated with falls or sudden unexpected moves during sexual intercourse. It has also been reported with direct blunt trauma. A sudden intense pain associated with a snapping noise and immediate detumescence usually occurs. Most authors support surgical intervention in an attempt to restore normal function and prevent angulation.

13. What is the role of ultrasound in the evaluation of testicular trauma?
Ultrasound is a valuable tool in assessing the integrity of the testicles. Adequate palpation may be prevented by hematoma formation. Ultrasound can distinguish between simple hematoma and disruption of the parenchyma. Failure to suspect and diagnose testicular rupture may result in subsequent loss.

CONTROVERSY

14. What is the diagnostic approach to asymptomatic microhematuria in the patient with blunt trauma?
Any trauma patient with gross hematuria or with penetrating injuries and any degree of microscopic hematuria requires further radiographic evaluation. There is, however, no consensus regarding the significance of microscopic hematuria in the otherwise asymptomatic patient with blunt trauma. The amount of blood in the urine does not correlate with severity of injury. Furthermore, the relatively low incidence of positive studies requiring surgery may not justify an extensive radiographic evaluation. Although no protocol is universally accepted, many now advocate close follow-up of these patients and repeat urinalyses, with additional studies only if the hematuria persists.

BIBLIOGRAPHY

1. Barbagli G, Selli C, Stomaci N, et al: Urethral trauma: Radiological aspects and treatment options. J Trauma 27:256–261, 1987.
2. Bretan PN Jr, McAninch JW, Federle MP, et al: Computerized tomographic staging of renal trauma: 85 consecutive cases. J Urol 136:561–565, 1986.

3. Callaham: Current Practice of Emergency Medicine, 2nd ed. Philadelphia, B.C. Decker, 1986.
4. Carroll PR, McAninch JW: Major bladder trauma: Mechanisms of injury and a unified method of diagnosis and repair. J Urol 132:254–257, 1984.
5. Carroll PR, Klosterman PW, McAninch JW: Surgical management of renal trauma: Analysis of risk factors, technique, and outcome. J Trauma 28:1071–1077, 1988.
6. Cass AS, Luxenberg M: Accuracy of computed tomography in diagnosing renal artery injuries. Urology 34:249–251, 1989.
7. Harwood-Nuss A, Linden CH, Luten RC, et al: The Clinical Practice of Emergency Medicine. Philadelphia, J.B. Lippincott, 1991.
8. Husmann DA, Morris JS: Attempted nonoperative management of blunt renal lacerations extending through the corticomedullary junction. J Urol 143:682–684, 1990.
9. Rosen P, et al (eds): Emergency Medicine: Concepts and Clinical Practice, 3rd ed. St. Louis, Mosby–Year Book, 1992.
10. Trunkey DD, Lewis FR: Current Therapy of Trauma–2. Philadelphia, B.C. Decker, 1986.

104. FOREIGN BODIES

W. Peter Vellman, M.D.

1. What is the generic initial approach to a patient with a foreign body?

First, attempt to visualize it; secondly, palpate for it; and finally, if it is not visible or palpable, order appropriate diagnostic studies to determine its presence and location.

2. What is the best approach to evaluating and removing superficial foreign bodies from the eye?

Patients generally report a foreign-body sensation associated with tearing and conjunctival injection. Meticulous examination of the eye is performed under magnification (i.e., loupes or slit lamp), including eversion of both lids to look for foreign bodies in the conjunctival sacs. If a foreign body is not visualized, the inner aspects of the lids are swept with a moist cotton swab, or the eye is irrigated gently with normal saline. Fluorescein staining and examination under blue light should reveal corneal abrasions, which may present with the same symptoms as a foreign body. The safest way to remove corneal or conjunctival foreign bodies is with an eye spud or moist cotton swab under direct magnification. Rust rings may require removal with a hand-held burr.

3. How can you avoid missing an ocular foreign body?

The physician must always have a high index of suspicion for an ocular foreign body, particularly with orbital trauma, sudden eye pain with or without a history of trauma, and/or visual loss. A hyphema may be the only clue to a penetrating ocular foreign body. Physical exam must include visual acuity testing and meticulous inspection of the eyelids and globe. Careful funduscopic examination should be performed but may prove difficult in the presence of hemorrhage or cataract formation. External pressure on the globe should be avoided. Small high-velocity missiles that penetrate the orbital soft tissue or globe may leave no sign of entry. If there is any suspicion, plain films, ultrasonography, or CT scan should be performed. Missed ocular foreign bodies with subsequent loss of visual acuity are a leading source of malpractice losses.

4. What is the best way to remove a foreign body from the ear canal?

There is no one correct answer. The physician must use his or her knowledge and experience to optimize patient comfort and to limit injury to the ear structures when extracting the foreign body. Techniques vary from simple irrigation or suction to forceps extraction under direct visualization. Conscious sedation may be required, especially in children. Fine right-angle forceps, a right-angle hook, or small suction cups may be particularly useful. If extraction cannot be accomplished readily, referral to an otolaryngologist for removal under anesthesia, with or without an operating microscope, may be required. After foreign body removal, the canal and tympanic membrane should be inspected. Any evidence of injury to the tympanic membrane should prompt acuity testing and referral to a specialist.

5. How is an insect removed from the external ear?
A 2% lidocaine solution is effective in immediately paralyzing live insects and facilitates their removal from the external auditory canal.

6. When should a nasal foreign body be suspected?
Always suspect a retained nasal foreign body when there is a history of persistent unilateral nasal discharge. Nasal foreign body is a common ED presentation, particularly in small children and the mentally retarded. Careful examination of the nasal cavity requires patience and the proper equipment.

7. How is a nasal foreign body removed?
Techniques of removal are based on the physician's experience and ability; safe removal occasionally requires general anesthesia. There is always a risk of airway compromise if the foreign body dislodges posteriorly during attempted extraction or with forced inhalation.

8. How do you handle the adult with an esophageal foreign body?
A careful history is critical to the management of such patients. Over 80% of swallowed foreign bodies pass through the GI tract without incident. Sharp objects (e.g., bones, needles, wire) may impale the wall of the esophagus, whereas soft objects, such as meat, may obstruct the anatomic points of constriction of the esophagus: the postcricoid area, the aortic arch, and the gastroesophageal junction. Flexible esophagoscopy is the accepted method of removal for sharp, inert, radiopaque, or recently impacted foreign objects. Balloon catheter retrieval may be effective for removal of nonsharp objects, such as coins, but is controversial. Intravenous glucagon results in smooth muscle relaxation of the distal esophagus and may be useful in relieving obstructions at that level. Gas-forming agents have been used to propel a food-bolus impaction into the stomach from the distal esophagus.

9. Do children with possible coin ingestion and no symptoms need an x-ray?
Absolutely. A significant percentage of children with an esophageal coin are asymptomatic. Delayed diagnosis may lead to mistreatment and complications due to esophageal erosion, such as bleeding, perforation, and obstruction. In general, if the coin passes the gastroesophageal junction, it traverses the remainder of the GI tract without complication. Subtle symptoms, such as failure to thrive, eating complications, and wheezing secondary to tracheal compression, may be the result of unsuspected esophageal coins.

10. How do you evaluate the patient with a fish bone in the throat?
The dilemma of a fish bone in the throat is whether the symptoms are caused by a retained foreign body or mucosal abrasion. Tenderness on palpation of the neck is an unreliable sign, whereas pooled secretions on laryngoscopy are almost always associated with a retained foreign body. Careful physical examination with visualization and removal of the bone obviates the need for radiologic studies or specialty referral. Plain radiography is

rarely helpful; however, barium swallow may detect retained foreign bodies or demonstrate a perforation.

11. How do you remove a rectal foreign body?

The preferred route of removal is through the same orifice into which it was originally inserted. This may not always be feasible, however, because of the size or shape of the foreign body or because of fragmentation or possible breakage. Laparotomy is rarely required. Mucosal edema may also preclude easy extraction. Direct visualization with a vaginal speculum and extraction with a ring forceps or tenaculum, sometimes with the tip of a Foley catheter passed proximal to the foreign body in order to overcome suction, is a common technique. If this is unsuccessful, removal in the operating room under general anesthesia may be required.

12. What are the common foreign bodies found in the rectum?

The three leading categories of rectal foreign bodies, in decreasing order of frequency, are glass or ceramic objects, sexual devices, and foods, primarily fruits and vegetables. Obviously, the type of foreign body dictates the best approach for removal. Large-bowel injuries should be suspected with all rectal foreign bodies, and appropriate evaluation should be performed after removal of the foreign body.

13. Why are button batteries a cause of concern?

Most button batteries contain an alkaline electrolyte and a heavy metal such as lithium or mercury. Impaction in a mucosa-lined cavity (i.e., nose, GI tract, respiratory tract) may result in corrosive inflammation that leads to perforation. Injury may occur by one of the following four mechanisms: (1) electrolyte leakage, (2) alkali produced from external currents, (3) mercury toxicity, and (4) pressure necrosis. Early diagnosis and removal are crucial to preventing complications such as perforation of the nasal septum or GI tract. Button batteries lodged in the external auditory canal can result in caustic injury to the canal and erosive perforation of the tympanic membrane.

14. How do you determine whether a foreign body has been aspirated into the tracheobronchial tree?

Patients may give a history of aspiration, but peak incidences for aspiration occur before the age of 3 and after the age of 50 and in patients with altered mentation. A clinical history of choking with a subsequent spasmodic cough should lead the physician to further investigation. Up to half of young children with aspirated foreign bodies are asymptomatic. Hoarseness or stridor indicates a tracheal or laryngeal obstruction, whereas unilateral wheezing and decreased breath sounds imply a bronchial obstruction. Delayed presentation is the rule in children, with only one-third of patients presenting within 24 hours. If plain radiographs are unrevealing, then fluoroscopy should be performed. Positive findings include a mediastinal shift away from the side of the foreign body and obstructive emphysema. Foreign bodies are rarely spontaneously expulsed and generally require removal with the rigid bronchoscope. Bronchoscopy is indicated if the index of suspicion is high despite the absence of symptoms and x-ray findings.

15. Which radiologic studies are helpful in elucidating subcutaneous foreign bodies?

Plain radiographs should be used as an initial screening device. Although some foreign bodies are radiopaque (e.g, metal, glass with and without lead), many, including wood, are not. If plain films are unrevealing, ultrasound should be used to detect superficial foreign bodies. Although controversial, xeroradiography does not seem to offer any advantage over standard radiography and requires much larger doses of radiation. For deep foreign bodies not detected by plain films or ultrasound, CT scan is indicated. CT and MRI are useful in studying the complications of retained foreign bodies.

BIBLIOGRAPHY

1. Busch DB, Starling JR: Rectal foreign bodies: Case reports and a comprehensive review of the world's literature. Surgery 100:512–519, 1986.
2. Flom LL, Ellis GL: Radiologic evaluation of foreign bodies. Emerg Med Clin North Am 10:163–177, 1992.
3. Fritz S, Kelen GD, Sivertson K: Foreign bodies of the external auditory canal. Emerg Med Clin North Am 5:183–192, 1987.
4. Hodge D III, Tecklenburg F, Fleisher: Coin ingestion: Does every child need a radiograph? Ann Emerg Med 14:443–446, 1985.
5. Holt GR, Holt JE: Management of orbital trauma and foreign bodies. Otolaryngol Clin North Am 21:35–52, 1988.

105. TRAUMA IN PREGNANCY

Jedd Roe, M.D.

1. What is the one concept I need to take away from this chapter?
Fetal outcome is largely related to maternal morbidity. Therefore, the best fetal resuscitation is aggressive maternal resuscitation.

2. How common is trauma in pregnancy?
It has been estimated that 6–7% of pregnancies are complicated by trauma. In blunt abdominal trauma, the usual causes are direct abdominal blows, falls, and motor vehicle accidents (MVAs). However, 80% of falls occur after 32 weeks of gestation. One study showed that serious MVAs accounted for a 7.2% maternal mortality rate, whereas the fetal mortality rate was more than double this value at 15%.

3. Is physical or sexual abuse seen frequently in pregnant patients?
Definitely. One large study reported a prevalence of abuse in the urban, pregnant population of 17% (1 out of every 6 patients). Sixty percent of physically abused women reported two or more episodes of assault. Injury was more common to the head, neck, and extremities, and a four-fold increase in the incidence of genital trauma was noted in this population.

4. How do physiologic changes in pregnancy affect the evaluation of the trauma victim?
First, decreasing blood pressure and rising heart rate might indicate hypovolemic shock in a nonpregnant woman, but in pregnancy this may merely reflect physiologic changes or supine positioning. Because of increased blood volume, signs of shock may not be clinically apparent until as much as 35% of maternal blood volume is lost. Given the markedly increased blood flow to the uterus, there is a new potential source of blood loss that will require aggressive investigation. Finally, because changes result in a decreased maternal oxygen reserve, tissue hypoxia develops more rapidly in response to a traumatic insult.

5. How do physiologic changes of pregnancy affect laboratory values?
A physiologic anemia is seen as the plasma volume rises by more than twice the amount of red blood cells. Thus, it is not unusual for one to see hematocrits of 32–34% by the third trimester. Fibrinogen levels are double those seen in other trauma patients. Therefore, disseminated intravascular coagulation (DIC) may be seen with "normal" fibrinogen levels.

Because of hormonal stimulation of the central respiratory drive, PCO_2 falls to approximately 30 mmHg, and thus injury sufficient to cause a respiratory acidosis might be manifested by what would ordinarily be considered a normal PCO_2 of 40 mmHg.

6. Are serious maternal injuries required for fetal injury to be present?

Not always. Although in utero damage is often associated with maternal pelvic fractures, up to 6.7% of maternal cases of minor trauma have been associated with poor fetal outcome. Direct injuries to the fetus in utero are unusual, but given the size of the fetal head, when direct trauma occurs, fetal head injury is by far the most common injury. The most common causes of fetal death are maternal death, maternal shock, and placental abruption.

7. How does placental abruption occur?

Abruption results from the separation of a relatively inelastic placenta from an elastic uterus due to a shearing, deceleration force. There may be little or no external evidence of such a mechanism. Classically, the clinical findings of abruption have included vaginal bleeding and abominal and uterine tenderness. Unfortunately, in a large number of cases, fetal distress may be the only presenting sign, as the reduction in placental blood flow to the fetus causes hypoxia and acidosis. A consumptive coagulopathy may occur with placental injury, and evaluation for DIC should be performed in all instances of suspected abruption.

8. How often does ultrasound detect cases of placental abruption?

Because a large separation must be present in order for the ultrasound to be diagnostic, it detects only about half of cases. In many instances, fetal distress is present prior to the clear visualization of an abruption by ultrasound. Fetal mortality from abruption is as high as 35% in some tertiary care centers. Usually, an abruption large enough to place the fetus at risk will declare itself within 48 hours. Detection of fetal distress mandates prompt delivery of the fetus.

9. Are radiologic investigations harmful to the fetus?

Fetal organs are maximally sensitive to radiation under 8 weeks of gestational age. Growth retardation and susceptibility to malignant change can be seen at later gestational ages. Most authorities would agree that a radiation dose of under 5–10 rads carries no significant fetal risk. For instance, the pelvic radiation dose of a chest radiograph is 3 mrads and a view of the cervical spine is <1 mrad, whereas CT of the head results in a dose of <1 rad. However, a pelvic CT scan may carry a radiation dose as high as 9 rads. In general, all radiographic studies should be undertaken with appropriate fetal shielding. However, clinically indicated studies (e.g., pelvis and lumbar spine studies) should be performed. Consideration should also be given to nonradiographic alternative evaluations such as diagnostic peritoneal lavage (DPL) and ultrasonography.

10. How should these patients be managed in the field?

Given the reduced maternal oxygen reserve, oxygen therapy is of critical importance. Intravenous volume resuscitation with crystalloid and blood should proceed as with other trauma patients. Avoid compression of the inferior vena cava by transporting the patient on her left side, or if the patient is immobilized, elevate the right side of the backboard to 15 or 20 degrees.

In the later gestational ages, inflation of the abdominal compartment of the military antishock trousers (MAST) is contraindicated because this may reduce venous return and cardiac output by uterine compression of the inferior vena cava. Aside from early transport, the most important aspect of prehospital management is to notify the ED so that the appropriate obstetric consultants may participate on the trauma team.

11. How do I begin to evaluate the fetus?

First, determine the size of the uterus and the presence of abdominal and uterine tenderness. Uterine size, measured in centimeters from the pubic symphysis to fundus, provides a rough estimate of gestational age and potential viability. Carefully, inspect the vaginal introitus for evidence of vaginal bleeding. Next, assess for fetal distress, which may be the earliest indication of maternal hypovolemia. Abnormal fetal heart rates are those >160 and <110 beats per minute. Continuous fetal monitoring should be performed to ascertain early signs of fetal distress (e.g., decreased variability of heart rate or fetal decelerations after contractions). Ultrasound should be performed as soon as possible to confirm gestational age, fetal viability, and the integrity of the placenta.

12. Is DPL safe and accurate in pregnant women?

DPL has been reported to be both safe and accurate when using an open, supraumbilical technique. Although the cell count thresholds and clinical indications for DPL are the same, the physiologic changes that take place with pregnancy and the elimination of radiation exposure from abdominal CT provide persuasive arguments for aggressive use of DPL as a diagnostic tool.

13. What is fetomaternal hemorrhage (FMH)?

This is the hemorrhage of fetal blood into usually distinct maternal circulation. The incidence of FMH in trauma patients has been reported to be as high as 30%. With FMH, the complications of maternal Rh sensitization, fetal anemia, and fetal death can occur. Unfortunately, laboratory techniques are not sensitive enough to diagnose FMH accurately. The prudent course is to give Rh immune globulin to all Rh-negative patients who present with the suspicion of abdominal trauma since a 300-μg dose of Rh immune globulin given within 72 hours of antigenic exposure prevents Rh isoimmunization.

14. When is cesarean section indicated?

The first factor to be considered is the stability of the mother. If the mother has sustained serious injuries elsewhere and is critically ill, then the mother may not be able to tolerate an additional procedure and the blood loss it will entail. Next, fetuses whose gestational age is above 24–26 weeks or whose weight is estimated to be over 750 gm are predicted to have a 50% survival rate in the neonatal ICU setting, and are considered viable. The most common indication for cesarean section is fetal distress. Other indications are uterine rupture and malpresentation of the fetus. Postmortem cesarean section should be performed when uterine size suggests viability (i.e., above the umbilicus) and evidence of fetal life is confirmed by Doppler or ultrasound.

15. Which pregnant patients with abdominal trauma require admission for fetal monitoring?

Any viable fetus requires monitoring. Monitoring is recommended even for patients without external evidence of trauma because it has been well documented that these patients are at risk from placental abruption. One prospective study advised that these patients be observed for a minimum of 4 hours with a cardiotocograph. If any abnormalities were discovered, the observation period was extended to 24 hours.

BIBLIOGRAPHY

1. Drost TF, Rosemurgy AS, et al: Major trauma in pregnant women: Maternal/fetal outcome. J Trauma 30:574, 1990.
2. Neufeld JD, Marx JA: Trauma in pregnancy. In Rosen P, et al (eds): Emergency Medicine: Concepts and Clinical Practice, 3rd ed. St. Louis, Mosby–Year Book, 1992.

3. McFarlane J, Parker B, et al: Assessing for abuse during pregnancy. Severity and frequency of injuries and associated entry into prenatal care. JAMA 267:3176, 1992.
4. Pearlman MD, Tintinalli JE, Lorenz RP: Blunt trauma during pregnancy. N Engl J Med 323:1609, 1990.
5. Pearlman MD, Tintinalli JE, Lorenz RP: A prospective, controlled study of outcome after trauma during pregnancy. Am J Obstet Gynecol 162:1502, 1990.
6. Pimental L: Mother and child: Trauma in pregnancy. Emerg Med Clin North Am 9:549, 1991.
7. Rothenberger DA, Quattlebaum FW, et al: Diagnostic peritoneal lavage for blunt trauma in pregnant women. Am J Obstet Gynecol 129:479, 1977.
8. Satin AJ, Hemsell DL, et al: Sexual assault in pregnancy. Obstet Gynecol 77:710, 1991.
9. Scorpio RJ, Esposito TJ, et al: Blunt trauma during pregnancy: Factors affecting fetal outcome. J Trauma 32:213, 1992.
10. Sherman HF, Scott LM, Rosemurgy AS: Changes affecting the initial evaluation and care of the pregnant trauma victim. J Emerg Med 8:575, 1990.
11. Williams JK, McClain L, Rosemurgy AS: Evaluation of blunt abdominal trauma in the third trimester of pregnancy. Obstet Gynecol 75:33, 1990.

106. EXTREMITY TRAUMA

Peter O. Fried, M.D., and Bernard J. Feldman, M.D.

1. What is a "stress" or "fatigue" fracture?
Stress fractures are caused by repetitive small forces, any one of which is not sufficient to cause a fracture, but the repeated loading of a bone ultimately results in fracture. A good descriptive analogy would be the repetitive bending of a paper clip, back and forth, until it eventually breaks. Stress or fatigue fractures commonly involve the metatarsal shafts, the distal tibia, and the femoral neck.

2. Why is a fracture sometimes more visible on x-ray 10–14 days after injury?
Undisplaced/impacted fractures (e.g., carpal scaphoid, ribs, etc.) are frequently not apparent on initial x-rays. In the initial stage of fracture healing, specialized cells (osteoclasts) debride (phagocytize) the devitalized edges of fracture, and thus a lucency at the fracture line can be appreciated at 10–14 days.

3. What should be done with an amputated part that may be reimplanted?
1. Wrap the part in a sterile dressing.
2. Insert the wrapped part in a plastic bag.
3. Place the plastic bag into a container with ice.

4. Which bones are most prone to avascular necrosis?
The proximal one-half of the carpal scaphoid and the femoral head often undergo avascular necrosis following injury as a result of the precarious blood supply to these bones.

5. What are the key factors that contribute to joint stability?
Joint stability depends upon the reciprocal contours of the articulating joint surfaces, the integrity of the fibrous joint capsule and the associated ligaments, and the protective power of the muscles that move the joint.

6. What are the immediate treatment priorities in an open fracture?
Open fractures are orthopedic emergencies. Any break in the skin near a fracture site should be assumed to communicate with the fracture until proved otherwise. Immediate

care includes assessment for neurovascular damage, application of sterile pressure dressings to control hemorrhage if needed, splinting, irrigation, use of Betadine dressings to cover the wound, culture of the wound site, early institution of intravenous antibiotic (cephalosporins are most commonly used), tetanus prophylaxis, and immediate consultation with an orthopedic surgeon.

7. Which associated injuries may be present with a scapular fracture?
Considerable force is required to fracture the scapula. These fractures are frequently associated with underlying rib fractures and pulmonary contusions.

8. What are the incidence and common causes of posterior shoulder dislocation?
Only 5% of shoulder dislocations are posterior. Tonoclonic seizures, electric shock, and direct anterior trauma tend to cause posterior shoulder dislocations.

9. How is a rotator cuff tear diagnosed?
If a fall on or against the shoulder occurs, particularly in a patient >40 years of age, traumatic tears of the rotator cuff can occur, which interfere with the initiation and the power of abduction. After complete rupture, the patient cannot voluntarily perform the first 15 degrees of abduction. The strength of abduction is inversely proportional to the extent of the tear. Pain and localized tenderness are usually located over the greater tuberosity of the humerus. Following local anesthetic injection and elimination of pain, initiation of active abduction remains absent.

10. Describe the difference between anterior and posterior dislocation of a sternoclavicular (SC) joint.
Anterior dislocations are not associated with major complications and are easily treated with a clavicle strap. Posterior dislocation of the SC joint may put pressure on the trachea, esophagus, or great vessels, and thus constitutes a true emergency that requires reduction.

11. What neurologic deficit is most likely to be seen with a humeral shaft fracture?
The radial nerve may be stretched (neurapraxia) or lacerated (rare). Disability includes inability to extend the wrist and fingers at the MCP joints. Numbness occurs on the dorsum of the radial side of the hand. Interphalangeal joint extension is preserved because it is an intrinsic muscle function that is dependent upon intact ulnar and median nerve function.

12. What do Monteggia and Galeazzi fractures have in common?
A fracture of the proximal one-third of the ulna with a radial head dislocation, usually anterior, constitutes a Monteggia fracture. A radial shaft fracture with a dislocation of the distal radioulnar joint is a Galeazzi fracture. Both frequently are reducible but typically require internal fixation to maintain reduction.

13. What are the major complications directly related to pelvic fractures?
The two major complications are hemorrhage and urologic injuries.

14. What are the major management considerations of hemorrhage in patients with pelvic fractures?
Pelvic fractures can result in significant, even fatal, hemorrhage, especially unstable (type III) fractures. Aggressive administration of crystalloid and blood is required. Stabilization of the fracture fragments by early temporizing use of military antishock trousers (MAST), followed by external fixation, may be required. Continued hypovolemic shock, unassociated with other injury, may signal continued bleeding from the superior gluteal or pudendal artery. Arteriography with embolization or laparotomy may need to be considered, even though both are often unsuccessful in controlling bleeding.

15. What is the incidence and mechanism of injury of posterior hip dislocation?
Over 80% of hip dislocations are posterior and result from a posteriorly directed force applied to a flexed knee, as occurs when the knee hits the dashboard in a motor vehicle accident.

16. What are the complications of posterior hip dislocation?
Sciatic nerve deficit is found in about 10% of patients with a posterior hip dislocation. Avascular necrosis of the femoral head is directly related to the length of time the hip remains unreduced.

17. How is posterior hip dislocation differentiated clinically from a femoral neck fracture?
Fracture and dislocation both result in lower extremity shortening. In posterior dislocation, the hip is adducted and internally rotated. In a fracture, it is abducted and externally rotated.

18. What other injury should be suspecteed in an elderly patient who has fallen and presents with knee pain?
A patient may experience pain in the anterior aspect of the distal thigh and medial aspect of the knee from hip problems. The exact mechanism for this relationship is not well understood; however, the hip and knee joints share common innervation through the obturator nerve. When elderly patients fall, always suspect a hip problem, even if the patient complains exclusively about the knee.

19. What is a "locked knee"? What are the two most common causes?
Locking of the knee joint involves the inability of the patient to actively or passively extend the knee, which has usually become locked in 10–45 degrees of flexion. True locking occurs suddenly, and unlocking takes place with equal abruptness. The two most common causes are a tear of the medial meniscus and a loose body or "joint mouse" (osteochondral fragment) in the knee.

20. What other injuries are associated with a calcaneal fracture?
Because axial forces are transmitted from the lower extremities to the spine, this mechanism of injury may be associated with compression fractures of lumbar or lower dorsal vertebrae, which may be unstable.

21. What is a "torus" or "buckle" fracture?
Torus means "round swelling" or "protuberance." In children, compression fracture of the cancellous bone of the metaphysis may merely buckle, but not fracture, the overlying cortex, producing a torus fracture.

22. What is a greenstick fracture?
Children's bones have increased elasticity. A greenstick fracture is caused by an angular force applied to a long bone of a child, resulting in bowing of one side of the cortex and fracture of the other. Completion of the fracture is necessitated in proper treatment of these fractures.

23. What is the Salter-Harris classification? What is its clinical significance?
The Salter-Harris (SH) classification is a method of classifying epiphyseal injuries. Any epiphyseal injury may result in growth disturbance, and parents must be informed of this potential. Fortunately about 80% of these injuries are SH I and II, both of which have a low complication rate. SH III, IV, and V injuries have a poorer prognosis. Displaced type III and IV fractures may require open reduction to restore the normal relationship of the epiphysis and articular surface.

Salter-Harris Classification

	DESCRIPTION	DIAGRAM
Type I	Fracture extends through the epiphyseal plate, resulting in displacement of the epiphysis (this may appear merely as widening of the radiolucent area representing the growth plate)	
Type II	As above, in addition, a triangular segment of metaphysis is fractured	
Type III	Fracture line runs from the joint surface through epiphyseal plate and epiphysis	
Type IV	Fracture line also occurs in Type III but also passes through adjacent metaphysis	
Type V	This is a crush injury of the epiphysis; it may be difficult to determine by x-ray examination	

24. Describe the difference in treatment of displaced and nondisplaced supracondylar fractures?

As long as the elbow can be flexed so as to prevent further displacement, nondisplaced supracondylar fractures can be treated on an outpatient basis with a posterior mold and frequent neurovascular checks. Displaced supracondylar fractures require reduction, admission, and the use of traction to maintain the position of the fragments.

25. What is "nursemaid's elbow"? What is its management?

A longitudinal pull on the elbow of a 1–5-year-old may result in a subluxation of the cartilaginous radial head, or nursemaid's elbow. The child typically presents with pseudoparalysis of the injured extremity. X-rays are usually negative. Reduction involves gently supinating the forearm and flexing the elbow. A distinct click over the radial head is usually appreciated. The child often begins to use the extremity normally within a few minutes.

26. Which nontraumatic hip disorders cause a limp in a child?

Although all of the causes are uncommon, they include septic arthritis, transient synovitis (ages 2–12), idiopathic avascular necrosis (males, ages 5–9), and slipped capital femoral epiphysis (males, ages 10–16). Transient synovitis is probably the most common nontraumatic cause of painful limp in a child.

27. What are the early lateral radiographic findings of a slipped capital femoral epiphysis (SCFE)?

Any asymmetry of the relationship of the femoral head to the femoral neck should raise the suspicion of SCFE, even if it is evident on only one x-ray view. If AP and lateral films are normal, frog-leg views should be obtained. Comparison of the two hips may not always be helpful in discerning subtle differences because SCFE occurs bilaterally over 20% of the time.

28. What is the ED management of a child with injury and bone tenderness adjacent to an epiphysis, which is still open, and who has a "normal" x-ray?

It is best to assume that the child has sustained an undeterminable fracture of the physis (SH I or V). Immobilize the joint with a posterior mold and keep the patient nonweight-bearing if the lower extremity is involved. Parents should be notified of the possibility of this type of injury and the potential for growth disturbance. The need for prompt follow-up is emphasized.

29. What vascular injury must be considered with a knee dislocation (tibiofemoral)?

A posterior dislocation of the knee is especially likely to injure or compress the popliteal artery. Strong consideration should be given to postreduction angiography.

30. What are the symptoms and signs of limb ischemia following injury?

Limb ischemia is indicated by the five "P's": pain, pallor, paresthesias, pulselessness, and paralysis.

31. What are the most common sites of compartment syndrome?

Extremity injury may increase the pressure within a fascial compartment enough to compromise circulation to muscle and nerve tissue within that compartment. The most common sites of involvement are the volar compartment of the forearm and the anterior tibial compartment of the leg. Supracondylar fractures of the humerus in children, and both bone forearm fractures, are the injuries most commonly associated with this process in the upper extremity. Proximal tibial fractures are the most common cause of compartment syndrome in the leg. Crush injuries without fracture (i.e., "wringer injuries"), animal bites, burns, excessive pressure from tight casts, dressings, or elastic wraps, and prolonged use of the MAST suit have also been associated with compartment syndrome.

BIBLIOGRAPHY

1. Hamilton GC, Sanders AB, Strange GB, Trott AT (eds): Emergency Medicine: An Approach to Clinical Problem Solving. Philadelphia, W.B. Saunders, 1991.
2. Kennington RT, Dwyer BJ: Avoiding misdiagnosis with pediatric arm injuries. Emerg Med Rep 11:189–200, 1990.
3. Korkal SS, Waekerle JF (eds): Pelvic fractures: Prompt recognition and appropriate early management. Emerg Med Rep 10:57–64, 1989.
4. Miller MD: Commonly missed orthopedic problems. Emerg Med Clin North Am 10:151–161, 1992.
5. Tintinalli JE, Krome RL, Ruiz E (eds): Emergency Medicine: A Comprehensive Study Guide. New York, McGraw-Hill, 1992.

107. HAND INJURIES AND INFECTIONS

Michael A. Kohn, M.D.

1. Are hand problems important in emergency medicine?

Yes! More than 16 million hand injuries occur annually in the U.S., most of which initially present to emergency departments (EDs). More than 30% of all industrial accidents involve the hand. Hand injuries account for 75% of all partially disabling injuries.

2. What are the essential elements of the history?

Age; dominant hand; occupation; how, where, and when injury occurred; posture of hand when injured; tetanus status; and prior injury or disability of the hand.

3. What are the elements of a complete hand exam?

Initial inspection of skin and soft tissue; vascular exam; evaluation of tendon function; nerve exam (motor and sensory); and skeletal exam.

4. What is "topographical anticipation"?

Topographical anticipation involves looking at the skin wound and thinking about which underlying structure (vessel, tendon, nerve, bone, ligament, or joint) could be injured. Know the anatomy. Do not hesitate to consult an atlas.

5. What is the normal posture of the hand at rest?

With the wrist in slight extension, the resting fingers normally assume a "cascade," progressively more flexed from index to small. (See this by relaxing your own hand with the wrist in slight extension.) An alteration in the normal posture can lead to immediate diagnosis of major tendon and joint injuries.

6. Does dorsal swelling signify an injury or infection in the dorsum of the hand?

Not necessarily. Most of the palmar lymphatics drain to lymph channels and lacunae located in the loose areolar layer on the dorsum of the hand. Always check for a palmar wound when a patient presents with dorsal swelling.

7. What is the Allen test? How is it performed?

The Allen test verifies patency of the radial and ulnar arteries as follows: occlude both radial and ulnar arteries. Have patient open and close hand 5 or 6 times. Hand should blanch. Release ulnar artery; blanching should resolve within 3–5 seconds. Repeat test, releasing radial artery instead of ulnar artery. Again, blanching should resolve within 3–5 seconds. The most accurate form of the Allen test uses digital blood pressures rather than return of color to monitor reperfusion.

8. How is function of the flexor digitorum superficialis (FDS) tendon tested?

The FDS inserts on the middle phalanx and flexes the proximal interphalangeal (PIP) joint. The flexor digitorum profundus (FDP) inserts on the distal phalanx and flexes both the PIP and distal interphalangeal (DIP) joints. The FDS muscle-tendon units should be independent of one another, whereas the FDP tendons arise from a common muscle belly. Testing the FDS of a finger entails flexing it at the PIP while stabilizing the other three fingers in full extension, thereby taking the FDP out of action as a potential flexor of the PIP joint.

9. In which finger is the test of FDS function unreliable?

Because the FDP to the index finger can be independent of the other profundi, the FDS test is unreliable in the index finger. Flexion at the PIP may be due to the FDP, even with the other fingers stabilized in extension. Suspected index finger FDS injuries must be explored.

10. Why is the flexor or palmar aspect of the hand called the "OR side," whereas the extensor or dorsal aspect is the "ER side"?
Unlike the extensors, the flexor tendons run through delicate sheaths. Because of these sheaths, repairing flexor tendons requires more expertise and a more controlled environment than repairing extensor tendons.

11. How is partial tendon laceration diagnosed?
If the location of the skin laceration is suspicious, rule out an underlying partial tendon laceration by exploration and direct visualization under tourniquet hemostasis. Because a flexor tendon runs through its sheath like a piston through a cylinder, a sheath laceration implies a partial tendon laceration, which will be visible only when the hand is in the same posture as when injured.

12. How do I test the extrinsic extensor tendons?
The extrinsic extensors alone extend the MCP joints, whereas they combine with tendons from the interossei and lumbricals to form the extensor mechanism that extends the IP joints. To test the extrinsic extensor, lay the hand, palm down, on a flat surface and ask the patient to elevate the digit.

13. Can extensor function to a finger be intact despite complete laceration of the extensor digitorum communis (EDC) to that finger?
Yes! The juncturae tendinum interlink the EDC tendons at the mid-metacarpal level. Even if the EDC to a finger is completely lacerated in the dorsum of the hand, extension at the MCP may still be possible because of the junctura.

14. How do I test sensory nerve function?
Assess nerve function prior to the use of anesthesia. Test digital nerves by checking 2-point discrimination on the volar pad. The two points should be 5 mm apart and aligned longitudinally.

15. What are the sensory distributions of the median, ulnar, and radial nerves?

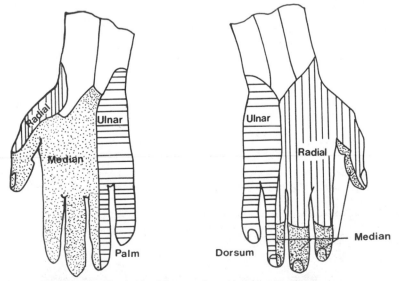

Sensory distributions of the median, ulnar, and radial nerves.

16. How is motor function of the median, ulnar and radial nerves tested?

Median: Abductor pollicis brevis (APB)—abduct the thumb against resistance while palpating the APB muscle belly.

Ulnar: First dorsal interosseous—abduct the index finger against resistance.

Radial: (No intrinsics) Extensor pollicis longus (EPL)—extend the thumb IP against resistance.

17. Which is the most frequently dislocated carpal bone?

The carpal bones are:

　　Proximal row—scaphoid, lunate, triquetrum, pisiform

　　Distal row—trapezium, trapezoid, capitate, hamate.

The lunate is most frequently dislocated. Its blood supply comes through the volar and dorsal ligaments from the radius. If both ligaments are ruptured, avascular necrosis results.

18. Which is the most frequently fractured carpal bone?

The scaphoid. Its distal blood supply increases the likelihood of avascular necrosis in the proximal segment after fracture.

19. What is the classic sign of a scaphoid fracture?

Snuffbox tenderness. Even without radiographic evidence of a fracture, the patient with tenderness on palpation of the anatomic snuffbox gets a thumb spica splint and a repeat x-ray in 2 weeks.

20. How do I control hemorrhage from a hand injury?

Direct pressure and elevation should control hemorrhage from the hand. Rarely, an incomplete arterial laceration requires a proximal tourniquet for temporary control, followed by sensory exam, anesthesia, scrub, and exploration under good light and magnification to tie off the bleeder. **Never blindly clamp a bleeder.**

21. Why the rule, "no blind clamping of bleeders"?

In the hand, the arteries run in close approximation to the nerves. Blindly clamping an artery may irreparably damage the associated nerve. Also, the clamp may damage a section of vessel vital to successful reanastomosis.

22. What should be done with an amputated digit?

Gently clean with sterile saline, wrap in moist gauze, place in sterile container, float container in ice water. (Avoid direct contact between ice and tissue to prevent freezing.)

23. What should be done with a devascularized but still partially attached digit?

Leave part attached (preserves veins for reimplantation), gently wrap in moist gauze, and apply a bulky dressing.

24. What are the indications and contraindications for reimplantation?

Indications: multiple finger injury, thumb amputations (especially proximal to IP joint), single finger injury in children, clean amputation at hand, wrist, or distal forearm. (A clean amputation at the wrist is easier to reimplant than multiple-digit amputations.)

Contraindications: severe crush or avulsion, heavy contamination, single-finger amputations in adults, severe associated medical problems or injuries, severe multilevel injury of amputated part, willful self-amputation.

Bottom line: Give the hand surgeon the opportunity to decide.

25. Which are the most deceptive of all serious hand injuries?
High-pressure injection injuries (from paint guns, grease guns, or hydraulic lines) may initially seem innocuous, often involving just the fingertip. However, in some reported series, 70% of such injuries resulted in some form of amputation and an average of 7 months lost work time, even with early radical treatment.

26. What are Kanavel's four cardinal signs of flexor tenosynovitis?
(1) Slightly flexed posture of digit. (2) Uniform swelling. (3) Pain on passive extension. (4) Tenderness along flexor tendon sheath. (Flexor tenosynovitis requires admission and surgery.)

27. What is a paronychia? How is it treated?
A paronychia is a common bacterial infection involving the folds of skin that hold the fingernail in place. In the absence of visible pus, treatment should consist of warm moist compresses, elevation, and antistaphylococcal antibiotics. If pus is present, do the minimum necessary to drain and maintain drainage. This usually consists of simply elevating the eponychial fold or making a small incision. Bilateral paronychia indicates subungual pus and necessitates removal of the proximal part of the nail plate.

28. How is whitlow different from a paronychia?
Whitlow is infection of the tissue around the nail plate with herpes simplex virus (rather than bacteria). The discharge is serous and crusting rather than purulent. The patient may also have perioral cold sores. Do not incise and drain herpetic whitlow.

29. What is a felon? How is it treated?
A felon is a painful and potentially disabling infection of the fingertip pulp. Treatment is controversial. Some clinicians argue for immediate drainage of the tensely swollen and painful fingertip pad. Others argue that early treatment with antibiotics, elevation, and immobilization may prevent the need for surgical drainage. Even if drainage is necessary, the best method is also a matter of controversy. Recommendations include the full fishmouth incision, the three-quarters fishmouth incision, and the simple lateral incision. Perhaps the wisest treatment is to start antistaphylococcal antibiotics, elevate, immobilize, and refer to a hand surgeon the next day.

30. What is a football jersey finger? How is it treated?
Rupture of the flexor digitorum profundus occurs commonly when a football player catches his finger in an opponent's jersey. The tendon is avulsed from its insertion at the palmar base of the distal phalanx, often taking a bone fragment along. Surgical repair within the next several days is indicated.

31. What is a mallet finger? How is it treated?
A mallet finger is the opposite of a football jersey finger; the insertion of the extensor tendon, rather than the flexor tendon, is avulsed from the dorsum of the distal phalanx, often pulling off a bone fragment. Appropriate treatment is to splint the DIP joint in extension (not hyperextension) for 6 weeks.

32. Describe a subungual hematoma. How is it treated?
A collection of blood under the nail plate can be very painful. Classically, this occurs when a weekend carpenter strikes his thumb with a hammer. Relieving the pressure by nail trephinization (poking a hole in the nail) will make you a hero to the patient. Use electrocautery, a red hot paperclip, or an 18-gauge needle (twisting it between your fingers like a drill bit). Removal of an intact nail plate is almost never indicated.

33. What is a gamekeeper's thumb?

A gamekeeper's thumb is a torn ulnar collateral ligament of the thumb metacarpophalangeal (MCP) joint. In 1955 Cambell reported the injury in 24 Scottish game wardens, arising from their technique for breaking the necks of wounded rabbits. The injury is more properly called skier's thumb because it most commonly occurs when a skier either catches the thumb on a planted ski pole or falls while holding a pole in the outstretched hand. The injury is potentially severely disabling. Complete rupture of the ligament always requires surgery. However, ED treatment consists of a thumb spica splint and referral.

34. What is a boxer's fracture?

Fracture of the fifth (small finger) metacarpal is common in barefisted pugilists. Because the small finger metacarpal is second only to the thumb metacarpal in mobility, large angles of angulation are tolerated without functional deficit. Nevertheless, attempts to correct significant angulation of an acute boxer's fracture are warranted. Any rotational deformity must be corrected. A laceration accompanying a boxer's fracture is assumed to be a fight bite.

CONTROVERSIES

35. What is a fight bite?

The most notorious of all nonvenomous bite wounds is the fight bite. As the name implies, this injury occurs when the soon-to-be patient punches his adversary in the teeth, lacerating the dorsum of one or more MCP joints. Other names for this injury, such as "morsus humanus" or "closed fist injury (CFI)," have been proposed. However, "fight bite" is more compact, descriptive, and poetic. All such wounds require formal exploration, including extension of the skin laceration if necessary. They should be debrided, irrigated, dressed open (no sutures), and splinted.

36. Are human bites more dangerous than other animal bites?

Not really. The fight bite gave human bites their reputation for being more prone to infection than other animal bites. This probably has more to do with the location of the bite and the typical delay in treatment than with the mix of organisms in the human mouth. True human bites (occlusive bites rather than fight bites) have no higher infection rates than animal bites. If humans punched animals in the teeth, these animal fight bites would have high infection rates also.

37. Should persons with uninfected fight bites be treated on an outpatient basis?

For:

  1. Admitting every person with a fight bite, without evidence of infection, is extremely expensive.

  2. Two studies [Peeples (1980) and Zubowicz (1992)] support outpatient management with oral antibiotics of reliable patients who present within 12 hours (Peeples) or 24 hours (Zubowicz) of the injury.

Against:

  1. Treating a septic joint is more expensive both in terms of hospital costs and patient disability costs than admitting a person with an uninfected fight bite for IV antibiotics.

  2. All studies on the subject include both fight bites and true occlusive bites to the hand, thereby confusing the issue.

  3. Fight-bite patients are notoriously unreliable and poor candidates for outpatient management.

Addendum: No controversy exists regarding patients with *infected* fight bites: all are admitted.

BIBLIOGRAPHY

1. American Society for Surgery of the Hand: The Hand: Examination and Diagnosis. "Blue Book" (3rd ed). New York, Churchill Livingstone, 1990.
2. American Society for Surgery of the Hand: The Hand: Primary Care of Common Problems. "Red Book" (2nd ed). New York, Churchill Livingstone, 1985.
3. Cambell CS: Gamekeeper's thumb. J Bone Joint Surg 37B:148–149, 1955.
4. Carter PR: Common Hand Injuries and Infections: A Practical Approach to Early Treatment. Philadelphia, W.B. Saunders, 1983.
5. Kanavel AB: Infection of the Hand. Philadelphia, Lea & Febiger, 1925.
6. Lammers RL, Freemyer BC: Hand. In Rosen P, et al (eds): Emergency Medicine: Concepts and Clinical Practice, 3rd ed. St. Louis, Mosby–Year Book, 1983.
7. Lampe EW (with ill. by F Netter): Surgical Anatomy of the Hand. Clin Symp 40:3, 1988.
8. Peeples E, Boswick JA, Scott FA: Wounds of the hand contaminated by human and animal saliva. J Trauma 20:383, 1980.
9. Szabo RM (ed): Common hand problems. Orthop Clin North Am 23:1, 1992.
10. Welch C: Human bite infections of the hand. N Engl J Med 215:901, 1936.
11. Zubowicz VN, Gravier M: Management of early human bites of the hand: A prospective randomized study. Plast Reconstr Surg 88:111–114, 1991.

108. BURNS

Jeffrey S. Hill, M.D.

1. What types of burns are commonly seen in the emergency department (ED)?

Direct thermal injuries are undoubtedly most common, although solar (i.e., sunburn), chemical, electrical, and radiation are other major sources of burn injury.

2. How should thermal burns be assessed initially in the ED?

Rapid assessment of the type of and severity of burn injury is key. The most important factors to evaluate include severity (estimated depth of injury), body surface area (BSA), and location. Other important factors are associated injuries and coexisting or preexisting medical conditions.

3. So where do I start?

Do a physical exam. Severity is most easily estimated in this way. First-degree burns (those involving only the superficial layers of the skin) are erythematous and painful. Second-degree (read "partial thickness") burns extend to the deeper layers of the dermis and can have a varied appearance. Erythema or mottled skin, often with blistering or a wet shiny surface, is often present; however, deeper partial-thickness burns can be pale and colorless. These burns are extremely and exquisitely painful. Third-degree burn injuries look like what they are: dead tissue. Here the burn extends through all the dermal layers and the skin may appear translucent to off-color to frankly charred. Importantly, these areas are insensate.

4. What is body surface area (BSA)? Why is it important?

It is a rapid means of estimating the extent of injury in a relatively simple and commonly recognized format. It is a means of quantifying the injury and has important clinical and prognostic implications. The "rule of nines" is the most widely employed topographic measurement, and divides the regions of the body into approximate percentages of total surface area. These percentages differ between adults and children, and the differences are noteworthy.

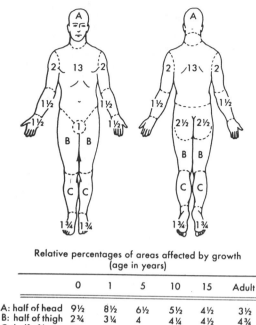

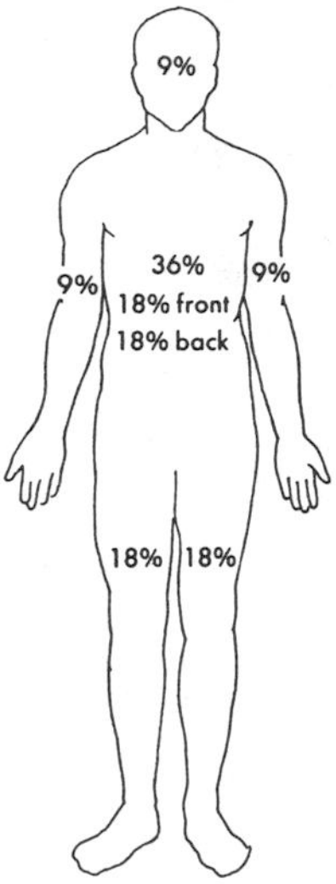

Above left, Percentages used in determining extent of burn by "rule of nines" (From Miller RH: Textbook of Basic Emergency Medicine, 2nd ed. St. Louis, Mosby–Year Book, 1980, with permission.)

Relative percentages of areas affected by growth (age in years)

	0	1	5	10	15	Adult
A: half of head	9½	8½	6½	5½	4½	3½
B: half of thigh	2¾	3¼	4	4¼	4½	4¾
C: half of leg	2½	2½	2¾	3	3¼	3½

Second degree _____ and Third degree _____ =
Total percent burned ____

Above right, Classic Lund and Browder chart. The best method for determining percentage of body surface burn is to mark areas of injury on a chart and then compute total percentage according to patient's age. (From Artz CP, Yarbrough DR III: Burns: Including cold, chemical, and electrical injuries. In Sabiston DC Jr (ed): Textbook of Surgery, 11th ed. Philadelphia, W.B. Saunders, 1977, with permission.)

5. What are the indications for surgical consultation?

Any significant burn (second degree or greater) involving the face, neck, hands, feet, or perineum mandates surgical consultation and, at a minimum, surgical follow-up. These vital regions are of special importance, as significant burn injury may be complicated by swelling or edema, which can lead to neurovascular or airway compromise. Surgical consultation should be sought immediately for any patient with a potentially life-threatening burn injury, preferably a surgeon familiar with the care of burn patients. Particular burns may require immediate surgical intervention. Specifically, circumferential burns of the neck are a true emergency, as rapid progression to airway compromise can develop. Aggressive airway management is mandatory. Circumferential burns of the extremities are also an emergency, as the neurovascular supply to the areas distal to the burn site can be impaired, and, as edema develops, tissue ischemia and frank compartment syndrome may develop. Early surgical intervention (escharotomy) may be limb-saving.

6. What are the criteria for admission?

General admission criteria state any infant or child with >10% BSA burn or any adult with >25% BSA burn must be hospitalized, but realistically these are loose guidelines at best and must be viewed in context with all other relevant clinical and social issues.

7. Are there special considerations in children?

Absolutely. The approach to the burned child must be as thorough and aggressive as for an adult, but consideration of nonaccidental trauma, conditions surrounding the home and social situation, and reliability of the parents must be considered before releasing any child with a minor to moderate burn for outpatient care. Burn patients at the extremes of age are at greater risk for morbidity and mortality, and children and infants less than 2 years of age with a major burn require hospitalization.

8. Are there similar modifiers for adults?

Victims at the extremes of age with major burns have greater morbidity, and burn victims greater than 60 years generally do poorly. Similarly, patients with underlying disease or debilitation should be approached with respect. Alcoholism, HIV illness or other causes of immunocompromise, diabetes, malignancy, cardiovascular or pulmonary impairment, etc. also require more aggressive inpatient care.

9. How are superficial thermal burn injuries treated?

First-degree burns. Care for first-degree burns is generally supportive; they usually heal quickly without scarring. Application of cool water or saline, adequate analgesia, and follow-up with one's primary physician as needed are reasonable. For sunburn, addition of an antihistamine may be helpful for associated swelling or edema (as occurs on the face). A short course of oral steroids may also be beneficial, although efficacy of this regimen has not been rigorously evaluated.

Second-degree burns. These burns are more complex and require more meticulous evaluation and care. After excluding any life- or limb-threatening injury, the burn should be gently cleansed with a mild antiseptic solution. When intact blisters are encountered, it is generally recommended they be left intact (controversial). Swain demonstrated that patients whose blisters were left intact had a lower incidence of bacterial colonization with microorganisms and less pain. Controversy also exists as to whether ruptured blisters should be debrided. If the ruptured blisters are debrided, the free, devitalized dermis is excised sharply. Outpatient care follows the usual tenets of basic wound care. Topical antibiotics should be applied liberally to the affected area. Silvadine may affect pigmentation of healing tissue and should be used with caution on the face. Interestingly, one study from India showed raw, unrefined honey to be an excellent covering for such wounds. A nonadhesive dressing and bulky bandage are then applied. If a joint surface is crossed, immobilization is appropriate. Aggressive pain control and follow-up in 24–48 hours for dressing change and reexamination are mandatory either in the ED or by a physician familiar with burn care.

10. What is artificial skin?

Skin substitutes (such as Biobrane) have been employed in burn units successfully as an alternative covering for burned regions of the body. Such coverings have advantages in terms of greater comfort, decreased rates of infection, and cost effectiveness. They may become a useful adjunctive therapy in the outpatient management of burns.

11. How about a potentially life-threatening burn?

The approach to a seriously burned patient should be appropriately aggressive and thorough. The basic tenets of patient care (the ABCs) must be strictly followed. Attention to airway management and respiratory support is essential. Establishment of adequate IV access is required (yes, you can place an angiocath through burned tissue if absolutely necessary). Because of the hemodynamic instability that may develop with major burns, central monitoring (including Swan-Ganz) is often used after the patient reaches the ICU. In the ED, central venous access is appropriate if indicated. Always consider conditions or circumstances that may have *contributed to* or *followed* the burn itself (e.g., toxic ingestion or exposure, alcohol, metabolic derangement, cardiovascular or CNS pathology). Remember, all patients who sustain a major burn are assumed to have carbon monoxide poisoning until proved otherwise.

12. What are the priorities in patients who have both multisystem trauma and burns?

In polytraumatized patients with major burn injuries, the traumatic injuries are a major contributor to death. Any patient who sustains traumatic injuries concomitantly with the infliction of the burn needs prompt resuscitation, with attention to life-threatening traumatic injuries taking priority. A trauma surgeon should be consulted.

13. What about thermal injury to the airway?

The physiologic mechanisms of cooling inspired air are remarkably efficient. With the exception of steam inhalation injuries, direct thermal injury to the subglottic structures is uncommon. Unfortunately, it is therefore the glottic and supraglottic structures that take the brunt of thermal inhalation injuries. There is little in the way of protective measures in the upper airway, and the most immediate life threat comes in the form of tissue edema in the hypopharynx. Aggressive airway management is the rule.

14. What other concerns must be kept in mind regarding smoke inhalation injuries?

Depending on the materials involved during combustion, additional toxic exposures may be sustained. These can be either local (i.e., pulmonary) or systemic. The most toxic is cyanide. Additionally, aldehydes, hydrogen fluoride and chloride gases, and nitrogen oxides may be present.

15. What are the indications for active airway management?

Evidence of progressive airway obstruction (especially changes in voice, stridor) should be acted upon immediately. Ongoing respiratory insufficiency despite 100% high-flow O_2 is also clear ground for support. Severe burns to the face and neck should be viewed with healthy respect and controlled anxiety; early intubation is appropriate (early airway management under controlled conditions is clearly preferable to hurried and potentially hazardous circumstances that develop later).

16. Which routes of intubation are appropriate?

If there is any concern about upper airway pathology or edema, blind nasotracheal intubation is contraindicated. Orotracheal intubation offers the clinician the ability to directly visualize the supraglottic structures and (hopefully) allows placement of the endotracheal tube atraumatically. In a stable patient, fiberoptic intubation via either nasal or oral route may allow further visualization of the respiratory tract. However, this may be unacceptably time-consuming in an unstable patient unless the operator is quite proficient in the use of the scope. Emergency cricothyrotomy is indicated if glottic edema will not allow passage of the endotracheal tube.

17. Are any anesthetic or induction agents contraindicated in burn patients?

Several texts still state that succinylcholine is contraindicated in the burn patient because of concerns about hyperkalemia. However, this is not relevant in the ED because it is a delayed response. This phenomenon manifests 7–10 days after injury and is related to up-regulation of certain muscle receptors. It does **not** happen acutely, and both succinylcholine and nondepolarizing muscle blocking agents are safe and may be used in any rapid-sequence intubation. The greater danger is the use of induction agents related to volume status. Depending on the time since the burn occurred, large intravascular fluid shifts occur and the patient becomes effectively volume depleted. Hypotension and cardiovascular collapse are real possibilities if fluid replacement has not been initiated. Further, judicious and careful use of induction agents that can cause or exaggerate hypotension such as barbiturates and narcotics is essential.

18. What is burn shock?

After a major burn, vascular integrity in the affected region is lost and significant amounts of fluid begin to leak from the intravascular to the extravascular spaces. These shifts are most pronounced in the first 8 hours following burn injury, and this "third spacing" of fluid can lead to profound intravascular volume depletion that results in hypovolemic shock.

19. How is fluid resuscitation carried out in the victim of a major burn?

Controversy exists as to the best solution for fluid resuscitation in major burns. Crystalloid (both hypertonic and isotonic saline) and colloids have been examined with mixed results. However, no one will argue with immediate fluid resuscitation using a balanced salt solution, i.e., lactated Ringer's or normal saline.

20. How much and how fast?

Many formulas have been devised for fluid replacement, but the Parkland formula is widely employed and easy to remember. It calculates the fluid requirements needed for the first 24 hours. One-half of the calculated volume is to be replaced within the first 8 hours postburn (coinciding with the time when initial intravascular fluid shifts are more pronounced). The formula is:

$$\text{Fluid required} = \text{Body weight (kg)} \times \text{BSA involved} \times 2\text{–}4 \text{ cc/kg}$$

This is a guideline. Clinical parameters, including vital signs, CVP (or PCWP), and urine output, should be monitored carefully. Ideally, urine output should be maintained at 30–60 cc/hr in adults and 1–2 cc/kg/hr in children.

21. Sounds simple enough. Anything else?

Yes. In most EMS systems patients transported usually have one or more IVs established and some fluid given before arrival. You must remember to include these fluids when calculating the fluid requirement and try to avoid overhydration early on. The fluid shifts seen in the first hours after burn injury are dramatic, but causing acute pulmonary edema in your patient is not helpful. Other considerations (pulmonary or CNS injury, for example) also complicate fluid management. Not so simple after all.

22. What about systemic pain control?

A common error is to undertreat pain. Appropriate and repeated use of narcotics, usually morphine, can be commenced in the field and should be withheld only if the patient is so hemodynamically unstable that these agents are life-threatening. Remember, paralyzed, intubated patients have a tough job letting you know how they feel. Be humane.

23. What about application of ice water for pain?

Covering the affected area with sterile sheets or bandages, then wetting them down with cool saline is a reasonable first step. Burned areas do not have intact autonomic or vascular function, and application of iced solutions further damages tissue and can lead to global hypothermia.

24. Is there a role for prophylactic parenteral antibiotics in the ED?

No.

BIBLIOGRAPHY

1. Baxter C, Waeckerle J: Emergency treatment of burn injury. Ann Emerg Med 17:1305–1315, 1989.
2. Erikson EJ, Merrell SW, Saffle JR: Difference in mortality from thermal injury between pediatric and adult patients. Pediatr Surg 26:821–825, 1991.
3. Gerding RL, Imbembo AL, Fratiannerb: Biosynthetic skin substitute versus 1% silver sulfadiazine for treatment of in-patient thermal burns. J Trauma 28:1265–1269, 1988.
4. Gunn ML, Hansbrough JF, Davis JW: Prospective randomized trial of hypertonic sodium lactate versus lactated Ringer's solution for burn shock resuscitation. J Trauma 29:1261–1267, 1989.
5. Kuehn CN, Ahrenholz DH, Solem LD: Care of the burn wound. Trauma Q 5:33–43, 1989.
6. Purdue GE, Hunt JL: Multiple trauma and the burn patient. Am J Surg 158:536–539, 1989.
7. Subrahmanyam M: Topical application of honey in treatment of burns. Br J Surg 78:497–498, 1991.
8. Swain AH, Azadian BS, Wakeley CJ: Management of blisters in minor burns. Br Med J 295:181, 1987.

109. WOUND MANAGEMENT

Daryl M. Turner, M.D., and Ann L. Harwood-Nuss, M.D., FACEP

1. Why is wound healing important?

Traumatic wounds constitute a significant portion of injuries seen in an emergency department (ED). Patients will judge the competency of a physician based upon their ultimate functional or cosmetic results and the development of complications.

2. What is the difference between functional and cosmetic closure?

Functional closure is closure of a wound in such a fashion as to return the body part to earliest full use of the injured part. A cosmetic repair is one that is performed in a fashion so as to result in the least visible scarring.

3. Which factors increase the visibility of scars and compromise wound healing? How are they minimized?

Factors that Increase Scarring and Compromise Wound Healing

CONTRIBUTING FACTORS	METHODS TO MINIMIZE SCARRING
Direction of wound, i.e., perpendicular to lines of static and dynamic skin tension	Layered closure; proper direction in elective incisions of wound
Infection necessitating removal of sutures resulting in healing by secondary intention and a wide scar	Proper wound preparation; irrigation, debridement, and use of delayed closure in contraindicated wounds
Wide scar secondary to tension	Layered closure; proper splinting and elevation
Suture marks	Remove all pericuticular sutures within 7 days
Uneven wound edges resulting in magnification of scar by shadows	Careful, even approximation of wound edges and top layer closure to prevent differential swelling of edges
Inversion of wound edges	Meticulous placement of sutures or use of horizontal mattress sutures
Tattooing secondary to retained dirt or foreign body	Proper wound preparation and debridement

Table continued on next page.

Factors that Increase Scarring and Compromise Wound Healing

CONTRIBUTING FACTORS	METHODS TO MINIMIZE SCARRING
Tissue necrosis	Use of corner sutures on flaps, splinting, and elevation of wounds with marginal circulation or venous return; excise nonviable wound edges before closure
Compromised healing secondary to hematoma	Use of proper conforming dressing and splints
Hyperpigmentation of scar or abraded skin	Use of no. 15 or greater SPF sunblock for 6 months
Superimposition of blood clots between healing wound edges	Proper hemostasis and closure; H_2O_2 frequent swabbing; proper application of compressive dressings
Failure to properly align anatomic structures such as vermilion border	Meticulous closure and alignment; marking or placement of alignment suture before distortion of wound edges with local anesthesia; use of field block

From Markovchick V: Suture materials and mechanical after care. Emerg Med Clin North Am 10:673–689, 1992, with permission.

4. What history should be obtained in a patient with a traumatic wound?

The time of injury, mechanism of injury, patient's current medications and immune status (AIDS, diabetes, chemotherapy, etc.), patient's occupation, and dominant hand if a hand injury has occurred. Also obtain the patient's tetanus immunization history.

5. What are the most important aspects of the physical examination?

The physical exam must be tailored to the underlying anatomy; therefore it is most important to be familiar with this anatomy, particularly as it involves the face, neck, hands, and feet. Proper testing of the neurosensory and motor function as well as the status of distal vasculature must be documented. If there is any concern about bony injury or deep penetration with a foreign body (example, glass into muscle), then proper diagnostic imaging studies should be obtained. Every examination of the wound must include in this final step control of hemorrhage and a direct visualization for the presence of any foreign body or deep structure involvement. For example, an 80% laceration of a tendon may result in normal motor function but has significant morbidity and complication if not recognized and treated.

6. What is the single most important thing I can do to prevent infection?

Irrigate, irrigate, irrigate. Irrigation with normal saline at approximately 8–10 psi, which is obtained by using a 19-gauge needle and 30-cc syringe, has proved to be the single most important procedure in decreasing the incidence of infection in traumatic wounds. In addition, exploration, debridement, hemostasis, and proper repairing, dressing, and immobilization are also helpful. Antibiotics have no proven prophylactic benefit unless they are administered prior to the wounding, which, of course, only occurs in experimental animals.

7. What causes the pain of local anesthetic infiltration?

Pain from the infiltration of xylocaine is caused by distention of tissue from too-rapid injection with too-large a needle directly into the dermis. Additionally, the other cause of pain is the fact that xylocaine is acidic. Pain can be minimized by very slow subdermal injection with a very small 25-gauge or smaller needle and buffering the xylocaine by adding 1 cc of sodium bicarbonate solution to every 10 cc of xylocaine.

8. What are the toxic doses of xylocaine?

One should not exceed 4 mg/kg of plain xylocaine or 7 mg/kg of xylocaine with epinephrine. A 1 cc of 1 percent xylocaine solution = 10 mg of xylocaine.

9. What are the contraindications to xylocaine with epinephrine?
Xylocaine with epinephrine should not be used on digits, the pinna, circumferentially around the penis, or in areas with poor or marginal blood supply such as flap wounds of the anterior pretibial area. Studies have shown that epinephrine decreases resistance to infection because of its potent vasoconstrictor effect. However, in areas of the body such as the scalp and face, the vasoconstriction and resulting hemostasis aid the exploration and repair of the wound and does not appear to increase wound infections.

10. What is TAC?
TAC is topical anesthetic that consists of tetracaine 0.5%, epinephrine 1:2000, and cocaine 11.8%. Cotton soaked with TAC is placed directly onto or into the open wound and will give excellent local anesthesia in very vascular areas such as the scalp and face.

11. What are the contraindications to TAC?
Contraindications to TAC are the same as for xylocaine with epinephrine, but TAC should never be used anywhere on or near mucous membranes because the cocaine can be rapidly absorbed and result in cocaine toxicity.

12. What is a contaminated wound?
A contaminated wound is any wound that has a high inoculum of bacteria. Some examples are full-thickness bites, wounds of the perineum or axilla in which there is a high normal skin flora count, and wounds that are exposed to contaminated water such as from ponds, lakes, or coral reefs.

13. Is a dirty wound the same as a contaminated wound?
Not necessarily. Studies have shown that "road rash," resulting from road gravel, has a very low bacterial count. In contrast, wounds that occur in a barnyard or are exposed to soil contaminated with fecal material have a very high bacterial count and therefore are contaminated.

14. What causes tattooing?
Tattooing is caused by the retention of foreign material and incorporation of it in the dermis during the healing process. In order to prevent this cosmetic complication, it is most important that all foreign material and dirt be removed through proper debridement, scrubbing, and irrigation at the time of the initial patient encounter.

15. What are the three types of closure?
Primary closure is closure within 6–8 hours of a wound on any part of the body except face and scalp up to 24 hours following injury. Secondary closure, or healing by secondary intention, is allowing the wound to heal by granulation without tape or sutures. Delayed primary closure is closure of a wound 3–5 days following the injury.

16. Which wounds should be closed primarily?
Any clean (not initially contaminated) wound may be closed primarily if it is less than 6–8 hours old and is located anywhere on the body except for the face and the scalp. Wounds of the face and scalp may be closed up to 12–24 hours following injury.

17. When should secondary closure be used?
Secondary closure should be used for contaminated wounds that penetrate deeply into tissue and cannot be adequately irrigated prior to closure. Examples of such wounds are puncture wounds of the sole of the foot and palm of the hand as well as stab wounds that penetrate into subcutaneous tissue and muscle.

18. When should delayed primary closure be used?

Delayed primary closure, an underutilized procedure, should be considered for all contaminated wounds that are gaping or have significant amounts of tension in order to decrease the risk of infection, optimize the cosmetic result, and accelerate the healing process.

19. How is a wound prepared for delayed primary closure?

The wound should be thoroughly examined, prepared, debrided, and irrigated. Hemorrhage should be controlled. A fine layer of mesh gauze should be laid in the wound, the wound should be packed open, and followed closely. At 3–5 days if there is no purulent drainage or wound-margin erythema, the wound may be closed in the same fashion as if it were being closed primarily.

20. How are bites treated?

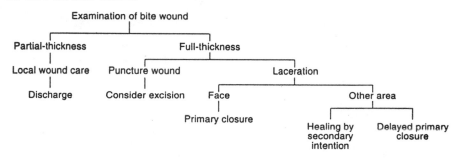

21. Which sutures are used, how is the wound repaired, and when do I remove the sutures?

Suture Repair of Soft Tissue Injuries

LOCATION	ANESTHETIC	SUTURE MATERIAL	TECHNIQUE OF CLOSURE AND DRESSING	SUTURE REMOVAL
Scalp	Lidocaine 1% with epinephrine	3-0 or 4-0 nylon or polypropylene	Interrupted in galea; single tight layer in scalp: horizontal mattress if bleeding not well controlled by simple sutures	7–12 days
Pinna (ear)	Lidocaine 1% (field block)	6-0 nylon 5-0 Vicryl* or Dexon in perichondrium	Close perichondrium with 5-0 Vicryl interrupted; close skin with 6-0 nylon interrupted: stint dressing	4–6 days
Eyebrow	Lidocaine 1% with epinephrine	4-0 or 5-0 Vicryl and 6-0 nylon	Layered closure	4–5 days
Eyelid	Lidocaine 1%	6-0 nylon or silk	Single-layer horizontal mattress	3–5 days
Lip	Lidocaine 1% with epinephrine or field block	4-0 silk or Vicryl (mucosa) 5-0 Vicryl (SQ, muscle) 6-0 (skin)	Three layers (mucosa, muscle, and skin) if through and through, otherwise two layers	3–5 days
Oral cavity	Lidocaine 1% with epinephrine, or field block; sedation may be necessary in children	4-0 Vicryl	Simple interrupted or horizontal mattress: layered closure if muscularis of tongue involved	7–8 days or allow to dissolve
Face	Lidocaine 1% with epinephrine or field block	4-0 or 5-0 Vicryl (SQ) 6-0 nylon (skin)	If full-thickness laceration, layered closure desirable	3–5 days

Table continued on next page.

Suture Repair of Soft Tissue Injuries (Continued)

LOCATION	ANESTHETIC	SUTURE MATERIAL	TECHNIQUE OF CLOSURE AND DRESSING	SUTURE REMOVAL
Neck	Lidocaine 1% with epinephrine	4-0 Vicryl (SQ) 5-0 nylon (skin)	Two-layered closure for best cosmetic results	4–6 days
Trunk	Lidocaine 1% with epinephrine	4-0 Vicryl (SQ, fat) 4-0 or 5-0 nylon (skin)	Single or layered closure	7–12 days
Extremity	Lidocaine 1% with epinephrine	3-0 or 4-0 Vicryl (SQ, fat, muscle) 4-0 or 5-0 nylon (skin)	Single-layer closure is adequate, although layered or running SQ closure may give better cosmetic result; apply splint if wound over a joint	7–14 days
Hands and feet	Lidocaine 1% (if field block with 2% lidocaine or 0.25% bupivacaine)	4-0 or 5-0 nylon	Single-layer closure only with simple or horizontal mattress interrupted suture, at least 5 mm from cut wound edges; horizontal mattress sutures should be used if much tension on wound edges; apply splint if wound over a joint	7–12 days
Nailbeds	Lidocaine 2% or bupivacaine 0.25% digital nerve block	5-0 Vicryl	Gentle, meticulous placement to obtain even edges	Allow to dissolve

*Vicryl and Dexon suture can be interchanged throughout the table.
From Markovchick V: Soft tissue injury and wound repair. In Reisdorff EJ, Roberts MR, Wiegenstein JG: Pediatric Emergency Medicine. Philadelphia, W.B. Saunders, 1993, pp 899–908, with permission.

22. What should be included in follow-up instructions?

In addition to local wound care, signs of infection, and time of suture removal, all follow-up instructions should include the facts that:

All wounds will heal with a scar.

All wounds may get infected.

All wounds may have retained foreign bodies.

23. Are there any controversies in wound care?

There are many; however, the primary controversy relates to the use of prophylactic antibiotics. The use of prophylactic antibiotics is widespread and has developed with little scientific support. Animal studies have shown that the only real efficacy of prophylactic antibiotics in contaminated wounds is if the antibiotics are administered intravenously prior to the injury and contamination of the wound. This never occurs in the real world, and to date there are no prospective controlled human studies that prove the efficacy of prophylactic antibiotics. Unfortunately, some have equated not using prophylactic antibiotics with malpractice. In addition, antibiotics may give a false sense of security (to the doctor and patient) and should never be a substitute for adequate wound irrigation.

BIBLIOGRAPHY

1. Markovchick V: Soft tissue injury and wound repair. In Reisdorff EJ, Roberts MR, Wiegenstein JG: Pediatric Emergency Medicine. Philadelphia, W.B. Saunders, 1993, pp 899–908.
2. Markovchick V: Suture materials and mechanical after care. Emerg Med Clin North Am 10:673–689, 1992.

XVII. Behavioral Emergencies

110. ACUTE PSYCHOSIS

Eugene E. Kercher, M.D., FACEP

1. What is acute psychosis?

Psychosis is a dysfunction in the capacity for thought and information processing. There is an incapacity to be coherent in perceiving, retaining, processing, recalling, or acting on information in a consensually validated way. There is a decreased ability to mobilize, shift, sustain, and direct attention at will. A major feature of the psychotic state is the failure in ranking the priority of stimuli. The ability to act upon reality is unpredictable and diminished, because the patient is unable to distinguish internal from external stimuli.

2. Define organic psychosis and functional psychosis.

Organic psychosis refers to a reversible or nonreversible dysfunctional mental condition that can be identified as a disturbance in the anatomy, physiology, or biochemistry of the brain. Functional psychosis refers to a dysfunctional mental condition identified as schizophrenia, a major affective disorder, or other mental disorders with psychotic features.

3. What are the types of psychoses?

Classification of psychosis is found in the Diagnostic and Statistical Manual of Mental Disorders (DSM III-R), and is appropriately divided into functional and organic varieties. The majority of organically caused acute psychoses result from dementia, withdrawal states, and intoxications. Schizophrenia and the affective disorders are the major contributors to functionally caused acute psychoses.

4. How does a patient in a psychotic state typically present to the emergency department (ED)?

Patients who are in a psychotic state act strangely (i.e., mannerisms, posturing), dress bizarrely, respond to hallucinations, harbor false and delusional beliefs, and consistently confuse the reality of events. They are frequently impulsive and in constant danger of acting on distorted perceptions or delusional ideas resulting in unintentional injury or death. The clarity of oneself and the environment is consistently blurred. The patient is unable to discriminate the stimuli that he or she perceives. Thinking is disorganized and incoherent, as evidenced from the patient's speech. Memory is impaired in registration, retention, and recall. Orientation may be impaired, especially for time. The psychomotor behavior may be hypoactive or hyperactive in regard to movements and speech. Emotions can range from apathy and depression to fear and rage.

5. Why does the psychotic patient come to the ED?

Psychotic patients are frequently brought to the ED by relatives or friends who can no longer safely control behavior. Frequently a psychotic patient is brought in by police or paramedics because the psychotic condition is considered potentially dangerous to self or others. Some patients come into the hospital in order to find refuge for their overwhelming fears.

6. Why is it important to immediately control psychotic behavior?
Patients who present in a psychotic state are impulsive and unable to prioritize stimuli and their reactions to them. Because of this dysfunction, they should always be considered a danger to themselves, a danger to others, and gravely disabled.

7. How can the potential for violent behavior be detected in the psychotic patient?
Clearly the best way to deal with violent behavior is to prevent it. Most emergency physicians recognize patients who are obviously confused, irrational, paranoid, or excited. The emergency physician must develop an intuitive vigilance in order to detect the possibility of violence in those patients who present more rationally and are less floridly psychotic. Any history or comment that suggests violence should be taken seriously. The potential for violence is, in general, directly related to the tone, volume, and character of the voice and body tension.

8. Are there behavioral controls that can be immediately used for the psychotic patient?
Yes. Recognizing the chance of violence and physical harm, the emergency physician is obligated to take definitive steps to avoid confrontation (1) Environmental—keep the environment simple and stimuli free and minimize staff changes. (2) Interpersonal—assume the role of patient advocate and engage the patient in a calm, self-assured voice.

9. What option can be exercised if the patient becomes increasingly disorganized and agitated?
Institute a formalized and rehearsed physical restraint plan. Upon summons by the physician, security guards should appear at the door, so the patient can see and feel their presence. This "show of force" indicates that any display of violence will not be tolerated and often helps patients to organize and regain control of their thoughts and behavior. Once the patient is physically restrained, thoroughly search the patient for any weapons or sharp objects.

10. Are there further methods of control if the patient continues to have psychotic turmoil?
Medication often complicates rather than accelerates the evaluation process of a patient in a psychotic state. The main indication for tranquilization is a persistence of behavior so disorganized or uncooperative that further evaluation proves impossible. An effective initial regimen is intravenous administration of 5–10 mg of haloperidol with 0.5 mg of lorazepam. If the desired effect is not achieved within 20 minutes, treat with repeat doses of haloperidol, 5–10 mg and lorazepam, 0.5–2 mg. Additional doses can be titrated at 30-minute intervals until sedation is satisfactory.

11. How should the priorities be set when an emergency physician first makes contact with a psychotic patient?
1. ABCs if necessary
2. Observation (quickly assess impulse control and tendency to physically act out)
3. Control and manage psychotic behavior (if necessary)
4. A history (gather from everyone who has been involved with the patient)
5. Differentiate between organic and functional cause through a formal mental status exam.
6. Physical examination (abnormal vital signs)
7. Laboratory (toxicologic and metabolic studies) and radiographic examination (CT scan) if clinically indicated
8. Consultation and disposition

12. What are the sources of information for psychotic patients who are usually historically unreliable?

Because acutely psychotic patients may be unable to adequately provide a history, emergency physicians must explore all avenues for obtaining information. This may include EMS personnel, family, friends, neighbors, law enforcement officers, and old medical records.

13. What historical information is important?
1. **Onset.** Did the behavior change suddenly or gradually?
2. **Longitudinal course.** Is this the first such event?
3. **Family history.** Do these symptoms or any other psychiatric disorders appear in the patient's family?
4. **Previous psychiatric disease,** organic brain disease, and medication, and history of drug use.

14. Which pharmacologic agents potentially cause acute psychosis?

Digitalis, corticosteroids, isoniazid (INH), antabuse, tricyclics, anticonvulsants, cimetidine, benzodiazepines, amphetamines and related drugs, antiarrhythmics, narcotics, barbiturates, methyldopa, nonsteroidal anti-inflammatory agents, anticancer agents, and recreational drugs.

15. How can a physical examination be tailored for a psychotic patient?

When performing the physical examination on a psychotic patient, defer the rectal and pelvic examinations and leave other parts of the physical examination that require undressing until the end. Start with those parts, such as the head, neck, and neurologic examination, that can be performed without undressing the patient. In most cases, emergency physicians will have built sufficient rapport with patients, in time, for the cooperation necessary for a more intimate examination. Tell the patient exactly what you are doing, what you are going to do, and what he or she should do during the examination. This helps to provide structure for the psychotic patient and avoids confusion or misunderstanding. Initially, check the patient's vital signs and observe his or her behavior.

16. Is laboratory screening necessary in an appropriate work-up of an acute psychotic patient?

Most laboratory investigations provide little help during the acute evaluation of a psychotic episode. The following tests are recommended if an organic etiology is considered: CBC with differential, electrolytes, toxicology screens, ABGs or oxygen saturation, chest x-ray, urinalysis, thyroid function tests, liver function tests, EKG, CT (with contrast if tumor is suspected), and lumbar puncture.

17. What are the key points to consider in the differentiation of organic from functional psychosis?

MADFOCS Mnemonic

		ORGANIC	FUNCTIONAL
M	**Memory deficit**	Recent impaired	Remote impaired
A	**Activity**	Hyper and hypo activity Tremor Ataxia	Repetitive activity Posturing Rocking
D	**Distortions**	Visual hallucinations	Auditory hallucinations

Table continued on next page.

MADFOCS Mnemonic (Continued)

		ORGANIC	FUNCTIONAL
F	**Feelings**	Emotional lability	Flat affect
O	**Orientation**	Disoriented	Oriented
C	**Cognition**	Some lucid thoughts	No lucid thoughts
		Perceives occasionally	Unfiltered perceptions
		Attends occasionally	Unable to attend
		Focuses occasionally	Unable to focus
S	**Some other findings**	Age >40	Age <40
		Sudden onset	Gradual onset
		Physical exam often abnormal	Physical exam normal
		Vital signs may be abnormal	Vital signs usually normal
		Social immodesty	Social modesty
		Aphasia	Intelligible speech
		Consciousness impaired	Alert, awake
		Confabulation	Ambivalence

18. Are there any other clinical "rules of thumb" in the work-up of the acute psychotic patient?
1. Fever and psychosis = meningitis
2. Acute psychosis and alcoholism = Wernicke's encephalopathy
3. Headache and psychosis = tumor or intracranial hemorrhage
4. Abdominal pain and psychosis = prophyria
5. Sweating and psychosis = hypoglycemia or delerium tremens
6. Autonomic signs and psychosis = toxic or metabolic encephalopathy

19. What are the potentially reversible causes of psychosis?
DEMENTIA Mncmonic

D	=	Drug toxicity
E	=	Emotional disorders
M	=	Metabolic disorders
E	=	Endocrine disorders
N	=	Nutritional disorders
T	=	Tumors and trauma
I	=	Infection
A	=	Arteriosclerotic complications

20. What three basic questions to answer concerning the disposition of the psychotic patient?
1. Risk of suicide or homicide
2. Realistic family support or supervision
3. Initial response to medication

21. When should hospitalization be recommended?
1. This is the patient's first psychotic episode.
2. The patient is a danger to self or others.
3. The patient is unable to appropriately care for himself or herself.
4. The patient has no social support system.
5. The functional psychotic patient is not sufficiently clear following initial ED tranquilization.
6. An acute organic psychosis does not clear while the patient is in the ED.

BIBLIOGRAPHY

1. American Psychiatric Association: Diagnostic and Statistical Manual of Mental Disorders, 3rd ed, revised. Washington, DC, American Psychiatric Association, 1987, pp 103–107.
2. Anderson EH, Kuehnle JC: Diagnosis and early management of acute psychosis. N Engl J Med 305:1128, 1981.
3. Anderson EH, Stern TA: Psychiatric emergencies. In Wilkens EW (ed): Emergency Medicine: Scientific Foundations and Current Practice. Baltimore, Williams & Wilkins, 1989, pp 423–430.
4. Cassem EH: Approach to the patient with mental and emotional complaints. In Jeffers JD, Scott EJ, Ramoz-Englis M (eds): Harrison's Principles of Internal Medicine. New York, McGraw-Hill, 1987, pp 60–64.
5. Dubovsky SL, Weissberg MP (eds): Clinical Psychiatry in Primary Care, 3rd ed. Baltimore, Williams & Wilkins, 1986, pp 85–124, 231–255.
6. Fernandez F, Holmes UF, Adams R, Kavanaugh SS: Treatment of severe, refractory agitation with a haloperidol drip. J Clin Psychiatry 49:239–241, 1988.
7. Frame DS, Kercher EE: Acute psychosis: Functional vs organic. Emerg Med Clin North Am 9:123–136, 1991.
8. Jorden RD: Initial evaluation of the patient with altered mental status. Top Emerg Med 13:1–9, 1991.
9. Viner J: Toward more skillful handling of psychotic patients. Pt I. Evaluation. Emerg Med Rep 3:125, 1982.
10. Viner J: Toward more skillful handling of psychotic patients. Pt II. Disposition and management. Emerg Med Rep 3:131, 1982.

111. DEPRESSION AND SUICIDE

Douglas A. Rund, M.D., FACEP

DEPRESSION

1. What are the symptoms of depression?

The cardinal symptom of depression is a dysphoric mood. The term dysphoric implies sadness, usually including loss of interest or pleasure in most activities in life. To diagnose a major depressive episode, at least four of the following symptoms must have been present nearly every day for 2 weeks: loss of interest in usual activities, sleep disorder, appetite disturbance, inability to concentrate, decreased activity, feelings of guilt, lack of energy, or recurrent thoughts of suicide. A useful mnemonic to remember these categories is the following:

In	=	Interest	C	=	Concentration
			A	=	Activity
S	=	Sleep	G	=	Guilt
A	=	Appetite	E	=	Energy
D	=	Dysphoria	S	=	Suicide ideation

2. Why is depression considered an affective disorder?

The term affect describes mood or "prolonged emotion that colors the whole psychic life." Affect refers to the conscious subjective perception of emotion apart from the physical changes that accompany it. When such moods cause impairment of function or extreme pain, a mood (or affective) disorder can be diagnosed. Examples of such disorders include major depression and bipolar disorder. Bipolar disorder typically manifests with mood swings from depression to mania.

3. What is the difference between primary and secondary depression?
Major depression is classified as primary if the symptom complex appears before any other significant medical or psychiatric illness. It is considered secondary when it follows and is related to other medical or psychiatric illness.

4. What medical conditions might cause secondary depression?
Endocrine disorders that can cause depression include the following: hypothyroidism, diabetes mellitus, and Cushing's syndrome. Neurologic disorders include cerebrovascular accidents, subdural hematoma, multiple sclerosis, brain neoplasm, Parkinson's disease, seizure disorder, and dementia. Certain connective tissue diseases, such as systemic lupus erythematosus, are associated with depression. Various known debilitating diseases and neoplasms such as pancreatic carcinoma can also cause depression. Medications known to cause depression in certain individuals include antihypertensives (reserpine, beta blockers, methyldopa), hypnotics and sedatives (benzodiazepines and barbiturates), corticosteroids, cimetidine, and ranitidine.

5. What is the relationship of alcohol to depression?
Alcohol is associated in some way with 25–50% of all suicides. Alcohol is a depressant drug. In some cases the depressed person may be trying to "self-treat" the condition with alcohol. The result is typically an overall worsening of the depression. Alcohol withdrawal is also associated with depression.

6. When should one suspect depression when a patient presents with what seems to be a medical complaint?
The emergency physician who is prepared to zoom in quickly on a specific physical complaint, such as an injured ankle or lacerated finger, may have to pause and consider depression when confronting a patient with a nonspecific complaint such as "sick all over," "weak and dizzy," or "just feeling bad." Such patients, of course, require medical evaluation, but the emergency physician can also quickly screen for depression with inquiries about the nine symptoms, beginning with sleep, appetite, and weight change. The mood alteration associated with depression may be expressed as fatigue, exhaustion, or hopelessness. Certain chronic pain syndromes (nonspecific facial pain, for instance) may constitute the initial complaint of a patient with a major depressive episode. The patient with depression may also complain about feeling agitated, nervous, or anxious. Depression as well as anxiety disorders should be considered in evaluating such complaints.

7. Are psychotic features ever a manifestation of depression?
Depression is an affective disorder that can cause psychotic symptoms. The severely depressed patient may have mood-congruent delusions or hallucinations. The patient may report that his "insides are rotting away," for instance, or hear voices that say things which generate guilt. When psychotic symptoms such as these are detected (assuming that the organs are not *really* rotting away), psychiatric consultation and probably hospitalization are usually indicated.

8. What therapies are available for treatment of depression?
In general, the term depression is treated by various combinations of the following modalities: antidepressant medications, psychotherapy, and electroconvulsive therapy (ECT).

9. What antidepressant medications are used to treat depression?
Cyclic antidepressants, monoamine oxidase inhibitors (MAOIs), and lithium are generally used to treat depression. Cyclic antidepressants may improve sleep in the first weeks of treatment, but antidepressant effects do not typically occur until after several weeks of therapy. Certain cyclic antidepressants cause side effects, such as anticholinergic symptoms,

that may be uncomfortable for patients beginning treatment. Patients taking MAOIs require extensive counseling about diet and drug interactions. Foods containing tyramine, for instance, may precipitate a serious hypertensive crisis. Lithium therapy requires careful monitoring, especially in the early stages, as well as medical assessments such as evaluation of renal function.

10. When should the emergency physician begin antidepressant therapy?
Lithium and MAOIs should not be prescribed unless one is refilling an expired prescription after psychiatric consultation. The cyclic antidepressants can take from 3–4 weeks to become effective and require close supervision because the dosage may need to be adjusted upward during the initiation of therapy. In most instances, therefore, such agents should not be prescribed by the emergency physician. An exception might exist when, after direct consultation, the emergency physician and the referring psychiatrist agree to commence treatment with 2–4 day's supply of medication and prompt psychiatric follow-up.

11. What are the complications of depression?
The major and most serious complication of depression is suicide. An estimated 15% of patients with primary depression eventually commit suicide.

12. Which patients should be hospitalized for depression?
In most instances, depressed patients who express the intent to commit suicide require psychiatric consultation and admission. Continued suicide ideation and a feasible, lethal plan are dangerous aspects of the patient's thinking. Suicide precautions should be instituted while the patient is in the ED. Depressed patients who exhibit symptoms and signs of psychosis require psychiatric evaluation, admission, and usually treatment with antipsychotic agents.

SUICIDE

13. What is the proper approach to a patient who has attempted suicide?
Medical management of any life-threatening condition precedes psychiatric evaluation. It is important, however, that as the treatment proceeds, the ED team maintain a nonjudgmental approach. Punishment or ridicule is neither therapeutic nor proper conduct for medical professionals. Nearly all patients who attempt suicide are at least somewhat ambivalent about the wish to live or die. Demeaning or harsh treatment of such patients, especially by health professionals who are symbols of medical authority, worsens the already low self-esteem and makes more difficult subsequent psychiatric care.

14. What are suicide precautions?
Because some patients have been able to repeat a suicide attempt while in the ED, suicide precautions are necessary. Such precautions include the following: searching the patient and recovering weapons, pills, or other potential causes of self-injury; keeping the patient under close observation; recovering any potential dangerous items from the immediate care area (e.g., needles, scalpels, glass, razors); and not allowing the patient to go anywhere (e.g., bathroom) unaccompanied. When constant staff observation is not possible, physical restraints may be necessary to protect the severely suicidal patient from further self-harm.

15. Are "accidents" ever suicide attempts?
It is important to remember that victims of trauma may have attempted suicide. Single-victim accidents, such as a car driven at high speed into a concrete structure, a pedestrian hit by a high-speed vehicle, or a fall are classic examples of suicide attempts presenting as trauma. Medical management should be followed by an assessment of suicide intent, including a discussion with family members, and perhaps even psychiatric consultation.

16. What psychiatric disorders are associated with attempted suicide?
In addition to major depression, the most common associated disorder, patients with the following conditions have a higher incidence of suicide: schizophrenia, panic disorder, adjustment disorder, alcoholism, and substance abuse.

17. How do I evaluate the risk of a subsequent suicide in a suicide attempter?
The following elements are part of an emergency assessment of suicide risks: age, sex, marital status, social supports, physical illness, previous attempts, family history of suicide, risk of the attempts versus likelihood of rescue, secondary gain, nature of any psychiatric illness, alcohol or drug abuse, and attitude, affect, and future plans of the suicide attempter.

18. How does age relate to suicide risk?
Older individuals, especially those over 45 years of age, are statistically more likely to complete suicide than younger patients. Such patients may experience loss of spouse, loneliness, physical illness, or economic hardship as well as depression. However, worrisome increase in suicide among younger persons has emerged in the past 20 years. Suicide is now the third leading cause of death in children 5–14 years of age and the second leading cause of death in teenagers and young adults aged 14–24.

19. What role does gender play?
The rates of completed suicide in men are higher than those for women, whereas the rates of attempted suicide are higher for women than for men.

20. What is the relationship of marital status to risk of successful suicide?
Patients who are single, divorced, separated, or widowed have a higher risk of suicide than married persons.

21. What about other social support?
Unemployment, loneliness, loss of home, and relative isolation increase the risks of suicide. Church, family, or community support helps to mitigate suicide risk.

22. Is there a relationship between physical illness and suicide risk?
Patients with a medical illness, especially a painful, incurable one, may seek a way out through suicide.

23. Does a history of prior suicide attempts signify increased risk?
Unless the previous attempts have all been minor and considered to be manipulative acts, a previous history of suicide attempt is a positive risk factor, especially if each subsequent attempt escalates in severity.

24. What is the relationship of family history to suicide risk?
Patients with a family history of suicide, alcoholism, or depression have a higher suicide risk than patients without such a family history. A family history of suicide in first-order relatives (e.g., parent or sibling) should cause particular concern.

25. How does the risk of the suicide attempt and the likelihood of rescue affect a suicide evaluation?
In general, a more serious or risky attempt is considered a more likely predictor of subsequent risk than a minor attempt. An attempt performed in such a way that rescue is likely is associated with a lower risk of subsequent successful suicide.

26. What is secondary gain as it applies to suicide attempt?
Sometimes a suicide attempt seems to have a goal other than death. This goal, which is termed secondary gain, may be increased attention from parents, friends, or paramours, for example. In attempts with no expected gain other than death, the potential for subsequent successful suicide is great. Moreover, with the increase in successful suicides among the young, one must now be careful in ascribing suicide attempts to the desire for attention or secondary gain until a reasonably thorough evaluation can be completed.

27. What is the value of assessing the suicidal patient's attitude and affect?
The patient who appears exhausted, helpless, hopeless, or lonely represents high risk. The patient who attempts suicide because of anger or in an effort to gain revenge has a much better prognosis than one who appears quiet, sad, fatigued, or apathetic.

28. Why is it important to inquire about a specific plan?
One should never hesitate to ask the patient about any plans regarding suicide. The patient who expresses continued suicidal ideation after one attempt is at risk for a subsequent attempt. The risk is highest if the plan is detailed, violent, or feasible.

29. What is the SAD PERSONS scale?
In 1983 Patterson et al. used known high-risk characteristics to develop the mnemonic SAD PERSONS Scale (see table). The scale was designed to be used by nonpsychiatrists to assess the need for hospitalization in suicidal patients. Hockberger and Rothstein modified the scale to facilitate use in the ED. A score of 5 or less indicates that a patient can probably be discharged safely; a score of 9 or greater indicates the probable need for psychiatric hospitalization; and scores of 6 or greater require psychiatric consultation.

Modified SAD PERSONS Scale

MNEMONIC		CHARACTERISTIC	SCORE
S	Sex	Male	1
A	Age	<19 or >45	1
D	Depression or hopelessness	Admits to depression or decreased concentration, appetite, sleep, libido	2
P	Previous attempts or psychiatric care	Previous inpatient or outpatient psychiatric care	1
E	Excessive alcohol or drug use	Stigmata of chronic addiction or recent frequent use	1
R	Rational thinking loss	Organic brain syndrome or psychosis	2
S	Separated, widowed, or divorced		1
O	Organized or serious attempt	Well-thought-out plan or "life-threatening" presentation	2
N	No social supports	No close family, friends, job, or active religious affiliation	1
S	Stated future intent	Determined to repeat attempt or ambivalent	2

Scoring: A positive answer to the presence of depression or hopelessness, lack of rational thought processes, an organized plan or serious suicide attempt, and affirmative or ambivalent statement regarding future intent to commit suicide are each scored two points. Each other positive answer is scored one point.

From Hockberger RS, Rothstein RJ: Assessment of suicide potential by non-psychiatrists using the SAD PERSONS score. J Emerg Med 99:6, 1988, with permission.

30. In general, which suicidal patients should be hospitalized?
Absolute indications for the patient's hospitalization after suicide attempts (involuntarily, if necessary) usually include the following: presence of psychosis; a violent, nearly lethal

preplanned attempt; and continued suicidal ideation. Relative indications include age over 45; high risk/rescue ratio; serious medical illness; alcoholism; drug addiction; living alone with poor social support; hopelessness, helplessness, or exhaustion; and definite plans for a repeated attempt.

BIBLIOGRAPHY

1. Hockberger RS, Rothstein RJ: Assessment of suicide potential by non-psychiatrists using the SAD PERSONS score. J Emerg Med 99:6, 1988.
2. Patterson WM, et al: Evaluation of suicidal patients with the SAD PERSONS scale. Psychosomatics 343:24, 1983.
3. Rund DA, Hutzler JC: Emergency Psychiatry. St. Louis, Mosby–Year Book, 1983, p 144.
4. Schmidt T: "Suicide" chapter in Emergency Medicine: Concepts and Clinical Practice, 3rd ed. St. Louis, Mosby–Year Book, 1992.
5. Weissman MM, et al: Suicidal ideation and suicide attempts in panic disorders and attacks. N Engl J Med 209:321, 1988.

112. MANAGEMENT OF THE VIOLENT PATIENT

Jonathan Wasserberger, M.D., FACEP, Gary Ordog, M.D., FACEP, Eugene Hardin, M.D., FACEP, and Mickey Kolodny, M.D., FACEP

1. Is violence a problem in the ED?

Yes. Acts of violence resulting in death have occurred in 7% of major teaching hospitals.

2. What can hospitals do to decrease the risk of violence?

1. All unnecessary doors should be locked and access into the hospital limited to a few patrolled entrances.

2. Metal detectors are used to screen patients and visitors for weapons.

3. Continuous surveillance closed circuit television monitors help to assure safety in the parking areas and the immediate grounds of the hospital.

4. Multiple methods of summoning police or security must be available to the ED without having to go through the hospital operator.

5. Responding police or security officers should be appropriately trained and equipped.

3. What can be done to preempt a violent episode?

1. Be aware of early signs of impending violent behavior, such as agitation, abusive language, and challenges of authority.

2. Completely undress major trauma victims as soon as possible thereby removing any weapons on their person.

3. Do not leave any instruments that can be used as weapons near a potentially violent patient.

4. What can a physician do to control a violent situation?

1. Do not ignore aggressive behavior, hoping it will go away. Evaluate such patients immediately. The patient who feels ignored is the one who is most likely to strike out for attention. Be professional and respectful. Position yourself near an exit, staying more than an arms length from the potentially violent patient.

2. If it appears that the patient is going to lose control or explode, immediately move farther away from the patient. If the only two options are injury to the caregiver or allowing the patient to leave, let the patient leave.

3. Do not be a hero and attempt to disarm someone with a weapon—this is police work. If the patient produces a weapon, ask the patient to put it on the floor, and then leave the examining room with the patient. No attempt should be made to retrieve the weapon with the patient present.

4. If violence is imminent, summon security personnel and impose external controls immediately. When the decision is made to employ restraints:

- Use overwhelming force. This means approaching the violent patient with at least five persons, preferably but not necessarily police or security personnel, each with a preassigned task.
- Grasp clothing and large joints. Restrain at least two and often all four limbs. If possible, restrain the patient on his side to prevent vomiting and aspiration.
- Avoid pressure to the throat and chest. Keep hands away from the patient's mouth (they sometimes bite).
- When using physical restraints, *the minimal force necessary* is the maximum that ethical practice allows. The goal is to restrain, not to injure. The restrained patient should frequently be reevaluated, as such patients may deteriorate or develop complications.
- As soon as possible, after the patient has been mechanically restrained, obtain IV access and a blood sugar. If the patient is hypoglycemic, administer 50% dextrose in water.

5. What do I do after the patient is mechanically restrained?
If the patient continues to struggle and exhibit violent behavior, sedation is indicated. A body of literature and experience support the use of intravenous haloperidol, although it is not approved by the FDA for intravenous administration. Haloperidol, 5–10 mg IM, may be given initially, followed by 5–10 mg every 30 minutes. In the elderly, one should begin with a much lower dose (1–2 mg) of haloperidol. Lorazepam or another benzodiazepine, 4 mg IM or IV, may also be used but is not as effective. Diazepam, 10–20 mg IV, can be given with continuous monitoring of the cardiorespiratory status. Beware that benzodiazepines can cause hypotension or respiratory depression.

6. What are the contraindications to haloperidol?
Benzodiazepines may be used in patients with a fever, but it is best to avoid haloperidol in combative PCP- or cocaine-intoxicated patients who are febrile. Benzodiazepines, such as diazepam or lorazepam, are preferred in an agitated cocaine user, as the benzodiazepines reduce the CNS production of catecholamines.

7. How can control be achieved in the markedly agitated head-trauma patient?
In the patient with acute head trauma with combativeness, the approach is to get control of the patient to allow for an atraumatic intubation followed by ventilation. An effective means of airway control is rapid-sequence intubation with an intravenous benzodiazepine, intravenous lidocaine, and a neuromuscular blocking agent.

If active airway management is not needed, the combative head-trauma patient is restrained, IV access is obtained, and the patient is sedated using haloperidol, droperidol, or diazepam. Hypoglycemia should always be considered a possible etiology for combative behavior. A Dextrostix should be performed or glucose administered early in the patient's course. Paralysis is to be used only by a person highly trained in the use of neuromuscular blocking agents and endotracheal intubation. In unskilled hands, such agents are extremely dangerous.

8. Why did the patient become violent in the first place?
Once the patient is controlled, determine the underlying problem. Emphasis is on determining if the patient has one or more of the following:

Metabolic disorder	Acute withdrawal
Infectious disease	Trauma
Cardiovascular disorder	Environmental injury
Intracranial disorder	Psychiatric disorders
Acute intoxication	

9. What paperwork is required after physical or chemical restraint?
Clear documentation in the medical record should include justification for the application of restraints and administration of medication. Where applicable, "legal hold" paperwork should be completed. Ongoing observation of patients in restraints must be documented.

10. Does the ED staff need any treatment?
The effect of major unpredictable violence and mayhem on ED employees can be devastating. Physical and psychological trauma is only part of the long-lasting effects. Such episodes may affect future job performance. A comprehensive program patterned after the critical incident stress debriefing model should be established to provide immediate and long-term psychological support.

BIBLIOGRAPHY

1. Browning RG, Olson DW, Stuevan HA, Mateer JR: 50% Dextrose: Antidote or toxin? Ann Emerg Med 19:6:83–687, 1990.
2. Clinton JE, Sterner S, Stelmacher Z, Ruiz E: Haloperidol for sedation of disruptive emergency patients. Ann Emerg Med 16:319–322, 1987.
3. Engel F: Helping the employee victim of violence in hospitals. Commun Psychiatry 37:159, 1986.
4. Kurlowicz LH: Violence in the emergency department. Am J Nurs 90:35–40, 1990.
5. Lavoie FW, Carter GL, Danzl DF, Berg RL: Emergency department violence in United States teaching hospitals. Ann Emerg Med 17:1221–1233, 1988.
6. Redan JA, Livingston DH, Tortella BJ, Rush BF: The value of intubating and paralyzing patients with suspected head injury in the emergency department. J Trauma 31:371–375, 1991.
7. Schumaker HM: Rapid-sequence induction. In Callaham ML (ed): Decision Making in Emergency Medicine. Philadelphia, B.C. Decker, 1990, pp 4–5.
8. Van Hoesen KB, Martell MC, Rosen P: Management of the violent patient in the emergency department. Hospital Physician 28:12–32, 1992.
9. Wasserberger J, Ordog GJ, Kolodny M, Allen K: Violence in a community emergency room. Arch Emerg Med 6:266–269, 1989.
10. Wasserberger J, Ordog GJ, Hardin E, et al: Violence in the emergency department. Top Emerg Med 14:71–78, 1992.
11. Weisberg MP, Dwyer BJ (eds): Safe strategies for recognizing and managing violent patients. Emerg Med Rep 8:22:169–176, 1987.

XVIII. Cost Containment and Risk Management

113. COST CONTAINMENT AND RISK MANAGEMENT IN EMERGENCY MEDICINE

Stephen V. Cantrill, M.D., FACEP

COST CONTAINMENT

1. What is cost containment in emergency medicine?
Cost containment is an approach to limit expenses on medical care without sacrificing quality of care.

2. Why is cost containment so important?
Medical care currently consumes 14% of the gross national product (GNP). Health care costs have continued to increase at a rate far above inflation. The federal government directly or indirectly pays for 42% of health care, and thus is quite concerned about this ongoing increase. One study by the RAND Corporation concluded that up to one-third of medical care may be unnecessary. It is clear that if medicine continues to fail to address these issues, the federal government will step in and "help" us deal with them.

3. What is the area in emergency medicine over which ED physicians have the most control in terms of containing costs?
Ancillary tests (clinical laboratory and radiology) constitute 44% of patient ED charges—the single largest component. These tests are done at the request of the emergency physician, and therefore represent an area directly under our control.

4. What are some reasons for excessive test ordering in emergency medicine?

Peer pressure (e.g., wanting to please a consultant)	Out-of-date hospital policies
Ignorance of the costs of tests	Intellectual curiosity
"Defensive medicine"	Patient expectations
	Reflex ordering/old habits

None of these reasons is adequate justification for ordering tests that are not medically indicated based upon the patient's presentation.

5. What is the "golden question" to ask before ordering any test?
How useful will this test result be in establishing a diagnosis or assisting in treatment?

6. What are some additional strategies to reduce inappropriate test ordering?
1. Avoid ordering reflexively. Carefully consider the benefits before ordering a test.
2. Do not order a test because "it would be nice to know," unless, of course, you are willing to pay for the test.
3. Learn how much routine lab tests and radiographs cost. (Prepare for a shock.)
4. Establish guidelines for the use of new technologies. Medicine is notorious for developing and using new tests without discontinuing the old ones.

5. Avoid ordering studies for medicolegal reasons. Good medicine is good law. Order only those studies that are medically indicated.
6. Use patient education to reshape patient expectations when possible.
7. Cancel studies that were ordered but then found to be unncessary.

7. Shouldn't we order tests to "cover" ourselves?

No. As noted above, "good medicine is good law." The criteria for ordering studies should be strictly medical, not based on the physician's notion of what would be helpful to have in a court of law. In addition, laboratory studies should not be used as a substitute for a proper history and physical examination.

8. What are some commonly overordered tests?

Extremity radiographs	Urine culture and sensitivity
Chest radiographs	Throat culture (excluding strep. screen)
Electrolyte panel	Blood type and cross
Abdominal radiographs	Blood ethanol level
Complete blood count (CBC)	Arterial blood gases (ABGs)
Rib radiographs	

9. How much can be saved with no compromise in patient care?

In a multicentered study of 20 hospital EDs, both teaching and nonteaching, a cost containment educational program was used. Seventeen tests or groups of tests or studies (including those mentioned above) were targeted. A 12.5% decrease in targeted test charges was demonstrated. No decrease in the perceived quality of care could be demonstrated. This clearly shows that the costs of medical testing in the ED can be contained by careful, thoughtful ordering without sacrificing patient care.

RISK MANAGEMENT

10. What is risk management?

Risk management refers to efforts to identify (and, when possible, improve or rectify) situations that place a provider of a service in jeopardy. This section addresses emergency physicians and how they are placed at risk. Good risk management deals not only with situations as they arise (e.g., dealing appropriately with a patient's complaint about care), but also anticipates health-delivery problems before they occur (e.g., establishing in advance the procedures for how to deal with a patient who wishes to leave against medical advice).

11. Why are emergency physicians at high risk for malpractice lawsuits?

The primary reason is the lack of an established physician-patient relationship. The patient often feels little rapport with a physician unknown to the patient prior to the visit to the ED. The visit is usually not at the patient's wish, occurring at an unscheduled time and in a situation in which the patient is under stress and sometimes pain. All of these factors may contribute to feelings of anger and hostility, laying the groundwork for feelings of dissatisfaction about the provided care. A second major reason is that in emergency medicine, the decisions are often irrevocable. If a mistake or misjudgment is made on a patient who is admitted to the hospital, there usually exists a second chance to correct the error because the patient is still accessible. In patients wrongly discharged from the ED, sometimes no such second chance exists.

12. What must be proved in a malpractice case?

All of the following four points must be proved in any malpractice case:
    1. **Duty to treat.** Was there an obligation for the physician in question to treat the patient? In emergency medicine, this answer is almost always "yes." By working in an ED,

an emergency physician automatically assumes the duty to treat any patient presenting to that department and requesting care.

2. **Actual negligence.** Was the care provided actually negligent? This often involves demonstrating (to the jury's satisfaction) that the care provided fell below what is to be considered the "standard of care." This point is the one most often contested by the opposing sides in a malpractice suit. Negligence may result from acts of commission or omission.

3. **Damages.** Did the patient suffer actual damages? Unfortunately, this can include the nebulous "pain and suffering."

4. **Proximate cause.** Did the negligence cause the damages? It must be demonstrated to the jury's satisfaction that the alleged damages were truly the result of the alleged negligent care.

13. What are some examples of high-risk patients?

1. **The hostile or belligerent patient.** These patients are difficult to deal with and therefore sometimes get less than complete, careful evaluation. Intoxicated patients represent a significant subgroup of this class of patients. Demanding patients also fall into this class. When confronted with patients in this category, remember that "you don't have to love them to give them proper care."

2. **The patient with a problem that may be a potential life-threat.** With these patients, the challenge is to discover and address the life-threat (see Ch. 1). Discharging these patients often results in a risk-management problem.

3. **The returning patient.** The patient who returns unscheduled to the ED should raise a red flag. What problem is being missed? These patients deserve extra care in reevaluation. The threshold for admitting an unscheduled returning patient should be low.

4. **The "private" patient.** Patients may be sent the ED by a private physician for diagnostic studies or treatment but not to be seen and evaluated by the emergency physician. Any patient in the department becomes the responsibility of the emergency physician in the department. If something goes wrong with the care of these patients, the emergency physician may also be held liable. It is advisable to have an established policy that **every** patient who enters the ED will be seen and evaluated by the emergency physician.

14. What clinical problems tend to get emergency physicians into malpractice difficulty?

There is regional variation in clinical problems that tend to cause malpractice problems for emergency physicians, but the following entities are generally major causes: (1) FTD/FTT (failure to diagnose/failure to treat) myocardial infarction, (2) FTD/FTT meningitis/sepsis (especially in young children), (3) FTD fracture (including spine and pelvis), (4) FTD appendicitis, (5) FTD ectopic pregnancy, (6) FTD wound foreign bodies, (7) FTD tendon/nerve injuries associated with wounds, (8) FTD intracranial hemorrhage (subdural/epidural/subarachnoid hemorrhage), and (9) wound infections.

15. What is the most common error emergency physicians make with regard to their malpractice insurance policy?

The most common error is failure to read carefully and understand the conditions of the policy, i.e., what is covered, what is not covered, what is required for a malpractice occurrence to be covered, what are the settlement options, and what are the "tail" requirements to provide coverage for past patient encounters when the current policy is no longer in force.

16. What common deficiencies in the medical record exacerbate malpractice problems for emergency physicians?

In a malpractice case, your record of a patient's visit can be your greatest friend or your worst foe. The following problems will place the record on the side of the opposing team:

1. **An illegible record.** Think about how the record will look when it is enlarged to 4 feet by 4 feet by the plaintiff's attorney to show to the jury. Dictated/typed records avoid this problem.

2. **Not addressing the chief complaint or nurses' and paramedics' notes.** Make sure your evaluation addresses why the patient came to the ED and what others have observed and documented about the patient.

3. **Not addressing abnormal vital signs.** As a rule, patients must not be discharged from the ED with abnormal vital signs. Whenever this is done, the record must contain a discussion of why the physician is taking this action.

4. **An incomplete recorded history.** As with all other parts of the medical record, an attempt will be made to convince the jury that "not recorded equals not done." The history must include information concerning all potential serious problems consistent with the patient's presentation. Significant negatives should certainly be recorded as well.

5. **Labeling the patient with a diagnosis that cannot be substantiated by the rest of the record.** This not only may cause difficulty if the physician's "guess" is wrong, but it leads to premature closure on the part of the next physician to treat the patient, removing the slim chance of correcting the diagnostic error if the patient returns to the ED because of no improvement.

6. **Inadequate documentation of the patient's course in the ED** with inadequate attention to the patient's condition at discharge. Often the patient's condition may dramatically improve while in the ED justifying discharge, but this fact is not reflected in the record. If this case becomes a malpractice problem, it will appear that the patient was discharged in the original (unimproved) condition.

7. **Inadequate discharge (follow-up, after care) instructions.** The greatest risk in dealing with patients is being wrong in our judgment. The best insurance is careful and complete patient discharge instructions that include when and where to follow-up and under what conditions to return to the ED. It is striking how little effort is put into this component of the record. After completing your evaluation and treatment of a patient, ask yourself "what if I am wrong and what is the worst possible complication that can occur?" Address these possibilities completely in your discharge instructions and document them carefully in the record.

17. What "systems problems" often lead to lawsuits?
System problems are not necessarily those under the emergency physician's control, but can still cause difficulty. Such problems include inadequate follow-up on radiology re-read of radiographs, inadequate follow-up of cardiology re-reads of EKGs, inadequate follow-up of delayed clinical laboratory results (e.g., cultures), poor availability of previous medical records, inadequate handling of patient complaints (your chance to possibly head off a malpractice suit), and inadequate physician and ED staffing patterns (leading to prolonged patient waits and subsequent patient hostility).

18. When a patient refuses care, what are the two criteria that must be present?
If a patient desires to leave the ED against medical advice, the patient must (1) be competent to refuse care and (2) understand the possible untoward sequelae that could result from refusal of care. All patients have the right to refuse care if these two criteria are met. Common sense (and most risk managers) would tell you to err on the side of treating the patient if there is any doubt as to competence.

19. What clinical problem-solving approach is most helpful in avoiding lawsuits?
When dealing with any patient, make sure you address the life-threats: those major problems that could exist, given this presentation for this patient. The safe approach is to assume the presence of these life-threats, and then set about to disprove them (see ch. 1).

20. What physician behaviors may help avoid lawsuits?

Although a physician may be sued for any reason at any time (and lose), certain behaviors may help to decrease the chance of a lawsuit:

1. Be courteous and kind to the patient and to the patient's family.

2. Take time to communicate with the patient. It takes only seconds to tell the patient what is going on, what the results of any diagnostic studies are, and what you are thinking concerning their case. Make sure all patient questions and concerns are addressed.

3. Dress neatly.

4. Explain and apologize for inordinate delays in patient care.

5. Make sure the medical record accurately reflects the care provided and the thought processes behind the care.

This approach can be summarized in a simple statement: "treat every patient as you would want your mother treated." This, of course, assumes you love your mother.

21. How can writing admission orders for admitted patients cause problems for the emergency physician?

In many situations, writing admission orders for patients has made the emergency physician liable for untoward events occurring to the patient in the hospital before he or she is seen by the private physician. There is often significant peer pressure for the emergency physician to write such orders. This practice is potentially dangerous and is to be discouraged.

22. What are the criteria for reporting a physician to the National Practitioner Data Bank?

The National Practitioner Data Bank (NPDB) was established by the federal government in 1989 to track potential problem physicians. The criteria for reporting a physician to the NPDB are: (1) any payment made for a claim or judgment against a physician; (2) any action taken by a state medical licensing board against a physician; and (3) any disciplinary action lasting more than 30 days taken against a physician by a group or institution. A hospital must query the NPDB about any physician applying for staff privileges and at the time of reappointment of a physician to the medical staff.

23. How can clinical policies ("standards of care") actually decrease malpractice risk for the emergency physician?

Many groups and organizations are developing "standards of care." These go under several names: clinical policies, clinical guidelines, protocols, standards. If it can be demonstrated that a physician's care was consistent with an accepted standard, it may help to demonstrate the appropriateness of the care and therefore the lack of negligence.

24. How can clinical policies potentially increase malpractice risk for emergency physicians?

Malpractice risk can be increased by applicable clinical policies or other "standards of care" if the emergency physician is not aware of those standards that apply to his or her practice, or if he or she chooses not to follow a standard without carefully documenting the reasons for not doing so.

BIBLIOGRAPHY

1. Cost Containment Task Force: Guidelines for Cost Containment in Emergency Medicine. American College of Emergency Physicians, Dallas, TX, 1983. (Available from ACEP, PO Box 619911, Dallas, TX, 75261-9911 Phone: 214-550-0911).
2. Detsky AS, Naglie G: A clinician's guide to cost-effectiveness analysis. Ann Intern Med 113:147–154, 1990.
3. Henry GL: Emergency Medicine Risk Management: A Comprehensive Review. Dallas, American College of Emergency Physicians, 1991.
4. Karas S: Cost containment in emergency medicine. JAMA 243:1356–1359, 1980.

XIX. Medical Control and Disaster Management

114. MEDICAL CONTROL AND DISASTER MANAGEMENT

Daniel W. Spaite, M.D., FACEP

1. What is medical control?

Medical control is the means by which physicians give direction and authority to nonphysicians to provide emergency medical care outside of the hospital and in the absence of a physician. This concept is a relatively new one. Before the 1970s, ill and injured patients were transported by personnel who had little, if any, training. At that time there was essentially no physician input regarding the scope of practice or quality of care provided. Medical control may be characterized as either on-line (direct) or off-line (indirect).

2. Why is the medical control of prehospital care important?

The importance of medical control lies in the concept that nonphysicians can provide physician-level medical care safely and effectively only when under the authority and direction of a physician.

3. Describe indirect medical control.

Indirect, or off-line, medical control is the process by which a physician develops and maintains the structure that ensures proper patient care within an EMS system. This entails numerous responsibilities such as training personnel, designing and evaluating the system, developing medical standards/protocols/standing orders, reviewing prehospital care, and initiating a program of quality management. Maintaining high-quality patient care requires that the physician has not only the responsibility for indirect medical control but also the authority and organizational support to develop, alter, and maintain the medical care system.

4. What is direct medical control?

Direct, or on-line, medical control entails the direction, observation, and evaluation of prehospital medical care as the care is being rendered. In many systems, direct medical control is primarily carried out by radio communication between the prehospital personnel and a medical control physician (or designee). The concept also includes the direct observation of prehospital personnel during physician "ride along" encounters. The percentage of EMS calls that have direct medical control varies widely among different systems. In some systems essentially every call has direct medical control, whereas in others it essentially never occurs.

5. Have there been any practical problems with the development of proper medical control?

Although the sense of profound need for medical direction is essentially universal among physicians, there has not always been unanimous interest in close physician supervision by system administrators. Much of the hesitation has been based on the fact that many physicians have little administrative, budgetary, public safety, or legislative education or experience. For instance, a fire chief might be concerned that a system medical director would mandate improvements in a system that require financial resources beyond the ability of the agency to support alterations. This issue led to the development, on a national scale, of specialized physician education and has also spawned the development of postgraduate fellowships that provide subspecialization in prehospital care as an identifiable medical discipline.

6. Define the term "disaster."
A disaster is any event or series of events that outstrips the ability of a medical system to properly care for all patients in a routine fashion. It is important to note that this definition does not require a large-scale or globally catastrophic event (such as a train crash or hurricane). Rather, a disaster exists any time the available community resources are inadequate for either the number or the severity of casualties produced. The collapse of a section of bleachers at a public event that seriously injures 200 persons is clearly a disaster. The rollover of a car with five people in a rural or wilderness area that outstrips the ability of local resources to respond, although perhaps less apparent, also constitutes a disaster.

7. Why is there a need for disaster planning?
The quality of medical care in general is directly tied to the experience of the practitioner. Proficiency of a given medical intervention depends on the frequent performance of that intervention. Holloway defined a disaster as "many people trying to do quickly what they do not ordinarily do in an environment with which they are not familiar." No matter how experienced an individual is, the level of care, resources available, and entire framework for resource management undergo major alterations during a disaster. Thus the development of a clear plan for the management of multiple casualties is imperative to ensure optimal outcome for the victims, given the resources available. Disaster planning must not be conducted in a vacuum but rather must include the various pertinent agencies within the community, such as police and fire departments, emergency medical service agencies, Red Cross, Salvation Army, hospitals, public works departments, utilities, and volunteers such as ham radio operators. For example, no matter how well prepared a trauma center might be to care for multiple casualties, if the transportation of disaster victims is disrupted or misdirected, patient outcome is adversely affected.

8. How can prehospital care of disaster victims be optimized?
A recent concept that is believed to improve overall outcome during disasters is the **Incident Command System.** Such a system is based on the philosophy that various sectors (triage, communications, transportation) are under the command of a single authority that can appropriately disburse and control resources. The purpose of such a system is to decrease the likelihood of wasting precious resources on patients who do not need them (minor injuries) or will not benefit from them (victims of unsurvivable injuries, given the setting). The incident command system provides a structure that can prevent the misuse of resources (such as transporting patients before triage occurs).

9. What is triage?
Triage means "to sort." Although numerous systems exist for triaging victims of multicasualty incidents, the basic concept generally identifies four groups of patients: (1) minor illness or injury (walking wounded); (2) serious but not immediately life-threatening illness or injury (such as a patient with an intraabdominal injury who is currently not in shock); (3) critical or immediately life-threatening illness or injury (loss of consciousness); and (4) dead or unsalvageable. The actual categorization of specific patients is different in various types and magnitudes of disaster. Thus a critically injured patient who might receive the benefit of a comprehensive life-saving effort in a three-patient incident might be deemed unsalvageable in a disaster with a thousand victims.

10. When is it appropriate for a physician to respond to the scene of a multiple-casualty incident?

Although from a scientific perspective, the answer to this question is unknown, most prehospital disaster plans include the potential request for a physician to respond to the scene. This is based upon the concept that a well-trained and experienced physician can provide the highest level of patient assessment and care available. However, this concept has several caveats. First, very few physicians have substantial training and experience in prehospital care. A physician who is highly proficient in the care of critically ill and injured patients in the hospital setting may be a "duck out of water" in the field. Indeed, a physician who does not have significant prehospital experience may generally make a scene less efficient rather than more so. In general, personnel who deal with uncontrolled environments daily are best prepared to efficiently manage such situations. Second, a physician who is known by prehospital personnel within the system is likely to command significantly greater authority during a multicasualty incident than one who is unknown. Thus, in systems that do have a plan for physician response, it may be most appropriate to designate the system medical director or a small number of identified physicians who have participated in disaster drills to function as the on-scene medical authority.

BIBLIOGRAPHY

1. Burkle FM, Sanner PH, Wolcott BW (eds): Disaster Medicine. New York, Examination Publishing Co., 1984.
2. Feldstein B: Disasters and disaster medicine: An introduction and overview. Top Emerg Med 7:1–19, 1986.
3. Holroyd BR, Knopp R, Kallsen G: Medical control: Quality assurance in prehospital care. JAMA 256:1027–1031, 1986.
4. Kuehl AK (ed): National Association of EMS Physicians EMS Medical Directors' Handbook. St. Louis, C.V. Mosby, 1989.
5. Mitchell G: The triage process. Top Emerg Med 7:34–45, 1986.
6. Pepe PE, Stewart RD: Role of the physician in the prehospital setting. Ann Emerg Med 15:1480–1483, 1986.
7. Roush WR (ed): Principles of EMS Systems: A Comprehensive Text for Physicians. Dallas, American College of Emergency Physicians, 1989.
8. Stewart RD: Prehospital care: Education, evaluation, and medical control. Top Emerg Med 2:67–82, 1980.

INDEX

Entries in **boldface** type indicate complete chapters.